Cancer nursing:
care in context

Edited by

Jessica Corner and Christopher Bailey

*Centre for Cancer and Palliative Care Studies,
Institute of Cancer Research/Royal Marsden Hospital,
London*

Blackwell
Science

© 2001 Blackwell Science Ltd
Editorial Offices:
Osney Mead, Oxford OX2 0EL
25 John Street, London WC1N 2BS
23 Ainslie Place, Edinburgh EH3 6AJ
350 Main Street, Malden
    MA 02148 5018, USA
54 University Street, Carlton
    Victoria 3053, Australia
10, rue Casimir Delavigne
    75006 Paris, France

Other Editorial Offices:

Blackwell Wissenschafts-Verlag GmbH
Kurfürstendamm 57
10707 Berlin, Germany

Blackwell Science KK
MG Kodenmacho Building
7-10 Kodenmacho Nihombashi
Chuo-ku, Tokyo 104, Japan

Iowa State University Press
A Blackwell Science Company
2121 S. State Avenue
Ames, Iowa 50014-8300, USA

The right of the Author to be identified as the Author of this Work
has been asserted in accordance with the Copyright, Designs and
Patents Act 1988.

First published 2001
Reprinted 2001, 2002

Set in 10/12pt Garamond and produced by
Gray Publishing, Tunbridge Wells, Kent
Printed and bound in Great Britain by
Alden Press Ltd, Oxford and Northampton

The Blackwell Science logo is a
trade mark of Blackwell Science Ltd,
registered at the United Kingdom
Trade Marks Registry

DISTRIBUTORS

Marston Book Services Ltd
PO Box 269
Abingdon
Oxon OX14 4YN
(*Orders*: Tel: 01235 465500
              Fax: 01235 465555)

USA
Blackwell Science, Inc.
Commerce Place
350 Main Street
Malden, MA 02148-5018
(*Orders*: Tel: 800 759 6102
                  781 388 8250
              Fax: 781 388 8255)

Canada
Login Brothers Book Company
324 Saulteaux Crescent
Winnipeg, Manitoba R3J 3T2
(*Orders*: Tel: 204 837-2987
              Fax: 204 837-3116)

Australia
Blackwell Science Pty Ltd
54 University Street
Carlton, Victoria 3053
(*Orders*: Tel: 03 9347 0300
              Fax: 03 9347 5001)

A catalogue record for this title is available
from the British Library

ISBN 0-632-03998-1

Library of Congress
Cataloging-in-Publication Data is available

For further information on
Blackwell Science, visit our website:
www.blackwell-science.com

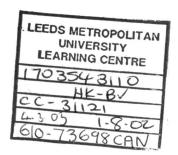

Contents

Part 4: The Management of Cancer-related Problems

Part 5: Needs and Priorities in Cancer Care

Foreword

This book has as its title *Cancer nursing: care in context*. But what is the context? What is it that will influence the care that is provided to cancer patients and their families over the next few decades? What is it that will determine the way in which we continue to improve both the management and quality of life of cancer patients?

First, it is important to remember that cancer is not a single disease, but a whole group of diseases, which differ in the way in which they grow, spread, and respond to treatment. Thus, the context and the outcome will change, depending on whether or not the particular cancer responds to therapy. This can make a difference to the patient and to the approach adopted by professionals.

A second issue, which follows from this, is the possibility of very considerable changes and developments in diagnosis and management. Research is at the heart of this and it must be assumed that much will happen over the next decade to improve the quality of care, as has happened in previous years. A research and development culture is critical to this, and thus one of the contexts in which cancer nursing will develop relates to the need for a solid basis in research and evaluation. Curiosity, and the wish to know more and do better, are important skills for the nurse.

This takes us to the next important contextual issue, that of the education and continuing professional development of all staff caring for cancer patients. This is certainly a key issue, as the level of education and training will determine the skills and expertise that are available to provide care to patients. Education and training are not synonymous, and to coin a phrase, 'training is to have arrived, education is to continue to travel'. Nurses of the future will need to learn new skills and continue to travel and expand their knowledge base. The clinical practice evidence base is part of this, together with links to a wide variety of sources of information, such as the Internet. Patients of the future will have much readier access to such information and professionals will need to keep up with them. This is the beginning of a further revolution in education and learning, 'e-learning', which will change the context in which care is delivered. The management and delivery of care to an individual patient will no longer be judged in relation to the local circumstances but according to standards set nationally and internationally. The information is there and we need to learn to use it more effectively.

A further issue is the context in which the service is delivered and how the health care system operates. There are many differences in the way in which this is already done worldwide, and most countries are reviewing how best to improve the delivery of the care provided. There is therefore likely to be change ahead. One significant part of this is the link between primary and secondary care. The primary care setting will increasingly be a place where health care, even of a specialised nature, is delivered. This relationship is likely to change with time, but will determine much of what can and should be done in these different settings. Another facet of this is inter-professional and team working, which recognises the skills and expertise of the many professionals who work together for the benefit of patients and their families. As care may well be delivered more on a community basis in the future, it is important that we consider different models of service delivery. In the UK the Calman–Hine model is currently being evaluated; this is based on two important factors, the determination of patients' needs and the outcome of treatment, and these are used to assess what level of care can be delivered and in which setting. This process is beginning to change the way in which cancer services are organised, and nurses have a key role in this process at all levels.

The social context in which care is delivered is also changing rapidly. The public has greater expectations about what might be achieved for them and they are able to compare local results with those elsewhere. From a public health point of view, issues such as prevention, diagnosis, and screening are also very much in the public eye. Society and the public at large expect that such services are delivered with expertise and competence, and that they can depend on them. There are also significant social and economic variations in the population which can be observed across any country or region, and which are reflected in inequalities in health, cancer incidence, access to care and its delivery, and the clinical outcomes of cancer treatment. These variations are considerable, and of course are not only confined to the UK. One important consequence of this is that the discipline of cancer nursing needs to be pursued within a framework which seeks to remove inequity from the way in which cancer care is delivered, and which might affect the outcome of treatment and quality of care.

Patients and their families are of course a subset of society at large. They now expect, and indeed have a right to expect, greater involvement and choice in treatment, and in the way in which cancer is managed. They have greater knowledge and access to information, and it is becoming increasingly common for patients to bring their computer printouts to the clinic and to challenge the team on the way in which their own case is being managed. The rapid evolution of the Internet and

development of the knowledge base will only increase this, but this is something that we should welcome. Patients have a right to expect information about their own management programme to be discussed with them, and that communication, a two-way process, is a central feature of this. At the end of the day, the objective is to deliver a service which is based on care and compassion as well as the appropriate use of technology, and which improves not only survival, but also quality of life.

The final context, which underpins all of the others, is the values and beliefs held by professional staff and society at large. What is it that we want to deliver? What are our values, and how can we ensure that across the professions, these are achievable? In the management of the patient with cancer there are many ethical issues which arise. Our response to these, and our wish to do our best for our patients, must be at the heart of this. The 'my mother' principle is relevant to this. If it were your mother, son, husband, what would you want to happen? If the care provided is less than you would wish for your own family, how can we in the professions respond to this challenge?

This book is thus set in a very broad context in which change will be the only constant feature. As a profession, nurses have already responded rapidly and creatively to these changes, and will continue to do so. But there is a challenge left. Cancer care will not happen and improve without considerable imagination, drive, and energy. It will require leadership, and a commitment to providing the best service to patients and their families. That is where the nurse with a special interest in cancer can, and must, become an effective agent for change.

To conclude this foreword, a quotation from Martin Luther King sums it all up appropriately and catches the sentiment of these last remarks:

> Human progress is neither automatic or inevitable . . . Every step towards the goal of social justice requires sacrifice, suffering and struggle, and the passionate concerns of dedicated individuals . . . This is no time for apathy or complacency. This is a time for vigorous and positive action.

Kenneth C. Calman
Durham
March 2000

Preface

This book is something of a departure from the standard textbook. Most are a source of knowledge about a particular disease, treatments, and health care practices. The function of a textbook is to compile in a single volume the 'state of the art' and the latest research evidence; to create a source of reference for knowledge, offering a kind of 'truth' in relation to what is known about, and what might constitute best practice in a given area. There are many such texts on cancer, cancer treatment, and cancer nursing on library and bookshop shelves. This book is not intended to replace these excellent texts; rather, the intention is to offer a different perspective.

An attempt is made here to reveal cancer as an experience that is socially and culturally determined in unique and powerful ways. It is acknowledged that there are many discourses or knowledge systems that surround cancer; indeed, several contrasting discourses may be found within the pages of this book. At times these are made manifest by the author; elsewhere the text is less self-conscious in this respect and adheres to a particular tradition or language. In general, however, it is acknowledged that cancer discourses dictate society's, individual and collective responses to the disease and to the people who have it, and it is these that in turn shape our understanding of cancer.

To work effectively with cancer, nurses need to understand their reactions to the disease, and the reactions of others. Nurses need to move between biomedical and lay understanding of cancer and how it is treated, and to be aware of the failings of professional carers and health care in supporting people who have cancer. Complex dynamics within society, and within professional and organisational contexts, determine how cancer is managed and understood. Knowing that such processes are at large, and how these may affect one's own response to someone who is ill, or how treatment and care for a particular condition is constructed, is, we believe, the basis for caring. This book therefore offers a critical exploration of the forces that shape the delivery of cancer care, and this is given priority over the need to assimilate biomedical knowledge about cancer and its treatment. Access to the latter is offered throughout the book, and is set alongside a critical exploration of cancer care, personal accounts by people who have cancer, and reviews of research into care and treatment.

The stance taken is that change needs to happen so that the many and complex needs of people with cancer and their families are met more completely than at present; nurses have much to offer here, and may themselves be powerful agents of change. Perhaps this book takes a small step towards empowering nurses to develop alternatives for people with cancer, offering choices over how cancer is understood and promoting the role of nursing in managing the day-to-day experience of cancer and its treatment.

Contributions to the book are from different perspectives and there is no claim that they speak with a single voice; it is a collection of differing but convergent viewpoints. A number of recurring themes draws the accounts together. The text as a whole takes a critical standpoint; all is not right with how cancer care is currently managed, therefore questions are raised about existing practice and whether this serves the interests of those who require care. Through the themes selected, discussion takes one beyond established orthodoxy, though the perspective of caring and the contribution of nursing are central.

At the outset, it was decided that this book should help nurses to access experiences of what it is like to have cancer, to receive treatment for cancer, or to care for someone who has cancer, since these are life-changing and life-defining. Unless one is able to think about what it must be like to experience cancer, it is not possible to understand what is needed. This has been achieved through the use of personal accounts derived from a variety of sources. Through the accounts the book adheres to a belief that in caring it is essential that nurses draw on the personal narratives, or stories, of people who are sick. In using personal accounts the book offers the reader knowledge through experience, albeit somewhat vicariously. The personal accounts, and indeed parts of the text itself, could be used as a focus for discussion or guided reflection; this is, we believe, the foundation for developing and changing practice. The book does not represent a single or final version of knowledge in cancer care; throughout, core texts, seminal works, and research studies are introduced so that readers can access and read these for themselves. The book therefore could be seen as a springboard from which the reader may begin his or her own journey of caring and scholarship in this intensely challenging area of health care.

The book has been organised into five parts. In the first, entitled 'Cancer, care, and society' cancer is set in context and the notion of cancer discourses and the responses of society, health care, and health carers are introduced and explained, as are some suggestions for escaping the defensive dynamics engendered by these. This discussion is set alongside the science of cancer epidemiology. Part 2 deals with the experience of cancer from the perspectives of the person who is ill, family members, and health professionals. This is developed in Part 3, which offers detailed insight into the experience of cancer treatment, and the role of nurses in administering treatment and helping people with cancer to manage the effects of treatment. Part 4 explores the nursing management of problems related to cancer, redefining the more biomedically driven term 'symptom' as 'problem' and placing nursing in a central position in helping people to manage problems. Finally, Part 5 identifies and reviews a number of needs and priorities in cancer care, including perspectives on the needs of particular groups such as children and adolescents, the elderly and people from minority racial groups. The organisation of care for people with advanced cancer and who are dying, health service policy, and research in cancer care, are also addressed.

A project of this kind inevitably feels incomplete: many other areas could have been addressed and there are omissions of content and argument. In presenting a somewhat different perspective, new avenues for care and research may have been created; if we have succeeded then much will have been achieved.

Jessica Corner
Christopher Bailey

Contributors

Audrey Ardern-Jones
Clinical Nurse Specialist in Cancer Genetics
Royal Marsden Hospital
Sutton, Surrey

Christopher Bailey
Senior Nursing Fellow
Centre for Cancer and Palliative Care Studies
Institute of Cancer Research
London

Nicola Beech
27 Palmerfield Road
Banstead, Surrey

Mary Bredin
Macmillan Research Practitioner
Centre for Cancer and Palliative Care Studies
Institute of Cancer Research
London

Dr John Bridgewater
Senior Lecturer and Honorary
Consultant in Medical Oncology
Royal Free and University College
Medical School
London

Professor Jessica Corner
Director and Deputy Dean (Nursing)
Centre for Cancer and Palliative Care Studies
Institute of Cancer Research
London

Dr Alan Cribb
Senior Lecturer
Centre for Educational Studies
King's College London
London

Siân Dennison
Lead Cancer Nurse/Senior Lecturer
Plymouth Hospitals NHS Trust
and University of Plymouth
Plymouth, Devon

Lisa Dougherty
Clinical Nurse Specialist
IV Services
Royal Marsden Hospital
Sutton, Surrey

Julia Downing
Mildmay International Study Centre
Kampala
Uganda

Ruth Dunleavey
Clinical Nurse Consultant
Medical Oncology Trials
Westmead Hospital
Sydney
Australia

Dr Rosalind Eeles
Clinical Senior Lecturer/
Honorary Consultant
in Cancer Genetics and
Clinical Oncology
Institute of Cancer Research
London

Sara Faithfull
Leader in Cancer Care
Centre for Cancer and Palliative Care Studies
Institute of Cancer Research
Sutton, Surrey

Deborah Fenlon
Lecturer in Cancer Care
Centre for Cancer and Palliative Care Studies
Institute of Cancer Research
Sutton, Surrey

Dr Martin Gore
Consultant Physician
Department of Medicine
Royal Marsden Hospital
London

Sue Hawkett
Nursing Officer
Department of Health
London

Danielle Horton Taylor
Epidemiologist
27 Thurleigh Road, London

Daniel Kelly
Senior Nurse
Research and Development
University College Hospitals NHS Trust
London

Meinir Krishnasamy
Senior Nursing Fellow
Centre for Cancer and Palliative
Care Studies
Institute of Cancer Research
London

Dr Anne Lanceley
Senior Research Fellow: Cancer Nursing
St Bartholomew's School of Nursing & Midwifery
London

Kay Leedham
Director of Nursing
Katherine House Hospice
Adderbury
Banbury, Oxon

Mary Wells
Clinical Research Fellow in
Cancer Nursing
Tayside University Hospital
NHS Trust and
University of Dundee
School of Nursing and Midwifery
Dundee

Jo O'Neill
Research Nurse
Neil Cliffe Cancer Centre
Wythenshawe Hospital
Manchester

Mary Pennell
Lecturer in Palliative Care
Centre for Cancer and Palliative
Care Studies
Institute of Cancer Research
London

Hilary Plant
Lecturer in Cancer Nursing
Centre for Cancer and Palliative
Care Studies
Institute of Cancer Research
London

Nancy Preston
Postgraduate Research Student
Centre for Cancer and Palliative Care Studies
Institute of Cancer Research
London

Dr Veronica (Nicky) Thomas
Consultant Health Psychologist,
Department of Haematology and
Honorary Senior Lecturer, Unit of Psychology
Guy's, King's and St Thomas's
United Medical and Dental School, London

Jenny Thompson
Freelance Lecturer and Writer
Moorbank Farmhouse
Old Forewood Lane
Crowhurst, Sussex

Angela Williams
Doctoral candidate
39 The Grove
Brookmans Park
Hatfield
Herts

Part 1

Cancer, Care, and Society

CHAPTER ONE

What is cancer?

Jessica Corner

'Cancer' is the term used to denote a group of diseases sharing common characteristics, represented by each site of the body from which these arise. Many are quite different in nature, rate of progression, sequelae, treatment and outcome. While at least one-third of people can expect to be cured of the disease, and important progress has been made in the management of cancer and palliation of symptoms, a diagnosis of cancer is known to hold grave consequences.[1] The effects of the disease process, the protracted nature of treatment, and the psychological impact of cancer, mean that the implications for the individual reach beyond other acute and chronic conditions. As Donovan and Girton[2] highlight:

> The magnitude of the problem of cancer in our society is only partially reflected by statistics on mortality and morbidity. These figures do not tell of the panic inherent in the mere thought of cancer, the role changes and conflicts that may arise when cancer is treated, or the dozens of other problems encountered by the person who faces a diagnosis of cancer. Since cancer is frequently a chronic disease with periods of acute intensive illness interspersed with the constant threat of death, the patient with a diagnosis of cancer must face the problems of each of these kinds of illnesses.

In being used to describe disease, cancer serves only as an umbrella term to draw together a large group of diseases (more than 200) with certain characteristics, rather in the way the term 'arthritis' is used. The difficulty with the term 'cancer' is that it is loaded with meanings for people and these are inevitably negative. Understanding 'what cancer is' is therefore complex.

One way of understanding cancer is to explore how it is manifested within the population. The science of disease within populations – epidemiology – is discussed by Danielle Horton-Taylor later in this section. Cancer is a common condition: one in three people will develop cancer at some point in their lives. More than 250 000 people in the UK develop cancer each year. Although cancer can develop at any age, most people with cancer are over 65 years old.[3] At least 7.5 million new cancers are diagnosed each year in the world; cancer thus represents a huge burden of disease.[3]

In the UK, four cancers account for over half of all cases: these are lung, breast, colorectal and prostate cancers. Figure 1.1 shows the 10 most common cancers in the UK, and Figure 1.2 shows a comparison between common cancers for developed and developing countries of the world, since these are different and reflect environmental factors contributing to cancer. Liver cancer is common in developing countries, where it is related to hepatitis B virus and food contaminated with aphlatoxin. In contrast, breast cancer is most common in developed countries.[4]

Table 1.1 shows the risk associated with developing the most common cancers in men and women. These are somewhat different, with lung cancer the most common for men, and breast cancer for women. Figure 1.3 shows the relative percentage of people who survive 5 years after diagnosis; this is an indicator of the chance of being

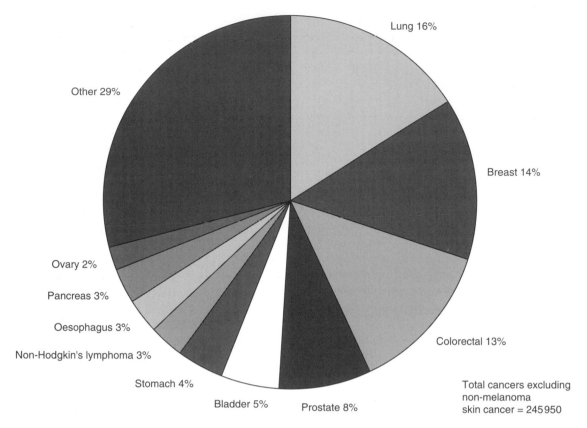

Figure 1.1 Ten most common cancers, persons, UK, 1995 (reproduced with permission from *Cancer Research Campaign Factsheet 1.1,* 1998).

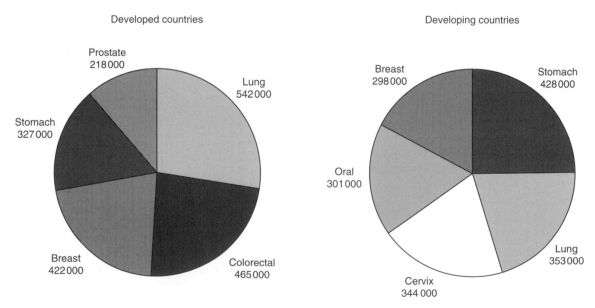

Figure 1.2 Number of new cases of the five most common cancers in developed and developing countries, 1995 (reproduced with permission from *Cancer Research Campaign Factsheet 22.1,* 1995).

cured of any particular cancer. Some cancers, such as skin cancer, if melanoma is excluded, have a very high chance of cure, whereas others, such as cancer of the lung and pancreas, have very low 5-year survival rates. Stage of the disease at diagnosis is an important determinant of survival. Survival for cancers detected and treated early is invariably better.[5] In the UK in 1994 there were 161 000 cancer deaths: lung cancer accounted for 23% of these and is the most common cause of cancer death; breast cancer accounted for 9% and is the leading cause of cancer death in women. In developed countries cancer is the cause of one in four deaths.[6]

Interestingly, cancer is unusual among diseases, in that in professional discussion in oncology, 'survival' is used as a benchmark for measuring

Table 1.1 Estimates of the % out of a cohort who develop cancer by age 65 and over a lifetime, England and Wales (reproduced with permission from *Cancer Research Campaign Factsheet 1.1*, 1998)

| Site | % of cohort who develop cancer by age group: | | Lifetime risk |
	0–64	0–85+	
Males			
Lung	1.9	8.4	1 in 12
Prostate	0.6	7.0	1 in 14
Colorectum	1.3	5.3	1 in 19
Bladder	0.7	3.2	1 in 31
Stomach	0.4	2.1	1 in 48
Non-Hodgkin's lymphoma	0.6	1.4	1 in 71
Oesophagus	0.4	1.4	1 in 71
Pancreas	0.3	1.1	1 in 91
Leukaemia	0.4	1.1	1 in 91
Kidney	0.3	1.0	1 in 100
Females			
Breast	5.0	9.5	1 in 11
Colorectum	0.9	4.7	1 in 21
Lung	1.0	4.3	1 in 23
Ovary	0.8	1.8	1 in 56
Uterus	0.6	1.3	1 in 77
Stomach	0.2	1.2	1 in 83
Bladder	0.2	1.2	1 in 83
Non-Hodgkin's lymphoma	0.4	1.1	1 in 91
Pancreas	0.2	1.1	1 in 91
Cervix	0.6	0.9	1 in 111

outcome and the effectiveness of treatment. Individuals and tumours are discussed in terms of an individual's chances of survival, measured formally as relative 5-year survival rates. Treatment choices are made on the basis of assessment of an individual's survival chance offset against attendant levels of toxicity for any given course of treatment. The possibility of death is immediate, and avoiding this as a goal predominates, reinforcing and responding to social and cultural images of cancer.

Biological understanding of cancer has become much more detailed in recent years owing to discoveries in molecular biology and genetics. These discoveries in turn suggest new avenues by which treatment may be targeted at specific points in the natural history of cells in which cancer may originate. Weinberg[7] eloquently describes the defining features of cancer at a cellular level:

Almost every tissue in the body can spawn malignancies; some even yield several types. What is more each cancer has unique features . . . the basic processes that produce these diverse tumours appear to be quite similar . . . 30 trillion cells of the normal, healthy body live in a complex, interdependent condominium, regulating one another's proliferation. Indeed, normal cells reproduce only when instructed to do so by other cells in their vicinity. Such unceasing collaboration ensures that each tissue maintains a size and architecture appropriate to the body's needs.

Cancer cells, in stark contrast, violate this scheme; they become deaf to the usual controls on proliferation and follow their own internal agenda for reproduction. They also possess an even more insidious property – the ability to migrate from the site where they began, invading nearby tissues and forming masses at distant sites in the body. Tumours composed of such malignant cells become more aggressive over time, and they become lethal when they disrupt the tissues and organs needed for the survival of the body as a whole [p. 3].

This description immediately transports us into a world deep inside the body, to a kind of internal city of citizen cells. Cancer is the sinister anarchistic force that threatens this internal society, and signals its ultimate demise; pictured in this way, fear of cancer and feeling the need to fight cancer seem natural responses.

A closer look at this deep internal world reveals a far less sinister sequence of mechanical or system failures, which, when they occur together, lead to

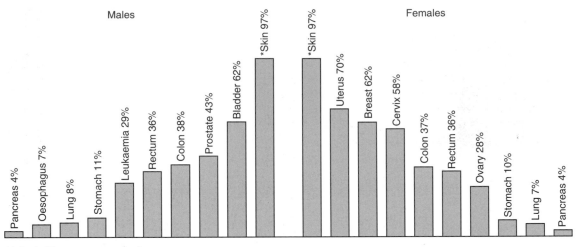

*Adjusted for non-cancer deaths.

Figure 1.3 Five-year relative survival %, England and Wales, 1981 (reproduced with permission from *Cancer Research Campaign Factsheet 2.1,* 1998).

the formation of a cancer. The aim of cancer science is to understand fully these mechanisms and eventually to find ways of correcting the mechanical failure, or to counteract the deleterious effects of it. The steps in the biological development of cancer outlined by Weinberg[7] are shown in Figure 1.4.

There is a number of mechanisms that either alone or in combination causes abnormalities in cell growth and multiplication. For a cancer to develop, it probably requires several to occur together. Alterations, or mutations, in genes within human cells contribute to abnormalities in cell growth. The mutations occur through errors in the replication of deoxyribonucleic acid (DNA) during cell division and may occur after exposure to a carcinogen. Mutations that activate the normal functions of the cell are called proto-oncogenes.[8] Mutated proto-oncogenes can cause excessive cell multiplication and through this contribute to the formation of a cancer. In contrast, tumour suppressor genes inactivate cell proliferation and if they fail to do this cell growth may continue when it is no longer needed.

Growth-stimulating proteins produced by proto-oncogenes bind to receptor sites on the cell membrane and pass a signal to proteins within the cell; these in turn pass signals in a cascade from protein to protein to the cell's nucleus, where transcription factors (regulatory proteins that bind to DNA sequences)[8] either stimulate or inhibit genes, producing important proteins within the cell. The result may be activation of the cell's own growth cycle and with it the chance of cancer forming. The cell may itself produce excessive growth factors. If this process is also accompanied by a loss or absence of tumour suppressor gene activity, cell growth and proliferation will be further enhanced, again increasing the likelihood of a cancer forming (see Figure 1.5).

The cell cycle is the name given to the process of cell division and is likened to a kind of clock that is set to a particular speed and rhythm.[7] The cell cycle proceeds in a series of phases; this results in the cell's DNA being replicated and the cell, and its DNA, dividing and becoming two daughter cells. Initially, the cell increases in size and prepares to copy its DNA ready for cell division. Then the chromosomes are replicated and the cell prepares to divide. Finally mitosis, or cell division, occurs. The cell then rests until it prepares to divide again. This cycle is controlled within the cell by cyclins and cyclin-dependent kinases or enzymes.[9] Mechanisms of control prevent cells within the body continuing to divide and proliferate unless this is required. Tumour suppressor proteins within the

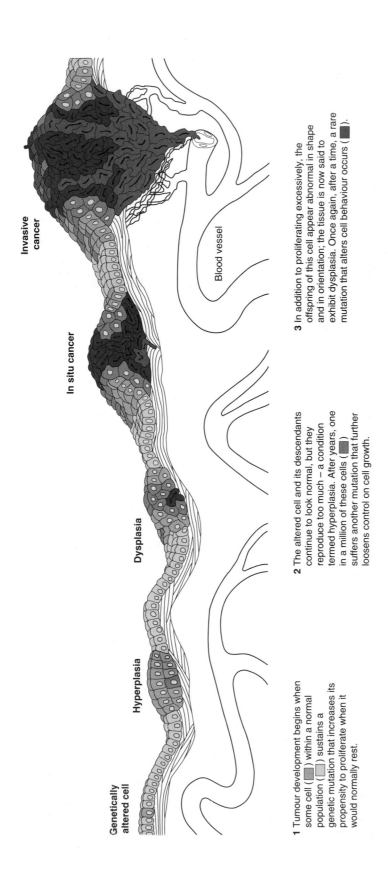

Genetically altered cell

Hyperplasia

Dysplasia

In situ cancer

Invasive cancer

Blood vessel

1 Tumour development begins when some cell (▨) within a normal population (▨) sustains a genetic mutation that increases its propensity to proliferate when it would normally rest.

2 The altered cell and its descendants continue to look normal, but they reproduce too much – a condition termed hyperplasia. After years, one in a million of these cells (▨) suffers another mutation that further loosens control on cell growth.

3 In addition to proliferating excessively, the offspring of this cell appear abnormal in shape and in orientation; the tissue is now said to exhibit dysplasia. Once again, after a time, a rare mutation that alters cell behaviour occurs (▨).

4 The affected cells become still more abnormal in growth and appearance. If the tumour has not yet broken through any boundaries between tissues, it is called in situ cancer. This tumour may remain contained indefinitely; however, some cells may eventually acquire additional mutations (▨).

5 If the genetic changes allow the tumour to begin invading underlying tissue and to shed cells into the blood or lymph, the mass is considered to have become malignant. The renegade cells are likely to establish new tumours (metastases) throughout the body; these may become lethal by disrupting a vital organ.

Figure 1.4 Tumour development occurs in stages. The creation of a malignant tumour in epithelial tissue is depicted schematically. Epithelial cancers (carcinomas) are the most common malignancies. The mass seen here emerges as a result of mutations in four genes, but the number of genes involved in real tumours can vary. (Reproduced with permission from Weinberg RA, *What you need to know about cancer, Scientific American*, special issue, 1997.)

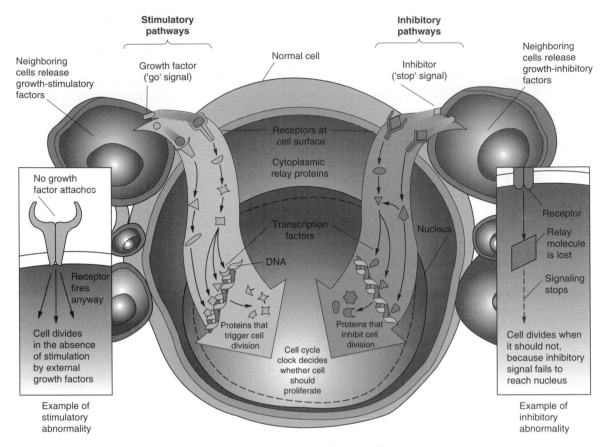

Figure 1.5 Signalling pathways in normal cells convey growth-controlling messages from the outer surface deep into the nucleus. There, a molecular apparatus known as the cell cycle clock collects the messages and decides whether the cell should divide. Cancer cells often proliferate excessively because genetic mutations cause stimulatory pathways to issue too many 'go' signals or because inhibitory pathways can no longer convey 'stop' signals. A stimulatory pathway will become hyperactive if a mutation causes any component, such as a growth factor receptor (box at left) to issue stimulatory messages autonomously, without waiting for commands from upstream. Conversely, inhibitory pathways will shut down when some constituent, such as a cytoplasmic relay (box at right) is eliminated and thus breaks the signalling chain. (Reproduced with permission from Weinberg RA, *What you need to know about cancer, Scientific American,* special issue, 1997.)

cell can either block the activity of these cell cyclins, and therefore cause the cell cycle, and therefore cell division, to pause; or, if excessive amounts of cyclins are produced by the cell, then cell division may proceed unchecked. Further cellular mechanisms exist to prevent uncontrolled cell division, for example, a process known as apoptosis. This is a mechanism whereby an abnormality in the cell's DNA is recognised within the cell and its own death is brought about as a consequence. The p53 protein is involved in apoptosis; disruptions in the gene involved in the production of p53 may mean

that abnormal cells can avoid apoptosis. Cancer cells may also produce proteins that prevent apoptosis. If apoptosis is avoided then an abnormal cell will continue to divide and replicate itself, perhaps indefinitely.[7]

A mechanism exists within the body to regulate and monitor the number of times any single cell can replicate itself. Normally this occurs 50 to 60 times before a cell becomes senescent and eventually dies.[7] This is dictated by the length of telomeres or sections at the ends of chromosomes; these become slightly shortened each time a cell multiplies and once below a critical length the cell stops dividing. In cancer cells an enzyme, telomerase, is produced, which replaces the effect of the telomeres becoming shortened. This enzyme promotes excessive growth and cell multiplication; again, this may be part of the process by which a tumour forms. These various mechanisms involved in cell growth and multiplication, if disrupted or where normal control mechanisms alter or fail, will lead to abnormal tissue growth. Thus, according to Weinberg,[7] cancer occurs directly as a result of 'runaway cell proliferation'. He concludes:

> Still, despite so much insight into cause, new therapies have so far remained elusive. One reason is that tumour cells differ only minimally from healthy ones; a minute fraction of the tens of thousands of genes in a cell suffers damage during malignant transformation. Thus, normal friend and malignant foe are woven of similar cloth, and any fire directed against the enemy may do as much damage to normal tissue as to the intended target [p. 14].

Weinberg returns to using metaphor to explain cancer. This time the intercellular world is not likened to reproduction or architecture, but to 'war', to be waged against runaway cells in an attempt to control cancer. Science and scientists make use of such metaphors and other techniques more familiar in literature, as devices to help reveal and articulate scientific facts. In doing this spaces are created in which such facts can become material or real when they are not in themselves visible; for example, as in the complex activities within the cell already described.[10] What is important is to understand how these metaphors may also become part of a wider social or cultural understanding of cancer, and themselves create 'what cancer is'. There is an important cyclical process here. Cancer the 'killer disease' becomes understood as a monstrous aberration of anarchistic runaway cell 'beings', an antisocial process working against the collective organism with grave or even fatal results. This is a powerful image, real to some extent because cancer is common and many people die from it (although, in developed countries, not as many as die from cardiovascular disease, which does not seem to engender such negative images). The 'runaway, anarchistic monster' is also a powerful

and difficult image for people who have the disease to experience within themselves, when cancer is visible, in the main, only through physical, embodied sensations such as pain or fatigue. Perhaps, given this, scientists should be more careful with the metaphoric and narrative devices they use to explain complex, 'invisible' facts.

Cancer is part of our culture, understood as a dreaded disease, feared perhaps more than any other disease, associated with inevitable death, and a death that is painful and unpleasant. Stories of people with cancer, especially celebrities who have cancer, frequently appear in newspapers and magazines. Jackie Stacey[11] has explored how popular cultural narratives are used to tell people's stories of having cancer. These, like fictional tales, or screenplays, follow a path through time, usually involving a heroic figure who struggles to overcome difficulties in the name of truth, justice, or love. The stories, like those in films or books, often involve tales of monsters and heroic recoveries. While the stories are real, in that they are about real people and cancer, in the way that they are told, they are constructed to fit this familiar fictional form. She says:[11]

> Cancer never really invades the body as such, but rather reproduces itself from within. Malignant growths secretly proliferate. Like the monster of screen horror, it threatens bodily order and takes over its regulating systems. Horror films often tell tales of the conquering of monsters. Invaders from outside . . . threaten the order of human society and must be exterminated in the name of civilisation. More often than not, the monstrous threat invades the body. Occupied by an alien force or physical presence, the innocent human victims lose control of the body and its functions. Be it vampires, ghouls or monsters from outer space, the horror narrative explores the boundaries between human and non-human, between life and death and between self and other. Its resolution requires the expulsion of the alien from the physical and social body it threatens, and the reestablishment of human order and stability. The heroes (the good scientists, the decent citizens, the protective fathers – and very occasionally the Sigourney Weavers) fight the monster to its death and return the rule of law to its rightful supremacy. Stories of surviving cancer fit easily into these patterns of journey from chaos to control. They combine the masculine heroics of such adventure narratives with the feminine suffering and sacrifice of melodramas [p. 10].

These stories use language laced with metaphor; people with cancer 'battle' for their survival, and cancer treatment is represented as a military campaign; the oncologist is at war against a killer disease, and cancer treatments are his ammunition. It seems that society as a whole is at war with cancer. As Susan DiGiacomo states:[12]

> In a society that has declared 'war on cancer' the cancer patient is a victim, held hostage by a disease that has invaded his body, which becomes the battle field on which the war is fought. The dissimilar meanings of corruption and battle combine to promote medical paternalism and authoritarianism. No effort is spared to defeat so evil an enemy, and no general needs to explain his orders.

The metaphors surrounding cancer also reflect changing attitudes within society towards death.[13] Today, as a result of longevity, it is possible for death not to be experienced within a family for a generation. Death has become something that is not part of our daily lives; unlike in pre-modern times, our relationship with death has increasingly become one of denial of its possibility, rather than an ever-present reality. In this situation, cancer has become a symbol of death itself. On every occasion it presents itself to us it forces cracks into man's armoury that represses fear of death. As De Beauvoir concludes in her account of her experience of her mother's death from cancer:[14]

> You do not die from being born, nor from having lived, nor from old age. You die from **something**. The knowledge that because of her age my mother's life must soon come to an end did not lessen the horrible surprise: she had sarcoma. Cancer, thrombosis, pneumonia: it is as violent and unforseen as an engine stopping in the middle of the sky. My mother encouraged one to be optimistic when, crippled with arthritis and dying, she asserted the infinite value of each instant; but her vain tenaciousness also ripped and tore the reassuring curtain of everyday triviality. There is no such thing as a natural death: nothing that happens to man is ever natural, since his presence calls the world into question. All men must die: but for every man his death is an accident and, even if he knows and consents to it, an unjustifiable violation [p. 92].

If cancer is understood as a disease through the use of metaphor, it is also in turn a powerful metaphor. Cancer is a word that is ubiquitous; it is used to suggest many things, such as, all that is bad in society, or a pervasive fault in a machine, or a flaw in how an organisation is functioning. The cancer metaphor has developed a meaning within our culture that is both part and not part of cancer the disease; it develops a life of its own, and may or may not in the end reflect the disease in any direct way. The more established the meanings surrounding cancer become, the more these then shape people's expectations and fears of the disease; the process is insidious.

Cancer is all around us, quite literally because of the numbers of people who have cancer or who will be affected by cancer because someone they know has it. It is also all around us in the way in which it is part of our culture, and how we use what we believe about cancer to convey what we mean about other things; this in turn affects how we respond when we come across someone who has cancer. It is understanding this, and finding ways of responding to this complex interrelationship between disease and its various constructions for individuals, for professionals, and for health care, that is the foundation of caring.

What is cancer? This is an unanswerable question: it is many things, it is what you make it, and it is what others make of it.

References

1. Tiffany R. and Pritchard P. (eds.) (1989). *Oncology for Nurses and Health Care Professionals*, Vol. 1. *Pathology Diagnosis and Treatment*, 2nd edition. Beaconsfield: Harper and Row.
2. Donovan M.I. and Girton S.E. (1984). *Cancer Care Nursing*, 2nd edition. Norwalk, CT: Appleton Century Crofts, p. 15.
3. Cancer Research Campaign (1998). *Factsheet 1.1. Incidence – UK*.
4. Cancer Research Campaign (1995). *Factsheet 22.1. Cancer – World Perspectives*.
5. Cancer Research Campaign (1998). *Factsheet 2.1. Survival – England and Wales*.
6. Cancer Research Campaign (1995). *Factsheet 3.1. Mortality – UK*.
7. Weinberg R.A. (1997). How cancer arises. In *What You Need to Know About Cancer. Scientific American*, special issue.
8. Yarnold J.R. (1996). What are cancer genes and how do they upset cell behavior? In Yarnold J.R., Stratton M. and

McMillan T.J. (eds.) *Molecular Biology for Oncologists,* 2nd edition. London: Chapman and Hall.

9. Carr A.M. (1996). Cell cycle control and cancer. In Yarnold J.R., Stratton M. and McMillan T.J. (eds.) *Molecular Biology for Oncologists,* 2nd edition. London: Chapman and Hall.

10. Lenoir T. (1998). Inscription practices and the materialities of communication. In Lenoir T. (ed.) *Inscribing Science: Scientific Texts and the Materiality of Communication.* Stanford, CA: Stanford University Press.

11. Stacey J. (1997). *Teratologies: A Cultural Study of Cancer.* London: Routledge.

12. DiGiacomo S.M. (1987). Biomedicine as a cultural system: an anthropologist in the kingdom of the sick. In Baer H.A. (ed.) *Encounters with Biomedicine: Case Studies in Medical Anthropology.* New York: Gordon and Breach, p. 323.

13. Sontag S. (1977). *Illness as Metaphor.* London: Allen Lane.

14. De Beauvoir S. (1969). *A Very Easy Death.* London: Penguin, p. 92.

CHAPTER TWO

Knowledge and caring: a philosophical and personal perspective

Alan Cribb

Preamble

Most days after I got home from school I would sit on a stool by the kitchen work surface and talk to my mum. She would be making dinner for the family and I have particularly clear memories of her preparing vegetables – peeling and chopping them whilst I pinched bits. I was eager to report the details of my day and to give her the benefit of my opinion on all manner of things. I was very interested in science at the time, having been fired by the thought that everything is made of molecules! Not only did it not occur to me to help but I don't think it ever occurred to me to ask about her or her day (she would just have returned from work), or about whether she had anything on her mind. It was one-way traffic. She would listen quietly, sometimes asking questions; occasionally offering advice. I suppose if I know anything worth knowing about care I started to learn it at times like that – being cared for body and soul as a matter of routine, and scarcely appreciating it. So writing about caring seems a bit odd.

Knowledge is a different matter. Knowledge belongs in books. School was about knowledge and I carried some of it home in my physics and chemistry textbooks, shut away in my school bag. Many people think knowledge ought to be only written about in the third person, that it is something formal and impersonal. There are academic conventions to adhere to (Bloggs, 1997). If one is going to write about knowledge one had better be on one's best behaviour. Furthermore, one had

better sound like an intellectual. Epistemological analysis demands a rigorous idiom (that sort of thing).

So there is the problem – how to write about these two different concerns together; how to do justice to my mum and the science textbooks. I have to admit at once that I cannot. I am in a textbook and I will have to be fairly 'text bookish', but from time to time I may also have to rebel.

PART ONE – PICTURES OF KNOWLEDGE

Two worlds

I want to start by reinforcing some of the contrasts in the preamble, by drawing a tidy distinction between two worlds – the scientific world (or more precisely the 'world as known by science') and the 'human world'. No doubt like all such distinctions it should not be drawn too tidily, and it may even collapse under close inspection; but there will be time for qualifications later. I want to argue that the reason for emphasising this contrast is because it plays a very important role in so much of modern life. It shapes so much of what we do and think.

Consider the furniture in your home. Items of furniture will have stories attached to them. Simple stories: 'This was a present from x', 'This was a bargain from y'. Elaborate stories: 'Remember the first meal we had at this table, when I hardly knew you . . .', 'This bed could tell a few tales . . .'. But suppose we are asked whether these stories are *really* about the furniture. Are they not only projections of our concerns, which we 'tag' onto it? Surely, it could be said, if we want to know about tables we should turn to science. Chemistry can help us to understand the material constitution of a table, and physics its ultimate constitution. The table is *really* some sort of configuration of energy. It appears to our common-sense eyes to be brown and solid, but in itself it is not even these things. Appearances are deceptive.

Of course, for virtually all domestic purposes we do not need to concern ourselves with the 'science of furniture' (although we might note in passing that the furniture industry employs people with expertise in material sciences, ergonomics, etc.). We can manage very well with common sense or 'lay beliefs'. But at the back of our minds we know that, at least with regard to material things like furniture, common sense is second rate. Our lay judgements are unreliable and sometimes plain wrong. Most people could make sensible guesses about which materials are most hazardous in a fire, but most people would get some of it wrong. This is one of many ways to 'die of ignorance'. What applies to furniture is certainly true for microwave ovens and television sets, and all the paraphernalia of modern life. The lay realm is one of opinion, guesswork, and myth. It is part of the real world but it is also shaded from it by various degrees of scientific ignorance.

None of this would be of much consequence if it only applied to domestic furniture, but it is possible to see this as a mere instance of a general truth. The modern world is, according to many perspectives, one in which lay beliefs have been eroded, demoted, replaced, and transformed by scientific knowledge. Secularisation is perhaps the most significant example of this change. A cosmos that has a personal creator at its heart has been superseded by a Godless, 'cold' universe. Human beings do not have an exceptional place in the meaning and the mystery of the world, they have emerged 'ordinarily' out of the processes of evolution, and they are biological rather than theological creations. Many other parallel and allied

shifts have taken place. Weber calls this process, by which the 'magic' is taken out of the world by a modern, scientific, rationalistic spirit, 'disenchantment'. When we see lambs or daffodils they may speak to us of hope and renewal, of an underlying sense of purpose, of belonging. But we also know that they are just natural 'blind' phenomena, and in a sense meaningless ones, and that our metaphysical interpretations of them are misleading. (I am deliberately overstating this. Of course it is possible, indeed probably the norm, to entertain both 'scientific' and 'lay' beliefs at the same time, to live, as it were, in two worlds. I will come back to this shortly.)

Furthermore, what I am calling the human world is being displaced and colonised not only by the natural sciences, but also by the social or 'human sciences'. Every facet of our lives is subject to increasing quantities of sociological and psychological research. Here also, personal and common-sense opinion is set beside 'more expert' analyses. An individual struggling with an incident of crime, or divorce, or illness will make their own interpretations of events. But much of the social scientific research will be designed to transcend these interpretations, to identify the underlying explanations, the underlying reality. A wife may go to the doctor on behalf of her husband because 'He's too busy at work'. But a sociological eye will see that the couple are acting out gendered roles. Over time, as with the natural sciences, these social scientific lessons will become incorporated into a changed set of lay beliefs. Thus, for example, someone suffering from grief might anticipate that their experience may come in certain well-documented packages – in complex and contradictory feelings, in waves, in stages and so on.

It seems to me that most of us live in two worlds. The 'scientific world' has not expanded to fill every corner of our experience, and even in those areas where it is generally deemed to uncover the real nature of things many people do not regard it as sufficient. So even in the most secularised and scientifically minded cultures people still live in a relatively enchanted world. This may be experienced as a source of tension or 'dissonance' in individuals' lives. They may, for example, be aware of a gap between their relatively 'tough minded' public persona in which they account for the behaviour of others in sociologically and psycho-logically informed ways (say as 'rational economic consumers') and their 'tender minded' private self (who takes romantic love seriously and sees their loved one as someone of unique and infinite worth). They may rely on the predictability of a scientific and technological infrastructure, while pursuing scientifically dubious or even anti-scientific belief systems. We cannot but acknowl-edge the explanatory power and the usefulness of scientific ways of thinking but we do not want to live in a cold world. Disinterested rational abstract inquiry helps us to gain mastery over our envi-ronment but in doing so it makes it less hospitable. How will we be better off if we gain control of the world but lose our soul and our home?

As I've already indicated, this contrast between the scientific and the human worlds is in many ways too simplistic, and it is tempting to overstate the dominance of a scientific perspective. I there-fore want to make some remarks designed to qualify and challenge the impression I have given up to this point. But I will also insist that something like this crude picture is a crucially important ingredient of life in the modern world.

Commentary 2.1

Reading through this chapter some time after it was drafted, I think I see what I am trying to do and say in it. It is very much a personal piece (maybe a self-indulgent one); I am not trying to say anything original but simply to sort out ideas about knowledge and caring, some of which have come from studying philosophy and some from my personal life. I want to take issue with the view that knowledge and caring are two entirely different things, the former being 'clever' and the latter 'natural'. I am starting by looking at some ideas of what real knowledge is. The aim is to prompt the reader into reflections on their own ideas about knowledge and caring, and the relationship between them.

Real knowledge (mark 1)

Here are some objections to the picture set out in the last section. First, why speak of 'science' when really I am drawing a contrast between expert knowledge and lay beliefs? Surely most forms of knowledge are not scientific, and am I not stretch-ing a point even by parcelling sociology and psy-chology in with the natural sciences? Second, the various sciences have not had such indisputable suc-cess. At best they offer one kind of explanation of one aspect of the world – they are not a substitute for theological, historical, or cultural accounts of the world. Third, many people – even in the 'most advanced' societies would, as I have hinted, see science as something on the margins of their life, as something largely irrelevant to their central con-cerns. How can this be reconciled with the picture of the scientific world inexorably displacing and colonising the human world? All these objections have merit, and they help to add some confusion to what is, after all, a confusing scene.

The rationale for starting with the tidy dis-tinction, and the crude picture, is that it reflects a powerful current (arguably *the* current) of modern-isation – the idea that human progress comes from the growth and application of knowledge, and that above all *real* knowledge is scientific knowledge. This is one of the ruling ideas of modern societies. Constant attempts are made to dethrone it and to kill it off, but it is not easily dislodged.

The philosophical version of this ruling idea is called 'positivism'. There are many variants of philo-sophical positivism, and many internal and exter-nal controversies about them, but it is worth briefly sketching out some of the key components of what might be called classical, or naive, positivism.

(a) *Methodological monism* – a fancy name for the idea that there is only one kind of method suitable for the production of knowledge. The natural sciences are typically taken to be paradigms of knowledge. Many traditional belief systems (especially metaphysical theories about transcendent realities but also 'this-wordly' ideological, moral, or aesthetic judge-ments) are seen to be without warrant or even without meaning. In general, a sharp demar-cation is made between real knowledge, which satisfies appropriate methodological rigours, and mere belief, superstition, and plain nonsense, which falls beyond the line.

(b) *The quest for generalisations and structures* – the most favoured method involves the discovery, formulation, and testing of law-like generali-sations that describe particular cases or events as instances of some general phenomena. (For example: this bucket of water conducts electricity because substances with such and such properties conduct electricity; this economy is suffering from inflation because economies with such and such properties always do so.) So the generalising manoeuvre is accompanied by another one – the identification of the underlying combination of properties or 'structures' that help to explain the phenomena. We cannot understand the nature of water or economies, or anything at all for that matter, by looking at their surfaces. We need to understand their inner constitution, the reality beyond the surface appearance.

(c) *Prediction and control* – the value of law-like generalisations is that they put us in a better position to intervene in events with predictable results, i.e. they enable us to exercise greater control over events. The capacity for effective technologies (including both mechanical engineering and social engineering) is enhanced.

(d) *Reductionism* – the shift from surface appearances to underlying structures is sometimes called reductionism. Although this is principally about explaining things, it also suggests that something is 'taken away' by the explanatory move. All manner of things are rendered mere appearance, not fully real. There are many forms of reductionism, some of which are very radical and, if accepted, denude the world of all kinds of phenomena. 'Physicalism' is the thesis that everything can be explained by the laws of physics. This is the adult version of my juvenile enthusiasm about everything being made of molecules. If, as seems plausible, everything is made of matter or energy, why not try to explain everything (tea parties as well as tea cups) in purely physical terms? (Sociology also practises many types of reductionism; the most extreme being the predominantly anti-positivist 'social construction of reality' thesis. Here it turns out that many seemingly substantial things do not really exist in their own right but only as a product of human languages and practices.)

Whether or not positivism has been successful as a philosophical position (and a huge amount of work has gone into arguing that it has not), it has certainly been extremely influential both in the academic sphere and in the wider community. In the academic sphere its influence is shown, for example, by the incorporation of scientific methodologies into a wide range of subject areas. Indeed, in many areas 'research' is more or less equated with scientific style research. Some of its immense impact on the wider culture is indicated in the previous section.

Before considering some of the main anti-positivist arguments I will say a little more about the wider cultural associations of the sharp demarcation between real 'expert' knowledge and mere 'lay' belief. I want to summarise a conception of real knowledge that has widespread currency, which I will call 'the encyclopaedic picture of knowledge'.

In this picture, knowledge is represented by an encyclopaedia. It is something solid, substantial; something in which we can have confidence. It is also something that can be written down, that can exist in an impersonal form and can be used as a common resource. Of course, more would have to be added to complete a full drawing of this picture but the idea of an encyclopaedia will do for a thumb-nail sketch.

A similar picture is evoked by the idea of a non-fiction library. Here knowledge is arranged by subject as well as alphabetically. Time and space are mapped through the history and geography of the world, period by period, region by region. The natural and physical aspects of the world are covered by biological and physical sciences. We can zoom in to organs, cells, genes and so on, or 'zoom out' to solar systems, galaxies and beyond. Human culture is stored in all its religious, aesthetic, practical, and technological varieties. Some encyclopaedias are organised in a similar manner, and are, in effect, 'portable libraries'. We can imagine them as a record of all accumulated knowledge, organised into an interconnected and mutually supportive matrix.

If we operate with a picture like this we may also picture learning as 'studying'. There we are at the beginning of a course; over the horizon the exams are looming, and the problem is how are we going to get all the knowledge in the books on our shelves into our heads in time. When we go into the library and the stacks of books multiply it is natural to panic – our heads are so 'empty'!

But there is also something rather dead or inert about an encyclopaedia. We seem to be able to get along with life very well while it gathers dust. Many of the things we know we learn without recourse to books, and furthermore there are many things we would be foolish to try and learn from books. (This is the sense in which caring doesn't belong in textbooks.) Libraries are all very well but surely virtually everything that matters goes on outside libraries. Are we not right to regard someone who does not appear to realise this as rather foolish and callow?

Here I am only playing with impressions, and with vague outlines and contrasts. But I think there are important clues in these contrasts between the 'bookish' and the 'non-bookish' parts of life; clues that point in the direction of another picture of 'real knowledge', a picture that does not place our everyday, practical and personal knowledge in the box labelled 'seconds', and that helps to restore the primacy of the human world.

Real knowledge (mark 2)

'And now for something completely different.' This was one of the catch phrases of the Monty Python team. It was used – cleverly – to provide continuity when there wasn't any, but it will do for me as well, because I intend to say something about humour.

Nearly everyone knows how to be funny, and some people are very good at it. There are few people who go around being self-consciously and deliberately funny (and this is very difficult to carry off successfully and without causing annoyance) but we can all try to see 'the funny side of things'. Smiles and laughter are a very large element of the compound that makes life tolerable. Although they can be used divisively, their natural tendency is to draw people together. They are part of the warmth and the enchantment of the world. Even if we come to the conclusion that the universe is meaningless they help us to 'look on the bright side of life'.

But although we can perfectly properly say that someone knows how to be funny, or knows how to see the funny side of life, we would not expect to find this kind of knowledge in a book. In fact, we know it is exceedingly difficult to theorise about

humour and that someone who does so might in any case (or as a result) be pretty humourless. Writing about humour is at best a small part of knowing about humour, and we are inclined to say that the real knowledge falls outside books. There are many sorts of things about which this is true. Perhaps the most obvious set is 'physical' skills such as swimming, typing, or driving a car. But there are other more general and more fundamental sorts of knowledge that fall into the same category, such as speaking English (or another natural language) or – equally important for our purposes – knowing how to conduct a conversation. Indeed, these relatively conspicuous examples are only the tip of the iceberg, or rather they are some of the prominent features of the human face obscured by the currency of 'encyclopaedic knowledge'.

These reflections serve as an introduction to a 'mark 2' picture of real knowledge, which I will call 'The Personal Resource Picture'. In some ways (but not all) this can be seen as the opposite of the mark 1 picture. According to this conception, knowledge is personal, not impersonal. Real knowledge *cannot* be written down; rather it can only exist as part of the outlook, dispositions, and skills of people. (Of course some 'shadows' of it can be written down, just as something of the knowledge of someone who is an expert cook can be written into cookery books.) This sort of knowledge is not acquired by studying but by doing, by living. Here experience and practice make all the difference and being able to recite 'knowledge' counts for little or nothing.

Similar distinctions are sometimes made by differentiating between 'knowledge' and 'skills', or between 'theoretical knowledge' and 'practical knowledge'. But these other terms can be misleading if they suggest that the former type of knowledge is intellectual or mind-centred and the latter is essentially technical or physical (and body-centred). Stupid divisions have often been made between 'working with one's brain' and 'working with one's hands'. These divisions are conceptually stupid because human activities (with very few exceptions) are not delegated to parts of persons, and because an individual is a single unified 'embodied intelligence', not a strange combination of a thinking disembodied executive with an unthinking physical workforce. And, as I have indicated, this division is also closely bound up with peculiar social divisions, which link kinds of work with personal and social status.

The Personal Resource Picture of knowledge, therefore, is not meant to pick out only practical skills, except in the sense that all knowledge involves 'skills that have to be practised'. These include thinking skills and theoretical skills. Thus it is not only being a good piano player or being a good listener that involves personal knowledge, but also being a good historian or physicist. In all of these cases, the real embodied knowledge cannot be written down. (This is not to dismiss completely the kind of knowledge that can be written down. But note that this does not consist entirely of the sort of abstract impersonal truths that the encyclopaedic picture would suggest; rather, much of it represents 'personal voices' with whom we, as readers, are in conversation.)

Commentary 2.2

My main preoccupation here seems to be with the relationship between 'book knowledge' and 'personal knowledge'. Is one more basic than the other? Is one more important than the other? How do they fit together? Perhaps this is only a personal preoccupation – something I've got a 'hang up' about. But I suspect it is something of general relevance. Everyone has to do more and more exams and assessments. More and more academic books are being produced and read. Yet it is clear to most people that there is much more to learning and development than the learning that takes place 'on paper'. These days, is enough emphasis placed on 'the university of life'?

Knowledge mark 2 belongs squarely to the human world rather than 'the world as known by science'. Indeed, it helps us to see how the latter is not independent of the former but is supported and sustained by it. The naive positivist would picture 'the world as known by science' as the real world, the solid foundation underpinning the 'apparent' world of everyday human affairs. But it is equally possible to see our everyday experience – of furniture, and friends and so on – as primary; as providing the frame of reference which makes possible the various abstractions of science and expert knowledge, and as providing the only real context in which these abstractions can be applied

and tested. This is the message of the most influential anti-positivist philosophies of knowledge, such as the 'phenomenological' and 'hermeneutic' approaches. This is not the place to do justice to these approaches, but a short summary of their central tenets will serve to sum up much of the ground I have covered so far.

These approaches emphasise the distinctiveness and the priority of the human world, the world of our consciousness and language. If we had to do an inventory of the kinds of things there are, we ought to be struck by the immediacy and all-pervasiveness of some apparently non-physical things – namely, states of mind and meanings. (Some thinkers would argue that these are the only things whose existence we can be sure of!) Human history and culture is made up of meanings and stories, as are our individual lives, and all of these things can only be properly understood and known about by taking these meanings seriously, rather than dismissing them in favour of some spurious 'science'. In fact, the stories which weave our domestic furniture into our lives indicate a reality just as substantial as the stories which scientists tell about the material of which they are made.

This suggests a different relation between expert and lay 'knower'. Instead of seeing the lay person as 'falling short' of knowledge, as essentially ignorant, these approaches see the processes of 'everyday knowing' as entirely continuous with, and the basis of, more specialised forms of knowledge. Many important forms of expertise are simply more practised, more disciplined, and hence more developed versions of so-called ordinary 'lay' practices. In these instances there are differences of degree rather than kind. The basic (and perhaps also the highest) form of expertise, which is open to all, is to know how to operate as a member of the human community, to be able to understand what others are saying, to have a sense of what matters, and to be able to contribute to one another's lives and well-being.

Parenthesis

I remember the shock when Dad rang to say Mum had got cancer the first time. It was a few minutes before I reacted. I sat down and kept looking in the direction of the television programme I had been watching. Outwardly the world was the same but it had been transformed. After a few minutes the first signs of this began to trickle through in waves of messy and contradictory feelings. Of course, I had no idea about the long years of upheaval ahead – the activity, the waiting, the uncertainty, the drama and the routine that would dominate our lives, a flood that would sweep us and all our lives along, hurling the familiar aside, ripping up our bearings, and yet demanding sanity and steadiness. In that first few days it was relatively simple: there was concern for Mum and Dad, there was the imperative to be 'OK', there was hurt and fear to be kept at bay, and there was the urgent need to understand what was happening at the hospital; what the successive tests indicated, what the implications were, what was being done, what more could be done.

Those early hospital visits had two aspects. Here was the site of intervention, here were drips and dressings, here was technical expertise. Yet there was my mum, out of place, and with her spirit quietened. She was also determined to be OK, but with a burden she couldn't quite displace from her face. The face of health care and my mum's face locked together. With the foolishness of a young man, I wanted a quick technical fix; I was impatient for progress, I wanted to reassure everyone (not least myself) that everything would soon be alright. But, of course, even if a relatively quick fix had been possible it would not have met Mum's immediate needs. Her life was overturned, she was away from her home, surrounded by strangers and strangeness, the 'taken for granted' gone, and she was alone.

PART TWO – CARING KNOWLEDGE

What are the connections between knowledge and caring? There are many, and they depend, of course, on what we mean by 'caring'. I will sketch out two possible connections by way of an introduction to this half of the chapter.

First, *caring can be seen as an application of knowledge* – in order to care for someone (assuming a health service context for now), there are a great many things we need to know. Some of these things fall clearly into the category of scientific and technical knowledge. Diagnostic procedures from pulse rates and temperatures to sophisticated imaging techniques are one example. They enable us to look below the surface, to get beyond the individual's subjectivity. Someone may feel perfectly well, with no desire to be a patient, but a routine screening procedure or the investigation of some apparently trivial anomaly might uncover a 'problem', and a whole clinical journey begins. Despite proper concerns about the medicalisation of life most of us, most of the time, are grateful for the instruments and techniques of clinical science. However, most of us, most of the time, are in some respects 'squeezed out' by clinical science. When we are unwell we are both the centre of attention and also 'on the margins' – hanging around in the waiting room of science. There are clearly other non-scientific sorts of things we need to know in order to care for someone. We may need to know a great deal about them (depending on how extensive our interactions with them are), e.g. how they feel, what their hopes, fears, memories, beliefs, opinions are; we may need to know about their home life, friends and relatives, work, leisure, cultural and religious life. In short, we need to get to know about them as a person, and the social and cultural network that shapes their identity.

But this takes us into a different realm, and a second sort of connection between knowledge and caring. Up to now the implication has been that knowledge is a mine of general and specific 'information' that we deploy when we care for someone, and that we need different sorts of knowledge because people are complex beings. This is to rely on an encyclopaedic picture of knowledge. But as we have already seen, this is an inadequate picture for many purposes. What is crucial is not knowing in the abstract but embodied knowledge, or know-how. To care for someone, even if that someone is construed as an object of scientific knowledge, I have to be prepared to work *with* that person. To care for someone *as a person* I have, to some extent, to get *to know them,* and not just 'about them' in the abstract. Indeed, a substantial component of caring for someone is precisely paying attention to, and concerning oneself with, the person for whom one is caring. This is one of the respects in which caring can be seen as a form of knowledge, and not merely the application of knowledge. This may seem an odd way of talking but it serves to emphasise a number of things, which I will merely assert here.

Caring is not some warm, 'wishy-washy' feeling but an exacting and demanding set of skills, which exercises all of our faculties and judgement (including our 'emotional judgement'); it is a form of know-how that admits of degrees of expertise and is developed through practice and experience as well as reflection. To be 'a caring person' is not an alternative to being an intelligent person, it is necessarily an exercise of intelligence.

In what follows I hope to illustrate and defend these assertions, and also to indicate some of the challenges of caring as a form of expertise. In particular I want to look at: (a) the relation between technical and person-centred elements of caring, (b) the idea of 'emotional expertise', and (c) the ways in which cultural and institutional contexts affect the possibilities of caring. These issues are closely interrelated but here I will separate them out as far as I can. But I will start with another and different distinction, which could be a source of confusion. Caring has both a practical and an affective side. We can use the label '*caring for*' to indicate the practical dimension of caring. If I care for someone then I look after them, give them food or medicines, tend to their needs, make sure the environment is suitable for them, that they are comfortable or sufficiently stimulated, etc. I might also care for them by listening to them, by treating them with respect, by ensuring that they don't feel ignored, etc. We can use the label '*caring about*' to indicate the affective dimension of caring. If I care about someone then I have feelings of concern or regard towards them, and to some degree their welfare matters to me. If we care about someone we are inclined to want to look after them, but the two do not necessarily coincide. At least up to a point we can care for someone without caring about them, and vice versa.

Technical and person-centred caring

In drawing a distinction between technical and person-centred facets of care, I am not referring to the practical/affective distinction discussed above; rather, I mean to draw attention to two interconnected elements of practical care, or 'caring for'.

What I mean by technical care is all the care that derives from technical knowledge, or more precisely, knowledge that treats the individual as an object to which generalisations apply. What I mean by person-centred care is care that depends upon regarding the individual as a unique subject, as a particular person with a distinct biography, outlook and set of preferences. In the main, 'technical caring' and 'person-centred caring' are complementary.

Human beings can be seen quite properly as both part of the 'world as known by science', and part of the human world. They are made up of both matter and meaning. If we want to understand them, and care for them, we must take equally seriously those aspects of them that can be generalised about and those that cannot. It is not very easy to draw a definite line here, but some things are certainly appropriate objects for technical knowledge (e.g. blood, bones, and bodies generally) and some things certainly require a more person-centred approach (e.g. listening to someone's 'story'). Both these aspects of care are important. If we are interested in 'technical success' we are likely to focus on health 'outcomes'; if we are interested in 'success with persons' we might look at whether the person feels valued.

These two aspects of care are often complementary but there are also respects in which they can be in tension with one another. They are complementary because if we want to achieve good outcomes this itself can provide motivation to work closely with a patient and treat them with respect. Their compliance and/or their positive state of mind might contribute to the technical success we want. This gives us an instrumental and derivative reason to value people (although the real direction of derivation is the opposite – technical success is valuable because people are valuable). It is tempting to emphasise this complementariness, and indeed to go further and say that we should not even separate out these two elements of caring, that there is only good caring, which must integrate these elements. This may be true in practice but it is also necessary to be aware of the possible tensions between these elements.

A mind set, or a set of practices, which is geared to treating people as objects for technical intervention is not necessarily one well suited to responding to persons. Partly this relates to the costs of a 'conveyor belt' approach to human dignity and sensibilities but it has widespread ramifications. Many of the routine, but important, issues in health care ethics spring out of these tensions. For example, a specific drug may be routinely prescribed and regarded as optimal for a specific condition but should it be prescribed if the patient has a considered preference for something else and there are alternatives available? A father wishes to delay a critical operation on his daughter until after his partner flies in from overseas – how far should these wishes be respected? Whatever is for the best here, these alternatives may not even come to light unless the environment is relatively 'person-centred'.

Achieving the right balance between these two elements of care will serve as an example of why caring is an exacting business. Not only does it potentially call upon a wide range of knowledge but it depends upon integrating different sorts of considerations together. This means paying attention to both technical and personal factors, and gaining confidence and experience in making continuous practical and moral judgements. However, this example may give the impression that what I principally have in mind is some kind of cognitive or intellectual challenge – the difficulty of 'weighing together' different considerations. Although I am happy to see this as an intellectually exacting process, I also have in mind the fact that it is, at the same time, emotionally exacting, and that it is the need for 'emotional expertise' that marks out the real challenge, and the special intelligence, of caring.

Emotional expertise

I am using the expression 'emotional expertise' to refer to the know-how at the heart of caring. Some people will dislike the expression and the whole idea of emotional expertise. There is a common view that emotions are things that 'just happen' to us; that we 'suffer' them rather than 'do' them. This being the case, how does it make sense to talk of developing expertise with regard to them? In addition, does not talk of expertise imply that there are 'emotional experts', that some people are 'good at emotions' and other people 'bad at emotions', and is this not unnecessarily elitist and divisive? I have sympathy for these thoughts,

and I have deliberately chosen the label 'emotional expertise' because it provokes them, but on balance I see these reactions as misguided. I think that in some respects: (a) we are responsible for emotions, and (b) it is possible to be more or less skilful and conscientious in the exercise of these responsibilities. What is more, this is not just my opinion but it is a view endorsed by a great deal of ancient and modern thought and scholarship. Of course, 'emotional expertise' is an umbrella term and using it may obscure many complexities and controversies; there would no doubt be disagreement about its components and how they can be combined.

One tradition with bearing on this matter is discussion of 'the virtues', i.e. admirable and desirable qualities of character, such as courage or wisdom. Although 'virtues' may sound like an archaic term, we still operate with closely related ideas. For example, we write 'character references' for people, and in so doing we may talk of their honesty, loyalty, tenacity, fairness, balance and so on. We admire friends or acquaintances for who they are and not just for what they achieve. If we are bringing up children we typically want them to be 'good' – to be people whom others respect for their integrity and dispositions. In all of these cases, we are concerned with 'the virtues'. In Western academic philosophy the discussion of the virtues normally begins with reference to Aristotle's ethics but there has been a continuing thread of discussion on this theme, and virtue theory, including Aristotle's related work, has had a substantial revival during the past 20 years.

I cannot do justice to these academic debates here. But perhaps I can indicate a few important issues arising from them. First, we are inclined to hold people as *to some extent* responsible for their character (although, of course, many other factors outside an individual's control help to determine character). Both religious teachings and the huge self-improvement industry are testament to the belief that we can make a difference to the ways we think and act, to the kinds of people we are. Second, character is not just about how we reason at some abstract level but it is also about how we feel about things, how we respond to things, and what our inclinations and desires are. If both of these claims are true then it follows that we are to some degree responsible for our emotional life, that it is possible to conceive of emotional development, perhaps even of emotional education or learning. This, in broad terms, is certainly what is entailed by much of the literature on the virtues.

Commentary 2.3

I suppose what I am getting at here is fairly straightforward: there are people we admire because they are good with others. They may possess talents and skills in this regard that we may not. Do we think that these qualities are just part of life's lottery, or do we, to some degree, feel that these 'role models' have earned our respect? I think the latter. Furthermore, if we want to aspire to some of these admirable qualities I think we need to try to become more clear about what these talents are and how they can be developed.

Perhaps I can make this seem more plausible by using an example. Imagine a young man who is very jealous about his girlfriend. If he sees her talking for any time to other people he feels anxious and resentful, and these feelings can easily collapse into despair or anger. We might say that he 'cannot help' feeling like that, perhaps even that these feelings are 'natural'. We might feel sorry for him (and his girlfriend!) It is unfair to say that he should just 'snap out of it'. But notice what a difference the facts make. Suppose his girlfriend has never given him any reason to be jealous; suppose we have it on the best authority that nothing in her actions or in her heart should give him cause to worry. We would surely draw this to his attention. We would ask him to re-appraise the situation, and over the course of time we would hope that he would come to see things differently and as a result to some degree to feel differently. If we were speaking bluntly we might say, 'You've got to learn not to feel like that!'

Now this example works because so many emotions, including jealousy, are intimately related to our beliefs about the world. So if our beliefs are unreasonable (or irrational), then the emotions which relate to them will be, to use a neutral-sounding phrase, 'somehow inappropriate'. Of course you cannot just switch your beliefs or feelings on or off. It takes time and practice to change. Consider a visitor who is frightened by being close to a cancer patient, or a novice nurse who feels

nervous and inadequate when performing routine procedures. In these cases too we might be sympathetic while, at the same time, hoping that they would learn not to have these feelings. Notice that this is about emotional change and not just about covering feelings up, which is also a necessary, but different, aspect of managing our emotions. In all the examples above we might expect the individuals to attempt to cover up their feelings as a short-term strategy; in other instances, it may be necessary to learn to 'put up a front' in the longer term. (Managing our own emotions involves a combination of change and 'acting' – here I am discussing the former rather than the latter, but I ought to at least make reference to the need for some 'acting', and of course the inherent problems of inauthenticity and self-alienation.)

Virtue theory is based on the insight that our understanding, feelings and dispositions form compounds such that we cannot effectively develop these elements separately. Someone who is prudent (or honest, etc.) sees the world in certain ways, feels in certain ways, and acts in certain ways; this is what is involved in having a virtue. Of course there is room for debate about which set of virtues we believe people in general should aspire to (and also about the virtues most fitting for certain roles or positions). Similarly, it is unclear exactly how far, and in what respects, our character is capable of being shaped by our learning and practice. However, it would seem foolish and irresponsible (and fly in the face of our experience) to dismiss completely the notion of character development and with it the notion of emotional learning and growth.

This discussion of virtues has concentrated primarily on self development and on managing our own emotions, but what has this got to do with caring for others? Perhaps it is obvious. The jealous boyfriend is not in a good position to care for his girlfriend. The visitor who is frightened of cancer is not well placed to care for the patient. The nurse who feels self-conscious and inadequate is going to be less helpful to her patients than she might be. We cannot really aspire to deal with other people's concerns and feelings unless we are dealing with our own. I will not stress this point again but I hope that it will be seen as the backcloth to what follows.

As we have seen, a crucial aspect of caring for persons is to relate to them as persons and not as objects. There are other aspects of caring that do not depend quite so much on this. For example, we could say that a government cares – practically cares – for the population by introducing clean air legislation (or other health protection mechanisms). In the case of these interventions, people can be treated as biological creatures (although there will usually be accompanying processes of consultation and education as well). One way of bringing out the differences is to ask how far the technology in our hospitals and health centres could take over from human beings. There are, no doubt, areas where it makes little or no difference whether a machine or a human being does the caring, but there are others where it seems to make all the difference in the world. If we are in a room full only of technology we are still alone. Here, again, is the double-aspect of persons – we are made of both matter and meaning, of both stuff and subjectivity. If we are to be 'treated' properly then both components need responding to, and our subjectivity can only be recognised and responded to by another's subjective awareness. Of course, if a human carer behaves exactly like a piece of technology, like a sophisticated robot going through procedures, then the fact that they are a person makes no difference. What is this special ingredient of caring of which human beings are capable? I will borrow the term 'emotional labour' to describe it.

A number of social scientists and feminist scholars has used this term to indicate a substantial and vital, but typically neglected, sphere of human activity and relationship, i.e. the hard work that goes into acknowledging and meeting one another's emotional needs. Most of this work is unpaid, but it goes on in every setting and context. It is largely and characteristically undertaken by women. It is often informal and invisible – it tends to take place 'behind the scenes', to be off the official agenda (some parts of health care, and pastoral care in education are, to varying degrees, exceptions). In a climate in which measurable public 'outputs' are valued, emotional labour is likely to be grossly undervalued, if not unnoticed. (This is itself a good enough reason to adopt the term.)

Different scholars will write about different facets of emotional labour, and will continue, no doubt, to use the term to mean rather different things. It is, I think, a strength of the term that it can be used to refer to a wide range of things. But here I am borrowing it simply to help capture some of what is entailed by the affective aspect of caring. To think of caring as 'hard work' suggests not only that it is strenuous but also that it is skilful. To talk of 'caring' may sound wishy-washy to many people; to talk of 'emotional labour' sounds – I think helpfully – as if you might be indicating a form of expertise, a demanding discipline. (However, there is the danger that we might start thinking of the affective aspect of caring as if it were some technical and highly esoteric skill, which would be most unfortunate.)

One way of indicating some of the expertise required to be an effective 'emotion worker' is to consider the range of relevant factors. Clearly, affective care has to be responsive to circumstances and to individuals. There is something farcical about thinking one could go around indiscriminately caring for people. Furthermore, it is downright intrusive and disrespectful to assume a licence to work upon other people's emotional well-being. Most of the time all we need to achieve is what might be called 'good manners', by being polite, and hopefully reasonably kind and sensitive to the people we meet. As part of this process we may notice that they appear upset, or anxious, or cross and we may tailor our words and deeds to their manner to some degree, but it is not generally part of our brief to do more than that. Everything depends upon our relationship with them, and the circumstances under which we are meeting. Are they friends or strangers? Are we in a bus queue or in a self-help group?

The same applies within health care settings: just because we are in a professional role and are practically caring for someone, it does not follow that we should be paying any *special* attention to their specific emotional or psychological needs. Most importantly, they may not want that sort of attention; in addition, it may not be a fitting part of the task in hand. The 'emotional labour' required may be fairly circumscribed. Someone who is taking blood samples from a series of patients in a waiting room needs to be able to be as reassuring and as gentle as possible, while doing their job effectively and efficiently. It is also useful to be able to recognise, and to be patient with, individuals who are unusually frightened of that procedure. But it would be completely out of place for them to strike up a conversation about the patient's deeper worries. What is fitting will thus depend, amongst other things, upon (a) what the individual person needs and wants, (b) the nature of the professional role, (c) whether the relationship has a history and/or a future, and (d) the particular characteristics and personal styles of the two people involved.

Furthermore, 'emotional labour' rarely occurs on its own, and this makes even greater demands. Most of the time when we are caring for someone we are doing something practical or technical. As a necessary part of these practical interventions, we will have regard to emotional matters. We may choose to comfort someone physically, or to listen to their point of view, or provide some occasional companionship, but in order to do these things well we often need to be fully engaged with the whole of their care. If we are listening to someone who is about to be discharged home and is concerned about how they are going to cope, it helps if we have some insight into what they are saying (and in turn this may involve a knowledge of their clinical condition, their medication, their attitudes, their family, home services, etc.). This is not necessarily because we are in a better position to do something about their concerns (although we may be) but because we are better able to listen, better able to hear what they are saying and to understand it. Sometimes people just need attention and recognition, but often what they really value is 'informed attention'. It is this compound of technical and emotional expertise that is so characteristic of health care and particularly of nursing.

Supporting care

Until now I have concentrated on the difference that individuals can make, but it is not all a question of individual responsibility. In many respects individuals can only do what circumstances allow, and we all require the support of each other and of the right policies and cultures. There are some deep philosophical and practical questions raised here, which I will pass over very quickly. First, it is very difficult to separate out individual and collective responsibility. The debate about criminality is a familiar one – how far, and when exactly, should we hold individuals responsible for a crime rather than seek explanations in the various pressures and contexts that help to shape them? It is broadly the same debate with virtues as with vices. In professional roles we should certainly expect that individual practitioners will be motivated not to fall below certain minimal standards of practice, but can the wider society expect them to be motivated to aspire to, and strive for, ideals of best practice? I would argue that the latter is an unrealistic expectation unless a good deal of thought and effort is put into creating supportive contexts for professional work. This takes us on to a second set of puzzles, i.e. what counts as a 'supportive context'.

Commentary 2.4

In this final section I am trying to correct a possible overemphasis in the previous discussion. What I have called personal knowledge is essential but it cannot stand on its own. It is no good simply saying that everyone should 'pull themselves up by their own boot straps', and miraculously develop the caring virtues. We need to think hard as a society (and institutionally) about how we can support each other's development. We need to understand more about personal knowledge and 'emotional expertise' in particular. I think it is partly about putting these discussions firmly at the top of the agenda along with other important topics such as budgets, etc.

I will not try to solve these puzzles in this chapter (nor could I!) but I will try to suggest some factors that need to be borne in mind. These questions about fashioning the context of professional work can draw upon a variety of forms of knowledge. There is a lot of relevant work in management studies, organisational theory, economics, social psychology, social policy, sociology and so on, as well as practical expertise relating to leadership or team-working, etc. But, as always, it is vital that those who are developing or applying these forms of knowledge are asking the 'right questions'. It seems to me that all too often those voices that are most influential in policy making neglect important questions. Efficiency and health gain are most important but we also need to ask 'How can institutions and cultures be developed in ways that underpin and that foster "caring expertise"?' Health care is about health and care, and it is foolish to assume that these two are the same and that whatever delivers one will deliver the other. (Of course, some people may wish to develop the argument that at some level these two concepts converge in important ways – but that is a different matter.)

There are two related sets of reasons for this relative neglect of caring:

- a policy climate increasingly dominated by 'outputs', the language of audit and the use of performance indicators, which by their very nature are reductionist
- the ambiguities and complexities surrounding the notion of caring, which make it difficult to have a confident public debate about, let alone to accommodate this debate to, an 'output-orientated' policy climate.

Both of these sets of reasons are worth attending to and I will say a little more about the relationships between them shortly. But on this occasion I have concentrated more on this second set of reasons. I am conscious of the difficulties of treating caring with due seriousness. It is all too easy to retreat into sentimentality or wishful thinking, and to deal in vague generalisations. We are inclined to see it as a question of instinct or intuition, perhaps something it is counter-productive to theorise about (rather like humour). I think there is a lot to be said for this attitude; there is a limit to how far we should, as individuals, be self-conscious and analytical about dispositions and skills that need to become 'second nature' if they are to be truly effective. But I believe we do need to be self-conscious about these questions as citizens, or as professional groups and to ask how we, collectively, can create conditions under which this particular embodied form of knowledge can be acknowledged and nourished. One issue that can be used to illustrate this sort of question is the use of time. It is a crucial issue because underlying the output-orientated culture is the imperative to allocate public resources efficiently. The time of health professionals is, in every sense, the most valuable resource of health services and is itself necessarily rationed.

Anyone who has visited their general practitioner will understand how time creates certain caring possibilities. There is a limit to what can be done in a 5–10 minute consultation. A GP, especially if they are of a holistic persuasion, may well ask about your home or work circumstances – are you under stress, or do you have specific problems that are keeping you awake? They may also ask about your diet, exercise patterns and so on, and they will have to consider whatever condition or concern brought you there in the first place. All of this is good practice and may well throw up important clues to improving your health. But the time pressures on the consultation will powerfully shape the structure and the 'feeling' of the interaction. The process will nearly always be informed by the move towards some 'intervention' on the part of the GP, whether it be encouragement, advice, treatment or referral. Two things will rarely be possible: (a) the doctor simply listening to an extended account of this range of life-related problems, prompted by their questioning, and (b) a careful negotiation of a shared understanding of some of these factors. Yet both of these things can be, depending on the case at hand, vital foundations for certain forms of caring. This shortcoming is not necessarily a problem – the limitations on these particular consultations are widely understood and accepted. But if, under budgetary pressures, a predominantly instrumental style of interaction increasingly comes to be seen as the appropriate model of personal interaction across a range of settings, the potential for caring relationships in professional health services will be greatly diminished.

There are many other things we need to understand in more depth. For example, what sorts of professional support enable different practitioners to sustain person-centred caring over years? How can we effectively encourage practitioners to find their own style of 'emotional expertise' and to know when they are at the limits of their competence? How can we create settings with the right balance of generalist and specialist 'emotional expertise'? Above all, how can policy making give proportionate emphasis to both technical and person-centred facets of care, and to both 'health gain' and caring processes? The first step to a better understanding is to ensure that we give proper respect to, and consideration of, the whole range of forms of expertise that people possess. We should not take caring for granted; we should not assume that we understand it, we should not treat is as a fixed 'natural resource' that can be deployed in any set of circumstances. It is a precarious and priceless form of knowledge.

Postscript

I do not really want to say anything about my mum's death or dying. It still seems too private to talk about (especially in such a public place). And I certainly don't want to imply that there is some kind of wisdom, some kind of caring, that could 'make it right'. Suffering cannot be denied. But, of course, there are also good things and gratitude. All of those people who supported her, and us, through the upheavals of her last few years did something immensely precious. Friends, neighbours and colleagues spring to mind, but so do people who were once strangers, people who were 'just doing their job'. There were mistakes, misunderstandings, insensitivities, and general clumsiness mixed up in all of this, but what should we expect? Human beings are pretty imperfect creatures and caring is such a demanding business. Care has so many faces, and serves so many ends, and different compounds are needed from instance to instance.

I am grateful for the technical expertise, for the people who listened or provided companionship, for those who understood the practical routines, for the kind touches, for the opportunities for laughter and for many other things. It seems to me – and I admit I'm biased – that both my parents were exceptionally brave and good during these ordeals (although of course they 'failed' too sometimes) and they were lucky to have each other and their family around. There is a limit to what 'professional carers' can do and there is a limit to what can be expected of them. Yet, at the same time, within these limits there is scope for an infinite amount of good.

At the thanksgiving service for my mum, as before and since, people celebrated her. They spoke about her gentle and sympathetic nature. In my opinion gentleness cannot be overrated, but I don't see these good qualities as entirely passive or as just

'natural', such that they cannot be learned or practised. It seems possible for us to be more or less alive to other people's needs. Our capacity for this may vary from time to time and according to many other factors. But some people seem to be very good at it. They are able to generate a powerful current of attention that places other people at the centre of things. This is how my mum's friends and (albeit in different ways) her patients and acquaintances knew her and remember her.

Acknowledgements and further reading

First, I would like to say thank you to my mum, Joan Ashton Cribb. Thanks are also due to a few close friends and colleagues who encouraged me to write this chapter and gave me helpful comments on it. There are other debts unacknowledged in the text; indeed, I do not claim any originality for what I have written. I have no doubt been influenced by many things, only some of which I could even bring to mind. One of the more conspicuous influences (to those with an interest in philosophy) is Gilbert Ryle's discussion of 'Knowing how and knowing that' and subsequent work on the same theme [G. Ryle (1945) *Proceedings of the Aristotelian Society*, Vol. XLVI, 1–16; J.C. Nyiri and B. Smith (1988) *Practical Knowledge: Outline of a Theory of Traditions and Skills.* Croom Helm, London]. There are plenty of references to work on 'caring' in other chapters but I have explicitly drawn on two traditions of related work – virtue theory and work on emotional labour in health care [see for example, G. Pence (1984) Recent work on the virtues, *American Philosophical Quarterly* **21**, 281–297; P. Smith (1992) *The Emotional Labour of Nursing.* Macmillan Press, Basingstoke].

For those interested in thinking in greater depth about some of the issues raised in this chapter, I suggest a couple of possible starting points – M. Hollis (1994) *The Philosophy of Social Science, An Introduction.* Cambridge University Press, Cambridge; J. Oakley (1992) *Morality and the Emotions.* Routledge, London.

CHAPTER THREE

Cancer, care, and society

Christopher Bailey

Cancer probably affects most of us, directly or indirectly. We may, professionally or informally, provide care for someone who has cancer. We may have or have had cancer ourselves. Someone we know has probably had cancer. We hear about it and read about it; we see images that depict it. It is common to find cancer written about in our newspapers in terms characteristic of war, violent hostility, or killing, rather than of care or therapy:

> Surgery that immobilises cancer by freezing diseased cells to death could give new hope to patients with multiple liver tumours where surgery might not leave enough liver tissue needed for survival. In cryosurgery, tumours are frozen by applying liquid nitrogen via a probe directly to the affected area. Doctors . . . are studying the technique and report the case of a 76-year-old woman for whom a year of chemotherapy had failed to destroy four liver tumours. Since cryosurgery was performed in January this year she has been healthy and no new tumours have been found.
>
> *The Sunday Times,* 17 November 1996

Here cancer is 'immobilised' (disruptive prisoners are also 'immobilised' by wardens or police officers) by freezing cancer cells to death; other techniques have 'failed to destroy' tumours, but the death of the diseased cells restores health and order.

New cancer treatments are often described using military terminology, and sometimes emanate from institutions whose primary role really is military:

> Government scientists at Porton Down, the chemical and biological defence research centre, are working on

new anti-cancer drugs that avoid the toxic side-effects of chemotherapy . . . 'We are working on more effective delivery systems for targeting specific tumours' . . .
>
> *The Guardian,* 16 July 1998

Like chemical and biological weapons the new agents 'break open' the tumour and 'release the drug over it' (*The Guardian,* 16 July 1998).

'Hope' seems to depend on the outcome of this violent struggle, as if in some way we were drawing strength from and depending on the idea of being at war with the cancer, the enemy. At the same time, the word 'cancer' is applied outside the health care arena to express terror and destruction, the overwhelming of once healthy and vigorous social institutions:

> There is a terrible cancer devastating our national museums. One after another is being annexed by the entertainment industry . . . The introduction of museum charges . . . is undoubtedly having a grim impact.
>
> *The Sunday Times,* 17 November 1996

> Frank Field yesterday launched the latest salvo in his post-resignation fightback with an assault on spin doctors, whose activities he called a cancer at the heart of the Government . . . He said . . . 'In the long run, you can't run a government like this. It's a cancer that will eat away at the heart of our very existence and undermine the way ministers behave' . . .
>
> *The Guardian,* 4 August 1998

This is another side of the war, where cancer is attacking the social, rather than the physical body. Susan Sontag[1] believes that 'Cancer is a metaphor for what is most ferociously energetic, and these energies constitute the ultimate insult to the natural order' [p. 72]. That is to say, cancer is also a metaphor for what is antithetical to constructive social organisation and process. In health care, the 'war against cancer' continues, but the idea of health care is applied beyond the health care system: if parts of society 'have cancer', or are sick, they too need treatment to put them right. Health care provides a model for putting things right, which applies not only to our physical selves, but to our social selves, to us as members of society. The importance we place on the 'war against cancer' reflects a longing not just to make our bodies right, but also to make our society healthy.

Cancer is part of the everyday lives of thousands of people, yet it often seems not to be 'everyday' at all, but different, frightening perhaps. Every day thousands of people learn, or realise, or suspect, or fear that they have cancer; they learn that their mother or father, or son or daughter, or wife or husband or partner, or friend, or neighbour or aunt, cousin, niece or nephew has cancer. In one study,[2] which invited partners of women with breast cancer to express their feelings about the diagnosis, one man described how present experience can lead to the re-awakening of past trauma:

> What most worries me is the cancer itself – knowing [wife] has it. My mother died of cancer; that was a terrible time for me . . . I'm afraid of when [wife] goes to hospital for an operation to have cancer. I don't know if I can handle this because then everything comes back [p. 607].

Claudine Herzlich and Janine Pierret, French sociologists whose studies of illness are based on collections of personal experiences, refer to cancer as the 'most frightening illness of all'.[3] So frightening in fact that cancer is a word that sometimes cannot be spoken: a word that, if spoken, 'condemns the sufferer' (p. 57), as if by magic. In France, say Herzlich and Pierret, it is rarely publicly acknowledged that people have died of cancer; rather, they are said to have died after 'a long and painful illness' (p. 58). They record conversations that reflect the 'quasi-magic image' or the 'phantasms' (p.106) of contagion, which affect both people with cancer and those who are not ill themselves. Despite modern pathology, which has

transformed much of our understanding of illness, anxiety in our society still 'crystallises around one scourge of illness, which is totally associated with death . . . cancer . . . has become the very embodiment of physical suffering for us'; cancer is the 'specific illness of our society', 'THE illness of our time', so dominant that it sometimes seems to be the '*only* illness' (p. 55). Herzlich and Pierret believe that cancer is the 'modern equivalent of the age-old scourges, and that, like diseases in the past, it is 'fraught with phantasms of rot invading the body, and animals that gnaw and destroy it'; it is, they say, as if cancer had 'appeared only recently, at the very moment when the threat of the other ills was no longer as great' (p. 56). They point to two 'conceptions' or themes in the aetiology of cancer, which illustrate how cancer has become the 'prototype' of modern illness:

> One of them sees it as an illness of the individual, the other as a disorder of our way of life and of society. In fact . . . *cancer is the illness of individuals in their relations with society.* It is indeed an illness of the individual, but this individual can only be conceived of in relation with society as a whole. At the same time cancer is also an illness produced by society, but one that manifests the flaws of the present-day individual [p. 62].

Cancer is sometimes seen as a development of certain psychological characteristics, such as repressed or anaesthetised feelings, resignation in the face of life, lack of self-confidence, or an inability to express energy, particularly sexual energy, freely; the contemporary image of the 'cancer personality' being, Sontag[1] writes, a 'forlorn, self-hating, emotionally inert creature' (p. 57). Herzlich and Pierret[3] do not agree, though, that this 'schema' reflects the majority of people's ideas of 'cancer as an individual disease' (p. 63). Instead, they emphasise that people see themselves as predisposed towards the disease (for example, because they have relatives with cancer), or as 'favourable terrain' for it. People often believe, however, that their environment determines their individual behaviour: the ideas of cancer as an individual illness and cancer as an illness produced by society (for example, by pollution) co-exist. Herzlich and Pierret finally incline to the view that cancer is experienced both as 'timeless scourge' and as part of the dangers of modern life: ' "Is cancer a part of myself, or does it come to me from the outside world?" the sick person wonders' [p. 65].

Whether we experience cancer personally, as an individual who is given this diagnosis; or personally through a partner, friend, or relative; or personally, as someone whose responsibility it is to support and care for someone else who has cancer; whether we experience cancer indirectly, through the airwaves, on the screen, on the page, or on the billboard; however we experience it, we are almost always moved by it, and often we find ourselves feeling a need to respond, to shake off a mood, offer some form of help, or perhaps to avoid the subject altogether. It is difficult to see how we can avoid having some stance, some collection of thoughts and feelings, some mixture of the rational and irrational that is evoked by cancer.

My father, for example, has had a fear of cancer for as long as I can remember. When I told him about the research I was doing into older people with cancer of the bowel and the treatment and care they receive, he looked at me accusingly as if to say, 'You would pick that one, wouldn't you!' and was unable to discuss it with me. It was as if the coincidence was more than coincidence, something more fateful; as if being involved with the cancer he fears most and talking about people of his age who have this cancer was bringing it into his life; almost as if I was exposing him to the risk of developing it himself.

My mother, also, rarely asks me about my work, but every so often she asks me quietly, when no one else can hear, whether I think she is likely to have breast cancer. She seems genuinely afraid of this possibility, though she has no symptoms and is not in a high-risk group. Cancer can sometimes play on our fears, our worries about our safety and well being; it can be a focus for feelings of vulnerability and fragility we may not even know we have.

My own feelings about cancer and about working with people with cancer have changed over time. When I started out as a student nurse I found cancer a forbidding illness, and what sticks in my mind is a feeling that I didn't really know what it was, what kind of 'disease' or 'illness' it was. Caring for people recovering from abdominal surgery for cancer of the colon or rectum seemed to me, a raw recruit to nursing, to be almost impossibly complicated. People's bodies, after surgery, seemed so radically altered, pieced together, that I was quite disorientated. I marvelled at the dexterity and matter-of-factness of more experienced nurses (who were, in reality, probably only recently or only just qualified).

Cancer was a mysterious disease, and treatment sometimes left people scarred or permanently altered, bowel rerouted to the abdominal wall and protruding swollen and pink, purple or black into a large bag. Yet over time, with support from others, a sense of being orientated again, and of the wholeness of people, together with a consciousness of the effects of illness and surgery, returned, though it is probably true to say that a sense of the impact (or collision) of illness and treatment in cancer has remained with me. It is, overall, a feeling I welcome, because it is an incentive not to accept the status quo, a powerful message that we must always question whether accepted or 'normal' practice serves the interests of those who require health care.

Cancer, and sometimes treatment for cancer, can appear to elbow out the person at the centre who is experiencing it; it can be so intimidating, and cause such physical and mental upheavals. The treatment we provide for it is traumatic, and the feelings it evokes can weigh heavy on us. I wonder sometimes how those more experienced nurses acquired such sang-froid, such composure. Was it the composure of confidence or understanding, or did it sometimes include a kind of detachment? Do we sometimes push our feelings about a disease like cancer to the back of our minds? How often have we said, or heard our colleagues say, that if you thought about it all the time, you couldn't do it, almost as if this was a necessary skill for the job. But, don't we all 'think about it' a lot as well? Thinking about it, about cancer, about how it affects people, how it affects us, about how, as a society we respond to it, both in health care and more widely, in the media, across the dining table, may be vital to understanding. But thinking alone, about such a strange and difficult thing as cancer, may not take us far enough. Talking about it, with our colleagues, our family or friends, with the people we care for, may take us further if we can do it mutually and supportively. Indeed, dialogue may be one means of creating the mutual support and the opportunity to express ourselves that we need to be able to understand cancer, our feelings about it, and what we want to achieve professionally. Without this further mutual, exploratory dimension, how easy is it to review and build upon the joys and sadnesses of the day's or the week's events?

The status quo sometimes feels like the only possible way for things to be: we know that caring for people with cancer is physically and emotionally demanding – that is the way it has always been – so why do we need to go through all the effort of discussing things ad infinitum and 'being supportive', and all those 'touchy feely' politically correct strategies? For some, the answer is that it is difficult to make care happen if we don't take a reflective stance towards ourselves and our work; others point out that nurses as well as patients are disadvantaged by ways of organising ourselves that are too detached, and that leave little room for the personal issues, whether you are a patient or a nurse.

Chris Johns[4-8] has written a series of articles on the theme of enabling practitioners 'to learn through reflection upon lived experience with the intention of realising caring,'[5] essentially the same question I am raising about the importance of exploring and understanding our experience of cancer and our work with people with cancer.

The purpose of 'reflective practice', according to Johns,[4] is 'to enable the practitioner to access, understand and learn through his or her lived experiences and . . . take congruent action towards developing increasing effectiveness within the context of what is understood as desirable practice'.[4] In this version of reflective practice practitioners are given the opportunity to 'tell their stories of practice' and are introduced to 'structured reflection' through a 'constant process of analysing supervision dialogue', either individually or in small groups. The practitioner is able to reflect on his or her experience with a supervisor who helps to direct the process of exploration and is available during difficult or painful issues. In Johns[5] we are given an example of the dialogue between Caitlin, a team leader on a medical ward, and Johns, her supervisor. They are discussing the care of a patient whose drug therapy has been discontinued, and who will soon die, though not at home, as a decision has been taken to keep him in hospital. The dialogue focuses on the question of why Ray, the patient, has not been asked to participate in the process of reviewing his care, whereas his wife has. Johns, the supervisor, introduces some ideas about dying people and their need to communicate, which, he says, produce an 'a-ha' moment for Caitlin, an 'opening of shutters'. Caitlin takes the decision to be much more open with Ray about his care and treatment, and to become involved in his wife Lucy's unhappiness. Doing so enables Caitlin to facilitate the saying of goodbyes between Ray and Lucy. Johns comments:

> Choosing to give herself to these people is a momentous leap of faith for Caitlin, a metaphoric cocktail of emotions that were difficult to manage and threatened to sweep her away. Perhaps it would be easier for her to remain detached and task-focused so she does not have to concern herself with these issues. Yet, she can no longer do this within her concern for this family and her beliefs about caring [p. 37].

Within Johns' scheme, 'being available' or 'true presence' is at the heart of caring: Caitlin's 'leap of faith' is her decision to become more fully available to Ray and Lucy – to 'open the shutters'. It is through such presence or openness, Johns claims, that we can experience the 'energy' and 'joy' of caring: 'failure to become involved means that the relationship is not a caring relationship'. There are, it is acknowledged,[6] forces that 'squash' or 'minimise' caring values; for example, the low status and lesser rewards of nursing relative to medical practice may have led nurses to adopt the values of the dominant group. Caring, it is feared, may have been reduced to a 'sub-culture', and it is for this reason that effective means of 'creating the conditions whereby caring beliefs can be realised' are urgently needed.[4] It is within the context of a 'minimisation of caring values' that Johns seeks to develop reflective practice, and to establish it as an engine for the regeneration of care.

We must remember that Caitlin[5] is well supported throughout to enable her to take the steps she does. She has 'contracted' to meet her supervisor for 1 hour every 3 weeks; between meetings she keeps a reflective journal, in which she records her experiences and her responses, guided by a series of 'reflective cues'. Like Benner and Wrubel,[9] Johns believes it is a mistake to think that caring is the cause of 'burnout' and that we should therefore 'protect' ourselves from caring, as if it were a threat:

> Rather, the loss of caring is the sickness, and the return of caring the recovery . . . Although disengagement may numb pain, one is also numbed to the resources and support of others in the situation. Recovery requires rest and respite, but it also requires the reintegration of concern and involvement [p. 373].[9]

Rather than seeing caring as the cause of stress, we should hold institutions and systems responsible if they fail to provide the means of developing and sustaining caring practices.[4] Johns[5] explains:

> However profound this process of becoming may seem, it is dependent on the supervisor being available to work with the practitioner. My key role was to balance high challenge with necessary support, so Caitlin did not feel threatened, which would inhibit learning. This was helped by establishing our therapeutic working relationship over several months. How I interpret and respond to Caitlin was a role model of 'being available' for her patients [p. 38].

Johns is available for Caitlin through the process of guided reflection and supports her, in the same way that she is becoming present for people like Ray and Lucy, in a supportive, but exploring, therapeutic relationship.

It is now some considerable time since Isabel Menzies published her thought-provoking paper on the organisation of the nursing workforce in a London teaching hospital.[10] Some, myself included, would argue that it continues to influence our understanding of the forces that shape the way that nurses collectively arrange their working practices. Menzies believed that the nurses she studied were organised collectively (or socially) in a way that suggested they were trying to defend or protect themselves from anxiety.

Menzies, who was employed by the Tavistock Institute of Human Relations in London, was asked by the hospital for help in a project to facilitate organisational change within its nursing service. Trained nurses were, she says, employed to a large extent in 'administrative, teaching, and supervisory roles', while the student nurses were 'in effect, the nursing staff of the hospital at the operational level with patients' (p. 2). She describes a situation in which the demand for care within the hospital was

such that staffing needs took priority over training needs. The researchers from the Tavistock Institute set about exploring this situation by conducting a series of interviews with nurses, medical and 'lay' staff, and by carrying out observational studies in clinical areas. Over and over again the researchers encountered such high levels of tension, distress, and anxiety among staff that they found it hard to understand how individuals were able to tolerate it. In fact, Menzies reports, there was a great deal of evidence to suggest that nurses were not able to tolerate such anxiety, and, 'in one form or another, withdrawal from duty was common' (p. 4). Menzies explores the nature of the anxiety she believed she had identified in the nurses in this study from a psychoanalytic perspective; and even 40 years on, her powerful account thoroughly merits rereading. Nurses, she says, are:

> . . . in constant contact with people who are physically ill or injured, often seriously. The recovery of patients is not certain and will not always be complete. Nursing patients who have incurable diseases is one of the nurse's most distressing tasks. Nurses are confronted with the threat and reality of suffering and death as few lay people are . . . The work situation arouses very strong and mixed feelings in the nurse: pity, compassion, and love; guilt and anxiety; hatred and resentment of the patients who arouse those strong feelings; envy of the care given to the patient [p. 5].

The extraordinary context in which nursing takes place affects us in extremely powerful ways. The very nature of caring for seriously ill or dying people evokes feelings so strong that they may shape the pattern of work in ways of which we are only partly conscious. In other words, we may organise our care activities in the way we do to minimise the impact of the situation on us, restricting what we do rather than expanding and exploring the possibilities of care, which Johns describes as 'squashing' caring values.[6]

Menzies argues that a social organisation, such as the nursing service in a hospital, develops a mode of functioning that is influenced by a number of interacting factors; namely, its primary task, the technologies available for performing that task, and the needs of the members of the organisation, particularly their need for social and psychological satisfaction and for support in the task of dealing with anxiety. The latter need, she believes, is especially important. To some extent, indeed, the mode of functioning of a social organisation may be determined by the psychological needs of its members.[10] The way we care for people with cancer could be determined, or shaped, by what we feel about cancer, our experience of it: anxiety, as well as positive, constructive feelings, may be part of this experience, and may cause us to pull in our horns on a personal level and circle the wagons on an organisational level, in an attempt to protect ourselves from harm. Chris Johns' guided reflection is, in effect, one way of helping us to manage the experience of caring for people constructively and progressively, giving us the support we need to avoid 'pulling in our horns', or 'putting up the shutters' in situations where issues and feelings seem just too intimidating.

Isabel Menzies argues that when members of an organisation are struggling against anxiety, defence mechanisms develop and become part of the organisation. For example, if a nurse experiences anxiety as a result of the closeness and intensity of her relationship with people under her care, the nursing service 'may attempt to protect her by splitting up her contact with patients . . . This prevents her from coming effectively into contact with the totality of any one patient and his illness.' The feelings we experience in nursing, unmitigated and unsupported, may actually cause us to limit our contact with people, or to avoid certain difficult aspects of our relationships with individual patients. In a more recent language of caring, we are not 'fully present' or 'available'. It is interesting to reflect on the extent to which protective attitudes may still be part of the way that nursing is organised today. How much of nursing is a 'social defence system' established to help us avoid certain difficult feelings? And how may nursing change if our need for such strong defences were reduced by more genuinely supportive structures, by 'conditions where caring becomes possible?'[5]

Menzies[10] concludes that in the institution she studied,

> The characteristic feature of the social defence system . . . is its orientation to helping the individual avoid the experience of anxiety, guilt, doubt, and uncertainty . . . the potential anxieties in the nursing situation are felt to be too deep and dangerous for full confrontation, and

to threaten personal disruption . . . In fact, of course, the attempt to avoid such confrontation can never be completely successful [p. 24].

In her opinion, 'true mastery' of the feelings evoked by nursing is most likely to be achieved by 'a deep working-through' of intense situations, a theme familiar to us today, though it may be couched in terms of caring 'visualised and realised through guided reflection.'[6]

Benner and Wrubel[9] describe caring as 'the producer of both stress and coping with the lived experience of illness'. They explain that this is because what we care about *matters* to us and therefore is a potential source of concern to us; and because if we care about something it *means* something to us, and we commit ourselves to it and involve ourselves in it, laying the groundwork for coping. Nurses, they say, 'help patients to recover caring, to appropriate meaning, and to maintain or re-establish connection'.

'Making contact', or understanding the 'lived experience of illness' is at the centre of their account of nursing: it is this principle of openness to others (which they believe is inherent in the phenomenological philosophy of Martin Heidegger) that empowers nurses to grasp the 'daily consequences' of illness, to 'convey acceptance and understanding', and to work with 'thoroughness and attentiveness'. Like Chris Johns, Benner and Wrubel see the ability to be present in the special sense of being accessible and connected as the foundation of nursing as a caring occupation. In their example of 'presencing',[9] a clinical nurse specialist, Mary, describes an interaction with Dave, who has lung cancer:

> He was yelling that he wanted everything packed up. I felt a panic among the staff . . . I went into his room and he yelled at me: 'Are you listening?' I said yes pretty calmly, and he began crying softly and talking. He knew I was listening [p. 15].

Mary explains that it is because she is not 'walking out of the door as she walks in' that her relationship with Dave is right; we might say that this is a way of describing 'making contact', or 'being accessible'. Benner and Wrubel explain that it is this 'presence' that makes all the caring, nursing processes that Dave needs from Mary possible. As Mary says,

. . . during the following weeks we spent some intensive time going over what needed to be accomplished . . . We began concentrating on his issues: chemotherapy at home, volunteers coming into his house, pain management. It was great, because with support he made the most of his time [p. 15].

In *Anguish*,[11] the American sociologists Anselm Strauss and Barney Glaser give a description (a 'reconstruction of the salient events') of the hospital care and treatment of one woman with breast cancer, whom they call 'Mrs Abel'. They give us what could be called an 'alternative' view of hospital care. The account is an extraordinary one, something of a landmark in health care research, because long passages of description are given in the form of dialogue between two nurse researchers ('Shizu' or 'SY' and 'Susie' or 'SA') and their supervisor, Strauss. Interspersed throughout the dialogue between the nurses and the sociologist are theoretical commentaries, which are provided by Strauss and Glaser.

While *Anguish* can be read as an account of Mrs Abel's experience of hospital care for her breast cancer, she is not obviously included in the process of collecting information about her. Neither, it is true to say, are the doctors and nurses on the 'floor' or ward where she spends her time. Shizu, who works as a nursing student on the floor, and Susie, who is part of the research team interested in Mrs Abel, provide most of the first-hand details. Of the two, Shizu probably contributes the greater part of the material that is discussed in the dialogues and commented upon in the theoretical asides. Shizu reports what Mrs Abel, or the nurses, or doctors have said, and this is supplemented by contributions from Susie, who also visits the floor, but does not provide nursing care for Mrs Abel. In effect, therefore, *Anguish* is an account of Shizu and Susie's experience, passed through the theoretical filter of sociologists Strauss and Glaser. They decide what is to be included in the final account, what is to be retained and what is to be removed, and what wider conclusions are to be drawn from Shizu and Susie's observations. Nevertheless, it is a remarkable account of Mrs Abel's nursing and medical care. It is, however, an equally remarkable record of how Mrs Abel was 'researched' and of how Shizu, in particular, managed her caring role with support from two experienced colleagues, who

largely remained outside the immediate context of events on the floor.

In *Anguish*,[11] Strauss and Glaser present the idea of 'dying trajectories', which is used to represent situations in which it is acknowledged that a particular individual will die, and which is part of 'a substantive theory of dying in hospitals' (p. 3). A 'substantive' theory is, they explain, not highly generalised or formal or 'grand', but 'grounded in research into the substantive areas within which the case falls' (p. 5). 'Substantive areas' can be understood to mean 'key', or 'essential' areas, which represent the issue in question.

Because the length of time it takes for someone to die varies, along with the certainty with which we can say they will actually die at a specified time, there is a number of possible dying trajectories: 'a trajectory has shape: it can be graphed. It plunges straight down; it moves slowly downward; it vacillates slowly . . .' (p. 12). Dying trajectories are, Strauss and Glaser emphasise, what is *perceived* to be the course of dying, and may depart from the *actual* course of dying. They suggest that dying trajectories are an important part of the life of health care institutions: some areas, ITUs for example, are 'quick dying wards'; others, like the oncology unit, are 'lingering wards'. The number of deaths characteristic of a particular ward or unit, and the speed with which deaths characteristically occur, are factors that play a part in shaping the way in which nurses and doctors organise their work.

Mrs Abel, who is seen as sharing this characteristic with other cancer patients, has a 'lingering dying trajectory', or a long-term course of dying in hospital: death is acknowledged as certain, though the precise point in time at which it will occur is not known: 'The shape of this trajectory had two major features: it was of long duration, and it moved slowly but steadily downward.' Patients, say Strauss and Glaser, have a 'hospital career', a period of weeks or months during which their condition is continually assessed. The idea that we might have a 'hospital career' is interesting, because it suggests that while we are in hospital, we are involved in a much larger social process than we might imagine. In our day-to-day lives, we are involved in efforts to establish ourselves socially, to become this or that sort of person, with a particular position, and with access to a certain range of goods and resources. When we are in hospital, we are there because we have met the conditions set by our society to regulate access to health care. We are subject to conditions determining how much and what kind of care we will receive, and once we no longer fulfil conditions set, for example, by governments, by the health professions, or even by friends, we may find that we no longer 'qualify' for care in one of its various guises. Thus 'being ill', like having a career, is a social matter, as much about changes in our relationships – with nurses, doctors, friends, employers, officials – as it is about physiology or biology; and, like our working careers, our hospital careers may be influenced by the things we do to 'get on'.

Strauss and Glaser describe how on Mrs Abel's floor staff saw terminal care as 'work', and found the physiological and psychological care of Mrs Abel 'distasteful'. They preferred to concentrate on patients who were getting better, or who were dying less difficult deaths. Dying patients, they say, could 'unwittingly compete with other patients for attention': Mrs Abel, for example, 'continuously wished to talk . . . no matter how pressed they were'.

Work on the floor had many important 'temporal features'. There were schedules for feeding patients, bathing, turning in bed, dispensing drugs, administering tests, close observation, and giving treatments. In fact, say Strauss and Glaser, 'the total organisation of activity . . . during the course of dying is profoundly affected by temporal considerations'.

The story of Mrs Abel ties together an interest in 'temporal features' with another aspect of the organisation of care. Some aspects of care are termed 'non-accountable', which means that nurses and doctors have 'considerable freedom' or 'latitude' in these areas, and do not feel obliged to report, or account for *how* tasks or procedures are carried out. Strauss and Glaser feel particularly strongly that 'social psychological aspects' of care (for example, relationships with patients) fall into this category. Because psychosocial care is 'non-accountable', it is 'unnoticed', and, as in Mrs Abel's case, aspects of psychosocial care, like relationships with staff, can be allowed to 'disintegrate'. The *temporal* dimension is vital to any hospital situation because it is such a fundamental tool in the organ-

isation of care: nurses and doctors shape care through their use of time. Therefore when the temporal dimension of an aspect of care is 'non-accountable', the consequences are likely to be profound. This, say Strauss and Glaser, is exactly the case with psychosocial care: if less and less time is spent on it, it is unlikely that anything will be done to halt the consequences, because 'psychosocial time' is 'non-accountable':

> temporality of action – whether more or less accountable – is of the utmost significance in understanding what happens during the entire course of a patient's dying . . . the temporal organisation of care for Mrs Abel enforced more and more isolation upon her . . . the staff were non-accountable for such a situation and its consequences [p. 11].

There are several factors, according to Strauss and Glaser, that change the way in which care is shaped and organised. Diagnosis and prognosis, a patient's 'illness status', nurses' *expectations* are, they feel, particularly important influences. Care is disrupted, becomes problematic, when expectations (for example, 'approximations' of patients' dying trajectories) are not fulfilled. Patients are 'expected to die on schedule', and 'when progress turns out to be unusual, personnel may experience a disquieting feeling of having missed certain steps . . . miscalculations can cause havoc with the organisation of work'.

The picture of nurses and doctors we get from *Anguish* is of a group of people whose behaviour is stereotyped, predictable, conforming; the last thing we might expect is for someone to make a 'leap of faith', like Caitlin in Chris Johns' account. But the staff in *Anguish* are not so different from the nurses in Isabel Menzies' study, who sought refuge in detachment from their patients and each other from the powerful emotions evoked by illness. Most of us, like Caitlin, need a mentor figure to throw our most difficult feelings about nursing at, and a place to rehearse difficult, unfamiliar nursing 'moves'.

Mrs Abel, the central figure in Strauss and Glaser's account of medical and nursing care, provides a powerful example of how the image of 'the patient' can be constructed. For the researchers (with the possible exception of Shizu) Mrs Abel remains 'a case', upon which theory is grounded.

While it would be unfair to say that she is treated as if she were part of a laboratory experiment, she is the object of inquiry or investigation, and is not seen as possessing independence or as an autonomous participant in the process of research. She is not invited in, or given a footing in what is essentially her story. Unlike the patients in Chris Johns' accounts, Mrs Abel is never seen as a primary source of knowledge about her situation: rather, it is the researchers who know, and who exercise powers of analysis and illumination. In a similar way, according to Strauss and Glaser, Mrs Abel is seen by her nurses and doctors as having a certain range of behaviour open to her, and her illness is seen as having certain parameters, a certain scope, within which to unfold. When her behaviour takes a different course, or her illness unfolds in seemingly inexplicable ways, sanctions are applied that are designed to restore acceptable conditions. Mrs Abel is ostracised, bullied, cajoled, and ultimately operated on in an attempt to restore order. As long as she remains a particular kind of patient, her behaviour and her illness will receive (one imagines) dedicated medical and nursing care. If, like an unruly actor, she departs from the script, every effort is made to induce her to return to it. It seems, therefore, that illness and illness behaviour are subject to a kind of contract, agreed between members of a community or society, which stipulates that it is okay to act in certain ways, but not to act in others. A cancer like Mrs Abel's is not associated with the particular kind of pain she reports, for example, and crying and monopolising time like she does is not what patients are *supposed to do.* There is therefore something insubstantial and unconvincing about the pain, and something outrageous, even offensive, about the behaviour.

Of course, the idea that there is such a thing as a socially sanctioned *role* to be adopted when ill is not new.

In *The Social System,*[12] the American sociologist Talcott Parsons gives an analysis of 'an important sub-system of modern Western society', namely medical practice. He sees health as a 'ubiquitous practical problem in all societies' but points out that the influence of 'the therapeutic process' extends beyond health to 'problems of deviance and social control'. Medical practice is theorised as playing a part in the maintenance of balance in the social system as a whole. When we are ill, Parsons argues, we are unable to perform our social roles effectively. But because illness is not only something which happens to us willy-nilly, but also something towards which our unconscious may for various reasons impel us, it is also a factor in the functioning of the social system in the sense that it is part of our (consciously or unconsciously) willed (or 'motivated') interactions. There is a dimension of motivation to illness, so that:

> it becomes not merely an 'external' danger to be 'warded off' but an integral part of the social equilibrium itself. Illness may be treated as one mode of response to social pressures, among other things, as one way of evading social pressures. But it may also . . . have some possible positive functional significance [p. 431].

Parsons claims that illness is a departure from normal functioning both biologically and socially. Illness changes us biologically, but it also changes our sense of ourselves in relation to others.

According to this particular sociological interpretation, medical practice provides the social system with a means of coping with illness: coping, that is to say, which is achieved through the adoption of a series of defined and established roles (p. 423). The principal roles in question are: (1) the medical practitioner, and (2) the 'sick person'.

The medical practitioner's role is 'collectivity-oriented' and above all requires a high level of technical competence. He or she is an 'applied scientist', setting aside personal likes and dislikes when making a judgement, striving for neutrality and objectivity (p. 435).

Parsons identifies four groups of expectations associated with the 'sick role' (pp. 436–437):

1. The sick person is exempted from 'normal social role responsibilities'.
2. The sick person is in need of care and cannot make him or herself better.
3. There is an obligation to want to get well.
4. There is an obligation to seek help from a competent (that is medical) practitioner.

Crucially, the medical practitioner is seen as exercising a power of 'legitimation'; that is to say, the medical practitioner determines whether the 'sick person' is legitimately sick enough to be given exemption from normal responsibilities. The sick role is seen as involving not just exemptions but privileges, and Parsons argues that this may motivate individuals to attain or to sustain the status of sick person. From the point of view of the social system it is imperative that the sick person is 'motivated' to recover; as Parsons sees it control of the motivational balance, tipped in order to favour as efficient and brisk an exit from the sick role as possible, rests in the hands of the medical establishment. Perhaps, in Mrs Abel's case, we can see legitimation faltering and the sick person's exemption from responsibilities losing its effect. Because the power of legitimation is exercised one-sidedly, Mrs Abel cannot herself establish that her pain is real. She steadily loses both credibility and respect in the eyes of the majority of her carers. Parsons' interpretation of the role of medical practice in the social system acknowledges the controlling role of medical practitioners in the health care system; and identifies the 'sick role' as abnormal or deviant, with the sick person potentially motivated to remain formally designated as sick.

In effect, this interpretation of the sick role establishes inequality as a principle of health care and in so doing leaves medical practice and the general public on opposite sides of a conflict of interests.

Parsons' concept of the patient's role belongs to a branch of the sociology of health and illness known as functionalism. Functionalism, in contrast to some more contemporary perspectives, sees relationships in health care as having been achieved through consensus, and the stance of medical practitioners towards their patients as both benevolent and directive at the same time. Lupton[13] points out that in the functionalist model the relationship between doctor and patient is characterised by a preponderance of power in the hands of the doctor, but is not seen as conflicted: rather, the imbalance of power is seen as a necessary addition to medical knowledge, allowing medicine to exercise its benevolent function (p. 7). She comments, citing Turner:[14]

> While Parsons' work was ground-breaking in elucidating the social dimension of the medical encounter, the functionalist perspective has been subject to criticism based on its neglect of the potential conflict inherent in

the medical encounter. Critics argue that the functionalist position typifies patients as compliant, passive and grateful, while doctors are represented as universally beneficent, competent and altruistic [p. 7].[13]

In our encounters with medicine and health care we are expected to behave with self-discipline: thus, in addition to attending to our health care needs (narrowly defined), medicine and health care are a training ground for good, orderly citizenship; the self-discipline we express as practitioners of healthy behaviours has a broader significance in the maintenance of a 'healthy' society through co-operative productive endeavour and the acceptance of benevolent power inequalities. Herzlich and Pierret[3] suggest that medicine 'is not just one institution among others'; rather, it is a model for all present-day social institutions and therefore has a profound effect on our experience of our place in society. By the end of the nineteenth and the beginning of the twentieth centuries, they argue, the medical practitioner had come to represent science and its power, and 'medicine henceforth claimed the right to state the rules by which society should abide'.

In support of their thesis, they point to examples of medical regulation of sexuality, early childhood, and the relationship between health, the environment, and social conditions. We are, they say, 'firmly entrenched in the age of medicine': getting well has become an obligation. Herzlich and Pierret cite examples from their interviews which, they suggest, show how common it is for us to believe strongly in the positive value of medical treatment and how we tend to submit to it: 'The sick acknowledge themselves to be in the hands of others, objects of their knowledge and their action.'

While Parsons interprets our relations with medicine as entirely positive, others have put forward quite different views, to the effect that the medical establishment acts as a disincentive to autonomous action on the part of individuals in response to feelings about sickness. Herzlich and Pierret[3] quote an interviewee to this effect:

> 'One is being infantilized', said a 25-year-old young woman . . . 'In the relations with the nurses, you just feel completely infantilized. Above all, don't try to speak about your feelings, or about your desires, or anything

like that . . . just swallow your medications like a good
girl, smile a lot, and especially don't think that you know
what's good for you better than the nurse. That is to say:
she always knows everything, *you must blindly obey her
and not say anything* . . . just be there like a good girl'
[p. 198].

It has become increasingly difficult, given the
medical view, for us to attribute any positive
values at all to sickness and death, though these
experiences have in the past been given meaning
by communal social events and practices.[3] The
professional medical viewpoint tends to define
problems in its own terms and medical practice has
a vested interest in controlling the nature and extent
of the services it makes available. Thus, in effect the
patient's or the lay person's viewpoint is set to
one side and the physician–patient relationship
becomes, contrary to functionalist teaching,
inherently conflicted.

A further dimension of the view that health care
encompasses the competing viewpoints of professionals and patients is that both viewpoints are
socially constructed, emanating from medical and
lay discourses – shared beliefs and idioms – on the
body and health. Herzlich and Pierret[3] argue that
'as the specialization that defines the field of the
physician's intervention becomes more and more
narrow [it] increasingly ignores the total reality
perceived by the patient'.

An important effect of sociological frameworks
such as the social constructionism represented by
writers like Herzlich and Pierret, Deborah Lupton,
and Bryan Turner (in contrast to the functionalism
of Talcott Parsons) is to 'problematise' the
doctor–patient relationship; that is to say, a critical space is opened up, which enables lay and
professional participants in health care, as well as
commentators, to set new goals beyond established
orthodoxies. Social constructionism sketches out a
rationale for the inequality and loss of autonomy
experienced by individuals involved in formal
health care, but instead of endorsing it, interprets
it as a rather one-sided exercise of vested interests.
The autonomy (or 'agency') of the lay person,
together with a re-evaluation of his or her whole
experience, is brought into view and identified as
a necessary dimension of relationships in health
care. The legitimacy of an imbalance of power, even
attached to a rhetoric of philanthropy, is brought

into question. Having said that, it is important to
remember that Michel Foucault, the French cultural historian, while acknowledging medical
dominance in doctor–patient encounters, saw it as
a voluntary and necessary arrangement:

> When discussing power in the medical encounter, the
> functionalist and the Foucauldian perspectives . . .
> overlap to some degree. In understanding power relations
> as productive rather than coercive, Foucauldian theory
> restates the assertion of classic functionalism that
> medical dominance is *necessary* for practitioners to take
> control in the medical encounter to fulfil the expecta-
> tions of both parties, rather than a source of oppression
> . . . In this view, detachment, reserve, responsibility for
> the patient's well-being and an authoritarian stance must
> be maintained by the doctor, and the notion of patients
> being 'empowered' to take control in the encounter
> makes little sense, for such a change in the relationship
> calls into question the reason why the very encounter
> exists [pp. 112–113].[13]

Carolyn Featherstone[15] writes of today's society
as one in which 'the body has become an object of
obsession', in fact the body is a 'project', a means
through which we set out to achieve social or
material ends. Cancer, though, disrupts the
'body-as-project' through its power to stigmatise
and to fragment our image of our bodies both
physically and emotionally. Featherstone draws our
attention to the role of writers like Michel Foucault
and the symbolic interactionist Erving Goffman in
providing a critical perspective on the notion of
disease in Western culture. Naturalistic theories,
which suggest that relationships in society (for
example, between men and women, different races,
and different classes) are founded on the different
strengths and weaknesses of our bodies, legitimise
inequality because they deem such differences to
be part of a natural and unchanging order.[15] Social
constructionism, in contrast, looks upon the
meaning our bodies have for us as being determined by social structures and encounters with
others. When our bodies are affected by disease in
such a way that the flow of everyday encounters is
interrupted or they conflict with dominant social
representations of the body, the experience is
traumatic. We feel stigmatised.[15]

Featherstone[15] suggests that Michel Foucault's
development of the idea of 'discourse' (statements
emanating from authoritative social groups that

have the power to constitute reality of a kind) gives us the means to understand how medical practice is able to shape our sense of our bodies:

> 'Discourse' is a key concept in Foucault's writings . . . 'discourse' is concerned with expert statements of powerful groups, i.e. statements which are taken seriously by a community of experts . . . we are talking about a mental model of reality, as used by expert groups. It will include the language, concepts and criteria of evaluation which are seen as legitimate for discussion of, for example, medical issues . . . The power of the medical profession is located in its discourse or ideas. Much of our thought about our bodies, then, is constrained by medical ideas which change over time [pp. 166–167].

Our experience of our bodies in illness is constrained by medical discourse, which in fact changes over time, but affects us as if it were part of a permanent order of nature, difficult, if not impossible, to resist. Holding on to a sense of our bodies as 'us' in the midst of intense medical discussion and cancer therapy is often beyond our means; we may be overpowered without being fully conscious of the loss (see Spence[16]).

Some recent sociological writing has tended to see Western medicine in terms of its influence on (or 'medicalisation' of) the body. Bryan Turner writes of medicine as the 'key institution in the regulation of bodies':[17] the body is 'socially constructed', made real to us through 'scientific discourses in medicine'. Our bodies are controlled not just in health care but more widely in society, through the exercise of medical power, which encourages us to exercise discipline over ourselves. The body, in this view, is 'problematised', can no longer be taken simply as a biological entity, and is seen instead more as a text, something written or laid down by powerful forces such as science or medicine. The need for a regulated body, a body under control and well-disciplined, is seen as originating in the emergence of Western capitalism, which requires 'docile and productive' bodies. Medicine, it is argued, is directed at creating such bodies:[17]

> the growing importance of preventive medicine and the use of the concept of 'life-style' to regulate employees in order to manage corporate insurance demands have meant that there is a major intervention of medical ideas and practice into everyday reality – through diet, exercise, anti-smoking norms, sexual regulation of appropriate (that is 'healthy') partners, the regulation of childbirth, and the hygienic treatment of death [p. 18].

The social constructionist perspective emphasises that medical knowledge is, like lay knowledge, constructed by and dependent on a particular society. Such knowledge is relative, and can be 'renegotiated', or undergo structural change, which incorporates changes in the relations between those who share in it, as when the doctor–patient relationship undergoes fundamental change. Within health care we often behave in a way that suggests that medical knowledge represents essential truths; from the 'poststructuralist' social constructionist point of view, this is because our society gives doctors (and scientists) special power over truth (as it once gave the church such power). Our behaviour with regard to nursing knowledge suggests that it possesses fewer essential truths, as if nurses do not enjoy quite the same social power as doctors. Social constructionism is a way of exploring the relative nature of such socially powerful bodies of knowledge as medicine; a way of understanding the social and historical conditions that give them their truth value. Renegotiation, repositioning of less powerful social groups according to interests obscured by a dominant body of knowledge, can theoretically follow. Turner[17] argues that 'constructionist epistemology throws doubt upon the idea of theory-neutral medical facts and more importantly casts doubt upon the idea of unambiguous medical progress'. This it does through the 'notion that the emergence of a scientific fact is the effect of various thought-styles . . . which in turn are supported and maintained by a thought-collective'. Turner[17] believes that the 'scientific medical curriculum', with its 'emphasis on acute illness and heroic medicine', maintains the dominance of the natural sciences; and that psychological, sociological, economic, political, and environmental causes of illness are excluded from systematic study, despite changes in the character of disease and the needs of an increasingly dependent population. He suggests that health care should commit itself to an 'interdisciplinarity' based on the idea of the 'whole person as the focus of health care':

Scientific medicine is limited because it is based on a narrow, specialised and technical view of the human body as a machine which responds in a determinate way to the therapies derived from clinical experience and basic research [p. 139].

In her paper, 'An anthropologist in the kingdom of the sick',[18] Susan DiGiacomo describes her experience of medical practice when she is diagnosed with Hodgkin's disease. Much of her account is concerned with her encounters with the doctors supervising her treatment. She sets out to 'demystify' her disease and her treatment, both as a means of 'staying sane' and to 'restore some sense of control':

Treatments of indefinite length and uncertain outcome invariably inspire fear and rage, and rob the cancer patient of much of his personal autonomy. In such circumstances knowledge is the only kind of power available [p. 316].

Hospital staff, she says, disapproved of her curiosity; and the hospital culture defined 'categories and persons – doctors and their patients' and their relationship to each other. As a patient, DiGiacomo finds the dynamics of health care both controlling, and disapproving of knowledge and power in the hands of the individual, and she experiences this as detrimental to her care and well-being. As an anthropologist, she believes that orthodox Western medicine ('biomedicine') is a cultural system that creates, or attempts to create, the reality of those involved in it. Powerful forces, like language, authority, organisational rules, and valuing of certain types of knowledge (the 'discourse' of biomedicine) combine to form a cultural system that is experienced as normality, though counter-systems exist and may be the chosen systems of different individuals.

The way we use language to represent disease and our bodies can be said to reflect our beliefs about disease, held individually or as a group. Cassell[19] found that the patients he interviewed in New York saw disease as 'an intrusive object rather than as a part of themselves', much as modern medicine does. It seems particularly appropriate to us to refer to malignant tumours as 'its' or independent entities, as the people in Cassell's study did; though, he says, it is possible to conceive of a language for

tumours that treats them as part of us. Cassell argues that it is the diseases themselves (and not merely the tumours) that are seen as objects. He found that symptoms and organs involved in the disease were referred to in the same impersonal way. Though Cassell remains undecided about whether the mind's view of the body, reflected in language, is culturally determined, or whether this view is 'biologically inherent' (neatly reflecting the line separating social constructionist and naturalistic, sociobiological viewpoints), he inclines to the latter. While the effect of speaking of disease as an 'it' may be to place distance between the person and the disease, Cassell concludes that it may be of greater therapeutic value to use language to reduce that distance: 'words in their concrete reality may be a bridge through which the person can bring into his ken and perhaps even influence, parts of the body which until then reside in a mysterious inner world seemingly inaccessible to consciousness, much less to conscious action' (p. 146).

As a cultural system, DiGiacomo[18] argues, biomedicine can sometimes be 'renegotiated': if patients hold strong beliefs in a counter-cultural system, a different way of constructing health care, they may be able, through dialogue, to modify the way that health care is made available to them. Biomedicine, though, is very powerful, and can point to the many benefits and advantages it confers: it is often difficult, as an individual, to impose oneself upon this system, and doing so may carry the risk of being judged disruptive. Susan DiGiacomo's account in effect chronicles her own efforts to 'renegotiate' the terms of the system of biomedicine that puts forward her regime of care and treatment.

Mathieson and Stam[20] describe a different, but perhaps related type of 'negotiation' in their discussion of 'cancer narratives':

For cancer patients these stories have a special meaning. In negotiating their way through regimens of treatment, changing bodies and disrupted lives, the telling of one's own story takes on a renewed urgency. In the end, they are more than just 'stories' but the vehicle for making sense of, not just an illness, but a life [p. 284].

Thus 'renegotiation' can be seen as taking place both externally, in interaction with a system or culture, and internally, as a process of retelling or reinterpreting identity in the face of illness; a process of making sense, and of seeing the world around us as a proper reflection of momentous personal events.

Frankenberg[21] suggests that the world of biomedicine and the world of the patient diverge chronologically, especially in chronic disease, where the physician's involvement is much shorter than the patient's:

> the knowledge and understanding over time of the sickness trajectory enjoyed by technicians, nurses, and especially patients and their relatives may well be much greater than that of their physicians. In general, the physician may know more than the patient about acute disease in practical as well as in theoretical terms. He or she may have seen many discrete patients over a period of years; the chronic patient on the other hand has had the opportunity to study one patient over many years and continuously. A collection of such patients organised into a specific patient group may have much to teach not only about illness and sickness but also about disease [p. 19].

Frankenberg offers a distinction between 'disease' and 'illness' consistent with a social constructionist perspective. By 'disease', on the one hand, Frankenberg means 'disturbance of body functions and performance seen in biological terms of the kind that physicians are primarily trained to detect, diagnose, and treat'.

'Illness', on the other hand, is 'concerned with the perceptions of sufferers of that which physicians conceive of as a disease':

> Disease depends on the existence of the social organisation of biologists and the medically trained, and illness on a socially constructed sense of self which certainly does not exist in the same form in all societies [p. 17].

Our sense of the nature of disease and illness and our related behaviour is specific to the way that we have developed, individually and historically, within a society. Frankenberg, who is making room for a 'renegotiation' of some widely held cultural assumptions by pointing to the relative nature of phenomena such as disease and illness, takes issue with sociologists who approach 'deathandying' (sic) as if it were one word; this, he points out, implies that all but the final stages of life can be 'reasonably analysed without reference to its most universal and inevitable end, and shifts responsibility for

'deathandying' to specialists, such as hospice workers and social scientists. Instead, he uses the word 'lifedeath' to refer to the part of life in which death is 'part of the not yet conscious', and 'deathlife' for life that is accompanied by 'consciousness of its not too far distant end' (p. 18).

Arthur Kleinman[22] sees a contrast between patients' experiences of illness and the medical focus on disease, though he believes it is possible, indeed therapeutic, for clinicians to help patients to 'order' their experience. What illness means to people, he says, should be interpreted by patients, families and practitioners together; the medical system, though, tends to detach practitioners from the experience of illness.

The cultural shaping of the experience of illness is reflected in the characteristic way we perceive and monitor our bodies. We are very careful about what we allow into our bodies, what we try to exclude, and how we manage material expelled from our bodies. We have a particular sense within communities and societies of what it means to 'take care of ourselves', and of what it means to lead a healthy life. We have social rules to manage contagion, as the rules for dealing with coughing, sneezing, and washing show. There are areas where the difference between good and bad practices becomes blurred, as with the taking of drugs in sport: some sections of the sporting world are more prohibitive than others, with the result that our sense of how to regulate our bodies well becomes touched by ambiguity. Keeping our bodies in order, not too spotty, not too fat, carries a sense of obligation to others: our fellows, our communities may accuse us of 'letting ourselves go' if we put on weight, and failure to follow social rules of good bodily order may offend or threaten others, as is the case with spitting, or scratching ourselves.

Kleinman's explanation of disease (as opposed to illness) is that it is created when illness is 'recast' by the practitioner 'in terms of theories of disorder'; disease is an 'it', not a 'me' of personal experience, created within a specific system of names and classifications. From the point of view of biomedical culture, disease is defined as, and confined to, changes in biological structure or function, but from a 'biopsychosocial' perspective, Kleinman argues, disease represents an interaction between 'body, self, and society'. The strong cultural position of biomedicine in Western societies means that the mechanism of disease (the way it alters biological structure or function) often represents its meaning. Thus, Kleinman suggests, 'in cancer the meaning is often that we do not yet know the mechanism'.

He proposes an alternative approach to therapy, in which medical care is 'reconceptualised' and relations between medical practitioner and patient are renegotiated. This approach involves 'an empathetic witnessing of the existential experience of suffering' and 'practical coping with the major psychosocial crises that constitute the menacing chronicity of that experience'; it is offered as a counter-blast to the biomedical specialist who, Kleinman suggests, does not 'credit the patient's subjective account until it can be quantified and . . . rendered more "objective" . . . Illness experience is not legitimated by the biomedical specialist, for whom it obscures the traces of morbid physiological change'.[22]

Frankenberg,[21] for one, expresses reservations about whether Kleinman's 'reconceptualisation' of medical care is a fundamental as it might seem (it may, he says, be 'radical' rather than 'revolutionary'). He points out that drawing a distinction between disease and illness does not mean that concepts of disease are rejected. Frankenberg implies that Kleinman's 'empathetic witnessing' amounts to a proposal that 'the physician must learn the patient's interpretation and the nature of the illness, and then in turn, as part of the cure, teach the patient as much about the disease as is possible and necessary for treatment to be both carried out and complied with' (p. 16). Consequently, power and control in the therapeutic encounter is retained by medical practice, and the patient remains suppliant, petitioning for dispensations.

Frankenberg[21] sees hospital patients' time as routinised and inflexible, with 'almost total disruption' of 'the natural rhythms of bodily desires' like sleeping, eating, evacuating waste, and enjoying sexual experience. Healing and illness, he says, take place within a 'time view' that is the patient's own, and which is infrequently shared by physicians and nurses; medicine, analysing and treating the disease, is practised in another time, distant from the patient. In hospital, the argument goes, patients lose control over their own time to medical

and nursing staff, who maintain the power relations of organised health care. Radical change has occurred within health care with the formation of self-help groups, consumer advice, and patients' advocates, but Frankenberg sees such change as less than fundamental as it does nothing to affect the processes of formal health care services. Revolutionary change can only take place when patients 'take charge of their own time'. For healing to be established as part of our culture, medicine must 'renegotiate' its relationship with patients and other health care workers on the basis of equal partnership, and relinquish its control over the time of others, which enhances its power, diminishes the autonomy of others, and puts distance between it and the experience of illness.[21]

Susan DiGiacomo, who writes of cancer treatment as 'as brutally primitive as any inflicted by the leeches and barber-surgeons of old',[18] found her identity 'assailed' by hospital and by having cancer. Cancer, she says, quoting Erving Goffman,[23] is a stigma, reducing 'a whole and usual person to a tainted, discounted one', and as such affects the way that relationships between patients and their doctors are structured. She agrees with Susan Sontag[1] that cancer and cancer treatment are often referred to with military terminology, and that metaphorically speaking, cancer implies 'social deviance, social injustice, and political corruption'; the individual with cancer is caught up in the implications of catastrophe and evil. Having lost control of her work and her body, Susan DiGiacomo was determined to keep control of her identity, including 'anthropologist', her professional identity. Knowledge, asking questions, was a means of avoiding becoming a victim; but when she approached doctors as colleagues, rather than superiors, she found they were both surprised and disapproving, and that conflict occasionally ensued. She experienced the social power relations incorporated in the formal health care setting as detrimental to well-being (or as Frankenberg might say, contrary to healing).

DiGiacomo relates how an eminent oncologist supervising her care treated detailed information about Hodgkin's disease as too dangerous to pass on to her and as potentially damaging to her sanity; her anaesthetist and surgeon refused her husband access to the recovery room on the basis of custom ('pseudo-hygienic and pseudo-practical nonsense'); the purpose of attending for treatment simulation was misrepresented; radiation 'burns' were reclassified as radiation 'reaction'; and hair loss that was more extensive than predicted was explained as the result of increased 'traction' caused by her long hair.

She provides a number of examples of what Frankenberg[21] sees as the medical control of patient's time:

> I was told peremptorily to appear the next day for my first treatment. I got angry. I lived more than two hours' drive from the hospital and needed advance notice in order to organise my new commuter life. I refused to come in until the following Monday, and the reaction was one of surprise and indignation. It did not matter that no time frame had been specified, I should simply do what I was told without argument, regardless of the dislocation and inconvenience it caused me.

> I prepared for my weekly visits with my radiologist as I would prepare for any interview I would do as a field anthropologist. I thought out my questions beforehand, and conducted the interview from notes. I had to talk fast, because after the first five or ten minutes, my doctor began edging toward the examining room door, an indication she felt she had spent enough time answering my questions and had other important things to do. These visits were clearly for her benefit, so she could gauge my progress, not for mine [p. 323].[18]

Ultimately, Susan DiGiacomo comes to feel that she has been 'bullied into accepting more treatment . . . made to submit, to comply, through the strategic manipulation of information': she sees the counter-process of overcoming confrontation and submission as becoming possible through 'negotiation' with clinical practice.

Reviewing her experience of hospital care and treatment for cancer, she comments that her refusal to participate in roles ordinarily assigned by the health care system enabled her to redefine her relationship with her doctors, and made apparent the meanings or beliefs which give the system structure and shape. Cancer patients, DiGiacomo feels, are particularly subject to a process of depersonalisation, in other words, they 'become their disease'. Personal contact with the patient is, she says, 'highly routinised', and doctors share the belief that a patient's knowledge that she has cancer

'renders her so emotionally unstable that she is unable to confront and live with any reminders of the severity of her condition'. Patients are assumed to be unable to understand explanations, so information is withheld. Angry patients are seen as hostile or resentful rather than as having a legitimate grievance; responsibility for conflict is seen as that of the patient and not the doctor. Consultations do not allow time for questions, because they are dominated by the physical examination: the end of the consultation is indicated by a shuffling of papers or an opening of the door, making a private discussion public and therefore ending it.

DiGiacomo concludes that encounters between doctors and patients with cancer are structured as they are to keep the patient in a position of ignorance, leaving the doctor in a better position to secure the patient's co-operation with dangerous and unpleasant forms of treatment. The doctor emerges 'omniscient and omnipotent', which has the effect of reducing the ambiguity surrounding the patient's prognosis following treatment. 'Declaring a war on cancer' justifies the most extreme of measures, diminishes the necessity for openness and proportionality and obscures the rationale for genuine consensus called for in a 'negotiation model' for practice. Some sociological work may actually 'aid and abet' situations in which patients are kept in relative ignorance by ascribing difficulties in communication to patients' own psychological states. Beneath the successful, technological public image of biomedicine, DiGiacomo sees a reality of uncertainty, ambiguity, and contradiction; treatment decisions that rely on medical control of information lead to distrust and fear, and end with a sense of betrayal when treatment does not produce the desired result.

Negotiation and resolution begin when she is informed promptly of a change in her medical condition, and progress further as her GP begins to act in the role of advocate. According to her GP she is more afraid of 'being out of control and not in a position to make an informed decision' than she is of her cancer; her most urgent need is therefore to 'comprehend my disease and its treatment to the fullest possible extent'. A meeting, lasting for an hour, is held for her with both oncologist and radiologist, with questions submitted in advance, and a transcript of answers provided. She is given a copy of the full research protocol for an investigation of experimental treatments for Hodgkin's disease before beginning chemotherapy.

She questions the necessity for 12 cycles of chemotherapy, pointing out that the standard 'salvage' regime for patients who have 'failed' radiotherapy is six cycles. Her oncologist tells her that there is no way of knowing whether six cycles is sufficient, but DiGiacomo continues to believe that 'overestimating the required dosages might be as serious as underestimating them'. At the beginning of treatment, she experiences severe facial pains, gastrointestinal problems, immunosuppression, and fever, though no infection can be identified. She discusses the possibility of chemotherapy being ineffective, and is given details of her chances of survival if this were the case; talking about death with her doctor seems to demonstrate the value of a 'negotiation model' for clinical practice, which she glosses as 'each of us seeing the other in three dimensions instead of two'.

As DiGiacomo renegotiates the terms of her health care, insisting both that she is given detailed information and that her experience of treatment and illness, and insight into the effects upon herself, are fully acknowledged, we see practice turned 180° away from Mrs Abel's predicament. Whereas Mrs Abel remained stranded, without credence or credibility and ultimately acted upon (literally operated upon) blindly, in ignorance of her needs and wishes, DiGiacomo has fought hard to win recognition of herself and of the grounds for her well-being. In her later dealings with her oncologist, she seems to experience greater acknowledgement of her own 'time view', her own 'illness-time', her sense of living 'lifedeath' not 'deathlife' (see Frankenberg[21]). Collaboration on medical decisions becomes part of their meetings:

> He came to respect my ability to observe and report sensitively and accurately . . . as I began to negotiate more aggressively (and more successfully) for lower doses. This was no fiction of participation; it was based on mutual understanding of chemotherapy as a necessarily and inherently indeterminate process [p. 333].[18]

Being a 'collaborator rather than an object of treatment' provides Susan DiGiacomo with a sense of empowerment, which relieves depression and fear, though it also means that she has to share her oncologist's worries. She believes that her persistent fever is a symptom of the damage chemotherapy is doing to her body: she feels she is being 'destroyed in order to be saved'. Eventually, treatment is halted and she concludes that her own explanation of her condition, that her body is unable to tolerate chemotherapy, is more credible than her doctor's belief that she has suffered an undetectable infection. She implies that her doctor is forced to acknowledge the strength of her case, and thus in a sense a new position has been negotiated on what counts as credible knowledge about illness: the medical explanation (or discourse) is finely balanced in terms of credibility with the personal one.

A long and difficult struggle, in the course of which a model for negotiation in clinical practice is mapped out, ends with the final word on a clinical problem going to the patient. At the end of the struggle, in the course of which biomedical culture has in a local way accepted compromise, opened its borders, DiGiacomo's oncologist acknowledges her time view, where illness is not experienced as a number of courses of chemotherapy but as degenerating physical integrity and impending collapse. A degree of parity is achieved as the relevance and significance of the personal experience of illness is conceded.

Del Vecchio Good and her colleagues[24] believe that in America, oncologists have 'a cultural mandate to instil hope' in their therapeutic dialogues (or 'narratives') with patients. Like DiGiacomo, they identify a layer of uncertainty in medical knowledge about the outcomes of cancer and treatment that must compete with the cultural imperative to offer hope. Their experience suggests that oncologists respond with expressions of 'time without horizons or of highly foreshortened horizons' to:

> create an experience of immediacy . . . Time horizons, through therapeutic discourse and interaction, are distinctly foreshortened, and experience is consciously composed 'for the moment'. Endings, though palpably present for participants in clinical encounters, are unspecified . . . Instilling hope 'for the moment' becomes a legitimate and realistic task in the world of clinical oncology . . . [pp. 856–857].

Creating hope by focusing on the present is a source of anxiety for patients who are looking for certainty and lack of ambiguity about the course of their illness; but patients, Del Vecchio Good claims, often contribute to the process of generating commitment to treatment and hope for the future seen in their encounters with doctors. Hope, and compliance with medical regimens are values deeply rooted in Western culture. To begin with, Del Vecchio Good believes, consultations with oncologists are structured so as to avoid suggestions of crisis or 'threat to daily existence'. A sort of 'housekeeping' takes place in which the organisational aspects of getting to treatment appointments are sorted out, and the effect is to keep things 'unremarkable'. At the same time, metaphors of slow and patient struggle may be introduced, like 'climbing a mountain' and 'one step at a time', to suggest a process of steady achievement, which continues even when a dying trajectory is clearly underway. The mountain climbing metaphor implies a kind of protest; it is 'an image which suggests that the oncologist will pull the patient to safer, higher ground . . . a metaphor which taps into American concepts that through mobilizing personal will, the patient has resources to engage in the struggle for higher ground, for cure or remission' (p. 857).

When challenged to respond to concerns about prognosis, Del Vecchio Good finds that clinicians employ 'narratives of immediacy', which 'drew patients back into the everyday realities of living and of therapeutic housekeeping, of treatment schedules, of dealing with immediate side-effects, of assessing the current efficacy of the latest therapy . . . endings are rarely made explicit and progression is measured in calibrated bits, even though disclosure is considered to be the norm . . .' (p. 858).

Ultimately, when death or dying becomes an unavoidable reality, these 'narratives of immediacy and hope, struggle and progress' fragment and collapse. Unambiguous medical assessment of the stage or likely progress of an illness may, Del Vecchio Good suggests, come out into the open more frequently at this point, when other narratives fragment.

Perhaps this is the inevitable consequence of what Del Vecchio Good[24] calls 'the dominant American narrative', the cancer care story, which seems to offer frankness yet employs sub-plots of

hope and encouragement to a soldierly willingness to shoulder necessary hardships in the battle to survive. The brave and hopeful soldier is not prepared for the potentially shattering end of the narrative. We find it helpful to put our faith in the brave persona we project as providers of health care or are offered as recipients; but we would perhaps like to be able to care for people with cancer so that we and they can be ourselves as much as possible *and* manage treatment, care, and future, without the need for such precarious roles.

Neither Mrs Abel nor the nurses and doctors on her floor were able to express or acknowledge concerns freely. Mrs Abel was hemmed in by a vicious circle of unresolved difficulties; nursing and medical staff resisted to the last any modification of the clinical story of cancer as they understood it. Caitlin, in contrast, takes 'a leap of faith' and immerses herself as openly as she can in the needs of her patient, Ray, and his partner Lucy. Susan DiGiacomo fights doggedly to be given a seat at the table, to renegotiate the terms of her dialogue with health care and to be given a say in tipping the balance of decisions, even when 'expert' opinion is against her.

It is not just a matter of rebelling against the system or trendy theory: what Mrs Abel and her carers lack, and what Caitlin and Susan DiGiacomo are struggling to achieve is a way of being in the world that is open to experience (both your own and that of others) and discriminating about what has meaning or what matters. Patricia Benner's word for this is 'agency', which she interprets as openness to matters of significance.[25] Agency develops with experiential learning:

> . . . what is learned in practice by the practitioner is considered knowledge even though it contains puzzles and cannot always be fully located in the currently explicated science . . . the knowledge of the practitioner goes both before and after science because what occurs in the natural field of clinical experience is more variegated and complex than can be captured at any one time by scientific experiment. What is known sets up the questions and influences what is noticed, and the actual clinical experience alters, extends, or disconfirms what is known in the scientific discourse. Experience . . . requires openness to the new situation, but that openness is constituted by what has gone before; it is not naïve and undifferentiated [pp. 14–15].

Benner is interested in the agency of nurses as health care providers, in their 'sense of responsibility for the patient's well-being', which becomes more sensitive to possibilities as the skill of the practitioner increases, and which is manifested in 'negotiating and managing physician's responses to the patient situation . . . and . . . being responsive to and advocating for the patient and family concerns in ways that more closely match the actual concerns and needs' (pp. 26–27).

'Agency' thus conceived is the domain both of the caring professions *and* the recipients of health care, but comes into view as a possibility only when the traditional balance of power in health care is conceived of as contingent on cultural and social practices (and therefore relative) rather than as absolute and essential, a part of the natural order. How indispensable 'agency' is to caring, how much a part of well-being, in or out of health care, probably depends upon one's perspective, one's beliefs given all the historical, social, and cultural influences that bear upon them. For me, 'agency' and 'being available' are ideas that try very hard to give us a sense of the closeness, insightfulness, inventiveness, and commitment of caring. They share an intense focus upon the individual, the nurse, the mentor. Sometimes they might seem to involve an intensity of focus on the practitioner that somehow excludes wider considerations, including the voice of those on whose behalf care is provided. Structures in health care can be constructed to be more or less controlling of others, according to how much or how little control is seen as necessary to care or 'manage'.

Health care and illness take place in the larger, collective arena. We designate people as 'well' or 'sick' or 'patient' according to shared rules; we respond to people who are 'patients' according to the conventions and accepted practices of the roles we see as our own or the positions we take in the groups to which we belong. If 'agency' and 'being available' are about being committed to respond with discrimination to the experience of others, and are in some way central to the idea of caring, caring also encompasses the wider social or cultural arena where experiences of health and illness acquire their distinctive character, and health care organisations develop their formulas and structures, their distinctive ways of operating.

It is easy to see health care as a monolith, immovable and unshakeable, but if we shake up the bits and pieces of our sense of what health care is, new arrangements come into view, to be espoused or discarded in their turn.

References

1. Sontag S. (1977). *Illness as Metaphor.* New York: Farrar, Strauss & Giroux.
2. Gotay C.C. (1984). The experience of cancer during early and advanced stages: the views of patients and their mates. *Social Science and Medicine* **18**, 605–613.
3. Herzlich P. and Pierret J. (1987). *Illness and Self in Society.* Baltimore, MD: Johns Hopkins University Press.
4. Johns C. (1995). Reflection-on-practice: enhancing student learning. *Journal of Advanced Nursing* **22**, 235–242.
5. Johns C. (1997). Caitlin's story – realizing caring within everyday practice through guided reflections. *International Journal for Human Caring* Summer, **1**, 33–39.
6. Johns C. (1996). Visualising and realizing caring in practice through guided reflection. *Journal of Advanced Nursing* **24**, 1135–1143.
7. Johns C. (1996). Understanding and managing interpersonal conflict as a therapeutic nursing activity. *International Journal of Nursing Practice* **2**, 194–200.
8. Johns C. (1998). Caring through a reflective lens: giving meaning to being a reflective practitioner. *Nursing Inquiry* March, **5**, 18–24.
9. Benner P. and Wrubel J. (1989). *The Primacy of Caring: Stress and Coping in Health and Illness.* Menlo Park, CA: Addison-Wesley.
10. Menzies I.E.P. (1959). *The Functioning of Social Systems as a Defence Against Anxiety.* London: Tavistock Institute of Human Relations.
11. Strauss A.L. and Glaser B.G. (1970). *Anguish: A Case History of a Dying Trajectory.* London: Martin Robinson.
12. Parsons T. (1951). *The Social System.* London: Routledge & Kegan Paul.
13. Lupton D. (1994). *Medicine as Culture: Illness, Disease and the Body in Western Societies.* London: Sage Publications.
14. Turner B.S. (1988). *Medical Power and Social Knowledge.* London: Sage Publications.
15. Featherstone C. (1996). Views of the body, stigma and the cancer patient experience. In Parry A. (ed.) *Sociology: Insights in Health Care.* London: Arnold.
16. Spence J. (1986). *Putting Myself in the Picture: A Political, Personal and Photographic Autobiography.* London: Camden Press.
17. Turner B.S. (1992). *Regulating Bodies.* London: Routledge.
18. DiGiacomo S.M. (1987). Biomedicine as a cultural system: an anthropologist in the kingdom of the sick. In Baer H.A.

(ed.) *Encounters with Biomedicine*. New York: Gordon & Breach.

19. Cassell E.J. (1976). Disease as an 'it': concepts of disease revealed by patients' presentation of symptoms. *Social Science and Medicine* **10**, 143–146.

20. Mathieson C.M. and Stam H.J. (1995). Renegotiating identity: cancer narratives. *Sociology of Health and Illness* **17**, 283–306.

21. Frankenberg R. (1988). 'Your time or mine?' An anthropological view of the tragic temporal contradictions of biomedical practice. *International Journal of Health Services* **18**, 11–34.

22. Kleinman, A. (1988). *The Illness Narratives: Suffering, Healing, and the Human Condition*. New York: Basic Books.

23. Goffman E. (1963). *Stigma: Notes on the Management of Spoiled Identity.* Englewood Cliffs, NJ: Prentice-Hall.

24. Del Vecchio Good M.-J., Munakata T., Kobayashi Y., Mattingly C. and Good B.J. (1994). Oncology and narrative time. *Social Science and Medicine* **38**, 855–862.

25. Benner P., Tanner C. and Chesla C. (1992). From beginner to expert: gaining a differentiated clinical world in critical care nursing. *Advances in Nursing Science* **14**, 13–28.

CHAPTER FOUR

Cancer and epidemiology

Danielle Horton Taylor

A definition of epidemiology

Epidemiology is the study of disease in relation to populations and its aim is to prevent or control diseases or health problems. The information obtained from epidemiological studies can be used to explain the aetiology of a disease, to evaluate the consistency of epidemiological data with aetiological hypotheses developed either clinically or experimentally, and to provide the basis for developing and evaluating preventive procedures and public health practices.[1]

An understanding of epidemiological techniques and findings can aid assessment with regard to a patient's risk for cancer, or evaluation of a screening programme in terms of risks versus benefits. To facilitate this, several definitions and essential concepts are described.

Historical epidemiology

A good historical example of an epidemiological study was that undertaken by James Lind in 1747, which concerned the aetiology and treatment of scurvy. Lind allocated seamen with similar cases of scurvy to different diets, one of which included citrus fruits. He found that the men whose diet included the citrus fruits were much improved and some fit for duty 1 month later. Lind correctly inferred that citrus fruits cured scurvy and could also prevent the disease.[1] The British Navy finally acted on this in 1795 (nearly 50 years later), when

it decreed that limes or lime juice should be included in the diet of all seamen, thus solving the problem of scurvy and resulting in the expression 'limeys'.

Another example of the use of epidemiology occurred in London around 1849. John Snow, an epidemiologist, noticed that cholera rates were high in parts of London that were supplied with water from the Lambeth Company and also the Southwark and Vauxhall Company, both of whom obtained their water from a part of the Thames that was badly contaminated by raw sewage. The Lambeth Company then relocated the source of their water to a less contaminated part of the river. As households on the same street received their water from one or the other of the two companies, Snow determined the number of houses supplied by each company, calculated the cholera death rates in the area per 10 000 houses, and compared them with the rest of London. He found that the mortality rates in the houses supplied by the Southwark and Vauxhall Company were about eight times higher than those supplied by the Lambeth Company. From these findings, and his investigations into the Broad Street Pump cholera epidemic (where the handle of the pump was removed in an attempt to prevent the spread of further disease), Snow inferred the existence of a 'cholera poison' that was transmitted via polluted water.[1,2] Epidemiological methods are now used routinely in cases of food poisoning, for example, where the item of food and its source must be determined and located quickly to prevent further outbreaks. Epidemiology was for some years primarily related to infection control, but this has now changed and includes cancer.

A modern example of an epidemiological study, now considered seminal, is Doll and Hill's[3] study of smoking and lung cancer in British doctors. This study is extremely important as it resulted in the recognition of the causal link between smoking and cancer. It was set up in 1951 to investigate the relationship between smoking habits and mortality. A simple questionnaire on smoking habits was sent out to 59 600 men and women on the Medical Register. Replies were received from about 69% of the men alive at the time the questionnaire was sent out. Of these, 17% were classified as non-smokers. Further inquiries about changes in smoking habits were made in 1957, 1966, and 1972[4] (Doll and Hill's findings are addressed later in the section on attributable risk).

Epidemiological concepts

In order to understand the tools of epidemiology, it is essential to start with a solid foundation of concepts and definitions. Epidemiology is concerned with the occurrence of disease by time, place, and people. It has '. . . **causal** and **preventive** factors that can be identified through systematic investigation of different populations or subgroups of individuals within a population in different places or at different times'.[5]

Epidemiology of cancer is 'the study of the **distribution** and **determinants** of disease frequency' in human populations.[6] The distribution refers to where people with cancer live, and the determinants are what are thought to be the causes of the disease in that area. These two factors, along with frequency (the quantification of cases), cover all the principles and methods involved in epidemiology. Epidemiologists also use techniques from, and work closely with, practitioners of statistics, demography and other sciences.

The study of distribution of disease looks at **who** within a given population is getting a given disease, describing the distribution in terms of sex, age, race and other demographics, and when and where the disease is occurring. This allows comparisons to be made amongst populations, amongst subgroups

within those populations, and amongst different time intervals. The information obtained through these observations allows the description of the patterns of disease, and ultimately leads to the hypotheses, that once tested and proven correct (or preponderable, believed to be correct), result in an understanding of the causality of a disease and thus a definition of possible preventive measures.

Aetiology

Aetiology deals with causation and must be distinguished from the study of mechanisms (pathogenesis). Sufficient is known about the aetiology of some cancers for effective cancer prevention or control measures to be instigated. Clues to aetiology come from comparing disease rates in groups with different levels of exposure – for example, excess lung cancer and pleural mesothelioma in people exposed to asbestos. It is, however, very difficult to establish causality in an observational setting.

Aetiology can be and often is multifactorial. Known aetiological factors include: chemicals (tobacco, alcohol, drugs), radiation (ionising, solar), genetic or familial, viruses and/or parasites, and immunological deficiencies. Other influences include diet and nutrition, occupation, and air and water pollution. Aetiology is particularly useful when it allows us to practise primary prevention, which will be discussed later.

Determinants

These are what are considered to be the **causes** of disease in a geographical area. Determinants of the observed distribution involve 'the explanation of the patterns of the distribution of a disease in terms of causal factors'.[6]

Frequency

Frequency involves 'the quantification of the existence or occurrence of disease'.[5] These data are a prerequisite for further study into the distribution and determinants of a disease. Epidemiological measures of disease frequency require a **count** of the number of cases of disease occurring in a population, although this count is of little informative value without further clarification. Account must be taken of the **size** of the population and (usually) the **length of time** over which its members were observed.

Rates and proportions are some of the most commonly used tools in epidemiology for reporting disease frequency and to describe disease distribution. Here are a few of the most commonly used.

Point prevalence

Point prevalence (usually known simply as prevalence) is a measure that is often used in *planning* the allocation of health service resources on a national or local basis. It is the number of cases of disease in a population at one point in time, taken as a proportion of the whole population. Period prevalence considers the number of cases existing over a period of time, typically 1 year, and is more often used in cancer epidemiology. Prevalence includes new cases and previously diagnosed ones in persons who are still alive in the period being studied.

$$\text{Prevalence} = \frac{\substack{\text{Number of diseased persons in a defined}\\ \text{population at one point in time}}}{\substack{\text{Number of persons in the defined}\\ \text{population at the same moment in time}}}.$$

As prevalence includes both new and old cases of disease, it is typically of less value in aetiological research than incidence, as incident cases of a disease are those which *first occur* or develop in a defined period of time. (We say first occur as sometimes people experience the same pathological event more than once, but it is only the first instance that counts for a conventional incidence rate.)

Incidence is the number of cases of disease that occur in a defined period of time as a proportion of the number of persons in the population at the beginning of the period. This cumulative incidence both describes the *disease experience* of populations and the *risk* an individual has of developing the disease in the specified period of time.

$$\text{Incidence} = \frac{\substack{\text{Number of persons who become}\\ \text{diseased during the period}}}{\substack{\text{Number of persons in the population}\\ \text{at the beginning of the period}}}.$$

One way to relate incidence to prevalence is to understand that each new (incidence) case enters the prevalence pool and remains there until either recovery or death (see Figure 4.1).

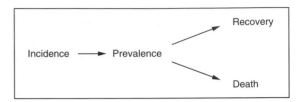

Figure 4.1 Relationship of incidence to prevalence.

If, however, the recovery and death rates are low, even a low incidence rate will produce a high prevalence, as chronicity is high (prevalence = incidence × average duration).

Crude incidence or prevalence refers to **whole populations,** without subdivision or refinement, whereas specific rates refer to selected groups (e.g. rates by age group). **Standardised** populations should be used when comparing incidence or prevalence so that disparities between populations do not skew the findings, i.e. comparing apples with apples and not with oranges. As the incidence of most cancers increases with age, it could be misleading to compare incidence rates of one country with those of another if the *proportions* of people of different ages in the populations being compared were not the same. Therefore, age-standardised incidence rates are used.

To use breast cancer as an example, Table 4.1 shows some age-standardised incidence rates (per 100 000).

The populations in this example were selected to demonstrate the wide variation in incidence rates that can exist between countries, ethnic groups, and socio-economic classes.

Table 4.1 Age-standardised incidence rates of breast cancer (per 100 000)

USA, Los Angeles: Non-hispanic white	103.7
USA, Los Angeles: Hispanic white	57.4
USA, Connecticut: White	93.3
USA, Connecticut: Black	84.5
Japan, Hiroshima	33.4
Japan, Saga	19.1
Sweden	72.9
UK (England and Wales)	68.8

(From: Parkin, D.M. *et al.* (eds.) (1997). *Cancer Incidence in Five Continents*, Vol. VIII.[3] Lyon: IARC).[7]

Relative risk

Relative risk (often abbreviated RR) estimates the magnitude of an association between exposure and disease and indicates the likelihood of developing or dying from the disease in the exposed group relative to those who are not exposed. It is the ratio of the rate of the disease (usually incidence or mortality) among those exposed to the rate among those not exposed, in other words a comparison of two incidences.

$$\text{Relative risk} = \frac{\text{Rate of disease among exposed}}{\text{Rate of disease among non-exposed}}.$$

Attributable risk

Attributable risk is the rate of the disease in those exposed that can be attributed to the exposure.

Attributable risk = Incidence or mortality rate of the disease amongst exposed people *minus* the corresponding rate in non-exposed people.

From Table 4.2, it can be seen that the relative risk of death from lung cancer in heavy smokers (2.27) as compared with non-smokers (0.07) is 32 times greater (2.27/0.07).

The calculation of the attributable risks is seen in parentheses in the third column, where, by definition, the non-smokers have a 0 attributable annual death rate, as compared with heavy smokers, who have a 2.20 attributable annual death rate. In other words, heavy smokers have 2.20 times the annual death rate of a non-smoker.

Standardised mortality ratios (SMRs)

Standardised mortality (or morbidity) ratios are used to discern whether the number of cases of disease or death is more or less than would be normally expected.

$$\text{SMR} = \frac{\text{Observed deaths (O)}}{\text{Expected deaths (E)}}(\times 100\%).$$

For example, say 58 cancer deaths were observed in a group of asbestos workers (O) and the expected number of deaths from cancer for that same age group, sex, etc., was 42.9 (E), then the SMR would be 58/42.9 = 1.35 × 100% = 135%. This SMR indicates that the mortality in the asbestos workers was 35% greater than other men in the population.[8] (Note that the SMR is the same as the relative risk if the populations are the same.)

Survival data

When determining and presenting cure data in cancer treatment, a graph of the proportion of patients alive at 5 or 10 years is often used. A **survival curve** is a plot of the proportion of patients surviving as a function of time (i.e. the x-axis is years). A **disease-free survival curve** is similar, but instead of the x-axis being years, it is time before the disease reappears. This is important in instances where patients are treated on relapse. How are survival data to be interpreted? A comparison can be made with patterns of survival of those who have not had

Table 4.2 Death rates from lung cancer attributable to cigarette smoking in British doctors, 1951–61

Cigarettes smoked per day (in 1951)	Annual death rate per 1000	Attributable annual death rate per 1000	
None	0.07	0	(0.07–0.07)
1–14	0.57	0.50	(0.57–0.07)
15–24	1.39	1.32	(1.39–0.07)
25+	2.27	2.20	(2.27–0.07)
Total	0.65	0.58	(0.65–0.07)

(Reproduced with permission from Doll, R. and Hill, A.B. (1964). Mortality in relation to smoking: ten years' observations of British doctors. *British Medical Journal* **I**, 1399–1410, 1460–1467).[3]

cancer [the **age-adjusted expected survival curve (E)**], and the **age-adjusted relative survival curve (R)** is calculated by dividing the observed survival curve (O) by the expected survival curve (E). Survival data can also be standardised by age, as survival does depend on age for many cancers.

Types of epidemiological studies

Epidemiological studies are either **observational** or **experimental**. In experimental studies, the epidemiologist can specify some of the conditions under which the study is to be conducted. These conditions are not controllable in observational studies.

Two types of analytical designs are used in observational epidemiology – prospective and retrospective.

Prospective or cohort study

In a prospective or cohort study, participants are selected who have had varying degrees of exposure to a suspected factor. These individuals have not experienced the particular outcome thought to be associated with the factor. They are then followed over time and observed to see whether the outcome being investigated occurs. An example of a cohort study of dietary fat and breast cancer would compare the incidence of the disease in those who ingest a high-fat versus a low-fat diet. Drawbacks to cohort studies are that they go on for a long time, patients often drop out, you need to be patient to wait for the results, they are often expensive and are unsuitable for rare tumours. Care must be taken to account for confounding variables (for example, diet is influenced by ethnic origin and social class, both of which are independently linked to the likelihood of developing breast cancer).

Retrospective or case–control study

In a retrospective or case–control study, study subjects are selected on the basis of a known outcome, controls are selected who are felt to be comparable to the cases, and the evidence of a factor being an antecedent to the outcome is sought. The number of instances in which the factor in question occurs in the affected group is then compared with the number of instances in which it occurs in the control group in order to determine whether significant differences exist. Thus, in oncology, case–control studies compare the characteristics of individuals with certain cancers and individuals with similar characteristics who do not have the cancer. For example, a case–control study of the possible connection between dietary fat and cancer would compare the diets of those with the disease (cases) with those without (controls). Case–control studies make feasible studies of rare cancers, as those exposed to the aetiological agent in question are followed and compared with those unexposed (or exposed to a lesser extent). Case–control studies solve the problems found in cohort studies of patients dropping out and having to wait for results, but introduce the potentially much more serious problem of selection bias. It is therefore essential (albeit difficult) to pick the right control group or groups.

Three case–control (retrospective) studies, in Nijmegen, Utrecht and Florence, were carried out, where characteristics of women with breast cancer (cases) were compared to those of women without the disease (controls). One of the great drawbacks of the case–control study is the risk of selection bias, where women with an especially high incidence rate refuse screening, and we have no way of knowing whether or not screened women have less chance somehow of dying from breast cancer.[8]

Experimental studies

In experimental studies, the epidemiologist controls the method of assigning subjects to either the exposed or non-exposed groups. This is usually done **randomly** to avoid bias, and is known as a **randomised controlled trial** (RCT) or clinical trial. Other types of experiment are known as non-randomised controlled trials, community trials, or field trials; in these trials, some of the attributes can be randomised, but not all.

An example of an RCT is the Health Insurance Plan of Greater New York (HIP) where 62 000 women aged 40–64 years who had been members of HIP for at least 1 year were randomly assigned to screening (experimental group) or usual care (control group). The experimental group was offered an initial screen consisting of mammography and physical examination followed by three follow-up examinations at yearly intervals. The control group was not offered the screening examinations, but simply their usual care. This study provided information about the sensitivity and specificity of breast cancer screening tools, as well as the effect of screening on reduction of mortality from breast cancer, as the study had a very long period of follow-up.[9-11] The HIP trial, as well as five other randomised controlled trials conducted around the world, found that the relative risk of breast cancer mortality in women invited for screening was significantly lower than for those not offered screening. (These studies compared different combinations of screening methods, as well as the effect of screening on different age groups.)

RCTs can be used to assess the efficacy of a drug or other treatment in the treatment of a disease, and can also be used to evaluate a prophylactic (preventive) agent such as a vaccine or a public health procedure such as screening. Randomisation is crucial as the experimental and control groups must be comparable in all factors except the one being measured. This experimental method corrects for nearly all biases, and RCTs are really gold-standard studies if properly administered and double-blinded.

Blinding is a method used to remove observer and participant bias and studies can be single-, double- or triple-blinded. In a single-blind study, the subjects have no indication whether they have been allocated to the experimental or control groups. In a double-blind study, in addition to the subjects, the observers do not know the subjects' allocation. In a triple-blind study, the subjects, the observers, and the analysts of the data all do not know the subjects' allocation.

Obviously, RCTs cannot be used in all cases, as it would be unethical to withhold a known efficacious intervention or treatment from a group of subjects, as it would be to subject a group to a known hazardous exposure. For this reason, no RCT has been conducted to assess the effectiveness of screening for cervical cancer, as it has been widely thought of as reducing mortality from the disease. Nor has an RCT been done to assess the link between lung cancer and smoking, as you could not make certain individuals smoke. It is in these sorts of situations that observational studies are necessary.

There are ethical considerations to be made in the case of an RCT or clinical trial.

- Is the proposed treatment safe for the patient (unlikely to bring them harm)? Is it safer than having the disease?
- For the sake of a controlled trial, can a treatment ethically be withheld from any affected patient in the doctor's care?
- What patients may be brought into a controlled trial and allocated randomly to any of the different treatments (i.e. who should be excluded)?
- Is it ethical to use a placebo treatment or standard treatment?
- Is it proper for the trial to be in any way blind? (It should be unless there are reasons that blinding is not feasible, e.g. surgery vs radiation treatment for prostate cancer).[1,12]

The relative strength of evidence, evidence-based medicine, and guideline development

The relative strength of evidence is ranked with prospectively randomised controlled trials the strongest level of evidence, down to observational studies as the weakest (the USPHS system is an example of this ranking of evidence). Trials and studies need to be evaluated as to their design and possible flaws in deployment, and the level of the study must be taken into account in order to put the conclusions into context and decide what weight to give them.

Evidence-based medicine has come to the forefront of care in many specialties. It is '. . . the conscientious, explicit, and judicious use of current best evidence in making decisions about the care of individual patients'.[13]

Evidence-based medicine has been described as:

The practice of evidence-based medicine means integrating individual clinical expertise with the best available external clinical evidence from systematic research. By individual clinical expertise we mean the proficiency and judgment that individual clinicians acquire through clinical experience and clinical practice. Increased expertise is reflected in many ways, but especially in more effective and efficient diagnosis and in the more thoughtful identification and compassionate use of individual patients' predicaments, rights, and preferences in making clinical decisions about their care. By best available external clinical evidence we mean clinically relevant research, often from the basic sciences of medicine, but especially from patient-centered clinical research into the accuracy and precision of diagnostic tests (including the clinical examination), the power of prognostic markers, and the efficacy and safety of therapeutic, rehabilitative, and preventive regimens. External clinical evidence both invalidates previously accepted diagnostic tests and treatments and replaces them with new ones that are more powerful, more accurate, more efficacious, and safer.[13]

Evidence-based medicine is related to guideline development in that the evidence is evaluated and then guidelines are developed based on that. It is now integral to the development of guidelines, which are used at both a national and local (e.g. office- or hospital-based) level. In addition to these, clinical pathways have been developed, which are aimed at improving care and reducing cost.

Clinical approaches to cancer

There is a number of clinical approaches to the management of cancer, including prevention, genetic screening, screening and early detection, diagnosis and staging, treatment, and support and rehabilitation. There are also three levels of prevention: primary, secondary and tertiary.

Genetic screening
This is used to predict high-risk groups who have a genetic predisposition to cancer. It is essential that counselling by genetic counsellors is given before any genetic testing is undertaken. Genes that have been identified and are being used successfully to identify those at high risk include the BRCA1 and BRCA2 genes for breast cancer, the HNPCC and FHP genes for large bowel cancer, and the RET gene in families with MEN 1&2 syndrome (multiple endocrine neoplasia) for medullary thyroid cancer. (Children are tested for the RET gene in those families.)

Primary prevention
Primary prevention prevents the occurrence of the disease in the first place by avoidance of known carcinogens/promoters or by active intervention. It is estimated that one-third of cancers could be

prevented in this way. Immunisation, nutrition, environmental control, vector control, disinfection and sterilisation, chemoprophylaxis, and health behaviour are all methods of primary prevention. These are all potentially highly cost-effective interventions.

Both tamoxifen and raloxifene have been found to be effective in reducing the incidence of new breast cancers in the contralateral breast of patients with breast cancer.[14,15]

Secondary prevention
Secondary prevention, which detects disease after the onset of pathogenesis and includes screening, contact tracing, and surveillance, has the goal of preventing the disease from developing further. It is estimated that one-third of cancers would be cured if they were detected early enough. Examples of cancers that are screened for include uterine cervix, breast, oral, and skin. Screening is not to be confused with early detection – screening detects *pre-symptomatic* disease, whereas early detection detects disease at its first clinical manifestation. There is, however, controversy about whether screening detects different types of cancers, which are so slow growing that the host is likely to die of old age before they succumb to the cancer.

Table 4.3 Cancers where primary prevention is possible through avoidance of known carcinogens and/or promoters and other areas of possible prevention

Cancers	Carcinogens and/or promotors
Lung, head and neck	Tobacco, alcohol
Bladder, kidney	Schistosomiasis, *B* napthylamine, tobacco
Pleura (mesothelioma)	Asbestos
Skin	UV radiation
Leukaemia	Radiation, drugs
Pancreas	Tobacco

Other possible areas of prevention:

Cancers	Methods of prevention
Colorectal cancer	Low-fat and high-fibre diet
Breast cancer	Anti-oestrogens or prophylactic organ removal
Liver cancer	Hepatitis B immunisation
Ovarian cancer	Oral contraceptives

Screening uses a test to assist earlier diagnosis of a disease process so than management of the disease can be more effective than it would have been if the disease had been recognised first by conventional clinical presentation. It can be defined as dividing the population into those who are test-positive, and who are likely to have the disease in question, and those who are test-negative, and probably without it. It is important to note that the screening test is not a diagnostic test – a positive screening test requires definitive testing in order for a diagnosis to be established.

How is it decided whether it is worthwhile to screen for a disease? In 1968, Wilson and Jungner published guidelines for a screening programme[16] with the following criteria.

1. The condition sought should be an important problem.
2. The natural history of the condition sought should be adequately understood.
3. There should be a recognisable latent or early symptomatic stage.
4. There should be an accepted and effective (early) treatment for patients with recognised disease.
5. Facilities for diagnosis and treatment should be available.
6. There should be a suitable test or examination available.
7. The test or examination should be acceptable both to the public and to professionals.
8. There should be an agreed policy on whom to treat as patients, including management of borderline disease.
9. Case-finding* (i.e. screening) should be a continuing process.
10. The cost of early diagnosis and treatment should be economically balanced in relation to total expenditure on medical care.

Colorectal cancer can be used as an example of the usage of the Wilson and Jungner criteria in investigating the plausibility of screening for disease (see opposite).

*Case-finding is nowadays defined as the opportunistic screening of people attending a doctor's surgery for some condition *other* than the disease to be screened for.

Box 4.1: The plausibility of screening for colorectal cancer

Is colorectal cancer an important problem?
Yes – it is the third most important cause of cancer mortality overall with an estimated 394 000 deaths worldwide in 1985.[17]

Is the natural history of colorectal cancer adequately understood?
Yes.

Is there a recognisable latent or early symptomatic stage in colorectal cancer?
Yes – most advanced colorectal cancers develop by progressing through the benign adenoma to carcinoma sequence.

Is there an accepted and effective (early) treatment for patients with recognised colorectal cancer?
Yes – benign adenomas are highly curable with surgical excision, but once visceral metastasis has occurred, few patients survive.

Are facilities for diagnosis and treatment available?
Yes.

Is there a suitable test or examination available?
Yes – faecal occult blood testing (FOBT) is easily done and haemoccult tests have been evaluated by RCTs. In addition, flexible sigmoidoscopy can be used and has been found effective.

Are the tests or examinations acceptable to both the public and the professionals?
Yes – FOBT is non-invasive, and flexible sigmoidoscopy is acceptable, although it is an invasive procedure.

Is there an agreed policy on whom to treat as patients, including borderline disease?
Yes – if polyps are found, they are removed, as is any other more extensive disease from *in situ* (Duke's A) onwards.

Can screening be done as a continuing process?
Yes.

Is the cost of early diagnosis and treatment of colorectal cancer economically balanced in relation to total expenditure on medical care?
Yes – it is considered to be within the bounds of reasonable expenditure.

Overall, having evaluated the disease with reference to these screening criteria, do you think the implementation of screening for colorectal cancer is appropriate?
Yes – it has been successfully implemented in many countries.

Of course there are pros and cons to all screening (see below). The objective of screening is the reduction of morbidity and mortality of the screened disease in those persons screened.

Box 4.2: The pros and cons of screening for breast cancer

Expected benefits from screening women for breast cancer include:

1. Mortality reduction.
2. Reassurance for women with negative results.
3. Less radical treatment for earlier cancers.
4. Avoidance of expenditure for advanced cancer.

Risks of breast cancer screening include:

1. False positives (resulting in unnecessary procedures, increased cost, and mental anguish).
2. False negatives (missed cancers).
3. Interval cancers.
4. Radiation exposure.
5. Emotional aspects.

Problems with screening include safety (the test is being applied to whole 'healthy' populations, on a recurring basis), cost, compliance (if compliance is too low, insufficient population coverage will render the screening test ineffective), false positives, false negatives, lead-time bias, length-biased sampling, and so on.

When evaluating the effectiveness of a screening test, pathological test, or any other test, the sensitivity and specificity of the test are measured and evaluated. **Sensitivity** can be defined as the ability to detect all those *with* disease (in other words, the proportion with the disease in whom the test gives a positive result). **Specificity** can be defined as the

ability to identify those *without* disease (in other words, the proportion without disease in whom the test gives a negative result). These are inversely related, so that as sensitivity increases, specificity decreases, and vice versa. Calculation of these is done easily using a two by two table, where positive and negative test results are entered, as well as the true reference (disease or no disease) (see Table 4.4).

Where a test result is positive and the reference is also positive, this is a true positive (TP). Where a test result is positive but the reference is negative, this is a false positive (FP). Where a test result is negative and the reference is also negative, this is a true negative (TN). Where a test result is negative and the reference is positive, this is a false negative (FN).

$$\text{Sensitivity} = \frac{\text{True positive}}{\text{True positive} + \text{false negative}} (a/a + c).$$

$$\text{Specificity} = \frac{\text{True negative}}{\text{True negative} + \text{false positive}} (d/d + b).$$

Suppose we have a population of 1000 people, of whom 100 have the disease (and 900 do not). A screening test is given to these 1000 to identify the 100 with the disease (see Table 4.5).

This screening test does not have a very high sensitivity or specificity and thus there are many false positives, which result in anxiety and unnecessary interventions, and false negatives, which result in false reassurance and delayed diagnosis. As sensitivity increases, specificity decreases and vice versa. Therefore, it is necessary to determine what the acceptable levels for each will be – that is, is it more important not to miss cases (higher

Table 4.4 Calculation of specificity and sensitivity using positive and negative results

	Disease	No disease
Test result	+	−
+	True positive (TP) or a	False positive (FP) or b
−	False negative (FN) or c	True negative (TN) or d

Table 4.5 Calculation of specificity/sensitivity for a population of 1000 people

	Disease	No disease	Total
Test result	+	−	
+	80 (TP or a)	100 (FP or b)	180
−	20 (FN or c)	800 (TN or d)	820
−	100	900	1000

Sensitivity = 80/80 + 20 = 80%; specificity = 800/800 + 100 = 89%.

sensitivity) but to have more false positives, or to be more specific and have more false negatives? This is generally specific to the particular disease and screening technique; for example, in a non-invasive test such as a blood test for HIV, the sensitivity would be higher and the specificity lower. However, if the test were a more invasive one, such as a biopsy, the specificity would be higher and the sensitivity lower.

In addition to its sensitivity and specificity, the performance of a test is measured by the **predictive value** of a positive or negative result. For positive predictive value, a/(a + b) represents the likelihood of a person with a positive test having the disease. When a disease has a low prevalence (or is somewhat rare) there is a greater proportion of true negatives (b + d) in relation to true positives (a + c) than when the prevalence is high, and the proportion of false positives (b) will be greater in relation to (a).

$$\text{Positive predictive value} = \frac{\text{True positive}}{\text{True positive} + \text{false negative}}(a/a + b).$$

$$\text{Predictive value of a negative test} = \frac{\text{True negative}}{\text{True negative} + \text{false positive}}(d/d + c).$$

Predictive value changes with disease prevalence. For example, a test with 99% sensitivity and 95% specificity would have a positive predictive value of 17% with a 1% prevalence, 29% with a 2% prevalence, and 51% with a 5% prevalence.

Table 4.6 Calculation of specificity/sensitivity for a population of 100 000 people

	Disease	No disease	Total
Test result	+	−	
+	990	4 950	5 940
−	10	94 050	94 060
Total	1 000	99 000	100 000

Sensitivity = 990/990 + 10 = 0.99 × 100 = 99%; specificity = 94 050/94 050 + 4 950 = 0.95 × 100 = 95%; RR = 1; point prevalence (per 100 000) = 1000; prior probability = 1%; positive predictive value = 990/990 + 4 950 = 0.166 × 100 = 16.6%; negative predictive value = 94 050/94 050 + 10 = 0.998 × 100 = 99.8%.

Another example uses a total population of 100 000 in which 1000 have the disease and 99 000 do not have the disease, where a screening test is applied to 100 000 people in order to identify the 1000 people with the disease (see Table 4.6).

Lead-time bias
Lead-time bias is the time by which screening advances the diagnosis of the disease (see Figure 4.2). If the diagnosis takes place *after* the critical point (B), where the cancer has already spread, then the interval between the diagnosis and the usual time of diagnosis (C → D$_1$) is the lead-time (say, 1 year), where it will appear that the cases diagnosed by screening survive 1 year longer even if there is no long-term benefit. If the diagnosis takes place *before* the critical point (D$_2$), cure is likely to result.

Length-biased sampling
Length-biased sampling has to do with the fact that people who develop rapidly progressive disease and are more likely to die than most people with disease are unlikely to be found in a population that presents for screening. This is particularly true for screening programmes of short duration and is why screening should be an ongoing process. However, in a population with two different types of disease with different mortality outcomes, screening will seem effective even when it is not.

Figure 4.3 shows a schematic representation of the prevalence of disease in a population, where 'X' represents death, short tails represent aggressive disease and long tails indolent (with the longest detectable phase or slowest progression), and S1,2,3,4 indicate when the screening programmes were performed, with the vertical lines intersecting (detecting) cancers.

The figure demonstrates that screening does need to be an ongoing procedure, performed at regular intervals. Indolent cancers are more likely to be detected than aggressive cancers, and detection varies depending on periodicity of screening. The screening at S1 detected two cancers, at S2 five cancers, one of them aggressive, and so on. At virtually any time, a one-time screening is more likely to select patients who live with the disease for the longest period of time – this represents length-biased sampling. Thus:

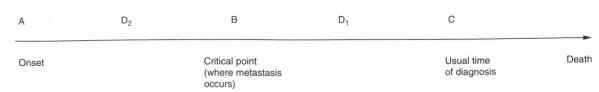

Figure 4.2 Diagram of lead-time bias.

The sine qua non of screening is that management of disease detected at an asymptomatic stage is more effective than treatment at the time of overt clinical presentation. In the absence of effective management, cancer screening may appear to be effective because it preferentially detects slower-growing neoplasms (length–time bias), thus advancing (in time) the diagnosis of incurable cancers (lead-time bias) and resulting in more years of life with cancer without lengthening life span. This is not the case with colorectal (or breast) cancer, for example, since effective therapy is available if cancers are detected early.[18]

(Bear in mind that, in general, screening will tend to look better than it really is due to these biases.)

The benefits, risks, and problems of screening need to be thoroughly investigated and measured before a screening programme is implemented. Questions as to when to start screening, when to stop screening, and how often to screen need to be addressed, as well as the cost-effectiveness of screening compared with other health care choices. Thus far, quite a few screening programmes have met the Wilson and Jungner[19] criteria and have been found to be effective in reducing mortality from the disease in question. Screening tests that have been found to be effective include breast, cervical, colorectal, skin cancer and some specific genetic syndromes. Conclusive evidence showing survival benefit from screening for prostate cancer is lacking, although PSA screening is being extensively used. Screening for lung and ovarian cancer has been found to be ineffective.

Policy and reasons behind screening
Sometimes cancer legislation is undertaken as a political platform, or as a potential vote-winning

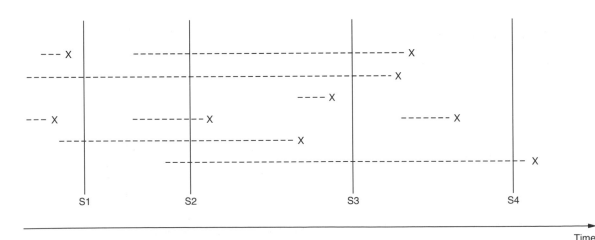

Key

X = death.
-- = disease course (short-tailed lines indicates aggressive disease, long-tailed lines indolent disease).
S = screening.
| = cancer detected.

Figure 4.3 Schematic representation of individuals with cancer in a population.

move. It could be argued that such was the case when breast cancer screening was investigated and implemented in 1987 in the UK under the Conservative government. The Secretary of State for Health and Social Security stated:

> In July 1985 the Government appointed a working group . . . to consider the position. The report has concluded that screening by mammography . . . will enable us to reduce deaths from breast cancer.

> The Government accept the proposals made in the report and accordingly have decided to implement a national breast cancer screening service . . . throughout the United Kingdom.

> . . . [with] all necessary back-up facilities . . . assessment . . . diagnostic . . . [and] treatment facilities, counselling and after-care and training for key groups of staff.[19–21]

Tertiary prevention

Tertiary prevention occurs after the onset of symptoms, and includes symptom recognition, diagnosis, and treatment, with the goal of preventing developed disease from killing the patient. Tertiary prevention is any intervention that limits complications from cancer after the disease is symptomatic. In the case of infectious diseases, tertiary prevention would include isolation (to prevent spread).

International cancer trends

The incidence of cancer is increasing for a variety of reasons. Most cancers have a positive age association, in that they are more prevalent with advancing age. In the developing world, as great strides are made in improving nutrition, containing and combating infectious disease, the incidence of cancer increases as people live longer:

> The steady increase in the world population (from 4.9 billion in 1985 to 6.3 billion in 2000) and its progressive ageing (6.0% aged 65 or more in 1985, 6.8% in 2000) mean that cancer will be of increasing importance as a cause of morbidity and mortality.[17]

The cancers most prevalent in the West are also increasing in developing countries, as risk factors associated with a Western lifestyle, for instance diet, reproductive habits, and industrialisation, are being replicated in developing countries as the diet begins to contain more fat, and women delay or avoid childbearing, or decide not to breast feed.

Worldwide, the most common causes of cancer death in men are lung, stomach, and colon/rectal (in developing countries they are stomach, mouth/pharynx, and oesophagus). Worldwide, the most common causes of cancer death in women are breast, cervix, and stomach, and they are the same three cancers in the developing world, except that cervix is most common (except in parts

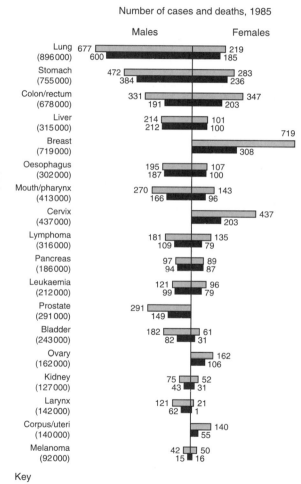

Key
▨ Estimated number of new cases.
■ Number of deaths.

Figure 4.4 Estimated numbers of new cases (grey bars) and deaths (black bars) (in thousands) of 18 cancers in men and women (Pisani *et al.*, 1993. Reprinted with permission from Wiley-Liss Inc., a subsidiary of John Wiley and Sons Inc.)[17]

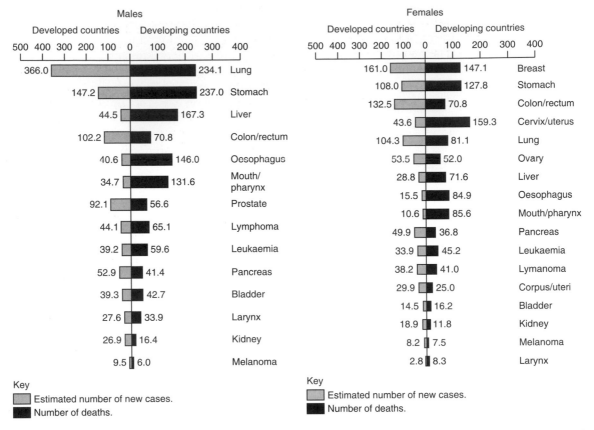

Figure 4.5 Estimated numbers of deaths (in thousands) from 14 cancers in men in developed and developing areas of the world (Pisani *et al.*, 1993. Reprinted with permission from Wiley-Liss Inc., a subsidiary of John Wiley and Sons Inc.)[17]

Figure 4.6 Estimated numbers of deaths (in thousands) from 17 cancers in women in developed and developing areas of the world (Pisani *et al.*, 1993. Reprinted with permission from Wiley-Liss Inc., a subsidiary of John Wiley and Sons Inc.)[17]

of Africa, Asia, and Latin America, where breast is more common than cervix). For both sexes taken together, lung cancer is the most frequent cause of death, followed by stomach (liver cancer ranks third in men, whereas colon/rectum cancer ranks third in women). 'Of the estimated 5 million deaths from cancer (excluding non-melanoma skin cancer), 56% occurred in developing countries.'[17] In developed countries, cancers of the colon/rectum and prostate maintain a high rank in men, and lung, ovary, and pancreas in women.

For comparison, in the UK the four most common causes of cancer death in men are lung (29%), prostate (12%), colon (7%)/rectum (4%), and stomach (6%). For women, they are breast (19%), lung (17%), colon (8%)/rectum (3%) and ovary (6%). For both sexes together, they are lung (23%), colon (8%)/rectum (4%), breast (9%), and prostate (6%).[22]

European Code Against Cancer

The 'European Code Against Cancer' is a campaign to encourage people to take action to reduce the number of deaths from cancer by 15%. A 10-point code that sums up the practical advice that is available to help reduce the risk of cancer is being publicised by countries in Europe, based upon current knowledge of prevention (primary and secondary) and early detection. The 10 points are as follows.

Prevention

1. Do not smoke.
2. Moderate consumption of alcohol.
3. Avoid excessive exposure to the sun.
4. Observe health and safety regulations at work.
5. Eat fresh fruit and vegetables and other foods high in fibre.
6. Avoid obesity and cut down on fatty foods.

Early detection

7. See a doctor for new lumps, changes in moles and abnormal bleeding.
8. See a doctor for persistent health problems, e.g. hoarseness, change in bowel habits.

For women

9. Have regular cervical smear tests.
10. Undergo mammography at regular intervals above the age of 50 years.

Each of these points is accompanied by an explanation of the relationship of the behaviour and the type of cancer, as well as figures on the magnitude of risk involved. Suggestions as to appropriate behaviour modification are given (for example, how much alcohol per week is acceptable, recommendations as to what constitutes a sensible diet and what preferable methods of cooking are).

Summary

In summary, epidemiology is integral to hypothesis generation, the development and evaluation of public health issues, the development of prevention and screening programmes and the assessment of clinical intervention trials.

Epidemiological studies of cancer have been instrumental in defining the aetiology of many cancers, and assessing their impact worldwide. Utilisation of epidemiological approaches and techniques will allow governments, institutions, and individuals to define the need for specific cancer-related programmes in prevention, screening, and care and also to assess the effectiveness of any programmes that have been developed.

References

1. Lilienfeld A.M. and Lilienfeld D.E. (1980). *Foundations of Epidemiology.* Oxford: Oxford University Press.
2. Snow J. (1936). On the mode of communication of cholera. In *Snow on Cholera.* New York: Commonwealth Fund.
3. Doll R. and Hill A.B. (1964). Mortality in relation to smoking: ten years' observations of British doctors. *British Medical Journal* i, 1399–1410, 1460–1467.
4. Doll R. and Peto R. (1976). Mortality in relation to smoking: 20 years' observations on male British doctors. *British Medical Journal* ii, 1525–1536.
5. Hennekens C.H. and Buring J.E. (1987). *Epidemiology in Medicine.* Boston, MA: Little, Brown.
6. MacMahon B. and Pugh T.F. (1970). *Epidemiology: Principles and Methods.* Boston, MA: Little, Brown.
7. Parkin D.M., Whelan S.L., Ferlay J., Raymond L. and Young J. (eds.) (1997). *Cancer Incidence in Five Continents, Vol. VII.* Lyon: IARC Scientific Publication No. 143.
8. Rodgers A. (1990). The UK breast cancer screening programme: an expensive mistake. *Journal of Public Health Medicine* 12(3/4), 197–204.
9. Shapiro S., Strax P. and Venet L. (1971). Periodic breast cancer screening in reducing mortality from breast cancer. *Journal of the American Medical Association,* 215.
10. Shapiro S., Venet W., Strax P., Venet L. and Roeser R. (1982). Ten-to-fourteen-year effect of screening on breast cancer mortality. *Journal of the National Cancer Institute* 69, 349–355.
11. Shapiro S., Venet W., Straw P. and Venet L. (1988). *Periodic Screening for Breast Cancer: The Health Insurance Plan Project and its Sequelae, 1963–86.* London: Johns Hopkins University Press.
12. Hill A.B. (1977). *A Short Textbook of Medical Statistics.* New York: J.B. Lippincott.
13. Sackett D.L., Rosenberg W.M., Gray J.A., Haynes R.B. and Richardson W.S. (1996). Evidence based medicine: what it is and what it isn't. *British Medical Journal* 312, 71–72.
14. Early Breast Cancer Trialists' Collaborative Group (1998). Tamoxifen for early breast cancer: an overview of the randomised trials. *Lancet* 351, 1451–1467.
15. Cummings S.R., Norton L., Eckert S. *et al.* (1998). Raloxifene reduces the risk of breast cancer and may decrease the risk of endometrial cancer in post-menopausal women. *Proceedings of the Annual Meeting of the American Society for Clinical Oncology* 17, 2a (abstract).
16. Wilson J.M. and Jungner Y.G. (1968). *Principles and Practice of Screening for Disease.* WHO: Public Health Papers 34.

17. Pisani P., Parkin D.M. and Ferlay J. (1993). Estimates of the worldwide mortality from eighteen major cancers in 1985. Implications for prevention and projections for future burden. *International Journal of Cancer* **55**, 891–903. Copyright © (1993 John Wiley and Sons Inc.). Reprinted by permission of Wiley-Liss Inc., a subsidiary of John Wiley and Sons Inc.

18. Levin B. (1996). Screening for colorectal cancer. *Cancer Control* **3**, 21.

19. Parliamentary Debates. Hansard 6 series, Vol. 3 1986–87. Report of the House of Commons, 25 February 1987, p. 272.

20. Forrest P. (1990). *Breast Cancer: The Decision to Screen.* London: Nuffield Provincial Hospitals Trust.

21. Her Majesty's Stationery Office (1987). *Breast Cancer Screening. Report to the Health Ministers of England, Wales, Scotland, and Northern Ireland by a Working Group Chaired by Sir Patrick Forrest.* London: HMSO.

22. Cancer Research Campaign (1995). *Factsheet 3.1. Mortality – UK.* London: Cancer Research Campaign

Part 2

The Experience of Cancer

Introduction

Benner and Wrubel[1] make an important point when they note that nursing and other caring practices have become paradoxical in a highly technical culture that seeks technological breakthroughs for all problems of illness. Taking the example of heart transplants as an important medical 'breakthrough', they remind us that:

> Few notice that the intensive medical and nursing follow-up – solving the day to day problems of living with a transplanted organ, treating sores in the mouth due to immunosuppression, coping with a new hormonal millieu, promptly recognising and responding to infection and rejection – were all caring 'breakthroughs' that led to the eventual success of heart transplantation. These essential day to day nursing-care issues had to be solved in order to make heart transplantation a viable therapy. Yet they are all overlooked in the scientific and popular media coverage of the transplant story [p. xv].

This book attempts to celebrate such caring practices in cancer care, while also providing insights into the areas where nurses need to direct their attention, and explore the demands and skills of caring practices, wherever they are found and whoever should practise them.

Much has been written about the experience of cancer; it is also the focus of an ever-increasing body of research. This section sets out to explore this experience, and to pursue themes that may receive less attention: families and carers, professionals as well as lay people, who experience the disease through others. The theme is to explore in some detail an insider perspective (at least to the extent that one can get near to this) on what it is like to have cancer, the problems and demands it brings, as well as the strategies people use to cope. The aim is to assist nurses to develop insight into what is needed in providing care.

People with cancer do not experience their illness alone. The experience of those close to them is of critical importance, for two reasons: first, because we know relatively little about the impact of cancer on relatives and friends, or for that matter on health professionals, and yet they are the most important sources of support for people with the disease. They will be responsible in many instances for a large proportion of the care and support that may be needed between episodes of formal treatment or institutional care. Cancer utterly disrupts people's lives; likewise, it disrupts in equal measure the lives of those around them. Second, those who are close to people with cancer, whether family members or friends, or health care professionals, determine through their actions and reactions the experience of cancer for the people who have the disease.

This section provides insights into these issues and also explores what goes wrong in care, and the possible reasons behind our occasional inability to care. Thoughtful ideas around how nursing and nurses might take on a greater therapeutic role in the emotional lives of people affected by cancer are offered. Mary Wells begins this section with a detailed overview of the impact cancer has on people who are diagnosed as having cancer. Hilary Plant draws on her research and the accounts of people experiencing the impact of a family member or friend having cancer to elucidate the experience of cancer within the family. In the concluding chapters Anne Lanceley begins to develop theory about nursing as a therapeutic endeavour in cancer care, the dynamics of therapeutic relationships in this context, and strategies and skills needed by nurses. She also exposes the barriers that exist for nurses working therapeutically; not the least of these is the sheer emotional burden that this imposes.

Reference

1. Benner P. and Wrubel J. (1988). *The Primacy of Caring: Stress and Coping in Health and Illness.* Menlo Park, CA: Addison-Wesley.

CHAPTER FIVE

The impact of cancer

Mary Wells

Care begins when difference is recognised. There is no 'right thing to say to a cancer patient', because the 'cancer patient' as a generic entity does not exist. There are only persons who are different to start with, having different experiences according to the contingencies of their diseases.[1]

Cancer is a disease with many manifestations, occurring at different sites of the body, and following a different course depending on the site and cell type. The variety in the disease itself is matched by the range of treatments that may be used to manage the disease. For this reason it is difficult to predict the effect a cancer diagnosis, or its treatment and aftermath, may have on an individual. The impact, for example, of mutilating surgery such as mastectomy for breast cancer, or the lingering concerns an individual with an early cancer of the larynx cured by radiotherapy may have, can vary considerably between individuals, and may not immediately reflect expectations by health carers. The apparent severity of the cancer, whether early or late stage disease for example, may not be reflected in an individual's emotional reaction to it or in their ability to adjust to living with the disease.

The emotional impact of cancer will depend on a variety of factors, such as the experiences leading up to the communication of a diagnosis of cancer, an individual's perception of cancer and its meaning, the disruption the disease causes to normal life, perceptions surrounding treatment and its effects, experiences of past traumatic events, and individual personality and coping styles. This chapter explores the ways in which cancer changes and influences the lives of those who are affected by the disease. The most important and meaningful descriptions of the impact of cancer are from people who have the disease, and wherever possible these have been used to illuminate the issues surrounding cancer and its impact.

The word cancer precipitates strong emotional reactions, be it fear, sorrow, shock, or secrecy. Many people find it difficult to use the word; even some experienced health professionals are more comfortable with using euphemisms such as 'growth', 'tumour', 'mass', or 'malignancy'. Historically, cancer has been associated with contagion, suffering, pain, and death, generating what has been termed 'cancerphobia'.[2–4] For many these associations are deeply embedded and, despite evidence for both improved survival and better quality of life through advances in treatment and symptom control, there remains a common perception that cancer is invariably fatal.

Benner and Wrubel[5] argue that in order to overcome the negativity that cancer engenders, there is a need for wholesale cultural redefinition of the disease, so that it is understood instead as a chronic or potentially curable disease. The concept of the chronic illness trajectory[6] could provide a meaningful framework for understanding cancer as a chronic disease that has a variable course and changes over time. The ever-increasing number of treatment modalities and approaches available, including surgery, radiotherapy, chemotherapy, hormonal therapy, immunotherapy, and peripheral stem cell and bone marrow transplantation, may mean that a variety of therapies is likely to be experienced at different times during the course of illness. There may also be periods of disease remission where treatment is not required, and relative health and well-being exists. These may be followed by times when symptoms may be uncontrolled or new disease is discovered and further treatment is needed.

Living with cancer brings ambiguity, disruption, and uncertainty. Cancer is rarely a one-time illness event; even if cure is achievable, the psychological impact of the disease may leave a profound mark on an individual for the rest of their life. As Frank[1]

states, critical illness such as cancer 'leaves no aspect of life untouched'.

Cancer rarely takes a linear or predictable course from diagnosis to treatment, cure or death. More often cancer and its treatment produces episodes of acute illness and treatment with periods of relative health and normal life. However, for the purposes of this chapter the impact of cancer will be discussed in relation to critical and important phases of the disease trajectory.

Diagnosis is rarely the real beginning of the disease, which may have taken months or even years to develop before a diagnosis is actually triggered. However, it is a point at which cancer becomes a reality, and therefore this represents an appropriate place to start.

Diagnosis

Receiving a cancer diagnosis is shocking and overwhelming. The magnitude of this shock initially tends to produce profound feelings of disbelief, and sometimes outright denial. These reactions are often characterised by acute distress and fear, and have been likened to a 'fever' or 'psychic inflammation'.[8] Adaptation to a diagnosis of cancer is influenced by a number of factors: the way in which diagnosis is conveyed, individual beliefs about the causation of cancer, beliefs about the disease and any delay in diagnosis, and individual personality and coping style.[9,10] The accounts below illustrate the kinds of reactions experienced after hearing the news of a cancer diagnosis. The first is an extract from an interview with a 71-year-old man diagnosed with carcinoma of the larynx.

> When he told me I'd got cancer – he bloody frightened me to death, he did. I went out, didn't I, went out cold . . . frightened me to death . . . I remember going down, sitting down and thinking that was it.[11]

The following is an extract from *An Experience of Breast Cancer: A Patient's Personal View.*[12]

> This can't be happening. Not to me. Why? What have I done to deserve this? Numbness like a cold shroud has enveloped my body . . . The expression 'scared to death' weaves its way in and out of my mind like a python slowly crushing the life out of my senses. The words rattle about in my head. Bold capital letters like cinema credits roll in front of my eyes. I blink in an attempt to block

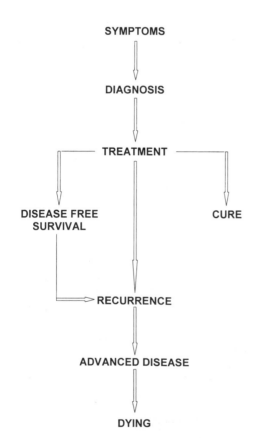

Figure 5.1 The disease continuum (reproduced with permission from Corner J. (1995). The scope of cancer nursing. In Horwich A. (ed.) *Oncology: A Multidisciplinary Textbook.* London: Chapman and Hall, Figure 17.1, p. 225).[7]

them out, but they dart back and forth like ghostly shadows taunting me.

The last is an extract from an interview with a 48-year-old woman diagnosed with carcinoma of the tongue.

> The first thing he more or less said was, 'I don't beat about the bush', he said 'what you've got, you've got a cancer,' and that's when it sort of hit me, because you're sort of mesmerised really, you sort of go into space, you think he can't be talking about me, he's probably wrong, he must be talking about someone else, but he said 'you have', he said 'you've got a cancer'. I think that was the worst time, because you come out of there thinking no, he's got it all wrong, he's got me muddled with somebody else . . . I was trying to work out where I could have got it from, you know that's the only thing you sort of have in the back of your mind, where do you get it from, I know they don't know, if they did there would probably be more preventatives but um, that's what I did wonder . . .[11]

Communicating a diagnosis of cancer is difficult for health professionals as well as for the person who is receiving the news. Frequently the diagnosis of cancer is communicated in a busy out-patient clinic where there may be few staff with specialist training and in-depth understanding of cancer and its treatment. Time is often limited; honesty and straightforward language are not always used, and those receiving the information may be too overwhelmed to understand or absorb what they are being told. Even in more ordinary circumstances most people forget over half of what is said to them during consultations with doctors.[13] The intense shock, fear, and disbelief experienced in a consultation involving a cancer diagnosis may mean that even less information is absorbed.

It is now advocated that people are given full information about their cancer, and the importance of truth telling at the time of diagnosis and throughout the cancer experience is felt to be important for adjustment.[14] This has not always been the case. In the past, many people were not told their diagnosis for fear of causing emotional harm. Telling the truth about cancer is often far from straightforward. It is not uncommon for members of the family to want to protect their loved one from the diagnosis, insisting that the truth is not told. Although there can sometimes be

tremendous pressure on health care professionals to maintain this charade, fear of emotional harm is rarely justified.[8]

It is normal to want and need to understand a disease or symptom that is being experienced, and it can be deeply troubling if there is no explanation for it. This may come from a desire to blame something or someone, possibly oneself, for the disease. For those who can legitimately 'blame' others (for example those with mesothelioma, an industrial disease associated with exposure to asbestos) it may be helpful to have a focus for their anger, although it may also foster bitterness, anger, or regret. Explanation may assist in making sense of what is happening and in coming to terms with illness. Care strategy 5.1 highlights some strategies that can be used in discussing difficult emotional issues surrounding a diagnosis of cancer.

Care strategy 5.1: Discussing difficult emotional issues, such as a diagnosis of cancer

- Check how much information has been given by the medical team, to avoid conflicting or inappropriate information being given.
- Listen to what the person is saying.
- Acknowledge the impact of what is being said.
- Find out what they already know and suspect, what conclusions have been drawn from this and what support is available from family or friends, as well as how much detail is wanted.
- Let them control the information as far as possible.
- Give information in simple language and in small amounts, so that it can be understood and digested.
- Ensure that you are both talking about the same thing.
- Define and interpret technical information as necessary.
- Be honest, straightforward and realistic, but be sensitive and do not destroy hope.
- Do not say anything that is not true or of which you are unsure.
- Give practical information and advice.

Delay in diagnosis

An individual's reaction to a diagnosis of cancer is to some extent dependent on the way in which the disease presents itself and is first acknowledged. A delay in diagnosis may be particularly significant.

This may be due to a failure by a general practitioner or other health professional to recognise symptoms suggestive of cancer, or it may have been particularly difficult to detect the cancer using diagnostic procedures; or the person may have delayed initiating the process of diagnosis due to fear, the stigma of cancer, denial, guilt, or not taking symptoms seriously.[9] The nature and length of delay prior to diagnosis may colour reactions to it, and an individual's ability to cope and adjust.

Where cancer has been detected through a routine screening test with little prior counselling, the diagnosis may be particularly shocking, because of its unexpected nature. Others who have suspected cancer for some time may be relieved to find out their diagnosis, since it ends some of the uncertainty. The example below illustrates this.

> He took a sample and after a week I had an appointment with him again, and then he told me it was malignant, that is was cancer. And to tell you the truth, I was very comfortable with it. He told me exactly how it was. And he told me how it was progressing and even if this is a disease that people don't like very much, I was very content to finally know what was wrong with me. Having been like this for a few years, I was always getting lower and lower. I was worse and worse all the time. I almost cheered up just to know what it was . . . You have been fighting some ghost that you don't know what is, nothing. That was absolutely the worst thing about the whole thing.[15]

Delays can be caused by lack of appropriate referral, failure to assess or recognise symptoms correctly, or even a doctor or other health professional finding it too difficult to confront the possibility that the person they are caring for may have cancer. Incorrect diagnosis or diagnostic delay occur quite commonly in older people due to the fact that concomitant disease is often present, and symptoms can be masked or interpreted wrongly.[16] Lack of awareness of the likelihood of cancer and delay in seeking help are common in older people. Edlund and Sneed[17] studied the attitudes and reactions of 133 people newly diagnosed with cancer of all ages and found that the older age group, that is those over the age of 70, were significantly less positive about the outcome of their disease, believing that nothing could be done. However, they were also significantly less psychologically distressed than other age groups. This may be because older people are more resigned to the idea of illness and death than younger people. This may also reflect the attitude of society and the health care system to the elderly; since they are no longer economically useful, older people may have a sense of time having run out.

For those who have delayed seeking help for signs of cancer, guilt and self-reproach may complicate acceptance of treatment, and psychological recovery.[18] Paradoxically, fear of criticism by doctors and health professionals may have played a part in extending delay. Family members may also feel responsible for not acting sooner, or may be frustrated in being unable to convince someone to visit their doctor.

For some, a conscious decision is taken not to seek treatment, and these people may delay their diagnosis until it becomes impossible to manage their symptoms, or until they need emergency care. This may occur, for instance, when an elderly woman with cancer feels she can no longer cope with the implications of her own illness in addition to nursing an already sick husband. Others may be too embarrassed to reveal their cancer, feeling that there is some stigma attached to it. It is not uncommon for an obvious cancer to be hidden from a partner for months or years, undressing in the dark and making other excuses for odour arising from the tumour. Fungating tumours in intimate places such as the breast, anus, vulva or penis, for example, may cause embarrassment, and therefore delay in seeking help for them. A mixture of guilt and relief may result when finally 'found out'.

As a professional carer it is sometimes hard to understand how someone could hide a cancer for so long, particularly when, in the case of a fungating wound, it is manifestly malodourous, weeping, raw and often extensive. Feelings of self-disgust, fear of rejection, judgement and blame, or anticipating punishment may be commonly experienced.[19] A supportive and non-judgemental approach is important in caring for such individuals. The case history of the school teacher presented in Personal account 5.1 features many of these issues.

Attributing personal responsibility onto illness can lead to feelings of guilt, self-blame, and shame.[20] Guilt and isolation can be felt because of a belief that cancer is a result of past wrongdoing or sinful behaviour, and cancer can be perceived as a 'punishment' and therefore deserved in some way. For example, lung cancer in someone who has smoked heavily can be accompanied by feelings of guilt and self-reproach; these may also be reinforced by unsympathetic health professionals. Guilt may also, however, be a means by which some individuals define themselves in order to preserve feelings of being in control. In this way guilt may permit protection from other more difficult emotions engendered by life-threatening illness.[21]

Personal account 5.1

A 44-year-old school teacher presented to his family doctor with a small rodent ulcer on his nose. He was referred to a dermatologist, and for whatever reason did not attend. Years later, the ulcer extended further, he did not go to his doctor, until his tumour had excavated his entire nose, upper lip and was beginning to extend into his eyes, and the smell and exudate were so bad he could not manage or bear it any longer. He had 'hidden' his tumour under a makeshift elastoplast 'nose', which he had made larger as the tumour grew. He had withdrawn more and more from his teaching responsibilities due to taunts from the children.

His doctor referred him directly to hospital, and when he arrived on the oncology unit, he was withdrawn, terrified and ashamed. He hid his face from sight whenever he could, and apologised almost continuously for how 'horrible' his tumour was, describing himself as a 'monster'. It seemed that his guilt at having delayed had become mixed up with a profound sense of self-blame and disgust. He saw himself as undeserving of any care or attention. His self-esteem had become so low that he was unable to bring himself to reveal what was really going on because it might make him even more of a monster to himself and others. He once wrote down a quote from the American playwright, Arthur Miller, which went some way to explain his feelings of guilt, and his ability to deny and delay: 'Guilt supplies pain without the need to act and the humiliation of contrition; by feeling guilt, in short, we weaken the need to change our lives.'

He stayed in his hospital room for a month, except when he had to go for his radiotherapy.

Dressing his face was an elaborate procedure which 'exposed' him in the most real sense, so the number of nurses involved in this care were kept to a minimum. His diagnosis of basal cell carcinoma was confirmed within a few days, and combined radiotherapy/chemotherapy commenced. Despite a lengthy course of treatment, which caused some unpleasant symptoms, he never complained about anything. Gradually, his tumour receded and he began to feel better and to be able to face people a little more. His confidence and self-esteem took months to restore and he found it difficult to sever his ties with the ward and department. However, he now wears a convincing prosthesis and was, when last heard of, alive and free of the disease.

Sontag[4] argues that recent psychological theories associating cancer with personality type may result in people feeling culpable for it. In addition, media attention surrounding prevention through diet and self-examination has encouraged notions of blame and fault in those who develop the disease. This is exaggerated by a health care culture that promotes a non-judgemental attitude towards consumers of care, yet at the same time strongly emphasises individual responsibility for health and illness. Thus, the health care system simultaneously both relieves and reinstates guilt.

Theories of adjustment and adaptation

The expanding field of 'psycho-oncology' has provided a large number of different theories of adjustment and adaptation to cancer and its treatment. While it is impossible to generalise about an individual's reaction to cancer, these theories may be useful in recognising common reactions and in helping to facilitate the expression of emotions surrounding the disease.

A number of the theories highlights stages that an individual may pass through in adjusting to the news of a diagnosis of cancer.[22,23] These include shock, numbness, and disbelief, lasting for days to weeks; acute distress, which may manifest itself as anger or anxiety, lasting for weeks to months, depression or despair and gradual acceptance, which may take several months or even years. While these theories are useful, they are also problematic in that they suggest that such emotional reactions are universally experienced and that progression through such stages of adjustment is always serial and in a forward direction, thus emphasising an overly constrained notion of what is 'normal' and 'healthy' adjustment.

Greer *et al.*[24] have identified five common adjustment styles in women with breast cancer and found these to be associated with survival after diagnosis:

- fighting spirit
- avoidance and denial
- fatalism
- helplessness and hopelessness
- anxious preoccupation.

A woman who adopts a fighting spirit towards her cancer may perceive the threat of cancer as a challenge that she is determined to overcome, expressing this with the following kinds of response: 'I'm not giving up', 'This is not going to get me', 'I'm going to fight it'. Greer *et al.* found that this kind of response was positively associated with longer survival. Interestingly, so too was the response in which women avoided or denied their disease. The conclusion drawn from their work was that 'fighting spirit' is a significant predictor of survival at 5, 10, and 15 years and active coping strategies should therefore be encouraged.

Research study 5.1

Greer S., Morris T. and Pettingale K.W. (1979). Psychological response to breast cancer: effect on outcome. *Lancet* ii, 785–789.

Aim of study

To assess psychological responses to breast cancer and their effect on outcome in a prospective 5-year study of 69 women with early breast cancer, most of whom had undergone mastectomy.

Method

Psychological assessment of 69 women with breast cancer was carried out prior to surgery. This included assessment of social adjustment (marital, sexual, and interpersonal relationships), depression, hostility, intelligence, personality, demographics, and usual responses to stressful events. Repeat assessments of depression and social adjustment were recorded 3 and 12 months after surgery, along with structured clinical interviews assessing psychological response to cancer. Interviews were repeated yearly thereafter. A pilot survey resulted in grouping of psychological responses into four mutually exclusive categories: denial, fighting spirit, stoic acceptance, and helplessness/hopelessness. Inter-rater reliability was tested as 85%.

Prognostic factors were also assessed: age, menopausal status, clinical stage, type of operation, post-operative radiotherapy, tumour size, and histological grade. However, oestrogen receptor and lymph node status were not available at the time of the study, and these are now considered to have an influence on prognosis.

Results

Initial psychological response was compared with 5-year outcome. A statistically significant association was found between the responses of 'fighting spirit' or 'denial' and recurrence-free survival, i.e. 75% of those who initially adopted one of these responses were alive at 5 years with no recurrence, compared with 35% of those who adopted 'stoic acceptance' or a 'helpless/hopeless' style.

This trend was reconfirmed by later analyses at 10 and 15 years, respectively.[25,26]

Conclusions

The responses of 'fighting spirit' and 'denial' are positively correlated with improved survival. A 'helpless/hopeless' response is associated with poor outcome.

Limitations

This was a relatively small sample on which to base such a brave conclusion. Although rating scales were used to assess depression and social adjustment, the categorisation of 'psychological response' at follow-up interviews was based on the interviewers' subjective assessment of the patients' mood and the meaning of verbatim statements. No account appears to be made of subsequent life events that may have influenced psychological response at later interviews. It is also difficult to make a judgement on a single response at a given time, as many patients will experience many different responses, perhaps simultaneously. A series of interviews at least 3 months apart is not necessarily sensitive to subtle changes over time, and it is impossible to say whether a stated 'response' on a particular day actually reflects that person's general attitude to their cancer. The results of this study, although very beguiling, are not necessarily generalisable to other cancer populations.

The basis of this study is problematic; it assumes that a single coping style is possible to identify, and that this is stable and durable over time. It also assumes that no other factors were influential to survival, and that these in themselves did not influence the type of coping style adopted by women. Taken literally, they imply that some attitudes are good and others are bad. What is apparent is that these two attitudes seem to represent forceful and definite opinions of illness, which may encourage feelings of being in control. It is perhaps this sense of being in control that is important. Subsequent studies have not always been able to replicate the findings of this highly influential study. A recent Norwegian study[27] of a more heterogeneous population of cancer patients found no relationship between psychosocial factors and survival. The authors point out that the assumptions about such a relationship are problematic, and the causal relationship may well be opposite to that put forward by Greer et al.[24,25]

How far health professionals should collude with or refute an attitude of denial is not straightforward. On balance it is considered unwise and possibly harmful to attempt forcefully to break through a patient's denial; however, to collude and encourage such denial might be equally harmful. Over-zealous health care professionals can insist on truth telling at times when a patient is not ready or able to deal with the impact of what they are being told. Careful and sensitive discussion in a safe, therapeutic relationship will often provide an opening for such dialogue, without removing the ability to hold on to control of the situation.

Those who are fatalistic about their disease, and do not believe they have any control, may express this through passive acceptance: 'You can't do anything and if you can't do anything about it there's no point worrying about it, so you have to make the best of it . . . I think you might as well make the best of it, otherwise you give up and get worried about it, no point in doing that.'[11]

'I'm in your hands' may frequently be said to doctors or nurses, by individuals who feel safer leaving any decisions to their professional carers. This fatalistic attitude may make it difficult for help to be accessed or for them to believe in their ability to influence the course of events, but it may also protect against the sometimes overwhelming burden of having cancer. There are probably times in most people's illness when placing responsibility and trust in others is an essential part of maintaining psychological stability.

As one man said, 'when you're not feeling well you don't feel very safe, you just want somebody to make it go away'.[11]

Someone who has 'given up' and is overwhelmed by the cancer and cannot see any way out may be said to have adopted a 'helpless/hopeless' adjustment style. Anxious preoccupation is a term used to describe someone who finds it difficult to think of anything other than their illness and looks for constant reassurance. They may seek alternative medicine or excessive amounts of information, worrying that every symptom is a sign of recurrent disease: 'I don't know what is going on . . . am I OK or am I not . . . I go over and over it in my mind.'[11] These adjustment styles are not necessarily pathological or negative, although they might indicate anxiety or depression, which could warrant psychological intervention. Many people will alternate between a variety of reactions to their situation, while others remain positive and in control throughout their illness.

The work of Greer et al.[24,25] has been criticised for creating a culture of blame in engendering assumptions about adaptive or maladaptive responses to cancer. What constitutes a truly maladaptive response is difficult to identify. Anger, anxiety, sadness, and other indicators of emotional distress are entirely appropriate responses to a life-threatening event, such as a diagnosis of cancer. These emotions are unlikely to go away completely unless the threat of the disease is also removed. However, studies of populations of people with cancer show a significant incidence of psychiatric disorder. It is estimated that about 30% experience an adjustment reaction and a further 20% some form of psychiatric illness.[28]

A number of studies also notes the remarkable capacity for individuals to adjust to a life-threatening illness such as cancer.[29,30] There are many theories surrounding the process by which adjustment takes place. A process of appraisal may help in making sense of the 'catastrophic threat' imposed by a cancer diagnosis. An individual's perception of the magnitude and consequences of this threat, as well as the extent to which one feels able to control the threat, will influence adjustment.[31]

The situational factors influencing this appraisal of threat following cancer diagnosis have been explored in a study using semi-structured interviews.[32] Factors found to be most strongly associated with an appraisal of severe threat were previous anxiety and depression, uncertain or pessimistic expectation about prognosis, and self-reappraisal following diagnosis. The authors of the study emphasise the need to elicit individual concerns about cancer early so that psychological interventions can be appropriately directed before maladaptive beliefs become entrenched.

A qualitative study[33] exploring strategies used in adapting to cancer found three main types of individual:

- *Preparers* – who created meaning by comparing themselves with those worse off than themselves, searching for a cause, or describing something positive that had arisen from their cancer.
- *Avoiders* – who believed that others made them have treatment, and did not acknowledge responsibility or involvement.
- *Suppressers* – who were dissociated from their cancer, thought about other things, or excluded anxiety-provoking thoughts.

The American cancer nursing literature concentrates on perceptions of health and illness and how these influence the adjustment process. One study found that women who perceived their illness as chronic rather than acute were more depressed, regardless of their actual stage of disease.[34] Another study[30] found that patients with poorer physical health also had lower levels of psychological well-being and demonstrated greater discrepancy between their perceptions of their 'ideal' self and their 'actual' self. The study suggested that those who can align these perceptions may be able to be more realistic about what they would ideally like to do and what they can actually do, and are therefore more likely to adjust and to have higher levels of well-being.

Psychodynamic theory

This view of adjustment is founded on the belief that early developmental processes influence personality resources and thus the defence mechanisms employed in coping with cancer. When faced with the loss of control and threat of dependence imposed by cancer, attempts at retaining control are unconsciously made through enacting defences learned in childhood. Common defence mechanisms include:

- denial
- projection – attributing own unacknowledged feelings onto someone else
- displacement – redirecting energy into something other than the cause of the distress
- sublimation – channelling primitive emotions into something creative; for example, anger or art
- regression – return to childlike behaviour
- intellectualisation – at the expense of emotional expression

- conversion – expression of emotional anxiety through a physical symptom.[9]

Psychodynamic theorists believe that these defences must not be destroyed, since they help to protect against unbearable anxiety. Bion[35] believes that the essential role of the psychotherapist is to act as a 'container', in the sense of 'holding' this unbearable anxiety, in the same way as a mother contains or holds the feelings of her baby, handing them back in a more manageable and bearable form. In the same way, someone with cancer may also need an external person to contain unbearable feelings, until the point at which they become bearable again. Thus, containing and holding distress is an essential part of the therapeutic relationship between nurses and people with cancer.[36]

A psychodynamic model has been applied to adjustment in bone marrow transplant.[37] This model identifies three levels of adjustment, based on the characteristics of the individual, family and social support available, and on previous life experience. This model can be used to identify an individual's psychological state at the beginning of treatment, thus providing a means of identifying those at high risk, who may not be able to adjust without psychiatric help.

- *Level 1* – those who demonstrate what the authors describe as 'appropriate affect', including anger, sadness, or fear in response to their cancer. They usually have a solid family support system and a previous history of coping effectively with adverse life events, and show a realistic balance of hope and concern for the future.
- *Level 2* – those who display limited resources for coping with their distress or discomfort, and have often experienced unresolved loss in the past, and demonstrate high levels of agitation and anxiety.
- *Level 3* – those who are usually characterised by a previous psychiatric history, often originating from a dysfunctional family, and display extreme agitation and often suicidal ideation.

The issues of identifying those at 'high risk' of difficulty in adjusting to a diagnosis of cancer have also been explored by Baider *et al.*,[38] who compared the coping abilities of people with cancer who had previously lived through a severe life-threatening situation (survivors of the holocaust), with a matched group of people with cancer who had not experienced a severe life event. They found that the holocaust survivors used significantly more avoidance strategies, but still found the cancer significantly more intrusive than the matched group. Their psychological distress scores were significantly higher, indicating that living through severe and traumatic life events may reduce a person's ability to mobilise the adaptive denial required to cope with cancer. It is important to be aware of any previously experienced traumatic life events, so that psychological distress can be appropriately assessed and interventions planned accordingly.

Frank[1] is critical of the emphasis in the psycho-oncology literature on adjustment, and suggests an alternative way of looking at living with illness.

> I want to emphasise mourning as affirmation. To mourn what has passed, either through illness or death, affirms the life that has been led. To adjust too rapidly is to treat the loss simply as an incident from which one can bounce back; it devalues whom or what has been lost. When an ill person loses the body in which she has lived, or when a caregiver suffers the death of the person he has cared for, the loss must be mourned fully in its own time. Only through mourning can we find a life on the other side of loss [p. 40].

The impact of cancer is largely felt through the losses experienced by the individual and family. As Frank's story demonstrates, cancer causes the future to disappear. Life is turned upside down; it is no longer possible to make plans or allow oneself normal expectations of life. Another important dimension of loss is that of time. Imposed absence from work and home, attending hospital for clinic appointments and treatment and waiting for results, all contribute to the loss of one's own routine, sense of time, and control over that time. Being ill may enforce a 'waiting culture of medicine',[39] which can dominate and control long periods of time.

Loss is felt in every aspect of life, and is often compounded by physical change. In a study[11] of the experience of cancer of the head and neck, feelings of being embarrassed to go out showing any visible signs of cancer or its treatment, being embarrassed to eat in a restaurant for fear of dribbling or needing to use a straw were reported. Several of those interviewed explained how they held back from normal activities, preferring to do nothing, rather

than be disappointed if they found they were unable to do what they had planned. Cancer and its treatment had knocked their confidence and caused withdrawal from many of the aspects of life that gave them their individuality, such as gardening, work, church, swimming, and going out socially. Withdrawal from these activities meant that these people experienced a loss of identity similar to a sense of 'loss of belonging'.[1] The following are excerpts from interviews with people following treatment for cancer of the head and neck.

> 'I dribble at the corner of my mouth and this upsets me, I've never got full control, the whole thing makes me feel as if I'm not functioning properly . . . I don't want to get into one to these things and then not be able to do it properly.'

> 'I didn't want anyone asking me uncomfortable questions at the time . . . I felt I couldn't go out, people I knew I'd see and I didn't want to have to explain, that sort of thing.'

> 'Didn't go to church – didn't want people surreptitiously looking at my burns.'

The meaning of cancer

Adjustment to cancer also depends on the personal meaning of cancer, and the perceived threat of death.[31,40] A phenomenological view of adjustment and cancer emphasises the inextricable link between coping and the meaning and context of the illness experience.[5] The individual construction of meaning is to a large extent dependent on personal beliefs, characteristics and events, past and present.[10,41]

A cancer diagnosis often initiates a search for meaning, motivated by a strong desire to make sense of the situation. This search may assist the adaptive process through helping the individual to regain control and mastery of the chaos surrounding them. The need to create new meaning may occur around the time of diagnosis or recurrence, or on completing treatment and being designated 'well' again. Taylor[42] has devised a conceptual framework for the search for meaning.

- Identifying causal explanations; these may change over time and differ according to cultural background.

- Selective incidence: 'Why did this happen to me and not someone else?'
- Responsibility: who or what is to blame? Identifying a behavioural cause may assist in feelings of reduced susceptibility to recurrence.[43] Perceiving the cause to be inherent to personality factors may not allow this.
- Significance of the experience; some individuals construe benefits from their cancer.

Individuals will respond in different ways to the need to identify and create meaning. These may be through resignation (passive acceptance), remonstration (lack of acceptance and discontent), and reconciliation (significance found and accepted). Nurses need to understand that this search for meaning may be important for the individual, and they must have the ability to facilitate psychological adjustment through a search for meaning.

The sociological and anthropological literature identifies that the meaning of illness is attributed as a result of socially determined cultural interpretations and networks, and that an individual's own interpretation and explanation for illness and its symptoms are highly significant to the 'legitimisation' of disease.[44–47] Saillant[48] tells a story of a woman with breast cancer who strongly believed that the pain in her hips was due to a previous stillbirth, rather than the bone metastases that were the logical cause of her pain. Because her own belief about her pain was not 'acceptable' to her health carers, she did not express this openly. Her own construction and legitimisation for her disease was therefore left unrecognised, leaving her feeling isolated and alone. Saillant points out that the acceptance of 'popular' explanation is important as it 'permits patients to satisfactorily integrate their illness in a context where the need for coherence in the face of a break with life is essential'. Assigning meaning to illness helps to reduce or even resolve suffering.[41] Nurses can greatly assist with the process of finding meaning, by letting an individual tell their own story surrounding their illness, and helping them place this in context, thus reinforcing an acceptance of the importance of their feelings and explanations. This 'illness narrative' has been recognised as an important

means by which understanding of the meaning of illness can be developed by an individual, and may be of enormous therapeutic value.[44,49,50]

Care strategy 5.2: Facilitating narratives

Helping someone to 'tell their story' acknowledges that the individual has an identity that has been disrupted as a result of illness. The construction of such a narrative enables the individual to make sense of what is happening, as well as to incorporate their illness into the context of their life in its wider sense. Time, space and privacy are important. Many patients will tell 'how it all started' without needing encouragement. However, asking about the following aspects of the experience may assist the expression of a narrative or story:

- describing how life was prior to their diagnosis
- describing their thoughts and feelings at the time of the diagnosis
- how things are different in life now compared with before the diagnosis of cancer
- how friends, family, and work colleagues have responded to them since they have had cancer
- how their relationships have changed
- what the treatment and its effects have been like
- what a 'normal' day or week is like now
- how they have changed since having cancer diagnosed
- what they think caused or contributed to their cancer
- how they view life now and in the future
- what has been the most significant change in their life as a result of the diagnosis.

Time to 'de-brief' is important, as retelling many aspects of the narrative may provoke feelings and reactions that require support within the safety of the therapeutic relationship. As Atwood (1997) describes, the story may only make sense afterwards, and there needs to be time to reflect on its meaning: 'When you are in the middle of a story it isn't a story at all, but only a confusion; a dark roaring, a blindness, a wreckage of shattered glass and splintered wood; like a house in a whirlwind, or else a boat crushed by the icebergs or swept over the rapids, and all aboard powerless to stop it. It's only afterwards that it becomes anything like a story at all. When you are telling it, to yourself or to someone else' [p. 346].[51]

Unfortunately, the biomedical model of illness does not incorporate this vital dimension of popular explanation and meaning, and instead concentrates on the pathophysiology of illness.[41] Both conceptualisations of illness have limitations, since the medical model focuses on symptoms as cues only indicative of underlying pathology, and the sociological and coping models focus on the human behavioural response to the disease process, but may ignore physical aspects of illness.[52,53] A more comprehensive 'illness constellation model' has been proposed,[53] which recognises the experience of illness for the individual and significant others. This identifies three stages in coping:

• uncertainty
• disruption
• striving to regain self and wellness.

Uncertainty is a prominent feature of the experience of almost anyone diagnosed with cancer and is discussed in more detail later in this chapter. Life is disrupted by emotional, physical, and practical factors, which may include repeated hospital appointments for treatment or follow-up, the need for specialist clothing or food as a result of cancer surgery, or inability to work or care for children due to treatment side-effects. Such disruption requires a re-evaluation of life in order to move towards wellness. This re-examination of life may be a positive experience, resulting in a shift in self-image and perspective, which can help to make sense of illness, maintain self-integrity and permit re-establishment in the world.[29,54,55]

Taylor's[29] theory of cognitive adaptation involves the notion of 'illusions', which enhance self-esteem and enable mastery to be regained over illness and life in general. These illusions may be critical to mental health and successful adaptation. If an illusion such as a belief that a certain diet will prevent recurrence of disease is shattered by the development of metastases, another set of illusions may be chosen in order that control can be regained. Evidence also exists that an individual may adapt their expectations of themselves, lifestyle or personal philosophy in order to cope with the disruption brought to life by cancer.[56]

A phenomenological study[57] undertaken in parallel to a randomised controlled trial assessing the effectiveness of a health promotion intervention with patients with chronic illnesses, including cancer, found the following strategies used to promote health:

• creating a sense of purpose (for example, making the day worth something)

• consciously attending to own attitude (for example, thinking positively, doing things for oneself)
• drawing on personal and family 'patterning' (ways of coping)
• setting and striving for goals
• talking (to oneself and others)
• allowing oneself to learn about and learn from experiences
• taking one step at a time
• maintaining control
• using friends to help out
• comparing oneself favourably with others
• creating alternative ways of being (for example, moving the bed downstairs to increase independence)
• re-framing expectations of life and self.

Wells'[11] study of the experience of radiotherapy treatment for cancer of the head and neck found that a number of these strategies was used during recovery from radiotherapy treatment. Creating a sense of purpose, and taking one step at a time were combined with a tendency to monitor and mark recovery. Going to the post office, doing some gardening, visiting the dentist again, all signified the return of normality. The kinds of achievement described in the following extracts[11] may seem small, but it is important that nurses acknowledge their significance and encourage the adoption of meaningful coping strategies.

'As for getting back to normal, I've made a start, I've been out this weekend, bought a load of seeds, some compost.'

'I shall know I'm back to normal once I've had my teeth done . . . just step by step really, isn't it?'

The use of narrative accounts and the importance of meaning have been described. Several other therapeutic strategies may be useful in the process of assisting individuals to adjust to and live with a diagnosis of cancer. Moorey and Greer[31] describe the application of Adjuvant Psychological Therapy (APT), where therapy is orientated towards problem solving, reappraisal and 'cognitive restructuring' (reality testing). The components of this structured approach include the following.

• Enabling the patient to air their feelings.
• Teaching behavioural techniques such as relaxation, distraction, and activity scheduling, to

maximise the patient's sense of control and ability to feel pleasure during daily life.

- The use of cognitive techniques, which assist the patient to recognise any automatic or negative thoughts and learn to challenge them in a number of ways. The patient is helped to consider the evidence for any negative fears and to search for more constructive or alternative explanations. A process of 'decatastrophising' encourages the patient to confront their fears in a safe environment and to consider whether these are realistic. Simple distraction techniques that 'break into the spiral of increasing anxiety' (p. 117) can be useful. Patients can also be taught to say certain positive things to themselves whenever they feel anxious or have negative thoughts, e.g. 'I am going to get well'.
- Working with couples – partners can be effectively involved in this process by reminding the patient of their strengths, remembering previous ways that the couple have coped with stressful events. While working with the couple, the therapist can facilitate and enhance their communication skills through the use of behavioural and cognitive techniques.

This approach is essentially a joint problem-solving exercise, which is flexible enough to be tailored to an individual's needs. The application of the techniques employed by Moorey and Greer can help to develop more constructive coping strategies, which can positively change the ways of responding and adjusting to living with cancer.

The impact of treatment

Once a diagnosis is confirmed and treatment is offered, this then means coping with the additional burdens of toxic and lengthy treatment. However, progression from diagnosis to treatment may not always be immediate. As David Izod[58] recounts, it can be weeks before being seen by an oncologist and a treatment plan initiated, and is like being placed in a 'twilight zone . . . a time of suspicion, rumour and possibility, and feeling utterly powerless'.

Cancer treatment can be particularly difficult, since it frequently causes symptoms and difficulties and can make one feel worse rather than better,

producing 'an unacceptable transformation from active, attractive independence to physically unattractive dependence'.[18] Cancer treatment is rarely a one-off event; a whole range of cancer treatments may be experienced during the course of the disease. The chronic nature of cancer often means that treatment is never really 'completed'. Surgery may be followed by chemotherapy and/or radiotherapy; individuals may then be maintained on hormonal therapies, and may perhaps require some further radiotherapy or symptom control at a later date. Faced with constant reminders of disease, it may be difficult to maintain hope.[59] Repeated hospital visits for treatment or follow-up can prevent the resumption of normal life, and the presence or emergence of symptoms serves as an unwelcome reminder of past experiences, as can media coverage of cancer. The impact of treatment must be seen in the context in which it is experienced. Someone who has never experienced chemotherapy or radiotherapy before, for example, may react to the treatment differently to someone who is 'experienced'. Figure 5.2 shows a map of the different trajectories that may be travelled by a person with cancer, and provides the basis for understanding the impact of treatment in different situations.

Those who undergo radical therapy and can expect a cure (that is trajectory A) are likely to be those whose disease has been caught early, possibly through screening or even through a chance investigation. These individuals may have been quite well prior to diagnosis and are only made 'sick' as a consequence of cancer treatment. A much quoted study, however, revealed that most regard considerable toxicity as acceptable when presented with the possibility of cure.[60]

Although one of the main aims of curative treatment is to minimise later effects, certain therapies will almost certainly produce lasting side-effects, which can compromise 'normal life' considerably. For example, cure for a haematological malignancy, teratoma, or cervical cancer may be at the cost of infertility. In these instances, the lasting effects of cancer therapy may never be forgotten.

There have been several studies examining the side-effects of different cancer treatments, or the ability to cope with individual treatments. Many of these studies tend to isolate the impact of a

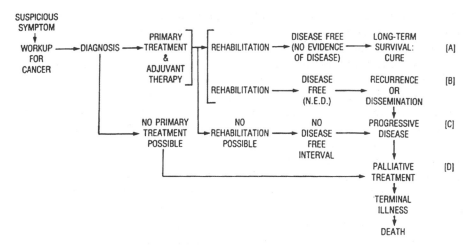

Figure 5.2 Clinical course and outcome of cancer (reproduced with permission from Holland J. and Rowland J. (1990). *Handbook of Psycho-oncology: Psychological Care of the Patient with Cancer*. New York: Oxford University Press).[8]

particular therapy, which although important in understanding the particular treatment, does not take into account the impact on the illness experience in its entirety. There is a need for more research studies to look longitudinally at the experience of cancer, taking into account the impact of a range of treatments, symptoms, and events in the context of a person's life.

Chemotherapy

Perceptions of chemotherapy may be clouded by memories of friends or family who were treated with cytotoxic drugs some years ago and experienced severe nausea and vomiting. Anti-emetics are now very much more effective and it is possible for most symptoms to be reasonably well controlled. The idea of toxic drugs entering the body may also be difficult, and may be perceived as poisonous. As well as nausea and vomiting, hair loss, sterility, mucositis, bone marrow depression, skin changes, diarrhoea, and damage to any of the major body systems are common side-effects of chemotherapy. Alopecia appears to be one of the most distressing of these. Frank's[1] experience of alopecia was one of discomfort and stigma. To him, baldness represented the person with cancer as a victim: the baldness being a visible symbol of the loss, suffering and fear of cancer. As well as causing overt side-effects,

chemotherapy removes the ability to take pleasure in everyday aspects of life. David Izod[58] remembers, 'I didn't feel like drinking, smoking, had no sex and ate only to stop myself from vomiting. I didn't laugh much and went to bed at 8 o'clock.'

Many studies of the impact of chemotherapy examine particular side-effects that are observable and quantifiable such as nausea and vomiting, rather than more subjective problems such as fatigue. A further limitation of such studies is that they concentrate on a given point in time, thus neglecting the day-to-day and cumulative impact of treatment. The inconvenience and disruption to normal life caused by repeated visits and admissions to hospital is significant, yet it is not often assessed.

A longitudinal study[61] was carried out in which 238 people with breast cancer or lymphoma were interviewed five times during a 6-month course of chemotherapy; individuals also completed daily diaries, which explored the severity and timing of side-effects, the emotional distress, and the disruption to social life and work resulting from chemotherapy. Disruption to work and social life tended to increase as more cycles of chemotherapy were completed. The cumulative impact of multiple side-effects appeared to outweigh any other single effect. Despite videotaped information and preparatory education sessions provided by nurses, the burden of side-effects, particularly tiredness, had been underestimated prior to commencing treatment (8% expected this and 86% experienced difficulties). One interesting finding was that there appeared to be much greater readiness to report distress or side-effects in the diaries than during interviews. This led the authors to conclude that reports of chemotherapy experiences given retrospectively to a doctor (or nurse) tend to under-represent the extent of problems actually experienced. They also found that nearly half had thought about discontinuing treatment, although few had discussed this with their doctor.

Continual communication throughout treatment is clearly necessary, to ensure that concerns can be voiced and the impact of chemotherapy on the individual assessed on an ongoing basis. There is a tendency for nurses and doctors to assume that if the first course of chemotherapy has been well tolerated, so will the rest. This is not always the case, and the cumulative effects can be very debilitating. As Love et al.[61] state, 'appraising a patient's treatment burden based only on the patient's initial response to treatment is inadequate because the experience of side-effects and subjective distress is continually changing' (p. 611).

As well as causing significant emotional and physical disruption, chemotherapy has been associated with an increase in psychiatric morbidity. One study[62] found that the incidence of anxiety, depression, and sexual difficulty was significantly higher in women who had undergone adjuvant chemotherapy after mastectomy, and that this was directly related to the degree of toxicity experienced. A proportion of patients also develops phobic reactions to chemotherapy; in particular, anticipatory nausea and vomiting, characterised as a learned or conditioned response to chemotherapy. This syndrome develops when certain events or stimuli are associated with treatment; for example, the journey to the chemotherapy clinic, the smell of alcohol wipes, with unpleasant post-treatment effects such as nausea and vomiting. This association induces nausea and vomiting *before* the chemotherapy is actually given, and is known as anticipatory nausea and vomiting. Studies have shown that teaching progressive muscle relaxation and imagery can reduce anxiety and nausea, although this is most effective when a therapist is actually present.

Radiotherapy

The technical and invisible nature of radiotherapy produces fear and misconception. Fears of the dangers of radiation are fuelled by disasters such as Hiroshima and Chernobyl. Radiotherapy can be perceived as a last resort,[63] despite the fact that over 50% of all patients will receive radiotherapy at some stage of their illness; many, however, do experience considerable toxicity and distress.

Little nursing research has been undertaken into the experience of radiotherapy. Studies have focused on symptoms, by measuring distress experienced from them at specific time points during and after radiotherapy.[64,65] An alternative and attractive approach is through the use of diaries, which appears to elicit information on the individuality of experience, often revealing intimate detail, which helps to create a picture of the impact of cancer and its treatment on everyday life.[61,66,67]

Attempts have been made to assess the emotional impact of radiotherapy, but most of these have 'assessed' anxiety and mood state,[68,69] uncertainty and adjustment to illness,[70] or information needs[71] using measurement scales that inevitably limit any interpretation of individual distress. Qualitative research on the impact of radiotherapy[65,66] reveals the extent of physical and emotional distress experienced with radiotherapy. The daily disruption of attending for treatment for up to 6 weeks is compounded by an often insidious build-up of symptoms, which cause a gradual deterioration, not always noticed by health professionals, or even by those undergoing treatment themselves. Radiotherapy symptoms tend to develop towards the end of treatment, or may develop after treatment is finished. As a result, there may be insufficient access to expert help, leaving many to try and cope on their own with extremely debilitating side-effects. The following is an excerpt from an interview with a 42-year-old man with parotid cancer.[11]

It happens so gradually that it sort of infiltrates slowly and you don't realise how ill you are actually feeling . . . you don't realise it's waiting for you to say . . . it's not bad enough to tell anyone about, and when it's bad enough to tell anyone about, the pills you're given aren't good enough to do anything about it . . . you think they should be working and if they're not working you must be doing something wrong because the doctor knows what he's doing and he's given you these pills, they're not having any effect but they must be helping the pain because he's given them to you.

Most specialist nursing roles and thus research and practice development have, up until recently, been concentrated in the area of chemotherapy rather than radiotherapy, perhaps because its side-effects tend to be more obvious and immediate. Those undergoing radiotherapy have been perceived as 'self-caring' or 'walking wounded', and have not been seen to require the same level of expert nursing attention as those undergoing toxic drug therapy. This is a misconception, and has led to the neglect of the development of nursing interventions in this area.

Surgery

The physical removal of a cancer through surgery can be reassuring, as it represents a cleansing and symbolic elimination of the evil within.[9] Izod[58] explains that his retroperitoneal node dissection following chemotherapy was 'violent, purgative, cleansing and . . . final'. The impact of surgery is dependent on the significance of the site of surgery and individual effects it may have on body image and concept of self. Surgery for cancer often results in some kind of disfigurement or mutilation, and may threaten social and sexual identity. Removal of part of the body such as a breast or limb induces a profound sense of loss as well as functional change, and the assault on body image and sexuality may also have an enormous impact on intimate relationships. Mastectomy or pelvic surgery threatens a woman's sexual identity and can also alter perceptions of them by others. Women can be made to feel ugly and deformed on account of their surgery. Helping a woman to come to terms with the changes in her body, while giving her control and choice is essential. One woman who actively decided not to wear a prosthesis following her mastectomy describes being approached before leaving the ward by a member of staff who wanted to know when she was coming in for her 'fitting'. When she said she was not, she was told she would have to, or 'she would make people feel uncomfortable'.[12] This kind of attitude gives neither control nor choice.

Sexual function as well as self-image may be affected by surgery. Urological or bowel surgery may result in loss of fertility, and cause impotence, nerve damage, and loss of libido. Gynaecological surgery may result in loss of fertility, shortening of the vagina, hormonal changes in pre-menopausal women, or external disfigurement after radical vulvectomy. An interview study of 105 women[72] who had undergone major gynaecological surgery for cancer of the cervix or vulva, up to 5 years following surgery, found that 31% were depressed and 41% were suffering from anxiety. Many had never resumed sexual intercourse following their surgery, 76% had encountered sexual problems in the first year after their operation, and 66% were still experiencing these difficulties at the time of interview. Partners of these women had not been involved in discussions with health professionals, which women would have liked. Nursing initiatives such as gynaecological support nurses and 'drop-in' clinics for women and their partners have been set up to meet some of these needs.[73]

The disfigurement caused by head and neck surgery may reduce the ability to control facial muscles, interfering with breathing, and the ability to kiss and communicate. Surgery to the head and neck attacks the most visible and arguably most expressive part of the human body. The identity of those who undergo such surgery can be profoundly threatened. Two studies have demonstrated that the psychological effects of treatment for head and neck cancer can be long lasting.[74,75] Extensive and disfiguring surgery has been shown to have a significant impact on self-image as well as on social and sexual relationships. The authors suggest that the need for rehabilitation programmes providing psychosocial support should be addressed.

The following is an excerpt from an interview with a patient and his wife following laryngectomy.[11]

It must be very embarrassing when you first use the artificial voice . . . the noise, people sort of look down to see where it's coming from . . . a couple of our grand-daughter's friends, they both stood there and laughed . . . sometimes when he's eating, he can't help it, he makes [imitates a loud gulping sound] type of noise. If we wanted to start up a conversation, we would just say hello, whereas he can only gape . . . we don't go out much, I think he would be embarrassed if he was sitting in a restaurant and had to drink with a straw.

One man who returned to the oncology ward 3 months after hemi-glossectomy and pectoralis major flap for cancer of the tongue explained that he had not kissed his wife since coming home from hospital. His tongue was deformed and his mouth had strands of chest hair growing inside it.

Recovery from treatment

Many presume that finishing treatment is a very positive experience. However, despite the fact that many will face the prospect of full 'recovery' and cure, this may not mean a return to the level of functioning experienced prior to cancer treatment, and this could affect employment, family and social relationships, or sexual expression.[41] Far too little attention is paid to the immediate period following the end of treatment, when side-effects may continue to be experienced, but also where there is loss of contact with the specialist treatment centre, which for many may have been a lifeline. Alby[76] describes the fear and uncertainty associated with this period of time as due to a combination of factors:

- the fear of leaving a protected environment with skilled, supportive staff
- the fear of facing life with a different body (for example, as a result of weight loss, surgery, alopecia)
- the constraints of treatment and diet (for example, immunosuppressive therapy following allogeneic bone marrow transplantation, steroid therapy, changes in diet following oesophagectomy or gastrectomy).

She concludes that 'discharge is feared just as much as it is wanted'.

Frank[1] and Izod[58] both describe the importance of 'ceremonies' and 'boundaries', which provide some structure to life *after* cancer. Frank describes how difficult it was for him to 're-enter' his world after the end of his treatment for testicular cancer. He believes that rituals are necessary to mark the end of treatment because they enable the process of re-entry to occur more easily. Even after 'cure' he described that his 'consciousness remained suspended between the insulated world of illness and the healthy mainstream'. When cancer treatment ends, it is some considerable time before a person

can know with any certainty whether treatment has been successful or that they have been 'cured', and is therefore similar to the experience of having a chronic illness that is in remission. This may mean that people have no 'socially sanctioned position on the health-illness continuum; they are neither sick nor well'.[55] Instead they may be in a liminal phase, which may be culturally unsafe, undesirable and even dangerous:[77,78]

> The period after treatment can be terribly hard for the cancer patient. For the previous six months, cancer, the treatment, and particularly the staff at the hospital had been the dominant factor in my life. And then all of a sudden nothing. I had been sucked in by the system as an ill person, treated by it and now it was spitting me out as a healthy person, but I was left with a very big hole. Although I hadn't been discharged, indeed I won't be for another 5 years, the intimacy had gone, there were other people more important than me, people whose treatment had just begun. And I didn't know what the hell to do with myself.[58]

Considerable difficulty may be experienced at the end of successful treatment since an individual's 'share of attention has been used up',[46] and they may feel that their problems are no longer legitimate. This may lead to self-doubt, a crisis of credibility, and the feeling that problems are not worthy of mentioning; a reluctance that may be reinforced by health professionals who make light of them.[52] An interview study of women with breast cancer, at or around the time of recurrence,[79] revealed that women felt supported up until the end of primary treatment, but they then experienced a lack of continuity of care and lack of interest in their case during out-patient consultations. They no longer felt treated as individual people and expressed an unfulfilled desire to talk about the future.

Emotional distress can also occur on completion of radiotherapy. In one study 80% were found to have a significant degree of anxiety after the end of treatment,[62] and an interview study of women before and after chemotherapy and/or radiotherapy for breast cancer found that 30% found the end of treatment upsetting, leaving the feeling that a 'safety net' had been lost.[34] Similar problems of emotional trauma, unexpected side-effects and a lack of information to equip people to cope after the end of treatment have been found in other groups of patients, such as those with cancer of the head and neck.[80,81] Wells[82] found that despite the level of distress at this time, there was also a reluctance to ask for help: as one woman said, 'you don't like to ring because there are other people still having treatment . . . you've finished your treatment, you ought to be fine'.

One problem for people completing radical treatment is that 'routine follow-up' practice does not always permit them to talk about their experiences, except in relation to the physical effects of therapy. The space and opportunity to explore meaning and the experience of cancer treatment appears to be reserved for those who are dying of their disease, rather than those who are in the recovery phase of illness. It is likely to be extremely helpful to talk through these experiences in order to make sense of them; it may even be necessary to provide some kind of psychological follow-up programme, to allow adjustment following traumatic cancer treatment. An important element of this programme would be to help people to 'let go of unsatisfactory aspects of the past in favour of focusing on the present, where positive change is still possible'.[83]

A recent phenomenological study[15] using in-depth interviews explored the 'lived experience' of nine men and women in remission from their cancer, enabling their stories to be told, with subsequent interviews developing a deep level of understanding about their experiences. An overriding theme of this experience was 'experiencing existential changes' encompassed by the five themes of uncertainty, vulnerability, isolation, discomfort, and redefinition.

In this study, uncertainty was experienced at all stages of the disease, about either the cancer itself, the efficacy of treatment, the threat of recurrence, or uncertainty about the likelihood of imminent death. The following is an extract from an interview with a 41-year-old man receiving phase I trial chemotherapy for metastatic cancer of the parotid gland following disease progression after radical radiotherapy.[11]

The uncertainty's the most difficult bit to deal with because there's uncertainty about whether or not the treatment you're having is doing any good, there's uncertainty about basically how long you've got . . . there'll always be uncertainty about how long I've got, I suspect, until I start getting symptoms that are very clearly demonstrating things.

The uncertainty is difficult . . . I don't know whether or not when I get switched off the drug next week, whether I'm going to be able to work next week . . . I'm planning to go to work on a day by day basis, I never know how I'm going to feel. I'm getting myself a second hand car to do up as a project but to be perfectly honest I don't know whether I'm going to be able to do it and I might just throw my money away. Then there's always the other bits you start worrying about, you know, money, my wife needs the money because I won't be around and there are those things as well . . .

In Halldorsdottir and Hamrin's study, vulnerability was another feature of having lived with cancer.[15] The impact of communications with health professionals at this vulnerable time was identified, in particular, the necessity for the latter to offer respect, warmth and understanding. Isolation and loneliness had been experienced by most at some point during their cancer, either because they perceived or actually experienced rejection by others, or because they had shut themselves off or withdrawn from normal life. As one explained, 'we cancer patients shut ourselves inside, draw the curtains, avoid people and feel poisonous'.[15] Physical and emotional discomfort was also a prominent theme in this study. Fatigue and weakness were particularly common, but pain, difficulty sleeping, and vomiting were also experienced.

All identified changes in themselves following the experience of cancer. Often these involved an alteration in their perception of the world around them, or of emotional relationships. Many felt they had become stronger or closer to those closest to them. Some did not feel so positive, regretting the incapacity imposed by the disease, or lamenting their changed role or position in society. The authors of the study recognise the limitations of generalising from a small interview study beyond the cultural and social group of Icelanders represented in their research. However, it does demonstrate the need for security, certainty, care, and respect, as well as support to maintain a feeling of control over their situation and find ways of redefining themselves or their lives.

Recurrence

The threat of recurrence is ever present, and the uncertainty it causes is central to the experience of cancer.[59] The dread that the disease may return is continuous, and if it does anxiety and distress can be greater than at initial diagnosis, because the threat of death is 'more real'.[84] Robinson's[79] study of women with recurrent breast cancer found that recurrence was experienced differently from their original diagnosis since it explicitly challenged confidence in a personal future. Robinson describes the process during which women suspected recurrence, experienced uncertainty and panic, then shock, devastation and threat when recurrence was confirmed. Many then felt disillusioned that they had not been able to prevent or detect the problem, and desperately sought an explanation, in an attempt to understand their situation.

The identification of recurrent disease causes the future to be viewed in terms of uncertainty, death and dying, and perceived loss. The psychological impact of the event is often compounded by a reduction in activity and stamina due to pain, weakness or debilitating symptoms. A prospective study of 269 women with breast cancer found that 61 (23%) developed recurrence within 3 years.[85] Thirty-eight of these were interviewed following this diagnosis, and overall, they reported feeling significantly worse than when they had been first diagnosed. Over 80% were very shocked when told about their recurrence, compared with half at original diagnosis. Levels of anxiety and depression were also significantly higher in these women than in those in the study who had no recurrence. The majority, however, claimed that they had been offered no support.

The discovery of recurrent disease has been found to be accompanied by feelings of anger, injustice, fear, emotional volatility, and the need to regain control.[86] Memories of the experience of initial diagnosis may return. Nurses need to understand these memories of the emotional and physical distress of diagnosis and treatment, and avoid making assumptions that levels of understanding, treatment preferences, or support networks remain the same as before. Careful assessment is needed of an individual's current condition, emotional or physical concerns, and support available. Case strategy 5.3 gives examples of the type of questions that might be asked during an assessment interview.

Care strategy 5.3: Examples of assessment questions at the time of recurrence or salvage treatment (adapted from Mahon[86])

How do you feel about the recurrence of your cancer?
What does it mean to you?
What problems are the recurrence or treatment causing for you?
How do you think you might handle these problems?
What do you remember about the treatment from last time?
Do you have any questions about your treatment or care now?
How are things at home and/or at work?
Do you have anyone you can turn to for help?
What is most important to you now?
How can we help you to cope with this situation?

Survivorship

The concept of survivorship derives from the USA, where self-help and coping strategies are actively promoted. Surviving cancer may be a mixed experience; while cancer survivors often say that they lead more fulfilling, meaningful lives through experiencing life-threatening illness,[87] they may also find it difficult to come to terms with the feeling that they do not deserve to be alive. This has been likened to post-war survival guilt.[18]

In a British study of 10 adults who had survived lymphoma, using semi-structured questionnaires,[88] some were found to feel that nothing had changed in their lives; however, most described survival as a process through which stages of adjustment took place, and changes had to be accepted. Many felt that the experience of cancer had produced positive outcomes. However, several had found it very difficult to forget and move on from the experience, and had flashbacks in which aspects of their life as a cancer patient were continually recalled and remembered. The authors concluded that although survival may be adequate reward for some, others may seek to improve, change, or adjust their lives, struggling with the effects of cancer long after cessation of treatment.

Dirksen's[89] study of 31 long-term survivors of melanoma in New Mexico, using the Search for Meaning Scale and Index of Well-being, found that over half believed in a specific cause for their cancer, and those who were younger, or who felt that it was their fault were more likely to search for meaning. Sixty-one per cent felt that their diagnosis had changed their life; 90% of these said it was for the better. It may be that these were untypical; however, positive reappraisal of life is emphasised in many studies of people who feel that the experience of cancer has enriched their lives in some way.

A survey of 687 cancer survivors[90] who were members of the National Coalition for Cancer Survivorship in the USA collected demographic and quality of life data. Although they were clearly a self-selected group – over three-quarters of the sample were women, and nearly half had breast cancer – the survey still provides an insight into the factors influencing quality of life in survivors. Psychological well-being was found to be lower than functional, social, or physical well-being, and this appeared to be affected by recall of initial diagnosis and treatment as well as fear of recurrence. Family distress and sexuality were reported as having the most negative influences on quality of life. Physical well-being was most severely affected by fatigue and aches and pains. The authors propose a quality of life model for cancer survivors (see Figure 5.3), which highlights aspects of well-being that might be positively influenced by nursing assessment and intervention.

Dying

When chronic illness becomes terminal illness yet another adaptation is faced and has been described as the 'crisis of the knowledge of death'.[91] Glaser and Strauss[92] describe four dying trajectories in which this crisis may be experienced.

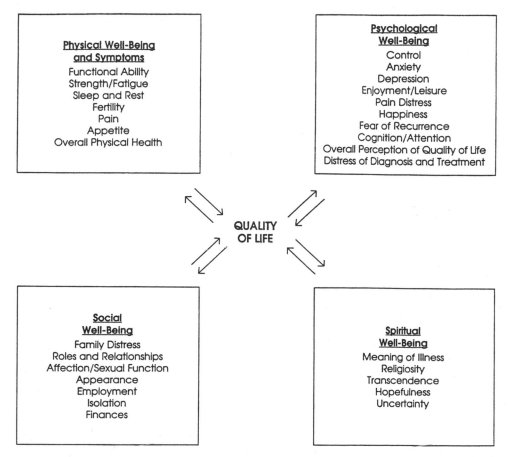

Figure 5.3 The quality of life model applied to cancer survivors (reproduced with permission from Ferrell B.R. *et al.* (1995). *Oncology Nursing Forum* **22**, 915–922).[90]

1. Certain death at a known time.
2. Certain death at an unknown time.
3. Uncertain death but a known time when the question will be resolved.
4. Uncertain death and an unknown time when the question will be resolved.

Many desire to know exactly when they are going to die, and ask questions such as 'How long have I got?' If death is inevitable, a time when death may be expected may be requested since such certainty may feel preferable in such a distressing and uncertain situation. However, it is unlikely to be possible to identify the trajectory of certain death at a known time until the last few days or perhaps weeks of life and, rightly, few doctors are prepared or able to make such precise predictions. If they do, it can produce a feeling of marking time and waiting for disaster to strike, which may limit the ability to enjoy the life that is left. Cancer is an uncertain disease and most live through the remaining three trajectories, as the following excerpt from an interview with a 42-year-old man with metastatic parotid cancer illustrates.

> I was told that I've got between 4 and 12 months, so you think, right, when was I told? So 6 months from then is then, therefore I've got to make sure this month I'm going to feel all right, this month I'm going to be in bed all the time, this month I've had it.[11]

Other personal experiences of death may give rise to expectations or preconceptions. This may make it difficult to face the prospect of one's own death. As one man who had been in the RAF explained, 'I've always been rather accustomed to sudden death . . . quite, quick bang, just like that . . . sudden not drawn out, I can't stand that . . . I don't like this at all.'[11] Thus he knew that he would die of his disease, but admitted that he was 'scared stiff', waiting for it to happen.

The fears of the dying have been described, and the importance of eliciting individual experiences of death so that such fears can be understood has been highlighted.[14] Most are understandably afraid of the unknown, of being separated from the people that they love and of suddenly ceasing to exist. Fears of dying in pain, or alone, losing control of bodily functions or mind, dying suddenly or violently, or being rejected by friends and family are all common. If these fears can be discussed, and

preferences about death are taken into account, this can at least give back some control and enable care to be focused on preventing these fears from becoming a reality.

Probably the most important aspects of caring for the dying are listening, allowing the person to retain as much control as possible, and providing optimum physical and emotional comfort. What this entails is very much dependent on a full assessment of the individual's needs and the flexibility and creativity of the caring team. If a person does have to die in hospital, nurses can do a great deal to integrate rather than separate the experience into the life of that person. Too often we stick to the rules and try to constrain the experience, or imagine that we can protect families from some of the realities of death. Sometimes families prefer not to be involved, but it can make a huge difference to both the dying person and their family if they are permitted to be part of the experience.

Conclusion

This chapter began with an acknowledgement that each individual is different, and will have a different experience of cancer. Adequate recognition of these differences is essential to understanding the impact cancer has on that individual. Examples have shown that the personal meaning of cancer and the context in which cancer is experienced may strongly influence a person's adjustment and adaptation to their diagnosis. Life can be profoundly disrupted at any stage of the cancer trajectory, disturbing physical, emotional, financial, social, and spiritual equilibrium. Fear and uncertainty can suspend any sense of future, and 'normal' life takes on a different interpretation. Living with cancer, however, is not always an overwhelmingly negative experience; for many, it precipitates a re-evaluation of priorities and relationships that may greatly improve life.

Many opportunities exist for nurses to contribute towards improving the experience of cancer. At every stage of the cancer trajectory, nurses can provide support and care that will enhance quality of life in its widest possible sense. This chapter has illustrated potential times of vulnerability during the trajectory, and demonstrated some of the many problems faced when living with a cancer diagnosis.

Nurses are in a unique position to anticipate and respond to these problems, and to develop care strategies that will help to reduce the impact of cancer in whatever sense it is felt. Assessing and understanding differences between individuals – their responses, support systems and interpretations of their illness – must be the starting place.

References

1. Frank A.W. (1991). *At the Will of the Body. Reflections on Illness.* Boston, MA: Houghton Mifflin.
2. Patterson J.T. (1987). *The Dread Disease. Cancer and Modern American Culture.* Cambridge, MA: Harvard University Press.
3. Dorsett D.S. (1991). The trajectory of cancer recovery. *Scholarly Inquiry for Nursing Practice: An International Journal* 5, 177–184.
4. Sontag S. (1991). *Illness as Metaphor.* London: Penguin Books.
5. Benner P. and Wrubel J. (1989). *The Primacy of Caring: Stress and Coping in Health and Illness.* Menlo Park, CA: Addison–Wesley.
6. Corbin J.M. and Strauss A. (1991). A nursing model for chronic illness management based upon the trajectory framework. *Scholarly Inquiry for Nursing Practice: An International Journal* 5, 154–174.
7. Corner J. (1995). The scope of cancer nursing. In Horwich A. (ed.) *Oncology: A Multidisciplinary Textbook.* London: Chapman and Hall.
8. Holland J.C. and Rowland J.H. (1990). *Handbook of Psycho-oncology: Psychological Care of the Patient with Cancer.* New York: Oxford University Press.
9. Guex P. (1989). *An Introduction to Psycho-oncology.* London: Routledge.
10. Barraclough J. (1995). *Cancer and Emotion: A Practical Guide to Psycho-oncology*, 2nd edition. Chichester: John Wiley.
11. Wells E.M. (1995). *The impact of radiotherapy to the head and neck: patients' experiences during and after completion of treatment.* University of London, Institute of Cancer Research, unpublished MSc. thesis.
12. Miller J. (1995). An experience of breast cancer: a patient's personal view. In Sheeran J. (ed.) *A Picture of Health: Paintings and Drawings of Breast Cancer Care by Susan Macfarlane.* West Royd: Sheeran Lock Fine Art Consultants.
13. Ley P. (1988). *Communicating with Patients: Improving Communication, Satisfaction and Compliance.* London: Chapman and Hall.
14. Stedeford A. (1994). *Facing Death: Patients, Families and Professionals*, 2nd edition. Oxford: Sobell.
15. Halldorsdottir S. and Hamrin E. (1996). Experiencing existential changes: the lived experience of having cancer. *Cancer Nursing* 19, 29–36.
16. Monfardini S. and Yancik R. (1993). Cancer in the elderly: meeting the challenge of an ageing population. *Journal of the National Cancer Institute* 85, 532–538.
17. Edlund B. and Sneed N.V. (1989). Emotional responses to the diagnosis of cancer: age related comparisons. *Oncology Nursing Forum* 16, 691–697.
18. Naysmith A., Hinton J.M., Meredith R., Marks M.D., and Berry R.J. (1983). Surviving malignant disease: psychological and family aspects. *British Journal of Hospital Medicine* 30, 22–27.
19. Priestman T. (1986). In Stoll A.B. (ed.) *Coping with Cancer Stress.* Dordrecht: Matginus Nijhoff.
20. Finerman R. and Bennett L.A. (1995). Guilt, blame and shame: responsibility in health and sickness. *Social Science and Medicine* 40, 1–3.
21. Rowe D. (1987). *Beyond Fear.* London: Faber.
22. Kubler-Ross E (1970). *On Death and Dying.* London: Tavistock.
23. Weisman A. and Worden J.W. (1976–1977). The existential plight in cancer: significance of the first 100 days. *International Journal of Psychiatric Medicine* 7, 1–15.
24. Greer S., Morris T. and Pettingale K.W. (1979). Psychological response to breast cancer: effect on outcome. *Lancet* ii, 785–787.
25. Pettingale K.W., Morris T. and Greer S. (1985). Mental attitudes to cancer: an additional prognostic factor. *Lancet* i, 750.
26. Greer S., Morris T., Pettingale K.W. and Haybittle J.L. (1990). Psychological response to breast cancer and 15 year outcome. *Lancet* 335, 49–50.
27. Ringdal G.I., Gotestam K.G., Kaasa S., Kvinnsland S. and Ringdal K. (1996). Prognostic factors and survival in a heterogeneous sample of cancer patients. *British Journal of Cancer* 73, 1594–1599.
28. Massie M.J. and Holland J.C. (1989). Overview of normal reactions and prevalence of psychiatric disorders. In Holland J.C. and Rowland J.H. (eds.) *Handbook of Psycho-oncology.* New York: Oxford University Press.
29. Taylor S.E. (1983). Adjustment to threatening events. A theory of cognitive adaptation. *American Psychologist* **November,** 1161–1173.
30. Heidrich S.M., Forsthoff C.A. and Ward S.E. (1994). Psychological adjustment in adults with cancer: the self as mediator. *Health Psychology* 13, 346–353.
31. Moorey S. and Greer S. (1989). *Psychological Therapy for Patients with Cancer.* Oxford: Heinemann Medical Books.
32. Parle M., Maguire P. and Jones B. (1996). Maladaptive coping and affective disorders. *Psychological Medicine* 26, 725–744.

33. Lev E.L. (1992). Patients' strategies for adapting to cancer treatment. *Western Journal of Nursing Research* **14**, 595–617.

34. Ward S., Viergutz G., Tormey D., DeMuth J. and Paulen A. (1992). Patients' reactions to completion of adjuvant breast cancer therapy. *Nursing Research* **41**, 362–366.

35. Bion W. (1962). Learning from experience. *Seven Servants.* New York: Jason Aronson.

36. Bailey C. (1995). Management of breathlessness. *European Journal of Cancer Care* **4**, 184–190.

37. Futterman A.D. and Wellisch D.K. (1990). Psychodynamic themes of bone marrow transplantation: when I becomes thou. *Haematology Clinics of North America* **4**, 699–709.

38. Baider L., Peretz T. and Kaplan De-Nour A. (1992). Effect of the holocaust on coping with cancer. *Social Science and Medicine* **34**, 11–15.

39. Frankenberg A. (1993). *Time, Health and Medicine.* London: Sage.

40. Krumm S. (1982). Psychosocial adaptation of the adult with cancer. *Nursing Clinics of North America* **17**, 729–737.

41. Cassel E.J. (1982). The nature of suffering and the goals of medicine. *New England Journal of Medicine* **306**, 639–645.

42. Taylor E.J. (1995). Whys and wherefores: adult patient perceptions of the meaning of cancer. *Seminars in Oncology Nursing* **11**, 32–40.

43. Loeshcher L.J., Clark L., Atwood J.R., Leigh S. and Lamb G (1990). The impact of the cancer experience on long term survivors. *Oncology Nursing Forum* **17**, 223–229.

44. Kleinman A. (1980). *Patients and Healers in the Context of Culture: An Exploration of the Borderland between Anthropology, Medicine and Psychiatry.* Berkeley, CA: University of California Press.

45. Good B.J. and Delvecchio Good M. (1980). The meaning of symptoms: a cultural hermeneutic model for clinical practice. In Eisenberg L. and Kleinman A. (eds.) *The Relevance of Social Science for Medicine.* Dordrecht: Reidel, pp. 165–196.

46. Bury M. (1991). The sociology of chronic illness: a review of research and prospects. *Sociology of Health and Illness* **13**, 451–468.

47. Wenger A.F.Z. (1993). Cultural meaning of symptoms. *Holistic Nursing Practice* **7**, 22–35.

48. Saillant F. (1990). Discourse, knowledge and experience of cancer: a life story. *Culture, Medicine and Psychiatry* **14**, 81–104.

49. Williams G.H. (1984). The genesis of chronic illness: narrative reconstruction. *Sociology of Health and Illness* **6**, 174–200.

50. Mathieson C.M. and Stam H.J. (1995). Renegotiating identity: cancer narratives. *Sociology of Health and Illness* **17**, 283–306.

51. Atwood M. (1997). *Alias Grace.* London: Virago Press.

52. Waxler N.E. (1980). The social labelling perspective on illness and medical practice. In Eisenberg L. and Kleinman A. (eds.) *The Relevance of Social Science for Medicine.* Dordrecht: Reidel, pp. 283–306.

53. Morse J.M. and Johnson J.L. (eds) (1991). *The Illness Experience: Dimensions of Suffering.* London: Sage.

54. Tishelman C., Taube A. and Sachs L. (1991). Self-reported symptom distress in cancer patients: reflections of disease, illness or sickness. *Social Science and Medicine* **33**, 1229–1240.

55. Kagawa-Singer M. (1993). Redefining health: living with cancer. *Social Science and Medicine* **37**, 295–304.

56. Heidrich S.M. and Ward S.E. (1992). The role of the self in adjustment to cancer in elderly women. *Oncology Nursing Forum* **19**, 1491–1496.

57. McWilliam C.L., Stewart M., Brown J.B., Desai K. and Coderre P. (1996). Creating health with chronic illness. *Advances in Nursing Science* **18**, 1–15.

58. Izod D. (1996). The patient's perspective. Plenary paper given at the *9th International Conference on Cancer Nursing,* 12–18 August, 1996, Brighton, UK.

59. Nelson J.P. (1996). Struggling to gain meaning: living with the uncertainty of breast cancer. *Advances in Nursing Science* **18**, 59–76.

60. Slevin M.L., Stubbs L., Plant H.J. *et al.* (1987). Attitudes to chemotherapy: comparing views of patients with cancer with those of doctors, nurses and general public. *British Medical Journal* **300**, 1458–1460.

61. Love R., Leventhal H., Easterling D.V. and Nerenz D.R. (1989). Side-effects and emotional distress during cancer chemotherapy. *Cancer* **63**, 604–612.

62. Maguire P., Tait A., Brooke M., Thomas C., Howat J.M.T., Sellwood R.A. *et al.* (1980). Psychiatric morbidity and physical toxicity associated with adjuvant chemotherapy after mastectomy. *British Medical Journal* **281**, 1179–1180.

63. Peck A. and Boland J. (1977). Emotional reactions to radiation treatment. *Cancer* **40**, 180–184.

64. King K.B., Nail L., Kreamer K., Strohl R.A. and Johnson J.E. (1985). Patients' descriptions of the experience of receiving radiotherapy. *Oncology Nursing Forum* **12**, 55–61.

65. Munro A.J., Biruls R., Griffin A.V., Thomas H. and Vallis K.A. (1989). Distress associated with radiotherapy for malignant disease: a quantitative analysis based on patients' perceptions. *British Journal of Cancer* **60**, 370–374.

66. Faithfull S. (1992). The diary method for nursing research: a study of somnolence syndrome. *European Journal of Cancer Care* **1**, 13–18.

67. Wells M. (1998). The hidden experience of radiotherapy to the head and neck: a qualitative study of patients after completion of treatment. *Journal of Advanced Nursing* **28**, 840–848.
68. Weintraub F.N. and Hagopian G.A. (1990). The effect of nursing consultation on anxiety, side-effects and self-care of patients receiving radiation therapy. *Oncology Nursing Forum* **17**, Suppl. 31–36.
69. Graydon J.E. (1994). Women with breast cancer: their quality of life following a course of radiation therapy. *Journal of Advanced Nursing* **19**, 617–622.
70. Christman N.J. (1990). Uncertainty and adjustment during radiotherapy. *Nursing Research* **39**, 17–20.
71. Johnson J.E., Lauver D.R. and Nail L.M. (1989). Process of coping with radiation therapy. *Journal of Consulting and Clinical Psychology* **57**, 358–364.
72. Corney R., Everett H., Howells A. and Crowther M. (1992). The care of patients undergoing surgery for gynaecological cancer: the need for information, emotional support and counselling. *Journal of Advanced Nursing* **17**, 667–671.
73. Jones B. (1994). Drop-in centre for cancer care. *Nursing Standard* **9**, 23–25.
74. Gamba A., Romano M., Grosso I.M. *et al.* (1992). Psychosocial adjustment of patients surgically treated for head and neck cancer. *Head and Neck* **14**, 218–223.
75. Rapoport Y., Kreitler S., Chaitchik S., Algor R. and Weissler K. (1993). Psychosocial problems in head and neck cancer patients and their change in time since diagnosis. *Annals of Oncology* **4**, 69–73.
76. Alby N. (1991). Leukaemia bone marrow transplantation. In Watson M. (ed.) *Cancer Patient Care.* Cambridge: British Psychological Society/Cambridge University Press.
77. Douglas M. (1966). *Purity and Danger: An Analysis of the Concepts of Pollution and Taboo.* London: Routledge.
78. Turner V. (1967). *The Forest of Symbols: Aspects of Ndembu Ritual.* Ithaca, NY: Cornell University Press.
79. Robinson L. (1994). *Cancer recurrence: a phenomenological study.* King's College, London, Unpublished MSc. thesis.
80. Eardley A. (1985). Patients and radiotherapy. 1. Expectations of treatment. 2. Patients' experience of treatment. *Radiography* **51**, 324–326.
81. Eardley A. (1986). Patients and radiotherapy. 3. Patients' experiences after discharge. 4. How patients can be helped. *Radiography* **52**, 17–22.
82. Wells E.M. (1994). *The first few weeks at home: patients' experiences of finishing radiotherapy to the breast.* University of London, Institute of Cancer Research, unpublished care study.
83. Cull A. (1991). Lung cancer. In Watson M. (ed.) *Cancer Patient Care: Psychosocial Treatment Methods.* Cambridge: British Psychological Society/Cambridge University Press.
84. Mahon S., Cella D. and Donovan M. (1990). Psychosocial adjustment to recurrent cancer. *Oncology Nursing Forum* **17**, 47–52.
85. Hall A., Fallowfield L. and A'Hern R. (1996). When breast cancer recurs: a 3-year study of psychological morbidity. *Breast Journal* **2**, 197–203.
86. Mahon S. (1991). Managing the psychosocial consequences of cancer recurrence: implications for nurses. *Oncology Nursing Forum* **18**, 577–583.
87. O'Connor A.P. and Wicker C.A. (1995). Clinical commentary: promoting meaning in the lives of cancer survivors. *Seminars in Oncology Nursing* **11**, 68–72.
88. Wallwork L. and Richardson A. (1994). Beyond cancer: changes, problems and needs expressed by adult lymphoma survivors attending an out-patients clinic. *European Journal of Cancer Care* **3**, 122–132.
89. Dirksen S.R. (1995). Search for meaning in long-term cancer survivors. *Journal of Advanced Nursing* **231**, 628–633.
90. Ferrell B.R., Dow K.H., Leigh S., Ly J. and Gulasekaram P. (1995). Quality of life in long-term cancer survivors *Oncology Nursing Forum* **22**, 915–922.
91. Pattison E.M. (1977). *The Experience of Dying.* London: Prentice Hall.
92. Glaser B. and Strauss A. (1965). *Awareness of Dying.* Chicago, IL: Aldine.

CHAPTER SIX

The impact of cancer on the family

Hilary Plant

The impact of cancer on an individual is invariably a profound and life-changing experience, the consequences frequently continuing long beyond the initial period of treatment. Likewise, the impact of this disease on the family and friends of someone with cancer may be equally disturbing, and is perhaps even harder to recognise or know how to support.

'Family' is difficult to define and will have a different meaning for each individual according to their personal situation. The concept of family may hold inherent connotations of its 'nuclear' form. For the purpose of this discussion, the term 'family' is broad and inclusive; the focus is on the defining relationships in a person's life, those with whom there is a degree of emotional attachment, however complex this might be. Thus the terms 'family' or 'relatives' are used to refer to those who are close to a person who has been diagnosed with cancer, and includes partners, parents, offspring, siblings, and close friends.

Family relationships are dynamic and the diagnosis of cancer in one member will resonate throughout the whole social group, changing the relationship with the person who has cancer and with one another. This will be influenced by the stage each individual has reached in their own developmental process. The experience of cancer is also mediated by factors such as the relationship an individual has with the person who has cancer, their own perceptions and understanding of cancer and other events or stressors that may coincide with illness.[1,2]

The major themes concerning the impact of cancer on families are interrelated and surround:

- the experience of cancer for families
- communication within the family
- living with cancer in the family
- interacting with health care professionals
- approaches to caring for families.

Each of these will be illustrated by comments made by individuals who took part in a study undertaken with the families of people diagnosed with lung or colorectal cancer.[3] These experiences were explored through in-depth interviews, undertaken over a period of 18 months. Participants who took part in the study were from diverse social backgrounds and all had established relationships with the person with cancer. Cancer is predominantly a disease of middle and older age and the focus of this chapter is on the impact that it has on adults. The experiences of young children whose parents have cancer, or those affected by childhood cancer itself are also be included through their experiences as reported in the literature.

The experience of cancer for families

The close family and friends of someone with cancer will experience distress. However, the extent of such distress is difficult to gauge. For many there is a deep 'existential' element to this, which can be difficult to understand or talk about, but that is in essence a fundamental loss of one's bearings and a sense of unreality created by the threat to the life of someone close. This is often accompanied by a tangible change in outlook; for example, in life's priorities or direction.

The news of a cancer diagnosis in a partner, friend or relative can cause intense emotional disturbance in the form of sadness, depression, anxiety, or anger. Day-to-day functioning can also be changed or impaired, for example with weight loss, tiredness, or insomnia. Just as for the person with cancer, the experience for families evolves over time as the illness progresses, so individual family members will feel the impact of cancer differently. This is illustrated by the comments of the following woman whose husband was newly diagnosed with cancer of the lung.

> But of course, when anybody sort of says the word cancer, the first thing you think about is, that's it, you've not got a chance in hell . . . you can't imagine the feeling until it actually happens . . . a very good friend of mine had cancer . . . so I mean I've been through the stages of it and it was pretty horrendous, but then it was a friend, not my husband . . . [now] it's like a blood relation . . . whatever Arthur was going through I was going through, I was going through the same with him.[3]

The threatened loss precipitated by a cancer diagnosis in the family causes the onset of grief since 'part of the social context for understanding, organising, validating, and defining feeling, action, values, and priorities is removed . . .'. Thus grief can be seen as arising not only because of a loss of a person but also because of losing a part of the foundation for dealing with loss and with all of experience,[4] as Anna Quindlen's fictionalised account of a daughter's experience of her mother's cancer illustrates.[5]

> I remember that the last completely normal day we ever had in our lives, my brothers and I, was an ordinary day much like this one, a muggy August-into-September weekday. Afterward I wondered why I hadn't loved that day more, why I hadn't savoured every bit of it like soft ice cream on my tongue, why I hadn't known how good it was to live so normally, so everyday. But you only know that, I suppose, after it's not normal and everyday any longer. And nothing ever was after that day.

A feeling of loss of security following the diagnosis of cancer in a partner can be experienced as the woman below expresses. She yearns for the time in her life when she felt safe and cared for:

> . . . the mental torture of it all. But I suppose it would be nice to have someone like your mum, it's stupid isn't it, but it's the comfort. You know when you are ill at home and you've been a young child, and your mum's there and it's lovely, but as you get older unfortunately you haven't got these people around you anyway. You *are* the person. It's the security you miss.[3]

Much of this loss of security must stem from the fact that for most, the immediate thought on hearing the diagnosis of cancer is that the person they love is going to die.[6,7] Partners may in fact express more fear of death than the person with cancer themselves,[8] as one husband describes when his wife was in hospital having surgery for bowel cancer. He was frightened for her but also very frightened for his own world without her. Many express the wish that it was they themselves who had the cancer, since this might make them feel more in control, or prevent them facing the prospect of being left alone:

> at the time I was really scared . . . of her dying, because again . . . it's self . . . it's giving way to yourself . . . just because somebody else is dying, you should be sorry for them, but no if you're honest, you're worried about yourself.[3]

Life may change quite fundamentally as a result of the diagnosis of cancer. For example, giving up work to care for the person with cancer, moving to live nearer them, or taking on additional household tasks. Important aspects of family lifestyle may be lost; for example, holidays are no longer planned, or there may be financial difficulties, sometimes to the extent of losing one's home if there is a substantial loss of earnings. In other instances there might be a less obvious change in daily life creating more of a sense of uncertainty and confusion about plans and hopes for the future. For example, a man whose wife had colorectal cancer reflected that:

> . . . you come to a sort of junction and you change . . . you go off a different way . . . it changes your whole life . . . there's no two ways about that.[3]

A young woman described her thoughts about how the loss of practical and emotional support from her mother would change her life:

all I could think of was . . . what's going to happen to me, who's going to look after me . . . she was going to organise my wedding and look after me when I have children.[3]

The parents of a child with cancer will invest everything in the child during the illness in the hope of recovery and all other aspects of life may become neglected.[9] The relationship between parent and child is an important source of security throughout life and disruption to this in childhood creates a vulnerability to psychiatric disorder in adulthood. Anxiety levels experienced by a child who has a parent with cancer are decreased when they have an understanding about the illness and are able to communicate well with their parents.[10]

Several studies indicate that distress in family members is as great or greater than in the person who has cancer themselves.[11] One study that attempted to identify the pattern of crisis experienced following discharge after surgery for bowel cancer found that there were few differences in the intensity of distress between the person with cancer and their spouse.[12]

Attempts have been made to assess the levels of anxiety and depression experienced amongst families where one member is diagnosed with cancer.[13] Helplessness, fear, and anger are reported as the most stressful emotions encountered amongst those who have family or friends undergoing chemotherapy.[14]

A man whose wife was in hospital with colorectal cancer and who was himself disabled commented:

> I could have gone off the deep end, one hears about people in hospitals who go and rush into the casualty and thump the doctors, I can sympathise with them . . . because to them why isn't somebody doing something, they don't know what is happening, they see you calm and quiet, I sympathise with them. When you don't know . . . this is . . . animal instinct. If you don't know you bite it or hit it or something, and I'm prepared to accept that . . . that when you're reduced to the minimum, all you do is act like an animal.[3]

Many relatives appear to find it hard to reflect on their own emotional distress. Sometimes it is easier to describe the physical manifestations of the emotional upheaval than more abstract emotions. For example, when relatives describe hearing the diagnosis they may recall reactions such as feeling 'dizzy', having a 'dry mouth', feeling 'cold', or unable to speak for some time. If these coincide with the moment when important information regarding the diagnosis or treatment is being communicated by doctors, or when they are asked if they have any questions, this may act as a barrier to full understanding of the news. One man who found it hard to express his worries described how he felt when he heard his wife's cancer had spread:

> I felt as though something had been stuck inside me . . . a knife or something, I don't know. That was the piercing blow I think . . . It was as though I had a sword stuck in me. It was like . . . that sort of feeling you get when . . . going to pass out . . . the hot feeling that goes right inside.[3]

These acute physical reactions experienced at times of stress such as on hearing the diagnosis or the news of recurrence, are usually short-lived, but they can contribute to longer term difficulties in functioning by causing fatigue, anorexia, or insomnia. The husbands of women with breast cancer have been found to report increased moodiness, loss of energy, and growing fears about their own illness and death. This has been attributed to the fact that these men deny their own feelings and place those of their wives at the foreground of their thoughts, intensifying deeper anxieties.[6]

During the course of her father's lung cancer, a woman commented on her own deterioration:

> . . . but I suppose really your health does deteriorate, you feel tired, you feel irritable, in my case you lose weight, you find it hard to put back on, you're tired, but you can't sleep, and it does catch up with you in the end.[3]

A man describing his home when his wife was in hospital with lung cancer commented:

> What was it like? Like a mortuary . . . fed up, I hardly ate, I hardly cooked anything. Well I didn't fancy it, know what I mean? . . . Even the whisky there, one night I had a good dose of it, it didn't make no difference.[3]

In brief, those close to a person diagnosed with cancer will experience a wide range of reactions to the illness. Their feelings will be complex and often difficult to express. They themselves may become unwell. These difficulties may not be readily apparent to the health professionals whose acknowledgement of the relative's situation, particularly around the time of diagnosis, might provide support and ease the strains that can exist between patient, relative, and professional.

Communication within the family

The social consequences of cancer on the family are many and varied, and are exacerbated by difficulties in talking about cancer. Communicating about the illness, changes in roles and coping strategies employed by different family members all have important social implications for family dynamics and functioning. The diagnosis of cancer in a family will have an impact on not only the internal world of each family member, but also on their relationships with the person who has cancer, and with others in their circle of acquaintances. Where relationships are strained, for example with an ex-partner or work colleagues, the tension may be heightened. People report that some (usually more distant) relationships are terminated entirely.

In Personal account 6.1, a young woman with ovarian cancer describes the impact on her relationship with her husband Paul,[15] illustrating how cancer may cause a slight but significant 'turning away', even in the most supportive relationships. Anne describes how she and her husband are adjusting together to the painful process they are going through. After 4 years of illness, it had become impossible to sustain the emotional closeness created at the time of diagnosis in the face of the prolonged uncertainty Anne's cancer had caused both of them.

While studies have shown that the reactions to cancer and the adjustment process are remarkably similar in both the actual person with cancer and family members, there are also important differences.[16] As in the case of Anne and Paul, cancer may confer some (albeit possibly unwanted) benefits to the person with the disease. However, this is less likely for the relative. Anne feels that Paul is 'holding back' or putting her first, attempting to protect her.

Personal account 6.1

Paul was so reluctant to tell me but I knew anyway. Fatigue has worn him down. The constant uncertainty, the ever present threat that I am going to die, has turned him away from me a little. It is so hard to remain com-

mitted to someone, not knowing whether they will be there in a few months or a few years time. I can understand that. And the uncertainty goes on and on. The tenderness when I was first diagnosed couldn't possibly be sustained without a break for nearly four years. I didn't expect or want it to. It would have been easier if I had either died or been cured quickly but it just isn't like that.

In a sense Paul is going through the same painful process of adjusting to this latest progression that I have had. The same resentment to the sharp cutting off of a relaxed attitude to life and an indefinite future. Anger at the possibilities we can't choose anymore . . .

It would be easier if I was less demanding, more oblivious, but I can't be. I have to be myself. More so perhaps now that I am under threat. I don't have the time, the patience to be untrue. That is part of the problem too. It hasn't been all bad. Cancer has given me opportunities for self development and I have taken them with both hands . . .

But Paul has been holding back, simply because I have cancer. I was angry when he said that, how could he be so patronising. I felt a little guilty too. I hadn't seen what was my advantage not to see.

Talking about cancer and its implications and uncertainties is difficult. Much of this difficulty arises from a desire (for all parties) to protect each other from any additional hurt or pain. In a study of the husbands of women with breast cancer,[13] few (less than 7%) were found to have discussed their worries with anyone, and an interview study with the families of people with lung cancer found that most spouses were not sharing their concerns with them.[11] Even couples who profess a very close relationship or who have similar coping styles can be set apart by cancer, however much they attempt to share their feelings about the illness. This will ultimately lead both to feel a sense of loneliness.

Many people with cancer and those close to them declare and practise a philosophy of being open about the illness and of talking about it together. Nevertheless, there are invariably some things that are very difficult to share. Communication may be open for the person with the disease, but not for the relative in terms of expressing emotions such as anger, fear, or disappointment. Relatives may not have a place to vent their own emotions and sometimes find that they are becoming the 'butt' for the emotions of the person with cancer, with nowhere to take them or pass them on themselves.

The following comments illustrate the difficulties of being a 'cancer relative'.

One man describes the week after his wife's diagnosis with breast cancer:

> I think almost every time after she had gone out and I was on my own doing something I would quite often break down and cry, but she didn't realise that.[3]

Another man explains how his wife complains about her treatment in hospital:

> I mean she comes home and she shouts off . . . spouts off at me so then I take the deflect on that, you know, I feel the same as she does then . . . in fact more.[3]

If there is a decision as a family that the illness will not be discussed, a wall of unexpressed emotion between the person with the disease and their family can be created. The exclusion of friends or family can be created by the person who has cancer if they refuse to talk about their illness, which may be very hard to bear. The implications of the cancer for siblings, adult children, or friends, those who are less publicly involved in the daily life of the person with cancer, may not be acknowledged by other social acquaintances or work colleagues or by health professionals. Friendships sustained by infrequent meetings are vulnerable, and can be disrupted or lost altogether, since the illness may make keeping in contact very difficult.

A sister comments on the distancing of her brother through cancer:

> You feel you've done everything you can and then you're just shut off from it when you feel you want to be there. And you want to say something but you're not being given the opportunity to sort of say the right words . . . I think one of the hardest things is that when you feel you could be there for somebody they put up a barrier against you . . . .[3]

Changes in roles at home, work, or socially have been found to occur in families, such as altered employment, household schedules, or curtailed social activities.[11,17] Social activities, finances if the person who is ill is the main source of income, and career plans may be severely disrupted. Sexual difficulties are common between partners where one has cancer. Fear and anxiety can decrease libido, as do many cytotoxic drugs. The fatigue experienced as a result of the disease or its treatment decreases interest in sex. Changed appearance may also cause embarrassment or physical difficulties.

Many relatives and friends have a conscious or unconscious desire to protect someone they love who has cancer from any additional hurt, both real and imagined. However well-meaning, this can add to problems in communicating. Wortman and Dunkel-Schetter[18] hypothesise that other people's reactions to a person's cancer are as a result of conflict between the essentially negative feelings about cancer and their beliefs about appropriate behaviours to display towards the person who has the disease, such as optimism and cheerfulness. They believe that this conflict results in responses that may be unintentionally damaging to the person with cancer such as physical avoidance, and avoidance of open discussion. While social support is potentially beneficial to well-being, those closest to someone with cancer may be unable to give it in the most helpful way. Anxiety and tension can result amongst family members who are constantly worried that they will say the wrong thing.

Buffering or shielding the person who has cancer from painful information and experiences is common. The most extreme form of this might be for the family to try to prevent the individual from knowing their diagnosis. This now happens infrequently, although families may still wish to protect the person from knowing the full extent of the severity of their illness and may not pass on any additional information that they have gleaned from health professionals. Hiding the full extent of the emotional distress the illness is causing and behaving in ways that they believe will be reassuring is also common and reflects the ways in which families deal with illness. Protecting the person with cancer from painful situations also allows the relative to avoid facing difficult emotions. However, this may create a barrier or distance between the person with cancer and those close to them.

A woman whose husband was concerned about how she would cope after his death comments:

> I try to hold it in . . . I suppose what I try to do a lot is make him feel that I can manage, 'cos that's what he worries about.[3]

A daughter who wants to protect her mother from distress about her son's illness comments:

> . . . when you are close to people you tend not to want to worry or upset them, there is this barrier, between close relationships.[3]

One relative may attempt to shield others in the family whom they feel are vulnerable, an elderly mother, for example. Nevertheless, even those perceived as most vulnerable, such as children or the elderly, are usually better prepared to cope if they are aware of what is happening. While parents of children with cancer may want to protect the sick child, other relationships between family members may become neglected. Siblings in particular may feel resentful about the increased closeness between their parents and the child with cancer.[9] The child's experience and ability to understand what is happening will obviously be dependent on their developmental stage.[19] Separation from a parent who is sick in early childhood will be followed by protest, despair and detachment, accompanied by possible bedwetting, constipation and sleeping difficulties. In later childhood the loss of a parent may commonly cause emotional and behavioural problems.[19]

Relatives may attempt to monitor the person's environment to ensure that they do not encounter something untoward to upset them; for example, avoiding media coverage of cancer that may include survival statistics. They also monitor the person themselves, checking for subtle changes in their well-being, such as in their eating or energy levels. The families of people undergoing radiotherapy have been found to monitor symptoms closely even though this was not requested by health professionals,[20] and this can be overprotective and frustrating for the person undergoing treatment. Others attempt to keep the sick person from 'dwelling' on their cancer, encouraging them to take up an activity and think about other things.

Thus, when cancer occurs within a family, adjustments in communication result – some conscious, some unconscious. Frequently these arise because open discussion of the disease and all its consequences is too difficult. The protection strategies employed by both the person with cancer and their relatives can sometimes exacerbate the problems consequent on opaque communication.

Living with cancer in the family

The social impact of the cancer and its effect on family relationships become part of day-to-day living with cancer. For example, the protection strategies just described are both a way of caring and a way of coping with the fear and uncertainty created by the illness.

There are many ways of defining care, and the amount of caring undertaken by families and friends will be variable. The extent to which families provide care for the person with cancer is dependent on their relationships, perceptions of the illness, and the extent of physical problems and level of dependency caused by the disease. Offering and giving care can be an important means of coping for some families. Some families may be so distant or dysfunctional that they will not take part in the course of the illness. This may be difficult for the person and the impact on absent relatives may be difficult to assess.

Many families will not actually perceive themselves as carers; rather they see themselves as dealing with changes in their daily routine brought about by the illness. Many people with cancer are quite well and are able to look after themselves. Nevertheless, some additional practical tasks are often required. For example, for some the biggest single problem may be fatigue, which can necessitate the family taking on extra practical duties. An individual will need supporting through major surgery or a series of toxic treatments with unpleasant side-effects. In the face of terminal illness, the family caring for their relative at home will have great demands placed upon them, and a large resource of emotional and practical support is likely be required:[21–24]

> . . . it's the watching, it tears you apart inside, because you can only do a certain amount for him, and sometimes I know I get on his nerves, I say 'Can I get you a drink?' . . . 'Can I get you this?' 'Shall I do that for you?' . . . 'What if you had this?' 'What if you have that?' And I know sometimes it does get on his nerves . . . but it's my way of trying to do something for him, and when I see him sitting there . . . really surviving as it were, and struggling, I just . . . I think 'Oh lord what are you doing . . . take him home now at the suffering.'[3]

'Standing by' and 'watching' as the disease progresses is an active process requiring intense emotional energy. The need to care and do something to help, even if this is not required, is intense. The physical demands of providing care while also struggling to make sense of the suffering observed are immensely demanding for families.[22,24]

The term 'caregiving burden' has been used to describe the caring activities of families of people with cancer.[22] McCorkle[23] conducted an interview study on the caregivers of people discharged from hospital who had complex care problems. Caregivers were interviewed three times over a 6-month period. Even though the person's condition stabilised or improved over the 6 months, caregivers continued to report high levels of burden. Caregivers of those whose mental state was poor and had greater responsibilities for physical care experienced greater impact on their daily life, finances, and health. Other studies have shown that caring for someone undergoing radiotherapy results in substantial time spent providing transport, undertaking extra household tasks, and giving emotional support.[20] For those caring for the terminally ill, the most frequently reported demand has been managing physical care and this is made more difficult by the family carer's lack of expertise in this role.[24]

The difficulties of caring increase with time, and in the case of cancer this may be prolonged over several years. The negative effects of caregiving have primarily been reported after the responsibility for care has continued for 2 years or more.[21]

A sister describes the long-term emotional drain of caring in the following terms:

> You do feel guilty and I suppose really if you are very honest with yourself after a while (and this is the hardest thing in the world to say) you resent illness. And this sounds awful but . . . when someone's ill for a long time like that you do somewhere deep inside you begin to think, you know, you're never going to get better or . . . It's hard to explain, I suppose it's almost an intolerance after a while which you then feel terribly guilty about.[3]

Caring is not always perceived as a burden by the relatives. In some instances caring is 'internally related' to self-identity.[25] The need to care is inherent within the person and is not something that is thought out or planned. Relatives may not comprehend any other option but to care.[26] The person concerned will not necessarily want to relinquish any of their caring role to outsiders and this may create problems for those who might believe that the family need help and would like to offer support.

A man who takes unpaid leave from work after his wife is diagnosed with cancer describes the following situation:

> And some people at work for instance have said, you know one person said 'You're being very unselfish about this.' And I said 'Well it's nothing to do with that and somebody else said 'You know it's very good of you to give up work rather than trying to bury yourself in the work.' And it was no more like that than flying to the moon. I thought about it over that night and there was no way I could vaguely think about going to work.[3]

One woman described her feelings about caring for her husband:

> What kind of a burden is it? If it is classed as a burden . . . I don't class him as a burden, not at all. I don't class it as a duty, not at all. I do it because I love him, I love him.[3]

Observers of such care may see this as 'heroic' but for the caregiver themselves, they are doing the only thing they can in the circumstances.[27] Caring may be an important means of coping with the emotional pain. For example, 'doing' things for the person to ensure their comfort can help to ameliorate feelings of grief about their illness. Concern to feed and nourish the person with cancer can be central to this. Large amounts of energy may be expended on searching out and cooking food, and attempting to present it in a way that is enticing. The activity of preparing and cooking food is a way of trying to do something constructive, bringing some normality to life and countering anxiety and deeper concerns, but this can also cause strain in the relationship. Cleaning and other household activities are also a means of maintaining order during times of stress for some people. Sustaining this level of caring over time, however, may become difficult. The relatives themselves may not perceive that they have needs of their own, which may be amenable to outside help.

Women continue to undertake the majority of care at home.[28] They have been described as 'invisible'[29] or 'forgotten'[28] and the considerable time spent caring or even just being available for the person with cancer may often compromise other aspects of their life. Sisters rather than brothers and daughters before sons become the closest support for the patient.[3] Place within the family, relationships and allegiances in childhood, personal circumstances and geographical distance are likely to play a part in who takes on the caring role. Teenagers may find it particularly difficult to provide support.[30] Their desire for independence may not fit easily with a possible requirement to take on more responsibility at home and they may find it hard openly to acknowledge their feelings about the situation.

Caring does not necessarily involve practical activity. Parents have been described as 'keeping vigil' over their hospitalised child. This is more than simply being in close proximity to the child at their bedside; it is 'more often an intense bearing witness with the child's plight'.[31] The parents of a child with cancer have been described as functioning as a 'protective filter' through which experiences may filter both ways.[32] The parent filters what goes through to the child and the child's experience of distress may be filtered back to the caring team through the father or mother. Although parents of sick children experience a particularly intense need to share their child's affliction, the need to be there and to be part of the experience applies to the families of adults as well.

For both the person with cancer and family and friends, cancer disrupts the way they see their life and future. In order to cope with the uncertainties brought by the disease, their view of the future may need to be reconstructed. In terms of organising the family's lives it is most often the desire of the person with cancer that is adhered to. Some (quite appropriately) begin to make plans for their death and the family's life after death; this is sometimes distressing for families. A husband's need to sort out his affairs while dying may be deeply upsetting to his wife, particularly if this means giving up precious possessions, or mementoes of their life together. Sometimes cancer precipitates a review of life, and a heightened awareness of mortality, or the decision to realise long-held ambitions. This is hard for a relative who has no such excuse and may not be included in the plans, who has to adjust their own to fit in with those of the person with cancer. It may no longer be possible for the family members to make plans of their own. This may create tension. For many, communicating the feelings of uncertainty that illness has brought, or the feelings surrounding the knowledge that there will come a time when they will be living alone, may be impossible.

Tension may also arise in the parents' relationship when a child has cancer because of the different roles and the separation that may occur during the illness. Women who tend to spend more time with the child appear better placed to cope with the illness than fathers, who are more likely to try to maintain life as it was.[9] Families are made up of diverse individuals with their own explanations and coping styles, and some families as a whole will create their own way of coping with the illness and its meaning.[33] Nevertheless, it is the individual diversity within the same family group that may create the most stress.

Making sense of the illness is difficult. The cancer itself may be explained by factors such as lifestyle, smoking or diet, but there is little attempt by the relatives to make sense of why this disruption happened to their own lives. The lack of opportunity to talk about and work through their own experience of the cancer may make it hard for the relatives to come to terms with it.

A diagnosis of cancer usually introduces into a family an onus to provide physical and emotional support. This may fall unevenly on the various members. For some it is accepted unquestioningly and the provision of physical care may be integral to a relative's coping mechanisms. Those close to the person with cancer may rarely spend time reflecting on their own needs and contemplation of their future may become very difficult.

Interactions with health professionals and the health care system

Research studies indicate that although the distress of the family and friends of someone with cancer is invariably high, it is inadequately addressed by health professionals, who frequently exclude them from care.[13,17,34] In Personal account 6.2 are two extracts from interviews conducted in the same week with a brother and sister who share a house. They were recorded 18 months after the brother was diagnosed with advanced colorectal cancer. The sister's life revolves around her brother's illness and she considered later in her interview when she would have to give up work to look after him full-time. Their attitudes towards the professional carers are strikingly different. The brother perceives the care he is receiving as good, but in effect this excludes his closest relative.

Personal account 6.2

When you're faced with an illness you can do nothing about and it has the potential to kill you, it's not like a broken leg which is going to get better, you are wholly in the hands of the doctors and their attitude is of paramount importance to your own feelings about what you're going through . . . And the attitude at the hospital was superb, it was all hopeful and you know, things to be done, and of course they were carrying on the treatment.

Brother

I still think the doctors and nurses are treated as if they're almost God, I still think that there is that feeling, although we're meant not to be impressed by these things . . . we are. You still tend not to think . . . of them as another human being who I can talk to . . . like you might talk to the ticket collector at the tube station . . . you do still tend to have this feeling that you should be looking up to them, you know they've descended from dizzy heights.[3]

Sister

The sister does not find the professionals either approachable or accessible. She has a need for information and later in the interview expressed the need for support for herself, although this is prevented by her situation. She is not married to the person with cancer, she is his sister, thus the professionals may not anticipate her needs to be great. She has at times a strained relationship with her brother who neither informs her of what is happening nor likes her to come with him to the hospital. Indeed, he does not want her to know very much. She, like many relatives, also has a full-time job and an elderly mother to care for. She thus remains on the margins of the medical care that her brother receives.

Most studies show that, whatever their own needs, relatives want good clinical care to be provided above all else, and where care is good most will declare themselves satisfied.[35] This overwhelming concern for the well-being of the person with cancer means that it is difficult for the family to consider or declare their own requirements for help as distinct from those of their sick relative.

Professional carers profoundly influence families' experience of cancer, for good or bad. For some

contact with health professionals is a key focus for the whole experience and there is great appreciation where care is perceived as good. However, distress may be high for those who have no contact with health professionals, and where staff are difficult to approach or information giving is poor.

Hull[35] interviewed family caregivers at home in the weeks before their relative died, to examine caregiving behaviours amongst people who were part of a hospice home care programme. Families identified four essential aspects of good care: 24-hour accessibility, effective communication, a non-judgemental attitude and clinical competence. These are likely to be equally important to families at earlier stages of the disease. Several studies report that the telephone is an important means of maintaining contact when the person has been discharged from hospital.[7] The following comments from the wife of a man undergoing chemotherapy show how reassuring a telephone link to health professionals can be:

It's that sort of relationship there . . . to know that you can actually phone them and you know who you are talking to . . . by face, is very important . . . particularly this problem, because you want to relate it to somebody that you know.[3]

A woman caring for her sick husband at home comments:

So I found myself reaching for the phone . . . getting ready to phone for the district nurse, but then thinking, 'Should I? Shouldn't I?' . . . I was worried, can I be doing any more for him? So if somebody had just like come or phoned, and said . . . 'how are things . . . It's three weeks since I last came. I know you said you don't need help, but how are things? Right?' and then I could say . . . 'Oh well by the way . . . he's got such and such thing at the moment, is that all in order' . . . Do you see what I mean?[3]

Lack of information or understanding of the care and treatment can be agonising. Parents of children with cancer have been described as experiencing 'heightened cue awareness', where the need for information creates a 'tendency to attribute meaning and significance to just about anything that is said or done by professionals'.[7] This 'over-interpretation' of the comments or behaviour of health care professionals is born out of a need for information and reassurance and is also likely to be experienced by all of those close to someone with cancer.

In the first 30 000 calls to the cancer information service of the British Association of Cancer United Patients (BACUP), more calls were received from relatives than from people with cancer themselves.[36] They required information in two key areas: medical information and support services. The need for honest, sensitively delivered information given at the appropriate time is crucial yet beset with potential difficulties, and the need to 'have questions answered honestly' has been ranked as the highest need amongst relatives.[36]

The family make themselves known to professional carers by their bedside vigil, attendance at hospital appointments, or requests for information. Relatives who, because of work or other demands, have difficulties in making themselves accessible to the health care system, remain invisible to health carers. The strategies people use for living with their cancer may inhibit communication between their families and health professionals. If someone is coping by knowing as little as possible, their relatives may also be denied information. Below, a woman describes how her husband prevented her from knowing that he was to be discharged following a thoracotomy, even though she would need to care for him and change his dressings.

> . . . the doctor told him he could come home, but he didn't tell me. I was going in three times a day, going in the morning, and then going in the afternoon and coming back and going in the evening . . . sometimes my daughter came in with me, but most times I was there, and he didn't say anything . . . and all of a sudden . . . The nurse came up to do something . . . and said, 'Oh anyway, you're going home tomorrow'. So I looked at him, you know . . . 'I knew three days ago' [he said], . . . he was frightened to say about it.[3]

It is not uncommon for someone to desire privacy about their disease and refuse to be accompanied on visits to the hospital. Just as relatives and friends attempt to protect the person with cancer from anxiety about the illness, the person themselves may desire to protect family from difficult news or from witnessing them being unwell; for example, while having chemotherapy. This is particularly pronounced for parents who wish to protect their children, even when they may be adults themselves. Alternatively, a relative's own anxiety about the situation may prevent them from attending hospitals and clinics. This can also hinder the recognition of their need for help. Some people do not want what they regard as interference from outsiders in their homes and this can also create barriers to the provision of adequate support.

Cancer is predominantly a disease of older adults and therefore close family and friends may also be elderly, with their own health problems, which prevent them from attending the hospital. For example, the daughter of a man with lung cancer described anticipating the day when her father would be taken into a hospice, which would mean that her mother who was housebound with cardiac failure would never able to see him again.[3] For a relative with a serious chronic illness or disability who is dependent on the person diagnosed with cancer, the consequences are likely to be serious since they risk losing the person who has supported and cared for them.

Lack of familiarity with the health care system can preclude the family from being able to speak to professional carers. A study in Britain revealed a lack of cultural sensitivity, which created deficiencies in access and provision of palliative care services to the black and minority ethnic communities.[37] For those who do not have English as a first language, information about services and diagnosis in the language of their choice was found to be unavailable.[37] The need for accessible support at diagnosis and information about symptoms was particularly emphasised.

Close family and friends may react to the illness in a way that professionals might not expect. Long-standing, unresolved differences with the person who has cancer may result in an apparent lack of concern, or in not attending the bedside of a dying relative, or refusals of help offered by professionals. Complicated relationships within the family may obscure the distress of some of those affected from the professionals; for example, ex-partners who share children. The difficulties of ensuring that adequate support is given to the whole family may be compounded by the geographical spread of modern families who live many miles apart.

Approaches to caring for families

Family distress is both substantial and complex.[38] The role of health professionals in helping this is much less well defined than in caring for the person with cancer. Early discharge and the increasing use of high-technology treatment at home is increasing the level of care.[23] Independent of any care they offer themselves, families require support. However, family members can be difficult to identify and many relatives are unable to express what their own needs or requirements from nurses might be. Caring for the person with cancer is sometimes a crucial part of living through the illness for families, therefore well-intentioned but insensitive outside support risks causing key coping mechanisms to collapse. The difficulty for nurses or even the person with cancer is to assess the needs of the family.[39,40]

A further issue is where the responsibility lies in providing family support, since family members are not usually physically ill. Hospital health professionals need to be more aware of the problems faced by relatives, and in cases of more severe distress be prepared to refer them to their family doctor or for specialist counselling.[38,41] Nurses who know the person with cancer and who come into contact with the family are well placed to be able to offer support, although it is not currently clear what the best form of such support might be.

Care strategy 6.1

- Do not pre-judge the situation.
- Identify key people who might constitute 'family'.
- Provide a contact telephone number.
- Listen to the relative's own story and acknowledge what is important for them.
- Be sensitive to the level of adjustment.
- Provide a supportive environment for the expression of distress.
- Be aware of the possible need to facilitate family communication.
- Be sensitive to individual requirements for information.
- Prepare for what might happen during the course of the illness.
- Attend important consultations with the family.
- Facilitate practical and financial support when required.
- Refer on to appropriate professionals where necessary.
- Assist attendance at support group if required.

Having the opportunity to talk about the experiences of having a member of the family with can-

cer and acknowledgement of these is helpful for families.[42] The most commonly cited concern for relatives has been reported as 'dealing with the symptoms'. While relatives may acknowledge the need for information, the need to express their fears and other emotions is often identified as a low priority.[43] A dilemma revealed in a number of studies of the needs of families has been:

> . . . . related to whether families wanted to share their feelings. If families needed to maintain control of their emotions and if the nurses encouraged them to ventilate their feelings, this was distressing and unsupportive. In contrast, if families wanted to discuss problems and share their feelings, the nurses' ability to explore these feelings was perceived as caring. The nurses needed to be sensitive enough to take the cue from what families were comfortable doing.[35]

Relatives need a calm unhurried approach by nurses, since it takes time to form a relationship of trust with individuals who may be anxious and frightened.

Children of people with cancer benefit from open and honest communication about illness. Parents will need support from early in the course of the disease about how to deal with their children's feelings, reactions and questions about the cancer.[10] Judd describes the role of the 'involved witness' in psychotherapeutic intervention with teenagers with cancer, a role that nurses can fulfil, even if intensive psychotherapy is not planned:[32]

> During the initial stage of the family's attempt to survive the shock of diagnosis, the therapist's usefulness is in being an involved witness: to feel, to hear, to register, and attempt to 'contain' the immediate as well as the far-reaching implications. This early position is important to subsequent work with the family or individual, without which it is difficult for the sufferer to feel, understood or be believed.

The need to have accurate and accessible information given sensitively at the appropriate time is clear. However, this may be a difficult task; Ball *et al.*[7] describe what was helpful to the parents of children with cancer:

> Skilled communicators are able to convey a sense of 'ifs and buts' and medical realism, while still holding out the possibility of a successful outcome to treatment.

It is important that professionals are knowledgeable about and sensitive to racial and cultural issues for the family.[37] If time and attention have been given to establishing a relationship with the family as well as with the person with cancer, some of these issues will become easier and nurses will be more attuned to the appropriate moment and style for communicating with an individual family.

Confidentiality for the patient creates dilemmas when working with families. Relatives may want to speak with nurses without the person with cancer present in order to glean more information, and to protect them from difficult news. Families need their own time to allow communication; however, in most circumstances they should not be given information that the person themselves does not know, and if they are this should be discussed with the person and family together. Some may want information withheld from the person. If this is an issue, the opportunity to explore feelings surrounding the desire not to communicate openly is important, as is the facilitation of more open discussion about the disease in families.

Both the person who has cancer and their family may need to know how future events might unfold, perhaps to make them less frightening. 'Therapeutic emplotment' has been described as a technique used by physicians whereby an attempt is made to provide continuity in discussions about illness; by agreeing together the likely course of the disease, this reduces uncertainty.[44] Families need the opportunity to prepare themselves as much as possible for what may ensue.

The need for information and emotional support has provided the impetus for the establishment of self-help and voluntary organisations over the last few years. While these organisations play a vital part in supporting families they do not excuse health professionals from providing information and explanation in the most appropriate way.[45]

One of the most frequently expressed unmet needs for families is a place to discuss their fears.[46] Long-term intensive psychotherapy is unlikely to be sustainable for families facing the trauma of cancer; instead, a supportive relationship, especially in the early days following diagnosis, is possibly the best solution:[32]

> . . . therein, the therapeutic ingredients are empathy, attempts at understanding the confusions around crisis

(some of which may echo earlier infantile traumas), understanding the ensuing losses, giving words to feelings and the facilitation of grief.

A study comparing death in a hospital with death in a hospice found that following death in the hospice where more open communication had been facilitated, surviving family members were less anxious and depressed, more involved socially, and less likely to be using tranquillisers.[47] An environment that allows the family open expression of grief, a resolution of unfinished business, and times for the person and family to talk about their life after the anticipated death is ideal.[47]

Support groups either exclusively for the family or that include the person with cancer are one way of enhancing the support available, and in some instances have been shown to improve communication within the family. A study of a support group offered to the male partners of women with breast cancer using 'sex role therapy' reported that the group members became significantly more communicative with their spouses about issues to do with mastectomy than members of a control group.[6] Wellisch *et al.* describe a group initially set up specifically for the families of people with cancer.[48] Among the aims were to enhance communication between people with cancer and their families, and to enable them to deal with intrapsychic conflicts concerning serious illness. This group was led by a clinical psychologist, but had a nurse as part of the team. After a few months the group was extended to include the person with cancer as well, and attendance by family members increased markedly. The authors found the group a safe arena for the expression of powerful emotions such as fear, rage, and sadness.

Support groups by no means suit everybody, and the availability of a support group does not necessarily mean that those invited will automatically attend and be supported. An evaluation of a support group for people with cancer and their families and friends at a London hospital showed that only a small number of those invited attended. For the people with cancer who attended, 80% felt happier and more relaxed, compared with only 46% of relatives who attended the group. A majority said that talking about cancer was easier after attending the group.[49]

Wortman *et al.*[18] discuss a family therapy programme which:

> . . . makes cancer patients and their family members aware of the complicated social environment in which they may be trapped, and which encourages more open communication . . . family members could be taught that their feelings of anger and guilt towards the patients are normal under the circumstances.

Relatively little attention has been paid to the impact of cancer on those close to a person with cancer, by either health professionals or researchers. It is apparent that a complex alteration in the emotions and patterns of communication between family members follows a diagnosis of cancer. These changes will accompany, and sometimes conflict with, the practical adjustments that might of necessity be made.

Health care professionals should view the needs of other family members as integral to those of the person with cancer. Acknowledgement that the illness will impact on relatives, and assuring that their individual need for support and information are recognised are key first steps. Nurses are often well placed to initiate and facilitate the process of meeting these needs.

One woman's feelings on the need for support was as follows:

> People need it, . . . I mean not to sort of go there for counselling, we had each other for that and I wouldn't have wanted anyone to invade our privacy, but just to sort of understand . . . what they're saying to you, for them to sort of talk to you in English . . . So people could . . . begin to understand, begin to think that there's more than this . . . and hope . . . things like that.[3]

References

1. Given B., Dwyer T., Vredevoogd J. and Given B. (1988). Family caregivers of cancer patients: reactions and assistance. In Pritchard P. (ed.) *Fifth International Conference on Cancer Nursing.* London: Macmillan Press, pp. 39–43.
2. Rolland J. (1989) Chronic illness and the family life cycle. In Carter B. and McGoldrick M. (eds.) *The Changing Family Life Cycle. A Framework For Family Therapy,* 2nd edition. Boston, MA: Allyn and Bacon.
3. Plant H. (2000). Living with cancer: understanding the experiences of close relatives of people with cancer. Unpublished Ph.D. thesis, University of London.
4. Rosenblatt P. (1988). Grief: the social context of private feelings. *Journal of Social Issues* **44**, 67–78.
5. Quindlen A. (1996). *One True Thing.* London: Arrow.
6. Sabo D., Brown J. and Smith C. (1986). The male role and mastectomy support groups and men's adjustment. *Journal of Psychosocial Oncology* **4**, 19–31.
7. Ball S., Bignold S. and Cribb A. (1996). Death and the disease: inside the culture of childhood cancer. In Howeth G. and Jupp P. (eds.) *Contemporary Issues in the Sociology of Death, Dying and Disposal.* London: Macmillan Press.
8. Gotay C. (1984). The experience of cancer during early and advanced stages: the views of patients and their mates. *Social Science and Medicine* **18**, 605–613.
9. Bignold S., Cribb A. and Ball S. (1996). *Families After Cancer: The Psychosocial Context of Surviving Childhood Cancer.* London: Cancer Relief Macmillan Fund and The Department of Health.
10. Kroll L., Barnes J., Jones A. and Stein A. (1998). Cancer in parents: telling children. *British Medical Journal* **316**, 880.
11. Cooper E.T. (1984). A pilot study on the effects of the diagnosis of lung cancer on family relationships. *Cancer Nursing* **August**, 301–308.
12. Oberst M. and Scott D. (1988). Post-discharge distress in surgically treated cancer patients and their spouses. *Research in Nursing and Health* **11**, 223–233.
13. Maguire P. (1981). The repercussions of mastectomy on the family. *International Journal of Family Psychiatry* **1**, 485–503.
14. Hart K. (1986). Stress encountered by significant others of cancer patients receiving chemotherapy. *Omega* **17**, 151–167.
15. Dennison A. (1996). *Uncertain Journey.* Newmill: Pattern Press.
16. Cassileth B., Lusk E., Strouse B., Miller D., Brown L. and Cross P. (1985). A psychological analysis of cancer patients and their next-of-kin. *Cancer* **55**, 72–76.
17. Oberst M. and James R. (1985). Going home: patient and spouse adjustment following cancer surgery. *Topics in Clinical Nursing* **April**, 46–57.
18. Wortman C. and Dunkel-Schetter C. (1979). Interpersonal relationships and cancer: a theoretical analysis. *Journal of Social Issues* **35**, 120–155.
19. Black D. (1998). Bereavement in childhood. *British Medical Journal* **316**, 931–933.
20. Oberst M., Thomas S., Gass K. and Ward S. (1989). Caregiving demands and appraisal of stress among family caregivers. *Cancer Nursing* **12**, 209–215.
21. Gaynor S. (1990). The long haul: the effects of homecare on caregivers. *Image: Journal of Nurse Scholarship* **22**, 208–212.
22. Carey P., Oberst M., McCubbin M. and Hughs S. (1991). Appraisal and caregiving burden in family members caring for patients receiving chemotherapy. *Oncology Nursing Forum* **18**, 1341–1348.

23. McCorkle R., Shegda Yost L., Jepson C., Malone D., Baird S. and Lusk E. (1993). A cancer experience: relationship of patient psychosocial responses to care-giver burden over time. *Psycho-oncology* **2**, 21–32.

24. Stetz K. (1987). Caregiving demands during advanced cancer. *Cancer Nursing* **10**, 260–268.

25. Cribb A. (1999). *Personal communication.*

26. Rose K.E., Webb C. and Waters K. (1997). Coping strategies employed by informal carers of terminally ill cancer patients. *Journal of Cancer Nursing* **1**, 126–133.

27. Benner P. and Wrubel J. (1989). *The Primacy of Caring. Stress and Coping in Health and Illness.* California, CA: Addison–Wesley.

28. Hicks C. (1988). *Who Cares: Looking After People at Home.* London: Virago.

29. James V. (1998). Unwaged carers and the provision of health care. In Field D. and Taylor S. (eds.) *Sociological Perspectives on Health, Illness and Health Care.* Oxford: Blackwell Science.

30. Larson P. and Dodd M. (1990). Caring – issues and patterns for the family experiencing cancer. *Sixth International Conference on Cancer Nursing,* Amsterdam, pp. 177–180.

31. Darbyshire P. (1994). Parenting in public: parental participation and involvement in the care of their hospitalised child. In Benner P. (ed.) *Interpretive Phenomenology.* London: Sage, pp. 185–210.

32. Judd D. (1994). Life-threatening illness as psychic trauma: psychotherapy with adolescent patients. In Erskine A. and Judd D. (eds.) *The Imaginative Body.* London: Whurr.

33. Thorne S. (1985). The family cancer experience. *Cancer Nursing* **8**, 285–291.

34. Northouse L. (1988). Social support in patients' and husbands' adjustment to breast cancer. *Nursing Research* **37**, 91–95.

35. Hull M. (1991). Hospice nurses. Caring support for caregiving families. *Cancer Nursing* **14**, 63–70.

36. Slevin M., Terry Y., Hallett N., Jefferies S., Launder, S., Plant R. *et al.* (1988). BACUP – the first two years: evaluation of a national cancer information service. *British Medical Journal* **297**, 669–672.

37. Iqbal H., Field D., Parker H. and Iqbal Z. (1995). The absent minority: access and use of palliative care services by black and minority ethnic groups in Leicester. In Richardson A. and Wilson-Barnett J. (eds.) *Nursing Research in Cancer Care.* London: Scutari Press.

38. Harrison J., Haddad P. and Maguire P. (1995). The impact of cancer on key relatives: a comparison of relative and patient concerns. *European Journal Of Cancer* **31A**, 1736–1740.

39. Hileman J. and Lackey N. (1990). Self-identified needs of patients with cancer at home and their home caregivers: a descriptive study. *Oncology Nursing Forum* **17**, 907–913.

40. Wingate A. and Lackey N. (1984). A description of the needs of noninstitutionalised cancer patients and their primary care givers. *Cancer Nursing* **12**, 216–225.

41. Fallowfield L. (1995). Helping the relatives of patients with cancer. *European Journal of Cancer* **31A**, 1731–1732.

42. Plant H. (1995). The experiences of families of newly diagnosed cancer patients – selected findings. In Richardson A. and Wilson-Barnett J. (eds.) *Nursing Research in Cancer Care.* London: Scutari Press, pp. 137–150.

43. Wright K. and Dyke S. (1984). Expressed concerns of adult cancer patient's family members. *Cancer Nursing* **October**, 371–374.

44. Del Vecchio Good M., Munakata T., Kobayashi Y., Mattingly C. and Good B. (1994). Oncology and narrative time. *Social Science and Medicine* **38**, 855–862.

45. Cull A.M. (1991). Studying stress in care givers: art or science? *British Journal of Cancer* **64**, 981–984.

46. Hinds C. (1985). The needs of families who care for patients with cancer at home: are we meeting them? *Journal of Advanced Nursing* **10**, 575–581.

47. Ransford H. and Smith M. (1991). Grief resolution among the bereaved in hospice and hospital wards. *Social Science and Medicine* **32**, 295–304.

48. Wellisch D., Mosher M. and Van Scoy C. (1978). Management of family emotion stress: family group therapy in a private oncology practice. *International Journal of Group Psychotherapy* **28**, 225–231.

49. Plant H., Richardson J., Stubbs L., Lynch D., Ellwood J. and Slevin M. (1987). Evaluation of a support group for cancer patients and their families and friends. *British Journal of Hospital Medicine* **38**, 317–322.

CHAPTER SEVEN

The impact of cancer on health care professionals

Anne Lanceley

The study of the impact of cancer and cancer care on health care professionals and the nature of nurses' strategies for working with people who have cancer shares a theoretical literature with other established investigations of therapeutic works, occupational development and stress. However, these texts, concerned with professionalisation, role, competencies, and strategies, share a history of limitations. For researchers and practitioners alike, nurses' therapeutic work needs to be understood in the context of the workplace and not only in terms of what the nurse practitioner does (forms of practice) but also why (professional and individual purpose).

Exploration of roles and functions, communications skills and competencies provides a useful starting point for understanding nurses' therapeutic work in cancer care. However, models of therapeutic practice need to be developed, not only to allow for the integration of different perspectives from other involved professional groups, but also offer an integrated social and psychological reconstruction of the nature of therapeutic nursing practice and that take account of conscious and unconscious processes.

This discussion is, in part, the product of research that began in 1991.[1] The verbatim accounts and care strategy commentaries are based largely on transcripts of tape recordings collected for this research, of cancer nurses talking with people they were caring for in acute and home care settings, and nurses' own reflections on these conversations.

The organisation of the chapter also owes a debt to this research, which acknowledges conscious and unconscious processes at work in nurses' encounters with cancer, and explores fundamental issues about cancer nursing, such as what the distinctive aspects of interpersonal work are, how nurses use their personality on behalf of people they are caring for, what the role imposes, what the irrational elements are, the ways nurses communicate with patients and colleagues, what the nurse and patient may represent to each other, and how nurses manage their anxiety in the face of relentless psychic pain and suffering.

The use and effectiveness of various nursing care strategies and approaches are considered alongside an evaluation of the impact the strategy may have on the nurse.

This chapter deals with the theoretical, professional, and organisational context of cancer nurse–patient relationships. Drawing on examples from the UK and the USA, it is concerned with the contentious issue of how far the concept of 'therapeutic nursing' is useful and appropriate to describe nurses' work with people who have cancer and their families. It explores the relationship between 'nursing as therapy', 'counselling', and more circumscribed ideas of cancer nurses' work, reflected in specific health promotional or support goals. Health care professionals' attitudes and defences to cancer are introduced as a way of understanding communication patterns in cancer care settings. Methodological issues in researching and evaluating the nature and impact of the nurse–patient relationship in cancer care are considered.

The theoretical context of nursing in cancer care

Within contemporary cancer nursing, the relationship between nurse and patient is perceived to be of central importance to emotion-focused interventions and the overall provision of quality care.[2,3]

This has not always been so and it is generally accepted that until recently the potential of nurse–patient relationships was limited. Medical diagnosis and treatment dominated cancer nursing's ideology and a person's physical body represented the primary focus of nursing work.[4]

Peplau was perhaps the first to emphasise the potential therapeutic value of the nurse–patient relationship, maintaining, in particular, that nursing is 'educative and therapeutic when nurse and patient come to know and respect each other, as persons who are alike and yet different; as persons who share the solutions of problems'.[5]

Her account conceives of the nurse as detached from the person being cared for and although she suggests that professional closeness shares some features with the physical closeness and interpersonal intimacy found in non-professional relationships, its focus is exclusively on the interests and needs of the patient. Effectively, she distinguishes 'professional closeness' as non-reciprocal, demonstrated by the nurse who can 'put herself aside and can bring all of her capacities and talents to bear upon the life of another person to the end that that person will grow a little, learn something new and, in effect, be strengthened in a favourable direction.'[6]

As Savage[7] notes, the closeness that Peplau refers to is 'not so much a matter of being closer to the person who is ill, but rather one of being "closer to the truth" of that person's possible life-threatening dilemma.' The cultivation of a special kind of detachment, demonstrating con-

cern, competence, and interest, while maintaining an emotional distance, is the hallmark of Peplau's model.

More recently, there is evidence of an alternative view and the themes of the patient knowing the nurse as a person and working in partnership have received considerable attention by nurses as part of effective cancer nursing practice.[8–11]

In 1991, McMahon and Pearson published their important book *Nursing as Therapy*. This did not offer a definitive explanation of what nursing as therapy is, since the role of the nurse depends on many societal and health care factors that are far from static. Instead, the authors set out their developing ideas, founded on the belief that a certain form of nursing, which involves deliberate nurse decision making, has a powerful effect on the patient and promotes adaptation, healing, and health.[12]

Areas in which nursing was considered to have therapeutic potential were:

- the nurse–patient relationship
- the interpersonal care environment
- providing comfort
- conventional and unconventional nursing interventions
- patient teaching.

The first two areas are the subject of this chapter.

MacMahon and Pearson believe that the ideal nurse–patient relationship involves mutuality or reciprocity. They consider the ideas of Muetzel,[13] who focused on three elements that coalesce in the encounter between nurse and patient: partnership, intimacy, and reciprocity. As key ingredients of a therapeutic nursing process, interaction between each pair of concepts generates three further concepts of atmosphere, spirit, and dynamics with concomitant defining characteristics.

What Muetzel is attempting to clarify through her therapeutic practice descriptors is the nature of the nurse's use of 'self' within the relationship. It is valid for the nurse and the patient to disclose their feelings and benefit from the relationship and she argues that the nurse who is 'self-aware' has a special contribution to make in the relationship, and that this self-awareness is a necessity for the achievement and evaluation of a subjectively therapeutic encounter. As Muetzel puts it:

> 'Being there' is that intangible and paradoxically difficult and very simple essence of the dimension of reciprocity and intimacy. It is simple because it is in the desire for closeness of the philanthropic vocation 'to help people'; difficult because a closeness that is mutually beneficial in a therapeutic relationship requires mature confrontation by the nurse . . . of the vulnerability of her own humanness [pp. 106–107].

People with cancer demand and help to evoke a particularly sensitive use of the self by nurses.[14]

The value of 'being with' the patient or providing 'existential presence' has been explored by other writers. Halldorsdottir[15] considers that there are five modes of being with another, each representing a qualitatively different degree of caring.

Box 7.1: Halldorsdottir's 'Five modes of being with another'

Life-giving	affirming the personhood of the other.
Life-sustaining	acknowledging the personhood of the other.
Life-neutral	where there is no effect on the life of the other.
Life-restraining	which is detached from the true centre of the other.
Life-destroying	which depersonalises the other.

Kitson[16] and Ersser[17] both explore the therapeutic dimension of nursing in their research, while Campbell[18] describes the companionship that nurses offer as a 'closeness' that is neither sexual nor deep personal friendship, but a bodily presence; it involves a 'being with' and not just a 'doing to'.

A therapeutic nurse relationship

The work of Carper[19] and Benner and Wrubel[20] helps in establishing a working definition of what a therapeutic nurse–patient relationship may be. Carper[19] describes fundamental patterns of nursing knowledge.

Box 7.2: Carper's patterns of nursing knowledge

- The scientific knowledge of human behaviour.
- The aesthetic perception of significant experiences.
- A personal understanding of the unique individuality of the self.
- The capacity to make choices within concrete situations involving particular moral judgements.

She stresses that none of the patterns is sufficient in itself and that if:

> . . . the design of nursing care is to be more than habitual or mechanical, the capacity to *perceive and interpret* the subjective experiences of others and to imaginatively project the effect of nursing actions on their lives, becomes a necessary skill.

The capacity of nurses to perceive and interpret the subjective experiences of others is the central tenet of the 'helping role' of the nurse as defined by Benner, who makes the fundamental point that 'the ability to interpret concerns enables the health care provider to help people deal with their illnesses'.[20] Since, in order to understand how someone feels, you must understand what they say, comprehending the meaning of the spoken word is a vital part of therapeutic nursing practice.

It is worth making a distinction between an identical expression of anxiety to a close friend during a 'heart-to-heart' and that which can take place between a nurse and the person being cared for. The difference lies in the imaginative, purposeful, and strategic use the nurse makes of the 'data' the person has offered. The nurse may use this to facilitate further disclosure or, if necessary, delay it. The heart-to-heart with the friend may be enormously helpful but is very different from a professional relationship, in which data 'about' the person and the experience of 'being with' them endorse each other and help the nurse to structure her interventions. The nurse practising therapeutically will create an emotional climate that will enable the person to explore their thoughts and feelings about their cancer illness progressively, to review problems and difficulties, and to have a sense of self-mastery.[21,22]

These theoretical ideas concerning the ideal therapeutic relationship are helpful in conceptualising the nature and range of relationships that may exist for nurses and the association between these and the experience or expertise of individual nurses. However, they do not consider the impact of the workplace organisation and ethos on nurses' professional relationships. Since they also overlook the collective nature of nursing work, any identified failure of the nurse to create a therapeutic relationship would rest firmly with the individual nurse.

Professional and policy context

UK health policy over the last 15 or 20 years can be seen as the bringing in of successive waves of rationality, with the government aim of calling various groups of health care professionals to account.[23] Rational approaches to manage health care were sought from within private sector organisations, a search that culminated in the introduction of general management and the 'internal market' into the Health Service,[24] ideas which underpin recent cancer and palliative care policy.[25]

Some claim that the impact of these changes on nurses' professional activity is minimal,[26] while others consider that moves such as the incorporation of professionals into management roles is an effective way of controlling their activity and thinking. The professional is a member of a team and beyond that an employing organisation and so subject to the rules, plans, and priorities of that organisation.

That accounting system initiatives, such as Resource Management, may have far-reaching effects upon both the practice and values of nurses has been noted by Bloomfield *et al.*[27] These systems develop standards of behaviour such that 'normal' practice can be not only defined, but also measured, and deviations and outcomes noted. What is also implied is that what is rendered visible, measured, and rewarded gains legitimacy. Conversely, that which is not recognised by the formal system may not be considered legitimate and consequently not rewarded. This is exactly the conclusion James[28] reached about the lack of value attributed to emotional care by nurses.

This raises several problems for the emotion-focused work of nurses where there can be no unequivocal answer about 'success' or about whether a particular intervention is 'good'. The nursing

Commentary 7.1: A possible reading of the nurse's comment above (after Traynor[30])

The nurse sets the scene, telling of the intrusion into nursing of a contrasting and alien set of values. While the way she lists the characteristics of this new value system – 'customer, computer, audit and budget' – are not intrinsically undesirable, we experience them as such, particularly when contrasted with the traditional and human terms 'empathy', 'bedside manner' and 'care'.

Perhaps by her use of the verb 'replace' and the words 'being replaced by' rather than 'are replaced', the nurse is enacting in words a passivity and powerlessness that she feels with her profession. As a consequence, we are encouraged to see nursing as the victim in this situation.

'Coming in' identifies the business orientation as a fad and reinforces the idea of an inappropriate intrusion, with nursing as the victim.

The third sentence can be understood in a number of ways. Its metaphor is one of the body. A possible reading is as a plea for a body (nursing), which is at the moment divided against itself to become integrated; for eye and hand to work together. Upper body organs are traditionally associated with rationality and so they are here with 'thoughtful eyes' needing to combine with the lower organs, hands. Atypically these lower organs are given a privileged position in the nurses' account as they are associated with the physical world of practical action, 'caring for our patients.' This is, at once, the end purpose of nursing and of her statement. The whole may be regarded as a desire for balance and integration; to reconnect and reground the rational, non-physical aspects of the organisation and profession that are becoming dominant and disconnected from physical, practical concerns.

strategy will be based on value and choice – without the freedom of that choice, no therapy based on self-mastery could ever hope to succeed. The very nature of the intervention makes it problematic to evaluate.

The roots of the managerialism described above are traced to the growth of bureaucracies by Davis,[29] who comments upon the way that formality and distance are not only valued within bureaucracies but seen as the only route to rational decision making.

Traynor[30] examines the impact of this managerial rationality on nurses' work. In his research study he explores the value systems of the new general managers and the nursing workforce of four first wave NHS community-based trusts through analysis of their talk. The managers' talk emphasises quantities, levels, numerical patterns; in short, it is disembodied knowledge, while embodied meaning and a language of closeness and human values haunt the nurses' talk. The conflict experienced by the nurses is distressingly evident, as illustrated by the comments of one staff nurse in a community hospital:

> I'm dissatisfied with 'simple is best' attitude in nursing being replaced by 'let's communicate', 'high tech' attitude coming in. Empathy, bedside manner, care. These words are being replaced by customer, computer, audit, budget. Why don't we start looking down at our hands with our thoughtful eyes and using common sense and intelligence; use those hands practically, to care for our patient?[30]

Traynor's view is that organisational strategies, which have emphasised continuity of care, camouflage extensions to the power of management control over the professional activity of nurses. However, the profession has responded positively to these developments. One response may reflect nursing's unique version of professional autonomy, characterised by moral agency and self-sacrifice.

The commitment to continuity of care is clearly expressed in what has been referred to as 'the new nursing',[31] typified by primary nursing, which explicitly aims to transform relationships with patients and promote their participation in care. As such, primary nursing is one example of an organisational mode in which communication is viewed as a central and legitimate aspect of nurses' work.[32] Underlying the 'new nursing' is a belief that the relationship between nurse and patient has the potential to be therapeutic and central to the process of recovery.

Professional debate about specialist and advanced practice roles is also driving theoretical discussion and practice initiatives concerning the therapeutic nature of cancer nursing. Questions that are emerging include whether it is possible for all nurses in cancer care to develop therapeutic relationships with the people in their care, what sort of environment or 'culture' is most conducive and supportive of this way of working, and what part might be played by an advanced nurse practitioner.

The role of advanced practitioner in cancer care encompasses more than expert nursing practice. Although there is no consensus view of such posts, they are generally considered to be multidimensional, integrating the sub-roles of educator, researcher, and consultant to promote and develop clinical nursing from clinical to strategic and policy levels, while simultaneously creating and sustaining a culture in which nurses and nursing strive for more effective patient and health care services.[33,34]

Manley[33] identified the skills and processes by which the advanced practitioner/consultant nurse fulfils each sub-role (see Figure 7.1). The processes bear a remarkable resemblance to qualities attributed to counselling relationships.[22]

Corner[2] takes up the debate and recasts the dimensions of the advanced practitioner role into 'cancer nursing as therapy'. This, Corner suggests, has the potential to operate on four levels to effect radical reconstruction of care, cancer services, and wider health care environments, so that they are more patient focused and offer 'nursing as therapy' as an integral part of cancer care. These levels include:

- fundamental knowledge and theory generation for therapeutic practice
- therapeutic interventions for individuals or problems
- developing and changing health systems or environments
- critique and reconstruction of care from a societal perspective.

Crucial to the accounts of Manley and Corner is the idea of radical change and facilitation of a 'transformational culture', which enables the therapeutic work of nurses.

This broad idea of 'cancer nursing as therapy' is offered as a contemporary vision of the necessary professional and organisational context for the concerns of this chapter, which are the emotion-focused interventions of cancer nurses working in one-to-one relationships with patients. It is for a variety of reasons that the nurse–patient relationship has come to be redefined. However, the extent and nature of the change required to realise the vision are likely to be immense.

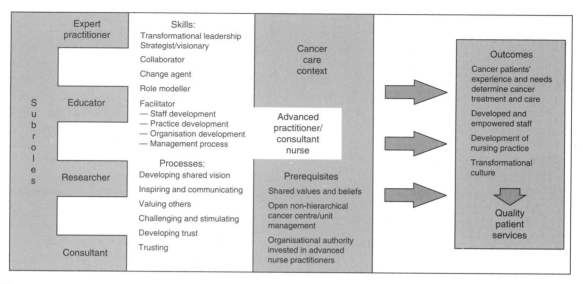

Figure 7.1 The sub-roles of advanced practitioners of cancer care and the skills and processes involved (adapted with permission from Manley K. (1997). *Journal of Advanced Nursing* **6**, 179–190, Blackwell Science).[33]

Organisational context

Glaser and Strauss[35] were the first to expose the profound emotional basis for the social organisation and context of care in relation to people with cancer and the dying. In their important study they not only identified the troubling reality of awareness categories in relation to a dying person but also described ways in which knowledge about diagnosis and prognosis was used to disallow or control feelings.

James[36] develops this theme of emotion management in her examination of the disclosure of a cancer diagnosis. She describes the management of emotions at this time by lay and professional carers, noting that many manage by denying rather than engaging with emotions. Differences in emotion management she attributes to different levels of involvement with the feelings associated with the cancer and competing forms of status and knowledge. These then influence the organisational and interpersonal mechanisms used to manage the feelings, such as the use of particular kinds of space and time, more or less public encounters, denial of the emotion, limiting the information released, formal and informal disciplinary rules, gender-divided labour and, most significantly, senior staff setting the context, routines, and rituals within which other staff and clients can express their anxieties and feelings.

In her study of nursing practices in a London teaching hospital, Isabel Menzies noticed that, far from responding in contextually sensitive ways to particular patients, nurses were task centred and, for example, awoke people in their care to give them drugs, regardless of need. Also, finding that nurses rotated frequently between wards, Menzies argued that these organisational procedures and practices became an end in themselves. They were rituals that were not designed to help people who were hospitalised, but rather enabled the nurses to contain the anxiety of working with the sick and dying.[37] The nurses did not have to think about what they were doing and, by not thinking, they could avoid feeling anxious. Menzies called such rituals social defences.

Menzies felt that 'although by the very nature of her profession the nurse is at considerable risk of being flooded by intense and unmanageable anxiety', the nature of nursing did not, by itself, account for the high levels of anxiety apparent in nurses. The very techniques used by nurses to contain and modify the anxiety appeared to constitute part of the problem. Not recognising the individual needs of people helped detachment, and led to minimising the mutual interaction of nurses with people in their care, since this might lead to 'attachment'. This trend was reinforced by an implicit operational policy of 'detachment', where the assumption was that a nurse would not mind moving form ward to ward, or hospital to hospital, without notice. The pain and distress of the moving, of breaking stable and continuing relationships, are implicitly denied by the system, although often stressed personally by people (including senior nurses who initiate such moves) within the system. In addition, nurses were encouraged to deny any disturbing feelings that arose within relationships. Those nurses facing difficulties were reprimanded rather than supported.

It is arguable that these social defence systems do not exist in cancer care today. If task allocation protected the nurse from anxiety, new organisational modes stressing continuity of care have stripped this defence away and pose new, personal challenges for nurses. There is compelling evidence to suggest that cancer nurses and their professional colleagues have generated various new 'systems' to organise their own work, the care environment, and cancer services in ways that may reflect a spectrum of techniques to defend against, contain, or modify what Menzies calls 'the unmanageable anxiety' of cancer care.

A study of hopelessness and how it is represented on a leukaemia ward is an example. The study revealed that 'hope work' was conducted within an objectifying medical frame as opposed to the person's own frame of reference. Not only was the legitimacy and credibility of the medical version of reality maintained but emotionally charged conversations were largely avoided.[38]

Another interesting example is research that was carried out on two wards where a high proportion of people with gastrointestinal cancers was nursed.[39] One ward used a primary nursing approach and the other patient allocation. The aim of the study was to explore ways in which nurses managed interactions and, in particular, their 'closeness' or intimacy while caring for people.

Data revealed that nurses managed deep, close, and consistent relationships with them, not only by expressive behaviours including the use of touch, body posture, and humour, but by transforming the

ward into a symbolic space in which the relationship became analogous with family relationships. Savage deduces that reconstructing the context of care in domestic rather than institutional terms enabled the nurses to deal better with the many anxieties and ambiguities of emotional closeness inherent in the 'new nursing'. The 'family' or the 'home' were not the only observed models for providing a context of care. It seemed that 'camaraderie' in the nurse team offered an alternative.

Another relevant finding from Savage's study is that the realisation of contexts for care deemed to have a therapeutic potential is less dependent upon the organisational mode of nursing on the ward than on the inter-relationship of this with specific local conditions of the hospital infrastructure including resource allocation, the approach of general management and the attitudes of other members of the health care team. The work of Smith[40] supports this.

The point is that feelings and how they are managed contribute to and reflect the structure and culture of the cancer care setting.[41,42] It is useful to consider communication patterns in this light.

Communication patterns in cancer care settings

Communication in cancer care settings is characterised by the avoidance of difficult or painful topics and misunderstandings that arise between the person who has cancer, their family, and the involved health care professionals.[43–48]

Sociologists attribute the cause of avoidance and misunderstandings to the nature of health care professional–patient relationships, which are largely dependent upon the power inherent in professional expertise and specialised knowledge.[4,49]

A considerable amount of the research on doctor–patient and nurse–patient communication in cancer care has been conducted specifically to analyse and to criticise the means, methods, asymmetry, and humaneness of the relationships.[50,51] The language doctors use in encounters with people with cancer has been shown repeatedly to reflect the non-egalitarian nature of the relationship.[52]

There is recognition from within the professions of the huge complexity of communicating with people who have cancer and their families.[1,53–56] Souhami highlights the particular difficulties for doctors who often have to deal with probability rather than certainty of treatment outcome, and repeatedly may be the bearers of bad news. The doctor also has to contend with the high expectations of team members, that these encounters will be good and that he or she will 'get it right'.

It is suggested in this book that cancer illness in Western biomedical culture is itself dependent upon this relationship, the encounter with the expert medical oncologist, radiotherapist, or cancer geneticist, for its definition. This emphasises the point that, whatever else it is, cancer illness exists as a social phenomenon, constructed through the interaction of the person with his or her relatives, the doctor, the nurse, and society at large.

Some studies of doctor–patient interaction have focused in recent years on problems of communication often caused by conflicting notions concerning the nature of this relationship.[57]

Mishler[58] considers the root cause of these difficulties to lie in the asymmetrical nature of medical consultations and presents the analogy of a struggle between *voices:* on the one hand the 'voice of medicine' and on the other the 'voice of the life-world' representing, respectively, the 'technical–scientific assumptions of medicine and the natural attitudes of everyday life'.

According to this model, the doctor is seen as pursuing a line of talk determined almost exclusively by biomedicine, which is often at odds with the person's own view, representing what Mishler terms 'life-world contexts'. Since the talk is dominated by the voice of medicine, argues Mishler, any contribution from the voice of the life-world is regarded by the doctor as an interruption. Conversely, any interruption by the voice of medicine when the person is speaking is not an interruption at all, but a return to reality, that is to the dominant medical techno-rational reality. The medical voice is clearly indicated within consultations by the typical patterns of:

Doctor: question
Patient: response
Doctor: assessment/next question.

The tendency of doctors to use closed rather than open-ended questions serves further to maintain the doctor's control of talk. This in turn strengthens the biomedical model as the framework of the

talk and permits the doctor to carry out the medical tasks of diagnosis and prescription, while avoiding discussion of the person's feelings and individual response to their cancer illness.[56]

This bias towards the 'voice of medicine' prevails in cancer care today, which is surprising considering the emphasis since the 1970s on the emotional needs of people with cancer, influenced in particular by the pioneering work of Kubler-Ross,[59] and also the beliefs about the ultimate benefits of:

- adopting a client-centred approach of open-ended questions
- explaining medical agendas
- the use of the person's own words in asking further questions
- listening with minimum interruption

to engender collaborative models of care based on desired right choice and self-determination for people with cancer.[60]

It may be that the coercive strength of medically orientated styles of talk is so entrenched in social attitudes that the style has become naturalised. Indeed, when ill, many people would feel uncomfortable without the asymmetry of the relationship with their doctor.

Silverman suggests that despite their pleas for humanism and equality, proponents of the client-centred approach are unwittingly reinforcing the central strategy of power in the doctor–patient relationship.[49] Attempts to conduct the relationship along the lines of an equal partnership would only be a simulation and would leave intact the essential nature of the power imbalance, which is based upon professional expertise and specialised knowledge. This situation is further complicated by the fact that recent technological advances mean that often oncologists and radiotherapists are working at the fringes of their own knowledge and the consultation is therefore forever threatened with becoming the domain of 'another expert', in which any progress towards interactional symmetry would have to begin again.

Other sociologists, in assessing the power relation within the medical interview, have been heavily influenced by the work of Foucault[61] and perceive the client-centred approach that has come to dominate first progressive and now mainstream thinking in cancer care, as little more than a placebo designed to obscure the real 'treatment' of an all-encompassing form of surveillance in which the medical gaze can roam freely.[62,63] They regard the arguments of the supporters of this approach as tenuous, relying as they do on the belief that liberation from the tyranny of conflicting and unequal power relationships can somehow be achieved by an incitement of the person to talk and by encouraging the doctor to listen.

These writings and research evidence present health care professionals with an impasse that must be negotiated if any meaning or credibility is to be salvaged. Silverman suggests that there is a way out and that it lies in individual practitioners rejecting pre-established roles and evading stereotyped talk with people, but instead constructing their own dialogues with them.[49]

Nevertheless, stereotyped interprofessional relationships account for some of the patterns of communication in cancer care. Nurses perceive that they often do not have sufficient clinical information to respond to the questions that are posed by people who are anxious about their illness, and that, even if they had, their own and others' expectations of their role may preclude further discussion.

According to some researchers, the positive effects of a good communication climate, in which there is open communication within the team, stimulates the 'therapeutic' interventions of individual practitioners and an attitude of openness to feelings.[64–66] This research has revealed that nurses take fewer risks in emotionally hazardous one-to-one conversations with people they are caring for than as members of groups. Certain characteristics of the group facilitate risk-taking and these include:

- extent to which risk taking is a norm of the group
- extent to which exchange of feelings is possible
- extent to which members of the group support each other
- extent to which responsibility can be shared.

Nievaard[67] examines power and attitudes of nurses, doctors and patients and cautions against solutions aimed towards improving emotional well-being, which are confined to the organisation of the nursing team or interventions solely reliant upon nurses. He concludes that improvement will depend on improving local working relationships between nurses, doctors, and management.

There is growing evidence not only that the expression of feelings may affect someone's ability to adjust to their diagnosis of cancer and cope with treatment, but that such disclosure may also influence recurrence and progression of disease.[68] Cancer nurses acknowledge this and also recognise the power of communication to arouse or assuage the fear that often accompanies cancer.[45,69] Yet numerous studies reveal that patterns of nurses' communication are dominated by routinised, stereotyped and overtly controlling forms of communication, which serve to maintain the conversation at a superficial level.

Avoidance of potentially difficult and emotional discussions of poor prognosis and death was identified by Glaser and Strauss in the seminal work, *Awareness of Dying*, as being surrounded by a 'conspiracy of silence'. They identified various forms of this, each dominated by secrets and silence: 'closed awareness' existed when health care professionals chose not to tell someone of their poor prognosis and impending death; 'suspected awareness', in which the patient has a hint of the truth; and 'mutual pretence', in which both parties, the health professionals and the patient, knew but chose to remain silent.[70]

Although there have been dramatic changes in the behaviour of health professionals with regard to telling someone their cancer diagnosis and prognosis, so that by the late 1970s most doctors said that they informed patients,[71,72] the reality is that uncertainty often exists about what has been said to whom and when. This affects team communication and requires constant vigilance by all members of the team.

Parkes recognised that questions may be asked of nurses that would not be asked of a doctor because a nurse can be more easily disbelieved if the information about the illness is given when someone is not ready to know. He acknowledged that the systematic investigation of such 'defended talk' is very difficult.[73]

The idea of 'defended' talk introduces an additional explanation for the patterns of communication existing in cancer care settings. This concerns the attitudes and levels of anxiety and the stress experienced by health care professionals working with cancer patients and includes the patient as one who can avoid and deny distressing thoughts and feelings as effectively as a nurse or doctor, thus 'blocking' professional help.

Health care professionals' attitudes and defences to cancer

Repeated reports to the Health Ombudsman[74] of insensitive, inattentive treatment, particularly of people who are dying and their families, have led to investigations into the importance of health care professionals' attitudes in the care of cancer patients,[75-79] and also to investigations of the levels of stress experienced by staff.

Attitudes

There is reliable evidence that nurses hold stereotyped, negative attitudes to cancer, which significantly affect their behaviour and communication with people who have cancer.[80, 81] Some more experienced trained nurses hold a more optimistic view of cancer, but they are in the minority. Elkind[82] found that most nurses considered it at least sometimes true that cancer treatment can do more harm than good and that they were pessimistic regarding the number of deaths caused by cancer, sharing the same fears as the general population.

The association of cancer with death and suffering held by many individuals is carefully analysed by Stacey,[83] who explores the cultural meanings of cancer. From her analysis, cancer emerges as a symbol of death and suffering, and the societal battle against cancer is then seen as the struggle to resist acceptance of the inevitability in life of death, decay, and decomposition. These overall trends play a significant role in the development of attitudes amongst individuals.

One well-documented danger in negative attitude, stereotype-governed health care professional behaviours is that people who have cancer may 'become' the stereotype.[84,85] For example, nursing staff guided by a strong prior belief that a diagnosis of cancer is hopeless and that all who have it suffer and die from their disease may, through their conversational approach, instill that belief in the person themself.

A study by Mood and Lick[86] designed to examine nurses' attitudes to the terminally ill provides some evidence for this. In their study, increased use of negative words (e.g. no, not, never, nothing, none), and substitution of the impersonal pronoun 'it' for death, were found in discussions of death as opposed to other topics. They concluded that such subtle encoding of the nurses' own fear, anxiety, and negative attitudes to death significantly altered the quality of the message communicated to dying people and their families, and would confirm feelings of helplessness and hopelessness.

Stress

Since the early work of Vachon,[87] there has been a recognition that health professionals who work closely with people who have cancer can experience stress from their work arising from the deterioration and death of patients, and from dealing with the emotional distress.[88]

A proliferation of reviews and research studies over the last 10 years, focusing on stress and burnout in those caring for the dying and people with life-threatening illness, has used quasi-experimental designs to attempt to delineate the specific variables of stress within predetermined categories using a variety of measurement scales (see Tables 7.1 and 7.2). Sources of stress consistently identified are:

- feeling overloaded with work and the effect of this on home life
- poor management support and resource/staffing limitations
- dealing with patients' suffering
- death and dying
- relationships with other health professionals
- lack of experience.

Findings also suggest that working with cancer may force health professionals to face their own mortality and that of their family and friends.[89,90] For those working in oncology settings, the conflict between the curative goals of medicine and the reality that many people will not respond to treatment in the long term, can lead to tensions between cancer care team members, as well as death being seen as a personal failure.[91]

Table 7.1 Selected studies of stress in cancer health professionals[90,92–96]

Study	Setting	Sample	Method	Findings
Ullrich A. and FitzGerald P. (1990)	13 cancer units	$n = 91$ nurses $n = 57$ physicians	Structured interviews. Questionnaire developed from this in four areas: conflict situations, background, institutional variables, health.	Strong associations between situational stressors and psychosomatic complaints. Nurses, interpersonal difficulties = physical distress. Doctors, job dissatisfaction = malaise.
Whippen D. and Canellos G. (1991)		$n = 1000$ oncologists randomly sampled	Questionnaire 60% response.	56% had experienced burnout. Significance between type of practice and burnout.
Cull A. (1991)	Academic oncology unit	$n = 11$ nurses $n = 6$ doctors $n = 4$ paramedics	Delphi technique. Poor response in third questionnaire = 6.	Need to discuss issues. Open problem solving group set up to maintain mutual support and communication.
Kent G. et al. (1994)	Oncology centre	$n = 125$ medical, university, nursing and support staff, randomly selected	Critical incident sheets. Maslach Burnout Inventory. Hospital Anxiety and Depression Scale. Intention to leave post. Response $n = 48$ (38%).	Perceptions of inability to help patients scored higher on MBI. 22% at risk of clinical anxiety. 33% recently considered leaving their job.
Ramirez A. et al. (1995)	National survey oncology centres	Medical and clinical oncologists and palliative care physicians	Questionnaire.	Prevalence of psychiatric morbidity of cancer clinicians similar at 32% among medical oncologists, 29% clinical oncologists and 25% palliative physicians, to that of consultants and junior house officers working in other acute hospital specialities.
Miller D. and Gillies P. (1996)	Seven HIV/AIDS and two oncology centres	$n = 203$ staff (all staff in unit for more than 6 months)	Structured interview. Maslach Burnout Inventory. General Health Questionnaire.	Low response rate for oncology. Few overall differences between staff in HIV/AIDS and oncology. 39% of sample's partners complained about commitment to work. 25% reported relationships had suffered as a result of their work.

Table 7.2 Selected studies of stress in cancer nurses[91,101–108]

Study	Sample	Method	Findings
Yasko J. (1983)	$n = 185$ oncology nursing specialists	Jones Staff Burnout Scale for Health Professionals (SBS-HP). Self-report questionnaire.	Burnout scores lower than other nurse samples. Burnout related to inadequate support, high levels of stress, feelings of apathy and withdrawal, dissatisfaction with role.
Stewart B. et al. (1982)	$n = 5$ out-patient oncology nurses $n = 40$ nurses from cancer, ITU, cardiac, theatres	In-depth interview questionnaire.	Oncology nurses experienced more enduring stress.
Ogle M.E. (1983)	$n = 22$ oncology nurses	Maslach Burnout Inventory.	Experienced moderate intensity of burnout. Subjects able to determine stage of burnout experienced.
Jenkins J. and Ostchega Y. (1986)	$n = 152$ Oncology Nursing Society randomised sample	SBS-HP. Yasko Survey Tool.	Oncology nurses are not at greater risk of burnout. Experienced moderate burnout. Variables correlating with higher scores: organisational problems, job stress, availability of support, level of job satisfaction.
Bram P. and Katz L. (1989)	$n = 29$ hospice nurses $n = 28$ hospital nurses	SBS-HP, Corwin's Nursing Role. Conception Scale, a work-related questionnaire.	Oncology nurses significantly more stressed. Different work-related variables correlated with burnout for each group, with exception of support.
Razavi D. et al. (1993)	$n = 72$ nurses (several institutions)	Nurses randomly assigned to 24-hr PTP or waiting group. Assessed 1 week before psychological training programme, 1 week and 2 months after. Assessment: semi-structured interview, Semantic Differential Questionnaire, Nursing Stress Scale, role play.	Significant change to self-concept and occupational stress related to inadequate preparation after PTP.
Hinds P. et al. (1994)	$n = 25$ paediatric oncology nurses $n = 9$ new nurses $n = 14$ experienced nurses	New nurses interviewed at 3, 6, '2 months, experienced interviewed once. Guided interviews.	Difference in stress between the two groups. New nurses fewer coping reactions. Most common reaction was resignation.
Papadatou D. et al. (1994)	$n = 217$ oncology nurses $n = 266$ general nurses	MBI, Hardiness Scale, Ways of Coping Scale, Life-style Scale, Type A Behaviour Scale, Job Stress Questionnaire, General Information Questionnaire.	No statistical difference in degree of burnout between groups. Personality greatest prediction of burnout. Sense of personal control in life and the work context found to protect against burnout.
Wilkinson S. (1994)	$n = 65$ cancer nurses, from six wards in two cancer hospitals	Self-administered questionnaire, Speielberger State-Trait Anxiety Inventory completed six times in 8 months.	General anxiety no different for working females generally. Newly qualified nurses more anxious. Most nurses reported job satisfaction. Statistical difference in nurses' anxiety between wards.

In palliative care, working with people who have incurable disease and who are dying is thought to barrage health professionals daily with suffering and tragedy.[97]

As a result of the particular demands made of them, cancer health professionals are perceived to experience high levels of job stress and to be at risk of developing work-related distress or compassion fatigue.[98] This may have repercussions for inter-professional work relations and organisational efficiency within the cancer care setting.[99,100]

However, according to this body of research, levels of distress do not appear to be uniquely high for those working with cancer compared to other health care professionals. It is nevertheless cause for concern that over one-quarter of senior cancer doctors report psychiatric morbidity at any one time and that levels among cancer nurses appear similar. The implications of this for care, in addition to the personal suffering of health professionals, give impetus to the need for action to reduce burnout and stress among those professional groups, and to support clinicians and equip them with the communication and management skills in which they feel insufficiently trained.[109]

A further cause for concern lies in the research findings themselves: the counter-intuitive finding that dealing with fatal illness and death does not emerge as a major source of job stress among cancer professionals.

Though it is often not explicit, in most cases a psychological approach to stress underpins research studies. Lazarus[110] is the main exponent of this. He maintains that stress occurs when there are demands on the individual that he or she cannot cope with or adjust to. Stress arises when the individual perceives and evaluates this situation as threatening. The model incorporates the concept of appraisal and reappraisal, together with the transactional view that stress can only be defined by the relationship between the individual and his or her environment. The premise of this model is that there is a 'right' way to cope and manage thoughts and feelings and a range of 'appropriate' responses to stress.

What this model largely omits, argue Benner and Wrubel,[20] is the view that stressful experiences and coping options are constituted by a person's unique involvement in a situation and their skills, concerns, meanings, particular history, and anticipation and projection of themselves into the future.

One explanation for the research findings could therefore lie in the mechanistic approach to the experience of stress in which an individual's stress is measured at a single point in time without thought for the changing nature of stress or the societal or organisational context of the stress. Both explanations leave unexplained the low levels of communication identified in some research studies between cancer care professionals and patients and the apparent endemic verbal 'blocking' behaviours.

Irrational processes highlight further possible limitations of classic stress theory. Theorists such as Lazarus or the more sociologically orientated Pearlin[111] have argued that all individuals face continuing stressors and that coping strategies and cognitive reappraisals are mechanisms for reducing stress. But because these theorists do not link the experience of stress to people's feelings of anxiety, they may have posed the issue of stress too narrowly and focused their solutions too narrowly on rational means.

When anxiety intrudes, rational thinking is distorted by irrational processes. For example, nurses in many oncology units 'fight' chronically with doctors over treatment policy, each blaming the other for the gap between expectation and treatment outcome. Because they feel anxious, they project their sense of blame and failure outwards, often scapegoating the person they need to work closely with, to reduce the stress they face.

Psychodynamic concepts, which highlight how people use one another to stabilise their inner lives and feelings and then how these psychodynamic processes within people help to shape the relationships between them, may be particularly helpful in understanding the stress health care professionals experience when working with cancer patients.[112]

Defences

Sometimes aspects of ourselves and our experience conflict with our consciously held ideals. These aspects of ourselves and our experiences cannot be easily assimilated into our conscious view of ourselves because of the anxiety or psychic pain they arouse. We may find it easier to function by suppressing and denying difficult or painful experiences and memories.[113,114]

When our work brings us into contact with cancer, it can be a very powerful experience because those in our care may be attempting to relieve their internal pains and distress by externalising them, and requiring us to contain and carry aspects of these. The difficulty for us is that we too have our own internal processes to contend with, such as our own unresolved conflicts and impulses, particularly those to do with death and destructiveness.

For brief periods we may be able to tolerate considerable anxiety and bear considerable mental pain and depression, for instance following a bereavement. Alternatively, we may try to ward off such emotional discomfort by employing a number of defence mechanisms (see Table 7.3). The defences

work through the processes of *splitting, projection,* and *introjection.*[115,116]

Menzies' interpretation of how nurses protect themselves against the anxiety caused by primitive feelings and impulses elicited by physical and psychological closeness to people in their care illustrates these processes.[117]

Menzies observed that nurses feel the anxiety and stress of helping sick people who might die and that they often engaged in physical care that by 'ordinary standards is distasteful, disgusting and frightening'. The nurses are unable to balance and integrate powerful and opposing feelings of compassion for the ill person and revulsion at their physical state. Unconsciously, the nurses welcome depersonalised care practices as a way of relieving themselves of contradictory feelings and keeping the good feelings separate from the bad ones. By *split-*

Table 7.3 Defences against anxiety commonly encountered in everyday clinical work

Denial	A defence mechanism by which either an aspect of the self is denied or some painful experience is denied.
Suppression	A conscious attempt to forget or deny and to avoid thinking about something.
Repression	An idea may be unconsciously repressed owing to its unthinkable nature. It may be an idea or feeling that conflicts with our view of ourselves and what is acceptable. It is prevented from coming to consciousness.
Splitting	Involves separation of good and bad aspects of the self and others, or between good and bad feelings.
Projecting	Externalising unacceptable feelings and then attributing them to others or an object.
Projective identification	Projecting not only feelings but important aspects of the self onto others so that that person feels and owns qualities and impulses that are otherwise not their own.
Reaction formation	Going to an opposite extreme to obscure unacceptable feelings, e.g. excessive calm to hide panic.
Rationalisation	Justifying an unconscious impulse or giving a good reason for something but it is not applicable to the situation.
Psychosomatic reactions	Unacceptable feelings may be converted into physical symptoms.
Phobic avoidance	Avoiding situations that arouse unpleasant feelings.
Displacement	Being too afraid to express feelings to the person who provoked them and deflecting them elsewhere.
Regression	If we feel unable to cope we may regress to more childlike and dependent ways of behaving.
Sublimation	Unconscious drives are allowed partial expression in modified, socially acceptable, even desirable ways.

ting off their sense of personal authority and agency from their own experience and *projecting* it outside – onto the ritual of drug administration, for example – they relieved themselves of the anxiety of the patient's experience. The nurses also psychologically took in, or *introjected,* the new authority of the rituals to justify their depersonalised relationship to the people in their care. Thus, through the linked processes of splitting, projection, and introjection, the nurses lent their individual and collective authority to ritual care, which in turn authorised them to behave in a depersonalised way.

The milieu and thrust of present-day cancer care challenges the defences of health care professionals by ever-increasing complex combination treatments, long illness trajectories, new technologies, increased specialisation and possible fragmentation, consumer expectations, and competition for patient contracts and research funds. As the risks of work grow, anxiety increases as well.

Menzies' work and other studies by psychoanalysts suggest that health care professionals may be deeply 'defended' against the stresses and anxieties of caring for people who have cancer. In a paper entitled 'The ailment', Main[118] considers that our choice to work with cancer has deep personal reasons and that it had abiding unconscious determinants, such as the need to heal sick parts of ourselves. There is therefore a range of feelings that may invade us as we work, including anxiety, guilt, depression, and compulsive reparative wishes.

Rather than being aware of our defences, which are developmentally normal and protect us from excessive anxiety, and ensuring they are reasonably flexible to enable us to remain open to distress, our defences can become immovable barriers to thoughtful, responsive practice. Institutional cancer care settings may actively contribute to this, since to keep the institution functioning and individual cancer care professionals functioning within it, time and other constraints only permit working at a superficial level.

This provides an alternative reading to the mainstream studies of stresses and burnout amongst cancer care professionals in which the comparatively low levels of stress found may be an indicator of the extent and effectiveness of staff's defences against the anxiety of their work, rather than an accurate indicator of their stress.

Methodological issues in researching and evaluating the nature and impact of the nurse–patient relationship in cancer care

Research is needed that will not only enhance understanding of the complex processes of communication between nurses and people with cancer but provide evidence of the value claimed, and indicate the nature of support and education required, to facilitate this therapeutic opportunity.

Almost all nurse–patient communication research to date has been carried out with a positivist psychological orientation. One consequence of this has been the focus on quantitative approaches concerned with the attributes of nurses or an enumeration of their communication skills (Table 7.4).[51,119] There has been a tendency in this research to establish operational definitions of 'facilitative' or 'blocking' nurse communications, which are then considered in relation to some idealised normative standard, or 'good' communication check list.[120] Though these works have provided invaluable insights into nurses' communication practices, the focus of such research has had adverse spin-offs. It has meant that linguistic and sociological issues such as language use, social context, and the conversation as a joint construction between nurse and patient have been downplayed. The therapeutic effectiveness of the communication has not been evaluated, and the role of nurse researcher, attempting to understand the complexities of nurses' therapeutic work and the stress of health care professionals in the field of cancer care, rather than exposing failures, has not been fully realised.

The challenges facing researchers are immense for it is proving difficult to establish ways to evaluate therapeutic work in health care.[128] Studies are required that will explore the nature and effectiveness of nurses' therapeutic work, as well as studies that go beyond individuals' communicative practice to address systemic and institutional influences. Such research will complement existing studies and reveal the limits of theoretical accounts of nurses' therapeutic potential, highlighting the education and support needs for practice.

A spectrum of research methods is necessary to explore fully the processes and impact of nurses'

Table 7.4 Examples of research exploring cancer nurses' practice in comprehending and responding to patients' concerns[1,46,48,51,119,121-127]

Study	Method	Findings
McIntosh I. (1977)	Non-participant observation.	Routinised forms of communication identified. Paucity of nurse-patient talk.
Bond S. (1978)	Non-participant observation in a radiotherapy department. Tape-recorded nurse-patient interactions.	Little evidence of conversation related to person's individual social or psychological concerns. Nurses controlled conversations. Less than 5% of conversations lasted beyond 3 min.
Macleod-Clark J. (1982)	Combination of audio and video recordings. Non-participant observation schedules. Field notes. Interviews with nurses.	Nurse interventions predominantly discouraging with widespread use of 'closed' or 'leading' questions. When open questions were used, often blocked by patient and/or nurse.
Drummond-Mills W. (1983)	Non-participant observation study.	Limited interaction. Nurses ignored person's cues and thus controlled the amount of emotion or personal information people could give.
Maguire P. (1985)	Tape-recorded nurse-patient interviews.	Nurses ignored signs of distress from people. No recognition of the person's individual voice.
Tait A. (1986)	Ethnomethodological case study of a single patient's 'career' as a breast cancer patient.	Nurse organised her talk with the woman, controlled the conversation and established it on her own terms.
Hunt M. (1989)	Extended case study within an ethnographic framework. Tape-recordings of nurse-patient conversations over 3 months.	Patients did not express wishes to discuss their feelings. Processes that promoted expression of feelings, the meaning of death or spiritual need were limited.
Wilkinson S. (1991)	Tape-recorded nurse-patient interactions followed by semi-structured interviews with the nurses. Coding frame used to categorise 'blocking' or 'facilitating' interventions by the nurse.	54% of nurses' verbal behaviours found to be 'blocking'. Psychological and emotional needs assessment largely ignored by nurses.
Booth K. (1993)	Prospective study of nurse-patient taped interactions before and after training and 9 months later. Researcher-nurse semi-structured interviews. Questionnaire re nurses' perceived level of support.	Blocking behaviours most evident when patients disclose feelings. These behaviours were less when nurses felt practical help and support was available.
Lanceley A. (1995)	Tape-recorded nurse-patient conversations. Nurse-participant reflective interviews. Discourse analysis, including analysis of figurative language.	Patients expressed their feelings to nurses. Conversations were jointly constructed. Nurses' response to patients' emotional expression was highly variable. The impact of cancer patients' expressions of feelings has been underestimated. Study revealed a depth and range of emotional expression to nurses.
Jarrett M. (1996)	Ethnomethodological study. Tape-recorded nurse-patient interactions. Nurse and patient participant accounting interviews. Communication skills analysis.	Patients' valued 'ordinary' conversation with nurses as well as talk about their illness.
Heaven C. and Maguire P. (1996)	Pre-test tape recordings of an assessment interview and nurses' list of patient concerns. Researcher-patient interview and administration of HADS and SA scale. 10-week training programme. 9-month nurse post-test.	Communication workshops based on 'skills' model provide necessary but not sufficient training to achieve sustained changes in nurses' communication behaviours.

therapeutic strategies in cancer care. Interpretative, figurative analysis needs to be incorporated into the more formulaic discourse analytic approaches, which have been used by some researchers to reveal the structures and general patterns of communication within therapeutic encounters. This innovation would reveal people's idiosyncratic, metaphoric ways of understanding and attributing meaning to their cancer illness and offer practitioners insights into how they might respond and work with these.

Put another way, therapeutic work, with its emphasis on feelings and motivations, as a subject of enquiry, invites research approaches that cross disciplinary boundaries.

Geertz[129] sees this 'blurring of genres' in research as part of a wholesale tendency towards de-categorisation:

> What we are seeing is not just another redrawing of the cultural map . . . but an alteration in the principles of mapping. Something is happening to the way we think about the way we think.

This blurring of genres means that the dividing lines between the humanities and the human sciences is now less clear,[130] and that more than one disciplinary or theoretical 'map' may be needed to explore the emotional 'territory' of cancer care. It is tantalising to speculate how far the assumptions of conscious intention and the transparency of language can be set aside, and research approaches that examine metaphor and personal imagery still produce sociologically and psychologically intelligible, clinically relevant findings.

References

1. Lanceley A. (1995). Emotional disclosure between cancer patients and nurses. In Richardson A. and Wilson-Barnet J. (eds.) *Nursing Research in Cancer Care.* London: Scutari Press, pp. 167–188.
2. Corner J. (1997). Beyond survival rates and side-effects: cancer nursing as therapy. *Cancer Nursing* 20, 3–11.
3. Smith M.E. and Hart G. (1994). Nurses' responses to anger: from disconnecting to connecting. *Journal of Advanced Nursing* 20, 643–651.
4. Armstrong D. (1983). The fabrication of nurse–patient relationships. *Social Science and Medicine* 17, 457–460.
5. Peplau H. (1952). *Interpersonal Relationships in Nursing.* New York: GP Putnam.
6. Peplau H. (1969). Professional closeness. *Nursing Forum* 8, 342–360.
7. Savage J. (1995). *Nursing Intimacy: An Ethnographic Approach to Nurse–Patient Interaction.* London: Scutari Press.
8. Bailey C. (1995). Nursing as therapy in the management of breathlessness in lung cancer. *European Journal of Cancer Care* 4, 184–190.
9. Davis B. and Oberle K. (1990). Dimensions of the supportive role of the nurse in palliative care. *Oncology Nursing Forum* 17, 87–94.
10. Froggatt K. (1995). Nurses and involvement in palliative care work. In Richardson A. and Wilson-Barnett J. (eds.) *Nursing Research in Cancer Care.* London: Scutari Press, pp. 151–164.
11. Thorne S.E. (1988). Helpful and unhelpful communications in cancer care: the patient perspective. *Oncology Nursing Forum* 15, 167–172.
12. McMahon R. and Pearson A. (1991). *Nursing as Therapy.* London: Chapman and Hall.
13. Muetzel P. (1988). Therapeutic nursing. In Pearson A. (ed.) *Primary Nursing: Nursing in the Burford and Oxford Nursing Development Unit.* London: Croom Helm, 1988.
14. Judd D. (1995). *Give Sorrow Words: Working with a Dying Child,* 2nd edition. London: Whurr Publishers.
15. Halldorsdottir S. (1991). Five basic modes of being with another. In Gaut D. and Leininger M. (eds.) *Caring: The Compassionate Healer.* New York: National League for Nursing Press, pp. 37–50.
16. Kitson A (1986). *Steps toward the identification and development of nursing therapeutic functions in the care of hospitalised elderly.* Ph.D. thesis, University of Ulster, Coleraine.
17. Ersser S.J. (1990). A search for the therapeutic dimensions of nurse–patient interaction. In Pearson A. and McMahon R. (eds.) *Nursing as Therapy.* London: Chapman and Hall.
18. Campbell A.V. (1984). *Moderated Love: A Theology of Professional Care.* London: SPCK.
19. Carper B. (1978). Fundamental patterns of knowing in nursing. *Advances in Nursing Science* 1, 13–23.
20. Benner P. and Wrubel J. (1989). *The Primacy of Caring: Stress and Coping in Health and Illness.* Menlo Park, CA: Addison–Wesley.
21. Cox M. (1988). *Structuring the Therapeutic Process: Compromise with Chaos.* London: Jessica Kingsley.
22. Burnard P. (1994). *Counselling Skills for Health Profesionals,* 2nd edition. In Campling J. (ed.) *Therapy in Practice Series.* London: Chapman and Hall.
23. Pollitt C. (1991). *The Politics of Quality: Managers, Professionals and Consumers in the Public Services.* London: Royal Holloway and Bedford New College, Centre for Political Studies.

24. Griffiths R. (1983). *Report of the NHS Management Inquiry.* London: Department of Health and Social Security.

25. Calman K. and Hine D. (1995). *A Policy Framework for Commissioning Cancer Services.* Cardiff: Department of Health, Wales.

26. Harrison S., Hunter D., Marnock G. and Pollit C. (1989). General management and medical autonomy in the National Health Service. *Health Services Management Research* **2**, 38–46.

27. Bloomfield B., Coombs R., Cooper D. and Rea D. (1992). Machines and manoeuvres: responsibility accounting and the construction of hospital information. *Accounting, Management and Information Technologies* **2**, 199–205.

28. James N. (1992). Care = organization + physical labour + emotional labour. *Sociology of Health and Illness* **14**, 488–509.

29. Davies C. (1995). *Gender and the Professional Predicament in Nursing.* Buckingham: Open University Press.

30. Traynor M. (1996). A literary approach to managerial discourse after the NHS reforms. *Sociology of Health and Illness* **18**, 315–340.

31. Salvage J. (1990). The theory and practice of the 'New Nursing'. *Nursing Times* **86**, Occasional Paper, 42–45.

32. Pearson A. (1988). Primary nursing. In Pearson A. (ed.) *Primary Nursing: Nursing in the Burford and Oxford Nursing Development Units.* London: Chapman and Hall.

33. Manley K. (1997). A conceptual framework for advanced practice: an action research project operationalizing an advanced practitioner/consultant nurse role. *Journal of Advanced Nursing* **6**, 179–190.

34. Knowles G. (1997). *Advancing Cancer Nursing Practice.* European Oncology Nursing Society, Brussels.

35. Glaser B. and Strauss A.L. (1965). *Awareness of Dying.* New York: Aldine.

36. James N. (1993). Divisions of emotional labour: disclosure and cancer. In Fineman S. (ed.) *Emotions in Organizations.* London: Sage, pp. 94–117.

37. Menzies Lyth I. (1988). The functioning of social systems as a defence against anxiety (1959, 1961,[1961b], 1970). In Menzies Lyth I. (ed.) *Containing Anxiety in Institutions: Selected Essays.* London: Free Association Books, pp. 43–94.

38. Peräkylä A. (1991). Hope work in the care of seriously III patients. *Qualitative Health Research* **1**, 407–433.

39. Savage J. (1992). *Implications of New Nursing Initiatives for the Nurse–Patient Relationship: An Ethnographic Study of Two Wards.* London: Bloomsbury and Islington College of Nursing and Midwifery.

40. Smith P. (1992). *The Emotional Labour of Nursing: How Nurses Care.* Basingstoke: Macmillan.

41. Fineman S. (ed.) (1993). *Emotion in Organizations.* London: Sage.

42. Obholzer A. and Roberts V.Z. (eds.) (1994). *The Unconscious at Work: Individual and Organizational Stress in the Human Services.* London: Routledge.

43. Frankel R.M. (1983). The laying on of hands: aspects of the organization of gaze, touch and talk in a medical encounter. In Fisher S. and Todd A.D. (eds.) *The Social Organization of Doctor–Patient Communication.* Washington DC: Centre for Applied Linguistics, pp. 19–54.

44. Di Giacomo S.M. (1987). Biomedicine as a cultural system: an anthropologist in the kingdom of the sick. In Baer H. (ed.) *Encounters in Biomedicine: Case Studies in Medical Anthropology.* New York: Gordon and Breach, pp. 315–346.

45. Lichter I. (1987). *Communication in Cancer Care.* London: Churchill Livingstone.

46. McIntosh J. (1977). *Communication and Awareness in a Cancer Ward.* London: Croom Helm.

47. Knight M. and Field D. (1981). A silent conspiracy: coping with dying cancer patients on an acute surgical ward. *Journal of Advanced Nursing* **6**, 221–229.

48. Bond S. (1978). *Processes of communication about cancer in a radiotherapy department.* Ph.D. thesis, University of Edinburgh.

49. Silverman D. (1987). *Communication and Medical Practice: Social Relations in the Clinic.* London: Sage.

50. Heath C. (1989). Pain talk: the expression of suffering in the medical consultation. *Social Psychology Quarterly* **52**, 113–125.

51. Wilkinson S. (1991). Factors which influence how nurses communicate with cancer patients. *Journal of Advanced Nursing* **16**, 677–688.

52. Fisher S. (1984). Doctor–patient communication: a social and micro-political performance. *Sociology of Health and Illness* **6**, 1–29.

53. Souhami R. (1978). Teaching what to say about cancer. *Lancet* **ii**, 935–936.

54. Fallowfield L. and Roberts R. (1992). Cancer counselling in the United Kingdom. *Psychology and Health* **6**, 107–117.

55. Maguire P. and Faulkner A. (1988). How to do it: communicate with cancer patients. Handling bad news and difficult questions. *British Medical Journal* **297**, 8–10.

56. Maguire P. and Faulkner A. (1988). How to do it: communicate with cancer patients. Handling uncertainty, collusion and denial. *British Medical Journal* **297**, 10–15.

57. Atkinson P. (1981). *The Clinical Experience: Construction and Reconstruction of Medical Reality.* Gower: Farnborough.

58. Mishler E.G. (1984). *The Discourse of Medicine: Dialectics of Medical Interviews.* New Jersey: Norwood Publishing Company.

59. Kubler-Ross E. (1970). *Death: The Final Stage of Growth.* London: Tavistock.

60. Byrne P. and Long B. (1976). *Doctors Talking to Patients.* London: DHSS.

61. Foucault M. (1973). *The Birth of the Clinic.* London: Tavistock.

62. Armstrong D. (1984). The patient's view. *Social Science and Medicine* 18, 737–744.

63. Arney W.R. (1982). *Power and the Profession of Obstetrics.* Chicago, IL: University of Chicago Press.

64. Bennis W. (1979). Emotional expressions in interpersonal relationship. In Bennis W. (ed.) *Essays in Interpersonal Dynamics.* Homewood, IL: Dorsey Press.

65. Cassee E. (1975). Therapeutic behaviour, hospital culture and communication. In Cox C. and Mead A. (eds.) *A Sociology of Medical Practice.* London: Collier-Macmillan.

66. Teger A.I. and Pruitt D.G. (1967). Components of group risk taking. *Journal of Social Psychology* 5, 189–205.

67. Nievaard A.C. (1987). Communication climate and patient care: causes and effects of nurse's attitudes to patients. *Social Science and Medicine* 24, 777–784.

68. Moorey S., Greer S., Watson M., Barvch J.D.R., Robertson B.M., Mason A. *et al.* (1994). Adjuvant psychological therapy for patients with cancer: outcome at one year. *Psycho-oncology* 3, 39–46.

69. Ley P. (1988). *Communicating with Patients.* London: Croom Helm.

70. Glaser B. and Strauss A. (1965). *Awareness of Dying.* Chicago, IL: Aldine.

71. Armstrong D. (1987). Silence and truth in death and dying. *Social Science and Medicine* 24, 651–657.

72. Cassileth B.R. (1980). Information and participation preferences among cancer patients. *Annals of Internal Medicine* 92, 832–836.

73. Parkes C.M. (1978). Psychological aspects. In Saunders C.M. (ed.) *The Management of Terminal Diseases.* London: Arnold, pp. 44–64.

74. Editorial (1993). News: complaints drop by 16%. *Nursing Times* 89, 6.

75. Baider L. and Porath S. (1981). Uncovering fear: group experiences of nurses in a cancer ward. *International Journal of Nursing Studies* 18, 147–152.

76. Brooks A. (1979). Public and professional attitudes towards cancer: a view from Great Britain. *Cancer Nursing* 2, 453–460.

77. Felton G., Reed P. and Perla S. (1982). Measurement of students' and nurses' attitudes towards cancer. *Western Journal of Nursing Research* 3, 62–75.

78. Rockliffe M. (1977). *A study to investigate nurses' opinions about the character of malignant disease and the factors that influence these opinions.* MSc thesis, University of Manchester.

79. Wegman J.S. (1979). Avoidance behavior of nurses as related to cancer diagnosis and/or terminality. *Oncology Nursing Forum* 6, 8–14.

80. Corner J.L. (1988). Assessment of nurses' attitudes towards cancer: a critical review of research methods. *Journal of Advanced Nursing* 13, 640–648.

81. Hanson E.E. (1991). *The Cancer Nurse's Perspective: Stress and the Person with Cancer.* Lancaster: Quay Publishing.

82. Elkind A.K. (1982). Nurses' views about cancer. *Journal of Advanced Nursing* 7, 43–50.

83. Stacey J. (1997). *Teratologies: A Cultural Study of Cancer.* London: Routledge.

84. Chaikin A.L. (1974). Non-verbal mediators of teacher expectancy effects. *Journal of Personal and Social Psychology* 30, 144–149.

85. Word C.O. (1974). The nonverbal mediation of self-fulfilling prophesies in interaction. *Journal of Experimental Social Psychology* 10, 109–120.

86. Mood D. and Lick C.F. (1979). Attitudes of nursing personnel toward death and dying: linguistic indicators of denial. *Research in Nursing and Health* 2, 95–99.

87. Vachon M., Lyall W. and Freeman S. (1978). Measurement and management of stress in health professionals working with advanced cancer patients. *Death Education* 1, 365–375.

88. Delvaux N., Razavi D. and Farvacques C. (1988). Cancer care–stress for health professionals. *Social Science and Medicine* 27, 159–166.

89. Gray-Toft P. and Anderson J. (1981). Stress among hospital nursing staff: its causes and effects. *Social Science and Medicine* 15a, 639–647.

90. Ullrich A. and Fitzgerald P. (1990). Stress experienced by physicians on the cancer ward. *Social Science and Medicine* 13, 213–218.

91. Stewart B., Meyerowitz B., Jackson L., Yarkin K. and Harvey J. (1982). Psychological stress associated with outpatient oncology nursing. *Cancer Nursing* **October**, 383–387.

92. Whippen D.A. and Canellos G.P. (1991). Burnout syndrome in the practice of oncology: results of a random survey of 1000 oncologists. *Journal of Clinical Oncology* 9, 1916–1920.

93. Cull A. (1991). Staff support in medical oncology: a problem solving approach. *Psychology and Health* 5, 129–136.

94. Kent F.G., Wills G., Faulkner A., Parry M., Whipp R. and Coleman R. (1994). The professional and personal needs of oncology staff: the effects of perceived success and failure in helping patients on levels of personal stress and distress. *Journal of Cancer Care* 3, 153–158.

95. Miller G. and Silverman D. (1995). Troubles talk and counselling discourse: a comparative study. *Sociological Quarterly* **36**, 725–747.

96. Ramirez A., Graham J. and Richards M. (1995). Burnout and psychiatric disorder among cancer clinicians. *British Journal of Cancer* **71**, 1263–1269.

97. Larson D.G. (1992). The challenge of caring in oncology nursing. *Oncology Nursing Forum* **19**, 857–861.

98. Weisman A.D. (1981). Understanding the cancer patient: the syndrome of the caregiver's plight. *Psychiatry* **44**, 161–168.

99. Cox T., Leather P. and Cox S. (1990). Stress, health and organizations. *Occupational Review* **February/March**, 13–18.

100. George J. (1990). Why stress is a management issue. *Health Manpower Management* **December**, 17–19.

101. Yasko J. (1983). Variables which predict burnout experienced by oncology nurses. *Cancer Nursing* **April**, 109–116.

102. Ogle M.E. (1983). Stages of burnout among oncology nurses in the hospital setting. *Oncology Nursing Forum* **10**, 31–34.

103. Jenkins J.F. and Ostchega Y. (1986). Evaluation of burnout in oncology nurses. *Cancer Nursing* **9**, 108–116.

104. Bram P. and Katz L. (1989). A study of burnout in nurses working in hospice and hospital oncology settings. *Oncology Nursing Forum* **16**, 555–560.

105. Razavi D., Delvaux N., Marchal S., Bredart A., Farvacques C. and Paesmans M. (1993). The effects of a 24-hr psychological training program on attitudes, communication skills and occupational stress in oncology: a randomised study. *European Journal of Cancer* **29A**, 1858–1863.

106. Hinds P., Quargnenti A. and Hickey S. (1994). A comparison of the stress-response sequence in new and experienced paediatric oncology nurses. *Cancer Nursing* **17**, 61–71.

107. Papadatou D., Anagnostopouros F. and Mouros D. (1994). Factors contributing to the development of burnout on oncology nursing. *British Journal of Medical Psychology* **67**, 187–199.

108. Wilkinson S.M. (1994). Stress in cancer nursing: does it exist? *Journal of Advanced Nursing* **20**, 1079–1084.

109. Ramirez A.J., Graham J., Richards M.A., Cull A. and Gregory W.M. (1996). Mental health of hospital consultants: the effects of stress and satisfaction at work. *Lancet* **347**, 724–728.

110. Lazarus R. (1966). *Psychological Stress and the Coping Process.* New York: McGraw-Hill.

111. Pearlin L.I. (1989). The sociological study of stress. *Journal of Health and Social Behaviour* **30**, 241–256.

112. Hirschorn L. (1988). *The Workplace Within: Psychodynamics of Organizational Life.* Cambridge, MA: MIT Press.

113. Freud A. (1993). *The Ego and the Mechanisms of Defence.* London: Karnac Books.

114. Klein M. (1937). *Love, Guilt and Reparation and other Works,* 1975 edition. London: Hogarth.

115. Brown D. and Pedder J. (1991). *Introduction of Psychotherapy: An Outline of Psychodynamic Principles and Practice.* London: Tavistock/Routledge.

116. Jacobs M. (1988). *Psychodynamic Counselling in Action.* London: Sage.

117. Menzies Lyth I. (1988). *Containing Anxiety in Institutions,* Vol. 1. London: Free Association Books.

118. Main T. (1968). The ailment. In Barnes E. (ed.) *Psychosocial Nursing: Studies from the Cassel Hospital.* London: Tavistock.

119. Macleod Clark J. (1982). *Nurse–patient interaction: an analysis of conversation on surgical wards.* Ph.D. thesis, University of London.

120. Booth K., Maguire P.M., Butterworth T. and Hillier V.F. (1996). Perceived professional support and the use of blocking behaviours by hospice nurses. *Journal of Advanced Nursing* **24**, 522–527.

121. Drummond-Mills W. (1983). *Problems related to the nursing management of the dying patient.* Unpublished M.Sc. thesis, University of Glasgow.

122. Maguire P. (1985). The psychological impact of cancer. *British Journal of Hospital Medicine* **34**, 100–103.

123. Tait A. (1986). The mastectomy experience: two interviews examined. In Stanley L. and Scott S. (eds.) *Studies in Sexual Politics.* Manchester: University of Manchester.

124. Hunt M. (1989). *Dying at home: its basic 'ordinariness' displayed in patients' relatives' and nurses' talk.* Ph.D. thesis, University of London.

125. Booth C. (1993). *Helping patients with cancer: putting psychological assessment skills into practice.* Ph.D. thesis, University of Manchester.

126. Jarrett N. (1996). *Comfortable conversation: nurse–patient communication in the cancer care context.* Ph.D. thesis, University of Southampton.

127. Heaven C.M. and Maguire P. (1996). Training hospice nurses to elicit patients' concerns. *Journal of Advanced Nursing* **23**, 280–286.

128. Silverman D. (1997). *Discourses of Counselling: HIV Counselling as Social Interaction.* London: Sage.

129. Geertz C. (1983). *Local Knowledge: Further Essays in Interpretive Anthropology.* New York: Basic Books.

130. Denzin N.K. (1970). *The Research Act: A Theoretical Introduction to Sociological Methods,* 3rd edition. Englewood Cliffs, NJ: Prentice Hall.

CHAPTER EIGHT

Therapeutic strategies in cancer care

Anne Lanceley

There is an increasing awareness amongst health care professionals and consumers of the painful issues surrounding cancer treatment and care. Receiving the diagnosis and negotiating subsequent treatment constitutes a psychic trauma and in this case professionals need to look into their own feelings, as well as attempting to be aware of those of the people in their care. An understanding of the need for not only quality medical care but also emotional care and support, including the right to express every sort of emotion as a response to the trauma of cancer illness, is well established.[1,2]

This interest and awareness has been driven, in part, by the idea that the way feelings are expressed and in particular active holding back from expressing feelings, not only may render a person 'cancer prone' but may affect the progress of the cancer illness.[3,4] This has been a powerful theme in the cancer literature and in the minds of some people who have cancer judging by patients' own accounts of their illness experience.[3-7] It continues to be a high research priority.

What is striking in this context is that cancer nurses, though generally accepting of the therapeutic potential of their role at some level, and while acknowledging that the people for whom they care may use the trusted relationship with them to explore their own feelings, in practice are pragmatic in their approaches to managing individual concerns. Put another way, nurses' actual practices are not generally theory driven and do not involve an explicit, mutually negotiated therapeutic plan.

Much of what follows is theoretical. This is not as a way of avoiding the feelings of uncertainty and the sense of vulnerability nurses experience when working with cancer but as a way of providing a variety of lenses through which the practice can be viewed. The use of theory and alternative frameworks for understanding this work enables us to see when processes are 'stuck'. It is hoped that the verbatim accounts will allow for contemplation and the pursuit of the reader's personal meanings in the light of their own clinical experience.

No essential right or wrong theories or practical ways of managing the concerns of people with cancer are advocated here. There are numerous texts describing ways of managing these practically.[8-12] At one level everything depends on how the particular nurse is attempting to work with an individual. There are, however, fundamental beliefs and questions that run throughout the chapter. They concern:

- the relative importance of nurses sharing awareness of their intent when working with someone with cancer
- how unconscious thoughts and feelings may influence work with cancer
- different levels and ways of helping individuals express and understand their feelings, deal with problems, adjust and make treatment decisions
- the ways nurses define themselves as 'listener', counsellor', or 'therapist'

- the belief that contact with the nurse is beneficial or 'therapeutic' if an individual feels understood and is thus helped to understand himself better.

The understanding alluded to in the last point may take an unspoken form in the case of a nurse who sits and bears silent witness to someone who is dying. Being with the person is an opportunity for them to 'be'. Allowing the person to be dying validates them, whereas to deny the person's dying life would be to deny their life. The nurse is communicating understanding and acceptance of the person's life and impending death.[13]

There are two styles of relating to someone with cancer, which can be placed along a continuum of therapeutic strategies: the first is concerned with the deciphering of meaning, whereas the second is in the nature of 'holding' and 'containing' the experience. The cancer nurse needs to strike a balance within these two broad types of functioning.

Structuring the nurse–patient relationship

In order for the nurse to do this and remain sensitive to the often chaotic emotional experiences during cancer treatment as well as recognising and helping with their information needs, Cox,[14] advocates structuring the relationship. The dimensions of time, depth, and mutuality, if thought about by the nurse, can help to locate her use of herself on behalf of the person and offers a means of monitoring the changing course of what happens in the relationship. Cox makes a useful analogy with the built-in range finder on a camera and the nurse's initiative in bringing what the person is saying into focus so that they are both operating at the same focal point. Like the personal qualities considered essential for nurses to relate and respond effectively – acceptance, warmth, genuineness, and empathy – the dimensions of time, depth, and mutuality are independent of any particular theoretical approach and are relevant, however brief or extended the encounter may be.

Time
The significance of time as a dimension is intensified for someone with a life-threatening illness and there is a shared awareness of this as the uncertainty of a limited prognosis is tolerated. This uncertainty gives an added poignancy to the maxim from counselling psychology: If the patient does not know when the end is, he cannot know when 'just before the end' is. This is important for thinking about the timing of someone's disclosures, and particular moments of insight within a talk when feelings are expressed and may be acknowledged and understood for the first time. The maxim is also relevant for a series of conversations and encounters that a person may have with a nurse over many months or years. It prompts the nurse to consider the beginning of her relationship with them and its likely duration, which may coincide with a treatment regime or commence at the palliative phase of the illness, ending with their death; it focuses attention on the length of time available for any single encounter, and on how boundaries may be set so that the time available can be used constructively. Holidays and other absences may become increasingly important and require managing.

A more subtle aspect of the time dimension is how aspects of the person's past, their present, and their plans and hopes for the future may be acknowledged and balanced so that there is momentum and sense of continuity in the relationship.

Depth
The second dimension concerns depth. This is related to levels of patient disclosure from surface to hidden aspects of their lives and themselves. It brings into play the complex interaction between unconscious and conscious levels of awareness, which has been one of the major contributions of psychoanalytic theory to the understanding of human behaviours and experience. Linked to this are the skills and activity of the nurse responding to different levels of personal disclosure. Cox[14] distinguishes between three levels of self-disclosure and offers them as a useful conceptual tool for practice, also suggesting that they can be used to assess the depth of the relationship.

First level disclosures are safe and relatively unimportant and act as 'feelers' in the relationship. Level two disclosures involve the disclosure of personal information but tend to be emotionally neutral. They are an indication that the relationship has developed to the point where the person feels confident and trusting with the nurse. Third level disclosures give insight into the personal, deep, existential concerns and by definition are unique to them. Things from the person's own private world that they may not have revealed before may be disclosed. The three levels can be used to assess the depth of the relationship, both on a session-by-session basis and within a longer term relationship.

While attempting to integrate depth and time structuring into a cohesive therapeutic strategy, the nurse must also be aware of the crucial significance of the place of mutuality and reciprocity within the nurse–patient relationship.

Mutuality

The third dimension of structure is mutuality, which describes the potential significance of the shared relationship. Mutuality refers to how much the nurse discloses about herself in order to share with the person the experience he is disclosing. This is not primarily about how much the nurse reveals about her own problems, which could be perceived as overburdening. It is about a mutuality of disclosure grounded in the here-and-now of the talk and physical care. The nurse may be very open in expressing her feelings in relation to this shared experience, which is very different from disclosing her own personal life experiences. Rather than emotionally withdrawing and hiding behind a professional mask, the nurse acknowledges the person's distress and the shared pain and distress inherent in the situation. This involves acceptance, warmth, genuineness, and empathy and, in addition, may develop through the nurse actively using transference and counter-transference.

Empathy is the ability to enter the perceptual world of another person and convey this identification of feeling to them.[8] As well as an empathetic 'looking in' through an exploration of inner feelings and meanings, empathy also involves 'looking out' on behalf of someone else; seeing the world, the context in which they live, work, and receive their treatment, through their eyes.

Some nurses have greater intuitive awareness than others, and a question that taxes nurse educators is how far empathy can be both taught and learned.[15] What seems clear is that it is the nurse's use of her own personality that sustains empathy. The quality that enables people who have cancer to risk what may amount to further reduction of self-esteem and distress, by emotionally exposing themselves still further, is if the nurse is empathetic and not only listens, but hears, understands and, most difficult of all, is able to convey that she understands. How is this done? Can one nurse do this for all those in her care?

One of the essentials for empathy is that of showing by word, gesture, and expression a de-trivialising, unconditional concern. The person believes that what concerns him is not trivial and he may to some extent test out the nurse, who may be presumed to adopt a 'trivialising' attitude to them by the very fact that he has become and is labelled a 'cancer patient'.

Therefore, mutuality is a measure of the depth of the relationship and of the nurse's commitment to the relationship.

Developing communication skills

The personal qualities of empathy, a non-judgemental attitude and even genuineness are considered essential for nurses to respond effectively to patients, and the use of communication skills enhances the nurse's ability to relate and to work confidently across the spectrum of functioning. The use of communication skills is independent of theoretical approach or the way in which the nurse and patient agree to structure their relationship.

Active listening
- Attending and being physically 'present'
- questioning: closed
                open
                leading
                value-laden
                'why', 'how', and 'what' questions
                confronting questions
- allowing expression of feelings
- prompting
- probing
- focusing
- clarifying
- reflecting
- paraphrasing

- challenging
- self-sharing
- summarising
- monitoring transference and counter-transference.

As this chapter is more a contextual exploration of nurses' strategies for managing cancer patient's concerns, knowledge and understanding of the skills needed to communicate effectively are not described in detail. A great deal has been written on this and numerous texts explain and give practical examples of the skills summarised above.[8,16–20]

Alternative frameworks for understanding nurses' work with cancer patients

Knowledge of a range of theoretical approaches (see Table 8.1) will open up a spectrum of possibilities for managing a person's concerns and is necessary if the nurse is to understand and work comfortably across the spectrum of functioning described at the beginning of the chapter, from 'holding' and 'containing' to helping to decipher the meaning of cancer illness.[12,21–35]

Table 8.1 Theoretical approaches for managing a person's concerns

Psychological approach	Theorist
Personal construct approach	Kelly (1955)
Gestalt therapy	Perls (1969)
Transactional analysis	Berne (1964)
	Harris (1973)
Person-centred therapy	Rogers (1951)
Rational emotive therapy (RET)	Ellis (1962)
Behavioural therapy	Krumboltz and Thorenson (1969)
Neuro-linguistic programmes (NLP)	Bandler (1985)
Reality therapy	Glasser (1965)
Psychosynthesis	Ferrucci (1982)
Psychotherapy	Freud (1938)
	Klein (1937)
	Bion (1962)
Cognitive therapy	Beck (1976)
Adjuvant psychological therapy for patients with cancer (APT)	Moorey and Greer (1989)
Logotherapy	Frankl (1959)

The meaning of illness and its therapeutic use

Cancer can disrupt virtually all aspects of a person's life. Everyday activities are affected, as well as short-term and long-term goals. A person is forced to reassess what is meaningful and to scrutinise values that have hitherto governed their life.

Silver and Wortman[36] suggest that a person's ability to find meaning or purpose in a crisis is associated with the ability to adjust to it. People need to see their lives as essentially meaningful, and as Brody[37] noted, 'suffering is produced and alleviated primarily by the meaning that one attaches to one's experience'.

The primary mechanism for attaching meaning to particular experiences is to tell stories about them. It is through hearing and telling stories that human beings have always come to organise and understand their experiences.[38] There are numerous important testimonies of personal struggles with cancer illness: *Diary of a Breast*, written by a woman with breast cancer,[39] *Cancer Through the Eyes of Ten Women*,[7] *Cancer in Two Voices,* co-written by partners facing cancer,[40] the intense descriptions by Ruth Picardie,[41] first in a series of newspaper articles and later in a book of the progress of her breast cancer, or *And When Did You Last See Your Father?* about a son's understanding of his father's cancer,[42] and the elegiac accounts of the experience of ovarian cancer treatment and illness by Anne Dennison,[43] to quote but a few. They provide crucial insight into work in the field and contribute forcibly to our clinical thinking. Stories and testimonies of illness are no different from other descriptions; we construct an understanding of illness by comparing it to things other than itself, to things found in the realm of our personal experience. It is all but impossible to conceive of illness without recourse to metaphor, if only because 'the objective world is not directly accessible but is constructed on the basis of the constraining influences of human knowledge and language'.[44] Lakoff and Johnson's seminal work provided evidence that metaphor was responsible for an individual's method of making sense of things.[45]

The metaphorical potency of cancer illness stories has been explored in the writings of Sontag[46] and is evidenced in recent studies.[47] By examining professional and lay expressions of cancer illness, Sontag revealed just how prevalent certain metaphorical descriptions are: 'cancer is war' and 'cancer is invasion' are two examples that sustain a host of other metaphorical expressions, such as 'they attacked it with chemotherapy', or 'his natural defences were low'. It is only recently that these ideas have begun to influence ideas for practice in cancer care.[48-50] Attention to the metaphors and personal imagery used by individuals is important in the therapeutic sense that an illness conceived of metaphorically might be coped with and responded to in the same way.[51]

There is a substantial literature concerned with narrative analysis of health and illness, much of it influenced by the seminal work of Kleinman and Mishler.[52,53] Kleinman suggests that individuals' explanatory models of illness originate in biomedicine but also from the construction of sustaining fictions that can make sense of the illness for the individual experiencing self. Kleinman insists that the patient's personal narrative does not merely reflect illness experience but rather it contributes to the experience of symptoms and suffering.

A nurse's ability to facilitate someone to find meaning in their illness and to help someone with cancer to arrive at explanations that sustain them are research and practice themes in cancer care.

This interest comes from an interweaving of various threads:

- an acknowledgement of the psychodynamic processes in which the patient comes to tell and then re-author his or her individual life story, thus throwing light upon their inner life
- the application of social constructionist philosophy and politics to health care, which places a sense of the person as a story-making, story-consuming, social being embedded in social, cultural, and historical conditions, at the centre of its conceptual framework
- the movement towards postmodern forms of clinical practice where the key characteristics are:
  - reflexivity
  - local knowledge replacing 'grand narratives'
  - multiplicity of meanings
  - patient empowerment
  - commitment to pluralism and multiplicity of meaning

- deconstruction of the idea of a singular entity – the 'true self' – in favour of the self as a construction.

How an individual nurse listens to a person's story and interprets it will depend on the broad theoretical approach of the nurse and decisions about the structuring of the relationship. There are many different ways in which a nurse and patient can work together to tell and then retrieve meaning from the story. If the nurse has a psychodynamic orientation, the interpretation of the story will be in terms of unconscious emotional processes, the functioning of psychological defences, and how the person's core life story repeats itself in different relations at different points in his or her life. If the nurse has a behavioural orientation then the story may be used to identify behavioural routines and if the nurse works cognitively, telling the story may be viewed as an act of problem solving and management. These broad approaches are summarised here:

Care strategy 8.1: Preliminary nurse strategies for narrative change

- Nurse listens for patient stories.
- Nurse uses communication skills to elicit the stories the person lives by.
- Nurse listens to *how* the story is told:
  - pauses
  - voice quality
  - phrasing
  - control of emotional distance by:
    - use of objectifying language, e.g. 'it', 'one'
    - absence of experiential detail and colour
  - emotional immediacy by:
    - descriptions of place
    - direct speech
    - present tense.
- Nurse gives close attention to the symbolisation of feelings in the stories and to the metaphors used as indicators of implicit meaning.
- Sensitive ear for differences and incongruities in story construction and telling.

Though it is recognised that there may be intrinsic value in the person telling their story to give voice to areas of experience that have previously been silenced, there is a difference between the nurse simply hearing the story and therapeutic storytelling described in Care strategy 8.1. In the former, the person may tell and retell the same story in the same way throughout their treatment experience and for years afterwards, and derive comfort and support from this. With therapeutic storytelling, the shared expectation for patient and nurse would be that the story can change. Through careful listening and sensitive interpretation of what the patient says the nurse facilitates the ability of the patient to make sense of their illness, with the possible emergence of a more satisfying and personally meaningful narrative.

Psychodynamic approach

An emphasis on the existence of unconscious processes and their role in communication lies at the heart of psychodynamic understanding, which differs from other theories concerned primarily with the conscious mind.

The approach focuses on early memories and feelings from the past that usually remain hidden from our conscious mind but that can be triggered by something in the present. The impact of past memories on present behaviour patterns can be a powerful one. A process of transference occurs when thoughts, feelings, emotions, and expectations belonging to a person in the past are transferred to a person in the present. That person is then reacted to *as if* they were the person from the past, which is often inappropriate.[53] An understanding of this process of transference may be an important tool for the nurse working to understand someone with cancer and other relationships within the work setting.

Behind the psychodynamic approach is the idea that meaning and the key to understanding a person's response to illness and ourselves lie beneath the surface and in the past, that what we are is the result of the dynamic interplay between past and present experience, between our conscious and unconscious, between our external and internal reality and our developing personality.

Internal reality, the part of the mind referred to as our 'internal world', contains many parts or representations of ourselves, as well as representations of relationships with important others and between parts of ourselves, i.e. our child self may

be in conflict with our parent self. The nature of these representations is influenced not only by our early external relationships with mother and father, but also by fantasies fuelled by impulses such as aggression, hate, love, with which children try to make sense of the world, when there is no way to check their perceptions against reality.[21]

These early imaginings are gradually modified, because we test them against reality as we progress through life. However, it is to these perceptions of people, ourselves, and the world that we often fall back or regress, when under stress. It is this inner world that informs and colours our perception of the outer world.[54]

When cancer strikes, usual ways of coping may not help and the person becomes vulnerable and regresses to reacting in more primitive ways. This might show itself through someone trying to cope with the severe anxiety of having cancer by temporarily transferring onto the role of the nursing staff qualities of an all-giving, warm, protective maternal figure.[54] Futtermen and Wellisch[55] provide some evidence for this. In their study, they observed how patients on a bone marrow transplant unit experiencing extreme distress and anxiety regressed to emotional levels of early childhood, relating to staff in the transference much as they did to their own parental figures.

Alternatively, the person with cancer may avoid struggling with ambivalent feelings by splitting them. They may need to keep hope and goodness separate so they do not get spoiled by more negative feelings such as rage and despair. In these circumstances when experience cannot be integrated, a nurse may be either idealised or denigrated.[54]

Another example of this is the kind of psychic splitting that facilitates the person's acceptance of impending death. Two opposite ideas are verbalised. One reflects a full realisation of the closeness of impending death, the other a faith in surviving, often expressed in vivid fantasies about the future.[54]

If nurses remain open to distress, holding onto feelings for a person until they can be made sense of or borne, broadly speaking they would be fulfilling the function a mother performs quite unconsciously for her baby. The mother allows herself to experience her baby's distress, to think about it and process it, so that she can think about and respond to the baby in a sensitive way. Our capacity to do this depends on the quality of our own mothering and the confidence we feel in our 'mother' institution to contain us.[54]

The idea of container/contained is another powerful idea for framing clinical work in which nurses may be needed to offer containment to cancer patients who cannot make sense of their experience for themselves and feel overwhelmed with anxiety as a consequence.[56]

In Bion's theory of container/contained, the capacity to think about emotional experience and develop emotional resilience to cope with difficulties in later life depends on a baby's earliest experience of being thought about and someone being attentive to him or her.[57]

Emmanuel[58] describes what happens according to this theory. A baby is bombarded by sense data that threaten to overwhelm him or her. The baby's mind is not developed enough to contain the powerful feelings and the baby is therefore totally dependent on the availability of an object into whom the powerful feelings can be put in order to get rid of them. Bion calls this object the 'container' and the incomprehensible painful feelings the 'contained'. The container, the mother or caregiver, then has to try and make sense out of the baby's experience by thinking about whatever the baby has made her feel. The mother has to decipher what the baby is communicating. By receiving the baby's feelings, i.e. the contained, and making sense of them, the mother can respond to the baby with understanding. The baby feels immediately more comfortable and is also able to take inside himself the idea that his mother has space in her mind for him and he feels understood. The baby begins to develop his own capacity to reflect on his experience and think. The relevance of this theory to nurses caring for cancer patients who may not be able to make sense of their experience for themselves, and feel overwhelmed with anxiety as a consequence, is clear: the nurse may be needed to offer containment to the person with cancer.

A nurse may gain crucial clues as to how far a person is requiring her to act as a container, and an understanding of the communication by the feelings aroused in him or her by the person. Counter-transference is the name given to the nurse's emotional response to the person, i.e. the conscious thoughts and feelings the nurse has when she is with them. This form of communication from the person can provide the nurse with valuable information as to their state of mind. When thought about by the nurse it can also inform him or her as to the most appropriate response to the person, since it prompts the question: 'What sort of feelings am I being asked to hold for this person?'

They may be feelings of vulnerability or feelings of anger, defeat, or overwhelming depression. When nurses have contact with a person's own unconscious in this way it is usually a very powerful experience. It is powerful because the person is attempting to relieve internal distress by externalising it and giving the nurse responsibility to contain aspects of the self.[54]

If the nurse can allow the person's feelings to sink in, this helps the person to explore the feelings in a personality powerful enough to contain them and perhaps to face something they previously viewed as unbearable. A further therapeutic skill lies in acknowledging the person's anxiety, naming it, and then deciding when and if to hand the feeling back to the person in a form that they can manage.

Cognitive approach

This approach relies on an understanding that behaviours and emotions are intimately linked with beliefs about the world. While beliefs influence feeling responses, they are rarely questioned; they lie beyond normal awareness but are not unconscious. In this approach it is not the appraisals, interpretations, and evaluations that the individual makes about their cancer symptoms or the effects of treatment per se, but the meanings they hold for the person involved. How a person *thinks* about the illness and his or her life is consequently central to their mental adjustment to cancer. As Moorey and Greer[12] note, if loss is the predominant meaning a person attributes to their cancer then the person is likely to feel depressed. If cancer primarily represents a threat to health, security, or life itself, the person is more likely to feel anxious.

In practice this approach aims to help people identify the relationship between cognitions, emotions, and behaviours, to increase their awareness of what seem like dysfunctional thoughts and alter them (Care strategy 8.2). This means challenging and confronting the person's beliefs and negative automatic thoughts. Negative thoughts may be enhanced and perpetuated by distortions in thinking and appraisal: for example, people may focus on only one part of their memory of a diagnostic consultation – the negative aspects – even though other parts contradict this. Habitual thinking increases a person's vulnerability to hearing certain information: someone whose usual style of thinking is very 'black and white' may think they face imminent death when they have been told that all diagnostic tests indicate that the cancer they have has a good prognosis.

Care strategy 8.2: Cognitive strategies

- Facilitation of emotional expression.
- Elicitation of automatic thoughts associated with the person's problems.
- Person is taught to identify his or her own negative thoughts.
- Person set task of monitoring own thoughts.
- Distorted, negative thinking is challenged by reality testing and examining evidence for a particular thought and belief. Searching for an alternative, decatastrophising and helping the person to think about what they fear to see.
- Practise and reinforce the use of more constructive thoughts and behaviours as a response to distressing thoughts.

The work is conceptualised as a joint problem-solving exercise in which the nurse collaborates with the person, seeking primarily cognitive or rational explanations in order to develop and try out strategies for coping with cancer. Therapeutic strategies are primarily educational and designed to foster a positive attitude so that insights gained will extend to future events. It is used extensively with people with cancer to reduce emotional distress and improve coping.[12]

Behavioural approach

This approach is based on the idea that since all human behaviour is learned through processes of positive reinforcement it can, if necessary, be unlearned.[28] The nurse working within this framework will be interested to identify with the person what they see as undesirable behaviours. Once these behaviours have been identified the next step is to organise a scheme of reinforcement whereby more positive behaviours will be encouraged. No attempt is made in the behavioural approach to understand the cause of behaviours or to understand current behaviours in relation to the person's past. Instead the focus is learning, unlearning, and relearning.

Cancer robs patients of a sense of control of their own bodies, and behavioural techniques are considered to help give a sense of mastery or control over the person's life and environment. Behavioural assignments can help the person to develop a sense of control over the illness through encouraging co-operation with treatment or self-help techniques such as visualisation and relaxation, distraction, graded task assignments, and activity scheduling. These behavioural assignments can also develop control in areas unrelated to cancer and indirectly foster a fighting spirit. The techniques are used in cancer to help with symptom distress, anxiety and depression, and notably as part of cognitive therapies, including Moorey and Greer's 'adjuvant psychological therapy'.[12]

Humanistic approach

Drawing heavily on the field of existential philosophy, humanistic psychology argues that people are essentially free and responsible for their own condition. We are not driven by an unconscious mind, nor are we simply the product of what we have learned. Essentially, we are agents. It is the fact of consciousness that gives us the ability to determine our own course of action through life and we are the best arbiters of what is and is not good for us. It was out of the humanistic school that the client-centred approach to counselling developed. The aim of working with the person, according to Rogers,[26] was not necessarily to explore their past, or to modify their behaviour or thinking, but to accept them and to help them progress through their difficulties by their own route, accompanying them on their own personal search for meaning.

Charting the work with cancer patients

Tschudin[10] and Burnard[8] argue that nurses need to make explicit the possible nature of their helping relationships with the person with cancer, based on the individual's needs. This is essential for the relationship to be consensual and collaborative. It may be that the nurse and patient explicitly agree to enter into a counselling relationship in which the nurse agrees to act in the capacity of 'counsellor'. Alternatively, the nurse and patient may agree to work on certain concerns while the nurse will continue to perform within her functional role as nurse. In this case, she will be using counselling skills to enhance her communication with the person. In either situation, a model for practice allows both the nurse and the individual to chart where the relationship is going and how it is progressing. As a result, work is likely to be more focused and more satisfying and goals will be identified, agreed and reached.

Different models for helping are presented in Table 8.2. They are broadly problem management models, which are underpinned by cognitive behavioural approaches to helping people with cancer. The primary sources give more information on these models.

How a nurse eventually does help a person to manage their concerns, how they incorporate a range of theoretical approaches into a personal repertoire of strategies for helping, and how they structure and model the progress of their work will depend on a number of things, including:

- skill level
- what he or she feels comfortable doing
- beliefs and value systems concerning people
- level of self-awareness
- mood at the time

Table 8.2 Different models for helping the nurse–patient relationship[8, 10, 17, 20, 59]

Egan (1994)	Carkhuff (1987)	Nelson-Jones (1993)	Burnard (1994)	Tschudin (1995)
Three-stage open systems model	Developmental model	Lifeskills helping model	Eight stage map	Four questions model
I Problem definition story: Present scenario Identify blind spots	Attending Responding to clients' feelings, thoughts	Developing the relationship, identifying and clarifying problems	1. Meeting the person	1. What is happening?
		Accessing problem(s) and redefining in terms of life-skills	2. Discussion of surface issues	2. What is the meaning of it?
	Personalising the experience Meaning		3. Revelations of deeper issues	3. What is your goal?
II Goal development possibilities: Preferred scenario Goals Objectives	Goals	Stating working goals and planning interventions	4. Ownership of feelings and emotional release	4. How are you going to do it?
			5. Generation of insight	
			6. Problem-solving future planning	
III Action strategies plan	Initiating action	Interventions to develop self-helping skills	7. Action by person	
		End and consolidate	8. Disengagement from the relationship	

- present life situation
- perception of what is 'wrong' with the person
- current workload
- nature of support and supervision available
- the context for the work
- lay and professional expectations of the therapeutic potential of the nurse–patient relationship.

Some of these influences will be evidenced in the extracts chosen to explore strategies for managing concerns below.

Managing concerns

This section of the chapter describes work with four people with cancer, using verbatim accounts of their experiences and how the nurse responded to their concerns. It is recognised here that there are times when the most important communication from the person is unspoken and that people with cancer often stir up feelings in the nurse. Nurses' own accounts of their interactions will be used to identify this unconscious dimension of their communication.

It is hoped that the clinical cases will provide useful learning material. All too often clinical examples either show the health professional in a good light or denigrate their skills. Nurses do not so readily share their difficulties but more can be gained if we are prepared to do so. The selection and permissions gained for the clinical material that follows keep faith with this.

Helping with fear and anxiety

Case examples

Joyce is a 58-year-old single woman who lives alone. The palliative care nurse who visits her on this occasion has known her for 2 years, since her breast cancer was first diagnosed. The nurse has been seeing Joyce weekly, for 3 months, either at home or at the hospital, after it was discovered that she had metastatic spread of her cancer. Joyce has been undergoing a course of chemotherapy but has become increasingly breathless, as the nurse discovers during this planned visit to her home the day before she is due to be seen by the doctor in the hospital clinic. This extract occurs 10 minutes into their half-hour conversation:

195 P. I'm really bad aren't I mmm (2.0) mmm (2.4)

196 N. I don't know Joyce I don't think you're getting better

197 P. No (5.2) oh God oh it's alright darling (6.0) sorry about this (sounding distressed)

198 N. That's alright (3.0)

199 P. What is it the doctor thinks I should do really

200 N. Uhm I don't think she's made a decision at the moment and I think she's waiting to see . . .

202 P. No, alright

203 N. . . . what the X-ray shows tomorrow . . .

204 P. Okay

205 N. . . . Joyce

206 P. But I'm getting worse

207 N. Mmm I think so (3.0) what does it feel like to you Joyce

208 P. It's very tight I know it's worse it's the breathing that worries me (.) like I feel as if I'm never going to breathe again

210 N. Mmm

211 P. They will be able to help me won't they (1.0) I can't go round like this you see not breathing (4.4)

213 N. I hope we'll be able to relieve the tightness in your chest but I can't promise that we'll be able to take the breathlessness away altogether

215 P. No

216 N. I think we'll be able to make it a bit better than it is at the moment

217 P. Moment

218 P. (6.2) but my life is limited isn't it (2.5) from the point of view of longevity (8.0)

220 N. I think so . . .

221 P. . . . Months years (8.0)

222 N. That's a really difficult thing . . .

223 P. Mmm (4.0)

224 N. . . . to answer Joyce I think probably the person to talk to about that with would be the doctor.

Joyce's breathlessness is a new and frightening feeling for her and induces fear of impending death. This prompts Joyce to seek reassurance from the nurse that something can be done to relieve her breathlessness. The nurse gives Joyce time to voice her fears (line 198) and gently explores the catastrophic understanding of her impending death (lines 196, 207, 213–214 and 220–224). Unbeknown to Joyce and the nurse the cancer has spread to the bones in Joyce's rib cage and shoulders and these have collapsed in on her lungs, causing her current breathing difficulties. In the next extract, Joyce gives a vivid description of her embodied experience of the metastatic spread of her cancer:

380 P. I can't can't unbend my shoulders either that's another thing I why's that

381 N. I'm not sure about that

382 P. . . . My shoulders are all hunched up and I can't

383 N. . . . Yeh I noticed that

384 P. I can't get them straight I have to do like a little old (.) hunch back. It doesn't straighten out that doesn't help either (.) it's uncomfortable for me (1.3) radiotherapy wouldn't help me really any more would it

387 N. On your lungs

388 P. no well on my sort of try to do something to my back

389 N. I'm not sure (3.8) possibly that's something else you could talk to doctor about tomorrow I really don't know what that is

391 P. You see I go like this (hunches her shoulders)

392 N. Mmm

393 P. I can't straighten out can I (4.0) I can't get straight

394 N. Mmm (7.5)

395 P. Oh God I don't know what to do (tearful)

396 N. Come Joyce (5.0)

397 P. I just want to lead my life

398 N. Mmm (2.0)

399 P. So *simple* I don't want I don't want to ask for very much you see (2.2) just want to lead a

(.) simple life go to I mean I've got it's a very mundane little job but I like it and (3.2) and a nice little flat I mean it needs a lot of money spent on it but I like it and I've got what I want and (.) and now all this happens (7.5) it's my mouth's so sore I can't eat properly (4.4.) I mean I suppose some of these ulcers are on my throat as well probably (.) which doesn't help

405 N. Mmm mmm

406 P. Mmm

407 N. That *will* get better

408 P. Mmm

409 N. I (.) can assure you that erm yeh (3.2.) mmm (7.0) know this is really hard for you (5.2)

410 P. I don't know what to do (1.0) or say or think (14.0) sorry it's uncomfortable for you here (leaning on the window ledge) . . . but it's the only way I can

412 N. . . . I'm fine (.) no don't worry I'm fine (28.2)

413 P. They'll probably give me something tomorrow do you think (2.0) mmmm

414 N. Yeh I hope so (1.0) try something (7.5) it might be that they could try some radiotherapy (4.4.) I don't know whether they'd be able to do that tomorrow . . .

416 P. . . . No . . .

417 N. . . . Its probably unlikely but erm that might help (4.0).

At first the nurse takes her cue from Joyce's description and considers with Joyce different treatment possibilities (lines 387 and 389). There is then a qualitative shift in the nature of Joyce's expression. From not being able to get her shoulders straight (line 384), she conveys very accurately her all-encompassing anxiety of not being able to 'straighten out' and understand her situation (line 393). This reading of the conversation is borne out in Joyce's explanation that she just wants to lead her life (lines 399–404). It seems that here, Joyce is attempting to reconcile wants for a 'simple life' with what is happening to her. Her anxiety and fear overwhelm her and unconsciously she wishes to rid herself of these feelings and for them to be 'contained' by the nurse. Joyce cannot bear speaking of her anxieties directly for very long and perhaps not surprisingly returns to describing her worries about her mouth ulceration and sore throat (lines 399–404).

This raises an interesting point about how far the nurse limits or engages her interpretive energy and skills in the face of the symptoms of cancer illness and treatment. In describing her sore mouth at this point Joyce is perhaps giving further voice to her overwhelming anxiety by associating primitive feelings and needs from childhood for feeding and being held. It appears very difficult for the nurse to receive Joyce's anxious communication at this point and she responds by acknowledging the symptoms Joyce is experiencing and reassures Joyce that these can be alleviated. It is distressing being with someone who is really upset and, just like the people we care for, we have ways of reducing the emotional discomfort. In her own reflection on the conversation the nurse described:

> The overriding thing is of erhm feeling absolutely helpless in the face of this extreme breathlessness and just and you know hoping against hope that they would actually be able to do something tomorrow but thinking probably they wouldn't. Poor Joyce. Poor woman, just lying there going 'huh huh' and it's just awful, you can't do anything.

The nurse continues to discuss the management of Joyce's symptoms and avoids directly addressing her anxiety. She fears causing Joyce additional distress and perhaps taking away hope. Joyce herself returns to her anxious thoughts after 5 minutes:

473 P. I don't know what to think I don't know what to do (34.0) miserable isn't it (laughs)

474 N. Mmm (5.1) you're doing really well Joyce

475 P. I'm not really it's it's just a miserable life I want to sort to breathe (4.2.) if I could just breathe a little is that *too* much

476 N. (6.0) Mmm (0.8) the tongue I think won't get better straight away but it *will* get better *that* I can assure you it won't always be like this (.) your breathing we might not be able to get back to normal but I hope that we'll be able to get it significantly better than it is now

480 P. Mmm (5.0) but the tight there isn't it

482 N. The tightness yeh

483 P. The bones is it in the bones

484 N. No it's inside the lungs themselves

485 P. Oh

486 N. Some sort of plaques

487 P. Yes tumour things (1.9)

488 N. Yeh

489 P. It won't go away will it

490 N. No they were hoping that they would be able to erase them with the chemotherapy . . .

491 P. . . . But I've only had two chemos so far

492 N. I know yeh there is a possibility that

493 P. I mean are you saying now that maybe the chemo's not going to do it

495 N. That's what they don't know

496 P. Mmm . . .

497 N. . . . but that's why doctor wanted to see you straightaway with an X-ray so she can . . .

498 P. Mmm mmm

499 N. . . . Have a good look at what's happening and see *you* at the same time

500 P. I mean it's only two weeks since I saw the consultant could it happen in such a space of time I suppose it could anything can't it

502 N. Mmm (20.2)

503 P. I'll just have to hope that tomorrow I can breathe (2.0) because if I can't I don't know what I'm going to do (4.2)

505 N. With regards to getting there

506 P. Oh no no no I mean just from the point of view of just being able to breathe again (.) oh no I'll get there (6.2)

508 N. But tomorrow they'll be able to do something is that what you're saying

509 P. Mmm uhm mmm (5.2)

510 N. I think it's quite important that you emphasise that to the doctor when you see her

512 P. Mmm uhm

513 N. That actually (.) the situation as it is right now (.) is (.) not something that you can live with.

In her long pauses and statements Joyce clearly gives the nurse an experience of what it is like 'not to know what to think or do'. The nurse's responses (lines 474, 476–479) indicate perhaps that she is at a loss to know what to do or think as well, in the uncertain context of Joyce's sudden deterioration. Joyce clearly wants the nurse to perform some thinking function for her. The nurse responds in practical ways and with clinical solutions, leaving unanswered Joyce's question, 'Is it too much to ask, to just breathe a little?'

It is important to consider the nature of reassurance in helping with fear and anxiety and whether, in the face of worrying evidence to the contrary, reassurance can leave the person feeling unsafe, and at risk of losing confidence in the nurse. It is also important to consider ways in which the nurse might have communicated more strongly her understanding of Joyce's predicament and feelings. The nurse recognised that the ability to receive the feelings that Joyce engendered in her was the key to future work in helping Joyce with her fear and anxiety. This led the nurse to communicate her understanding of Joyce's predicament and feelings more effectively than demonstrated in these extracts.

This example vividly demonstrates the dynamics of container and contained in attempts to understand.

Helping with guilt

Clarrie is 28 years old and has leukaemia. She is married and has three young children. Clarrie has been in hospital for 8 weeks because her disease relapsed after treatment. The nurse has been closely involved with Clarrie throughout her treatment. This extract is taken from an hour-long conversation they had together after Clarrie indicated to the nurse that she was feeling particularly 'fed up':

200 P. My mum scares me (.) she's the one really upsets me (cries)

201 N. She's your mum

202 P. Mmm (crying)

203 N. It's just her way of is she angry do you think that it's happened

204 P. I don't know (.) she's not saying (1.2) I mean she has said to me before that 'why why you'(.)

I mean I could ask the same question (giggles) I would not ask myself that (.) 'cos things like that happen all the time and you (.) just because you are not in it you don't know about it (.) you hear about it like on telly and things (1.8) and yeh you think I won't ask that I think I dread to ask that not towards me but towards other people (.) 'cos you're made to feel like rot (.) I think I've done this to them (her family)

301 N. You haven't done anything to them, Clarrie

302 P. What do you

303 N. You have got leukaemia through no fault of your own (.) through nothing you've

305 P. No you know what my sister-in-law said to me (.) she said to me that it was my fault

307 N. Why would it be your fault

308 P. . . . I don't know

309 N. . . . How could it possibly be

310 P. I told my sister that (cries) I thought why (.) and I couldn't understand (.) I *couldn't* understand why she said it I think thinking that I'd done something that's why I'd got it

313 N. There's nothing you could have done to make you get leukaemia little children get leukaemia

315 P. I know I kept thinking (.) what I kept thinking 'why'

316 N. Well believe me . . .

317 P. If she'd told my husband that can you imagine what he would then start thinking you know (1.2.) I probably caused it (sobbing)

319 N. Please believe me you've got nothing to reproach yourself about you didn't cause this leukaemia it just happened to you you had no say in the matter

321 P. A grown woman telling me that it's my fault if I had known something maybe I would have acted sooner

323 N. But that maybe wouldn't have altered anything anyway but *Clarrie* you didn't know you DIDN'T KNOW you had this last year and you didn't know when you just felt tired and unwell but . . .

326 P. Do you (9.5) (cries) when I think about that at the time (cries) I think about that and I'm trying to work out why it was my fault.

Clarrie is focusing on the consequences of what she has or has not done to get leukaemia and thus 'hurt' her family (lines 204, 311–312). Her sister-in-law personifies the persecutory, blaming part of herself that tells her that she is guilty of bringing the disease on herself and her family. The nurse recognises this self-blaming as a negative and faulty cognition (lines 301, 303) and wants to help Carrie see that her thinking is being fuelled by irrational beliefs and feelings, perhaps of excessive responsibility in relation to the cause of the cancer. The nurse directly challenges Clarrie's thinking (lines 307, 309) and reinforces less negative, 'right' thinking about the onset of her leukaemia (lines 313, 319).

It appears from the extract that the illness re-evokes painful needs in Clarrie's family relationships, which are mentioned but not fully articulated or discussed (lines 200, 204–300). Clarrie gives an indication that she is not experiencing her mother as supportive or nuturing and that she resents having to carry the emotional burden of her illness for her mother as well as for her own children. The nurse considered that Clarrie's negative thoughts had had a strange hold for some time and that she needed to work with Clarrie and some members of her family on this and a number of related issues over a period of several weeks. Together they decided to explore:

- how Clarrie first suspected she was unwell
- her partner's and family's immediate reaction to her diagnosis, including how they had been told and what they each now understood of the diagnosis
- what had changed for Clarrie and her partner and Clarrie and her mother and what they had discovered about each other since her diagnosis
- the impact of these discoveries on their relationships and parenting
- what they now wanted from each other.

Helping with anger and hostility

This is an example of low-key verbal aggression by a 45-year-old woman, Susan, in hospital for chemotherapy to treat a recurrence of her breast cancer. Susan's anger is directed first at the nurses caring for a dying woman on the ward and then at

doctors, who she does not perceive consider the individual communication needs of people in their care. She tells the nurse:

64 P. I've been a bit sort of upset at the way erhm (.) she's looked after very well in terms of being cleaned and turned and whatever but there's not an *awful* lot of time erhm that's devoted to all the little things I think she's very abrupt but then she has a right to be hasn't she (0.6) I mean if you're on your way out you can be any way you like (2.6)

69 N. It's not just . . .

70 P. . . . I sometimes think some people don't know how to approach someone they are very cheerful and 'how are you today' you know and 'those are nice flowers' but that's not what I think someone wants to hear they want to get down to the nitty gritty you know and talk about what's happening you know and I think the consultants are not very good at that either . . .

75 N. Some aren't always perhaps er I mean *you* saw Dr Thorn this morning and were you able to get down to the nitty gritty

77 P. Well it was all very cheerful in that he said I wouldn't expect it to come back and he said I'd be very unlucky if it did but I still don't know whether he's actually saying that because of all the years of experience or whether he's saying it because it's cheerful (laughs) you know and I would like him to talk to me as if he were talking to another doctor

82 N. What do you think he might have said about you to another doctor

83 P. And I think consultants are so erhm used to being jolly that sometimes they forget you want to talk you know brass tacks really

85 N. Yeh yeh.

86 P. You know I don't know everyone is different (.) but I think erhm maybe they should try and gauge what kind of a person you are

88 N. Yes . . .

89 P. . . . If you want to hear or not (2.7) I'm sure they do try but I think there's a lot of 'be better for her if I didn't' which makes me cross 'cos of the sort of person I am (.) I think when they are ill erhm they need special treatment and I think they need to be *really* asked how they are feeling

93   N.   Yes (.) yes

94   P.   You know and not just say 'oh how are you?'(.) 'good, fine' you know

95   N.   Well how are *you* feeling Susan

96   P.   Well I you know still have seeds of doubt in my head thinking there must be people here who've had treatment like I've had and then they've come back and that's why I'd like the doctor to be frank because I hate that sort of feeling of of er you don't have all the facts and I well I think I wanted to sort of make my feelings apparent (.) I was frightened I would appear grumpy and ungracious but if someone's ill I think then you have to sort of with (.) your yard's measure of people's behaviour has to go out of the window.

103   N.   My yard stick is away so can you tell me what sort of feelings you wanted . . .

104   P.   . . . You know without being rude or anything I did I am very I'm made (0.6) I feel very grumpy and cross.

What is immediately striking in this extract is how the language Susan uses portrays her self-identity. She is reluctant to describe herself in the first person preferring to use phrases like 'some people', and the words 'someone' and 'everyone' to distance herself from her experience and her feelings of anger, but also perhaps her uncertainty, fear, and anger in relation to the cancer itself. It may be that her anger is emerging, as denial and numbness of the news of her recurrence fade. Anger is often suppressed, perhaps unconsciously, by hospital staff in their attempts to make the environment as positive and cheerful as possible as this woman describes (lines 70–74, 77–81). It is then difficult for the person to express anger or negative thoughts and feelings, especially when staff are doing so much for them. Susan believes that more attention should be given to people's need and right to be angry and she is critical of false cheerfulness. Susan also seems to have mixed feelings of anger and dependency towards the doctors and nurses and this can make the role of carers more difficult, as it seems to here.

The challenge for the nurse attempting to help Susan to understand her angry feelings is first to help her to verbalise and own them in relation to her own situation. The nurse does this successfully

(lines 75–76, 82, 95, 103) and clearly provides a setting in which Susan feels secure enough to voice her dissatisfaction and angry feelings. The nurse does this by hearing her criticisms of care, not being defensive, and by channelling the energy of Susan's anger into asking for what she needs from professionals, all of which augurs well for Susan's emotional well-being.

Helping with a depressive response

An example of a nurse helping with a depressive response occurs when Tony, a 52-year-old man with myeloma, has been describing the problems he has been having walking with crutches and then using a wheelchair, and remarks to the nurse that 'I have to keep trying, I'm afraid, that's me'. He follows this with:

674   P.   I suppose in a way I'm worse off (2.0) I'm my own worst enemy in a way (1.2) well I don't know sometimes I ought to rest more than I do erhm I don't I keep getting into this model where I rest like I use the wheelchair and I stay in it all day long faithfully and then I try and walk (.) I've got stiff and stuff so I think well try being out of the chair a bit more and then you get tired and you want to sit in the chair and I don't know which end of the candle to put out

700   N.   Mmmm I see

701   P.   It's very difficult er whether it's just me getting worse this is what I was saying I get depressed I'm getting worse and worse and I don't know which way to go (sighs) erhm what I'd like to do is just sort of ignore the whole thing and just get on with life but I can't do that erhm (3.2) I'm no use to the kids or Dorothy (wife) I'm not sure whether I should just stay in bed I mean I've stayed in bed longer since I've been in hospital for the last two days erhm and I've never felt more tired than I do now I feel really strange so I'm not winning that either

708   N.   Yes

709   P.   I'm getting a bit tired of it all (1.2) I just want to be made better

710   N.   Yes

711   P.   I can't do much at all at the moment and I'm quite an active person normally in fact I'm

supposed to be organising a camp in two weeks' time

713 N. Are you? Where are you going to

714 P. In Sussex but I am getting quite stupified with all these pills I have been taking (1.9) it doesn't look as if I'll get there (1.2) and I feel very tired and well . . .

716 N. . . . Do you think it would be wise to have a period when you're resting and also a time when you get up and potter around

718 P. Mmm

719 N. Because then when you are resting it would be proper rest instead of just lying in bed

721 P. I've thought of that but what happens is my staying vertical is that my legs start to swell up and all my stockings start to cut in

723 N. But the other thing is you can sit out in the garden for a little while as long as you keep your feet up and er I can sort out a footstool

725 P. Oh (.) that yes would be helpful.

Tony uses the image of a candle (line 684) to represent the essence of his experience and his pronounced feelings of unhappiness. Instead of burning the candle at both ends, with its youthful connotations, Tony does not know which end of the candle to put out. The balance between fighting the illness and yielding to its implications has become dysfunctional for him. The nurse needs to work at Tony's own pace as much as possible, while being prepared to shift this balance when what is happening seems to be inappropriate. Tony is 'still trying' and the nurse encourages this (lines 716, 723–724) but perhaps does so by denying the seriousness of how Tony feels. It is the physical humiliation of the illness that disempowers Tony as he struggles to manage his pain and fatigue. For Tony to hold in his mind the incompatible images of his current state and his previous health is painful and the temptation for both him and the nurse is to switch the focus of attention on to something else or fail to take the implications on board, which avoids the distress (lines 715–716).

In this excerpt, the nurse recognised that he found it uncomfortable to confront what the physical changes of the illness meant for Tony's self-image, in terms of the value Tony placed on him-

self as a father of three young adults setting out on their careers, and as a husband. The nurse also recognised just how much Tony had revealed of his underlying concerns and sadness in this 45-minute talk. It is important to be aware of the ways we screen out pain and ask ourselves whether we inhibit the person exploring uncomfortable ideas by the methods we use to reduce our own exposure. In his future work with Tony, the nurse planned to empathise with Tony's concerns and to provide a comforting and supportive context so that Tony could be upset if he wished. Through more careful listening the nurse thought that, although he could not take away Tony's sadness and loss, he could work with Tony to shift the emphasis in his narratives from one of dependency to one of greater agency and sense of control. Tony placed considerable value on his expertise as an engineer, husband and father, and felt that helping strategies about acceptance and accepting his continuing responsibilities as a father and husband (his responsibility to help his wife and children face his illness, for example) may help to increase his sense of self-worth. The nurse considered how some of this work might take place with another family member, intrinsic to Tony's sense of self-worth.

Understanding how gender constructs our lives and our understanding of the meaning of care is growing. In this clinical example, a male nurse is talking with Tony and it is to this nurse that Tony is able to voice some of his worries. Tony's illness and incapacity presents an enormous challenge to his gendered identity. Bringing thoughts about gender overtly into discussions with Tony and his preconceptions about providing and receiving care, might provide an alternative lens through which to explore his situation. Therefore, it may be useful for the nurse to explore with Tony how being a man influences his response to cancer.

Helping when treatment fails

Phyllis is a 75-year-old woman with endometrial cancer. Phyllis suspects that the cancer might have spread:

442 P. I suppose I will find out when I'll get sorted out in the end

443 N. (0.2) Yes (0.6) but what would I mean what if they turned around and they said there's nothing really we can do about it

445 P. There's nothing I can do about it is there

446 N. No (.) 'cos I mean 'cos that 'cos that could be a possibility I mean 'cos you have been in a week and if there was anything they were going to do

448 P. That's what I mean yeh

450 N. They'd erhm (0.6)

451 P. I mean if I've got it somewhere else then it's

452 N. You've obviously thought about that

453 P. Yeh well you 'ave to don't ya (3.4) (clears throat) I mean it's hard

454 N. (2.5) Oh dear I know

455 P. (1.7) It's not that I'm frightened I *am* frightened but I'm not frightened if you know what I mean

457 N. (2.4) Yes

458 P. Err

459 N. What are you frightened of

460 P. Oh I don't know

461 N. It's the *not* knowing it's

462 P. I don't know what I am frightened of I mean (0.2) I mean I don't know if it's er (2.4) I don't know I really don't know

464 N. The uncertainty or

465 P. Well yeh in one way (0.2) erm but erm (3.2) depends what I am you know . . .

466 N. Yeh

467 P. . . . I think it's more that (1.2) *if* it has gone inside somewhere else

468 N. Yes

469 P. (0.2) How am I gonna feel how am I gonna get you know what I mean

470 N. Yes it's . . .

471 P. You know am I goin' to be *really* ill and in *pain* or you know what I mean

472 N. Yes

473 P. You know the things you you the things you you know what I mean

474 N. (3.2) There are things that we can deal with when they come

475 P. Yes yes I mean you know I think to myself I'm just going to end in a wheelchair that's it (.) a nice wee chat (laughs)

478 N. (laughs)

479 P. Your little machine (referring to the tape-recorder).

In this extract the nurse introduces bad news, i.e. news that materially alters Phyllis's view of her future. She does this in a supportive way (lines 443–444, 446–447). A person may temporarily block news they cannot take, but at least the information is made available so that they can use it constructively when they are ready. Here the nurse gives time for the idea she has raised to sink in and is not frightened of unleashing a reaction that might be difficult to deal with in the conversation. Phyllis does not block out the news by lightening the mood and changing the topic of the conversation until line 477. Up to this point she explores some of her thoughts about treatment failure. Even though the nurse tries to anticipate what Phyllis might be feeling (lines 461, 464), Phyllis does express her own particular concerns and uncertainty within the context of the supportive conversation with the nurse. Phyllis sets the agenda for subsequent conversations with this particular nurse. She wanted to talk more fully about what might happen to her as she got closer to death and how the family and friends could help her at home. The nurse agreed to do this in three half-hour conversations before Phyllis was discharged the following week.

Conclusion

Despite the urgency of the possibility of death for some cancer patients, it is important that nurses' therapeutic strategies proceed at a pace that feels safe, a pace dictated by the person and the nurse. Decisions about what feels safe to share rest with the individual and their family and this also influences the timing and pacing of the work. Creating space for the person to gain some understanding of their own response to cancer can help them to retain competence and integrity.

The extracts above are powerful reminders of the fear, anxiety, guilt, and humiliation that can disempower people as they struggle to manage pain, discomfort, fatigue, and disfigurement from cancer. It is therefore essential that we all examine what we can do in our different contexts to help and empower the people we meet in our work. This includes ensuring that our own authority and 'knowingness', manifest in a dogmatic application of our knowledge about cancer illness, do not lead to sterile, unhelpful interpretations of experience that unwittingly undermine the dignity of individuals.

All too easily we can find ourselves responding to people in terms of our familiarity with a certain theory or our clinical experience. We then attach to the person the understanding that we have gleaned elsewhere, even though it may not apply to this particular individual. We are most likely to engage in clichéd thinking about people when we feel insecure about our clinical understanding. By prematurely believing we recognise what the person is communicating, even if we don't, we can preserve the appearance of being competent. There is a danger in this: that we identify worries on the sole basis of similarity rather than from a genuine process of collaborative, consensual working with an individual.

The pitfalls of preconceptions are a hazard, and not only for the inexperienced nurse. A similar danger lies in wait for the experienced nurse who might have got into a rut with his or her thinking, or be a bit too sure. It is so tempting to use short cuts to insight based on what has made sense with other patients, particularly when we are working in very busy clinical settings.

Effective clinical supervision is an essential venue for prompting us to re-orientate our thinking and question assumptions we might hold about a person with cancer, so that we remain receptive and responsive to them and feel supported in our work.

References

1. Cooper C.L. and Watson M. (eds.) (1991). *Cancer and Stress: Psychological, Biological and Coping Studies.* Chichester: Wiley.
2. Barraclough J. (1994). *Cancer and Emotion: A Practical Guide to Psycho-oncology*, 2nd edition. Chichester: Wiley.
3. Greer S. and Watson M. (1987). Mental adjustment to cancer: its measurement and prognostic importance. *Cancer Surveys* **6**, 439–451.
4. Kreitler S., Chaitchik S. and Kreitler H. (1993). Repressiveness: cause or result of cancer. *Psycho-oncology* **2**, 43–54.
5. Doan B.D. and Gray R.E. (1992). The heroic cancer patient: a critical analysis of the relationship between illusion and mental health. *Canadian Journal of Behavioral Science* **24(2)**, 253–266.
6. Zorza R. and Zorza V. (1980). *A Way to Die: Living to the End.* London: Deutsch.
7. Duncker P. and Wilson V. (eds.) (1966). *Cancer Through the Eyes of Ten Women.* London: Harper Collins.
8. Burnard P. (1994). *Counselling Skills for Health Professionals*, 2nd edition. Campling J. (ed.) *Therapy in Practice Series.* London: Chapman and Hall.
9. Jacobs M. (1988). *Psychodynamic Counselling in Action.* London: Sage.
10. Tschudin V. (1995). *Counselling Skills for Nurses*, 4th edition. London: Baillière Tindall.
11. Altschuler J. (1997). *Working with Chronic Illness: A Family Approach.* In Frosh S. (ed.) *Basic Texts in Counselling and Psychotherapy.* London: Macmillan.
12. Moorey S. and Greer S. (1989). *Psychological Therapy for Patients with Cancer: A New Approach.* Oxford: Heinemann.
13. Judd D. (1995). *Give Sorrow Words: Working with a Dying Child*, 2nd edition. London: Whurr.
14. Cox M. (1988). *Structuring the Therapeutic Process: Compromise with Chaos.* London: Jessica Kingsley.
15. Gregory J. (1996). *The Psychosocial Education of Nurses: The Interpersonal Dimension.* Aldershot: Avebury.
16. Casement P. (1985). *On Learning from the Patient.* London: Routledge.
17. Egan E. (1994). *The Skilled Helper: A Systematic Approach to Effective Helping*, 5th edition. Belmont, CA: Brooks/Cole.
18. Murgatroyd S. (1985). *Counselling and Helping.* London: Routledge.
19. Mearns D. and Thorne B. (1988). *Person-centred Counselling in Action.* London: Sage.
20. Nelson-Jones R. (1993). *Practical Counselling and Helping Skills*, 3rd edition. London: Cassell.
21. Klein M. (1937). *Love, Guilt and Reparation and Other Works*, 1975 edition. London: Hogarth.

22. Kelly G. (1955). *The Psychology of Personal Constructs*, Vols 1 and 2. New York: Norton.

23. Perls F. (1969). *Gestalt Therapy Verbatim*. California: Lafayette.

24. Berne E. (1964). *Games People Play*. Harmondsworth: Penguin.

25. Harris T. (1973). *I'm OK You're OK*. London: Pan.

26. Rogers C.R. (1951). *Client-centred Therapy*. Boston, MA: Houghton Mifflin.

27. Ellis A. (1962). *Reason and Emotion in Psychotherapy*. New York: Lyle Stuart.

28. Krumboltz J.D. and Thorenson C.E. (1969). *Behavioural Counselling: Cases and Techniques*. New York: Holt, Rinehart and Winston.

29. Bandler R. (1985). *Using Your Brain – For a Change*. Moab, UT: Real People Press.

30. Glasser W. (1965). *Reality Therapy*. New York: Harper and Row.

31. Ferruci P. (1982). *What We May Be*. Wellingborough: Thorson.

32. Freud S. (1938). An outline of psychoanalysis. In Strachey J. (ed.) *The Standard Edition of the Complete Psychological Works of Sigmund Freud*, Vol. 23. London: Hogarth.

33. Bion W.R. (1962). A theory of thinking. *International Journal of Psycho-analysis* **43**, Parts 4–5.

34. Beck A.T. (1976). *Cognitive Therapy and the Emotional Disorders*. New York: International Universities Press.

35. Frankl V.E. (1959). *Man's Search for Meaning*. New York: Beacon Press.

36. Silver R.L. and Wortman C.B. (1980). Coping with undesirable life events. In Garber J. and Seligman M.E.P. (eds.) *Human Helplessness: Theory and Application*. New York: Academic Press.

37. Brody H. (1987). *Stories of Sickness*. New Haven, CT: Yale University Press.

38. Linde C. (1993). *Life Stories: The Creation of Coherence*. Oxford: Oxford University Press.

39. Segrave E. (1995). *Diary of a Breast*. London: Faber & Faber.

40. Butler S. and Rosenblum B. (1994). *Cancer in Two Voices*. London: Women's Press.

41. Picardie R. (1998). *Before I Say Goodbye*. London: Penguin.

42. Morrison B. (1993). *And When Did You Last See Your Father?* London: Granta Books.

43. Dennison A. (1996). *Uncertain Journey: A Woman's Experience of Living With Cancer*. London: Patten Press.

44. Ortony A. (1993). Metaphor, language and thought. In Ortony A. (ed.) *Metaphor and Thought*. Cambridge: Cambridge University Press.

45. Lakoff G. and Johnson M. (1980). *Metaphors We Live By*. Chicago, IL: University of Chicago Press.

46. Sontag S. (1991). *Illness as Metaphor*. Harmondsworth: Penguin Books (first published in 1978).

47. Stacey J. (1997). *Teratologies: A Cultural Study of Cancer*. London: Routledge.

48. Savage J. (1995). *Nursing Intimacy: An Ethnographic Approach to Nurse–Patient Interaction*. London: Scutari Press.

49. Bailey C. (1996). *Derrida, de Man, Habermas: implications for qualitative analysis of interviews in cancer care research. A methodological study*. M.Sc. thesis, University of London.

50. Froggatt K. (1998). The place of metaphor and language in exploring nurses' emotional work. *Journal of Advanced Nursing* **28**, 332–338.

51. Lanceley A. (1995). Emotional disclosure between cancer patients and nurses. In Richardson A. and Wilson-Barnett J. (eds.) *Nursing Research in Cancer Care*. London: Scutari Press, pp. 167–188.

52. Kleinman A. (1988). *The Illness Narratives: Suffering Healing and the Human Condition*. New York: Basic Books.

53. Mishler E.G. (1986). *Research Interviewing – Context and Narrative*. Cambridge, MA: Harvard University Press.

54. Gilbert A. (1994). *Personal Communication of Transference and Counter Transference*. London: Tavistock Centre.

55. Futterman A.D. and Wellisch, D.K. (1990). Psychodynamic themes of bone marrow transplant. *Haematology/Oncology Clinics of North America* **4**, 699–709.

56. Emanuel R.B. (1990). Counter-transference: a spanner in the works or a tool for understanding. *Journal of Educational Therapy* **3**, 3–12.

57. Bion W.R. (1962). *Learning from Experience*. New York: Jason Aronson.

58. Emanuel R.B. (1992). *Personal Communication on Containment, Cure, Care or Control*. London: Tavistock Centre.

59. Carkhuff R.R. (1987). *The Art of Helping*, 6th edition. Amherst, MA: Human Resource Development Press.

Part 3

The Experience of Treatment

Introduction

Cancer, its construction, and society's response to it, has been highlighted as pervasive and problematic. Characterised by fear and uncertainty, this response shapes the very environment in which people with cancer find themselves, and has been explored in the preceding chapters. The experience of having cancer treatment is much less evident in the cancer literature than the events surrounding being given a diagnosis of cancer. Instead, the focus has been on the efficacy of cancer treatment, measured as the proportion of people who will survive 5 years from the point at which they were diagnosed.

When oncology emerged as a medical speciality in the 1950s, survival from cancer of any type was relatively poor; few people would expect to survive their illness. A number of critical developments in cancer treatment has transformed the chances of surviving a number of cancers; from a situation of near certain death, to the possibility of cure. This has been particularly evident in childhood cancers, some of the leukaemias and in testicular teratoma. Early diagnosis, accurate staging, and multi-modal therapy (the use of multiple cancer treatments: surgery, chemotherapy, radiotherapy; and multiple-agent rather than single-agent chemotherapy) have made progress in cancer treatment possible. In other situations, cancer treatment is increasing in sophistication so that some of the side-effects and difficulties of treatment have been reduced. More recently, developments in molecular biology and genetics have made a vast new range of treatments possible (see Chapter 16); while most are experimental at present, many are likely to become part of mainstream treatment. These new treatments, and in particular issues around cancer genetics are already presenting challenges and dilemmas to those working in cancer treatment settings.

Advances in molecular biology have led to the understanding of cancer as a genetic disease (not to be confused with an inherited disease); although inherited cancers are the focus of a large research effort, these probably only account for about 1% of all cancers[1] and are discussed in Chapter 15. The genetic basis of cancer suggests a model whereby cancer initially develops from cells that have undergone a series of genetic mutations or alterations. As a result, cells become unable to respond to intra- or extracellular signals that control proliferation, differentiation and cell death. According to Hill,[2] cancer treatment can be thought of as adding negative signals to the cellular environment, and thus arresting or inhibiting tumour cell growth and multiplication. It is hoped that these will prevent the development of further cancer cells at the originating site or sites of metastatic growth at any other site in the body. The object of cancer science is to develop new and better methods of preventing the growth of cancer cells. The reality for people in cancer clinics is rather different, since it is impossible to detect cancer cells within the body once a tumour has been removed; cancer treatment is inevitably sometimes given where little is known about whether it is needed for any given individual. This can only be projected through estimates of risk, based on studies of cancer populations. Here lies a dilemma for the treatment team that is difficult to convey to people facing the devastating news of a cancer diagnosis; the personal accounts presented throughout this section convey the difficulty of living with this uncertainty for people.

Cancer treatment is an uncertain venture and is often experimental. The extent to which treatment will be effective in preventing future cancer spread is often unknown, yet it involves many side-effects both at the time of treatment, or in the long term, such as infertility or the risk of developing a second cancer, or permanent disfigurement or disability. Little is known about how people with cancer make choices about treatments in the light of their own risk of developing progressive cancer at some future date. This, when accompanied by the fear engendered by cancer, creates a cocktail of anxiety mixed with various personal and professional agendas, and makes genuine partnership in planning care and treatment difficult.

Studies of the quality of life of people undergoing cancer treatment have used questionnaires to evaluate the impact of treatment on the individual. The effects of cancer treatment on an individual's ability to function, the physical and emotional symptoms they may experience, and the social and psychological sequelae of cancer are reported by the patient, usually through a series of rating scales. These studies have documented the many effects of cancer and its treatment but, unfortunately, they have tended to be seen as simply an adjunct, or additional piece of data to be collected alongside survival data, for monitoring the side-effects of cancer therapies. By being combined with side-effect data, the relevance and impact of these data have been reduced in importance, so that insufficient information exists regarding the problems and difficulties that accompany cancer treatment. Studies of quality of life in people undergoing cancer treatment have offered little insight into the turmoil and confusion surrounding cancer treatment, or the sheer difficulty of living through the devastating effects that it can have on daily life.

The purpose of this section is to provide insights into the experience of cancer treatment through the use of personal accounts from people. Information is also presented on different treatment modalities and strategies for managing the problems people face while undergoing treatment. Nursing is presented as central to managing the experience of treatment, both emotionally and physically. An increasing number of nursing research studies is being undertaken into the problems caused by cancer treatment and findings from these studies are presented throughout. In time, it is hoped that nursing will make its own, unique contribution to the science of cancer treatment; in particular, in exposing the need for a more patient-focused culture in cancer treatment.

References

1. Bishop T. (1996). Genetic predisposition to cancer: an introduction. In Eeles R., Ponder B.A.J., Easton D.F. and Horwich A. (eds.) *Genetic Predisposition to Cancer*. London: Chapman and Hall.
2. Hill R.P. and Tannock I.F. (1998). Introduction to cancer biology. In Tannock I.F. and Hill R.P. (eds.) *The Basic Science of Oncology*, 3rd edition. New York: McGraw Hill.

The experience of treatment

Jessica Corner and Danny Kelly

The treatment journey with cancer (see Figure 9.1) is often long and arduous and may involve many stages and different treatments spanning months or years. This is illustrated by the personal accounts by Jackie Stacey.[1] The first account (9.1) describes her diagnosis following surgery, and the second the experience of undergoing months of chemotherapy.

Diagnosis

The process of receiving a diagnosis of cancer is not straightforward, as Jackie Stacey's account illustrates. Formal diagnosis within biomedicine requires the collection of data through a series of tests, investigations, acquiring tissue specimens from biopsies, needle aspirations or surgery, scans and histological or radiological reports. From the earliest moment when someone finds a lump, or reports some abnormality in the way their body is functioning, suspicions of cancer are aroused both for the person themselves, and for the health professional determining a course of action in response. Almost always there is a mismatch in time between the fear, anxiety, and confusion surrounding an increasing awareness that this might be cancer, and the biomedical system's confirmation that this is indeed the case. The battery of tests and investigations takes time to compile and interpret. A clear diagnosis is not always easy to determine, and even when this can be confirmed quickly, confusion and delay can occur as the exact type, stage, and location of the cancer is investigated to determine the

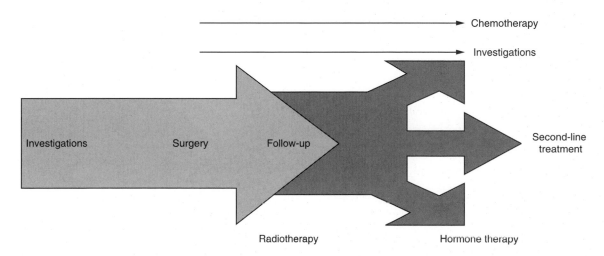

Figure 9.1 The treatment journey for cancer.

Personal account 9.1: The diagnosis

After surgery for an ovarian cyst I keep vomiting for several days.

'Why am I still being sick? Doesn't the anaesthetic usually wear off faster than this?'

Eventually I am told they've taken a biopsy of the bowel.

As in all good narratives, each answer leads to a new question.

'Why does a bowel biopsy produce continued vomiting?'

'The bowel is a very sensitive organ and stops working if interfered with. Vomiting is quite a common response.'

'And why have they taken a biopsy of the bowel?'

'To do some tests.'

What tests, no one will say. I am baffled.

The director of the hospital pokes his head around the curtain which surrounds my bed on the surgical ward. Unannounced, he robs me of my fragile privacy. He is the one I most dread dealing with. I saw him on my first visit to the ward. Mobile phone in hand, exuding paternalistic pride and arrogance, he had sped through this ward full of women recovering from hysterectomies, calling out to them one by one at the top of his voice to ask if they has 'passed wind' yet (a crucial sign of recovery after such surgery, I was later informed).

I am throwing up as he enters. Ignoring this he announces casually:

'You won't need further surgery but you may need further treatment. You've only got one child, haven't you? So we shall try to preserve your fertility in case you want another.'

'I don't have any children', I inform him.

'Have one of mine, I've got too many.'

And with this generous offer which amuses him enormously he leaves.

I am puzzled. I am not aware that there is any possibility of needing further treatment. What could this piece of information mean? My head and stomach spin. Waves of nausea are now accompanied by waves of panic and confusion.

Desperate to find out more, I ask for the doctor who performed the emergency surgery. Unlike her self-important boss, she sits down and at least pretends to have the time to talk. Though reluctant, she gradually lets slip a few more clues. I press her for an explanation. I may need further treatment, she confirms.

'What kind?' I ask, genuinely – incredibly – ignorant.

She hesitates and resents being put on the spot.

'Chemotherapy', she replies eventually . . .

'Do you mean I have cancer?'

'We're testing to see if the cyst was benign or malignant. I'm sorry. We've had to take biopsies from various organs to check – bowel, the ovary and so on. The cyst looked a bit nasty, but I can't tell you until the tests come back. You may need three month's chemotherapy. The test result will come back in a couple of days.'

She leaves. I am left with the news. Alone, but surrounded by strangers. I don't think they planned it this way. I don't think they planned it all. Perhaps that's the problem.

But the nurses are furious. They had plans. They had plans to keep it quiet until more definite news came. They are agitated. This unexpected revelation by a doctor had thrown them off course; they are left to deal with the fall out. They mutter to one another under their breath.

(Reproduced with permission from Stacey J. (1997). *Teratologies: A Cultural Study of Cancer*. London: Routledge, pp.104–105.)[1]

type of treatment that might be recommended, and most crucially an idea of the likely prognosis or course the disease might take. This time is fraught with difficulty. The uncertainty for all concerned leaves many dilemmas as to how much to reveal or withhold until confirmation of cancer is available.

As Jackie Stacey's account illustrates, how the process of diagnosis and determining the stage and type of disease is dealt with by the health care team shapes the experience, as well as the nature of the ongoing relationship that will be established throughout treatment and beyond. Biomedicine, while a powerful vehicle for identifying and treating disease, is also a means by which health professionals can find refuge from their own anxieties in dealing with the situation, leading to exclusion of the person undergoing investigation or treatment. This is not as straightforward as the debate surrounding 'to tell or not to tell' or even 'how to tell bad news' in the communication literature suggests. How information giving is constructed and managed, often in a situation where considerable uncertainty exists for the health care team, as well as for the person who has cancer, is one of the most challenging aspects of working in cancer care.

O'Mary (1997)[3] defines this stage in the illness as that of diagnostic evaluation, classification and staging. The goal is to determine the tissue type of the malignancy, its primary site (where the cancer originated), the extent of the disease, and the tumour's potential to recur in the future. This information is needed in order to determine therapeutic management.

The investigations needed for diagnostic evaluation vary according to the type of suspected cancer, the particular signs and symptoms, the person's general health, and the type of anticipated treatment. Simultaneously, a picture of the disease itself is developed, as well as an understanding of the general health of the person who has it, for example, a woman who is entirely well, who has discovered a breast lump, or the situation may be more complex, for example, someone who has presented with signs of advanced cancer, such as weight loss, pain, or bowel obstruction. In some cases it may prove impossible to determine the primary site from which a metastatic cancer has arisen.

Diagnostic tests used to guide decision making

As cancer can involve every organ in the body, and present as one of more than 100 different diseases, the diagnostic phase is crucial to gathering accurate data about the nature of the malignancy and how best the treatment available can be employed.

At initial presentation there is likely to be some history of worrying symptoms, which have guided the person to seek advice (although those diagnosed through screening programmes or a health check may be unaware of any changes at all prior to diagnosis).

The treatment decision-making process begins by the gathering of relevant data; this will commonly involve acquiring a detailed medical history before a range of diagnostic tests is undertaken.

The purpose of such procedures is to help to classify the cancer in terms of its pathology, range of spread and potential to put the person's life at risk.[3] Staging of cancer normally follows the internationally recognised TNM system.

Staging will thereafter remain a recurring feature throughout the treatment process and will provide ongoing data to direct decisions regarding the need for additional therapy. Investigations used in the initial diagnostic phase are often repeated if signs of the cancer returning or progressing are reported.

Box 9.1: TNM classification of malignant tumours[4]

The TNM system for describing the anatomical extent of disease is based on the assessment of the following components:

T – the extent of the primary tumour
N – the absence or presence and extent of regional lymph nodes
M – the absence or presence of distant metastasis.

The addition of numbers to these three elements indicates the extent of the malignant disease: T0, T1, T3, T4 N0, N1, N2, N3 M0, M1.

Two further factors may be added to the classification. The certainty factor or C factor reflects the diagnostic methods used to determine extent of disease (C1 is evidence from standard diagnostic means; C2 from special diagnostic means such as CT scans or MRI; C3 from surgical exploration such as biopsy and cytology; C4 evidence derived from surgery and cytology of resected specimen; C5 evidence from autopsy). The R factor indicates the presence or absence of residual tumour, indicating effects of therapy, and is strongly indicative of prognosis (Rx, presence of residual tumour cannot be assessed; R0, no residual tumour; R1, microscopic residual tumour; R2, macroscopic residual tumour).

Staging can be correlated with treatment to produce prognostic indicators for use with similar cases in the future.[3] The TNM staging system as a predictor of prognosis is illustrated in Figure 9.2, where the relationship between tumour size and the number of axillary nodes found to be involved at diagnosis has a clear relationship with the percentage of women diagnosed with breast cancer who will survive 5 years from diagnosis.

Important technological advances in imaging technology have allowed pictures of the human body to be produced with unprecedented resolution and clarity.[5] Improved methods to visualise tumours employ techniques similar to those used in geosciences and astronomy. Detailed three-dimensional pictures can now be produced to construct images that can be rotated, magnified, and panned to assist in distinguishing between tumour and normal anatomy.

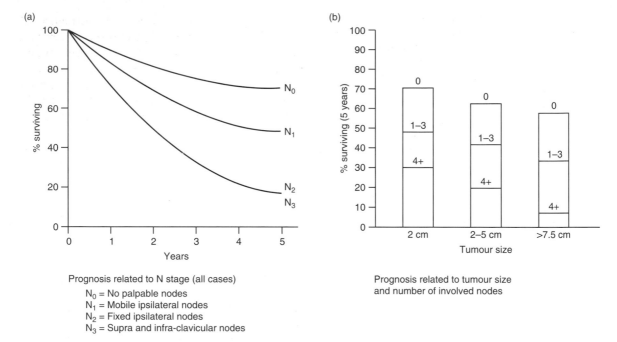

Figure 9.2 The TNM staging system as a predictor of prognosis (reproduced with permission from Souhami R. and Tobias S. (1995). *Cancer and its Management.* London: Blackwell Science Ltd).[5]

A crucial source of assessment data regarding the status of cancer will be obtained from the use of various clinical investigations. Eddy[6] provides a useful overview of these procedures; all are designed to enhance the accuracy of both cancer staging and the targeting of cancer therapies.

Box 9.2: Investigations used in cancer staging

1. **Surgical investigations**
   – biopsies, examination under anaesthetic, laryngoscopy, bronchoscopy, oesophagoscopy, mediastinoscopy, gastroscopy, colonoscopy, proctosigmoidoscopy, cystoscopy, laparotomy, colposcopy, and lumbar puncture.
2. **Haematological investigations**
   – full blood count, blood chemistry, assessment of tumour markers or electrophoresis. Different cancers can be identified through characteristic chemical alterations in the blood. Abnormalities may be seen in blood **enzymes** such as lactic dehydrogenase (elevated in 50% of patients with advanced cancer) or prostatic acid phosphatase (elevated in metastatic prostate cancer); **hormones** such as antidiuretic hormone (elevated in small cell lung cancer), human chorionic gonadotrophin (elevated in chorio-

carcinoma and testicular cancer); **metabolic products; proteins** such as IgA, D, and E, which are elevated in myeloma; **antigens** such as prostate specific antigen (PSA), a marker for the presence of prostate cancer and used for monitoring the progress of the disease, CA 125 elevated in more than 85% of cases of ovarian cancer, CA 19-9 and 72-4, indicators of gastric cancer and CA 15-3 in breast cancer.[4]
3. **Radiography**
   – chest X-ray, skeletal survey and mammography.
4. **Urine testing**
   – commonly carried out for the purposes of cytology, urinalysis, Bence Jones protein detection and screening for urinary catecholamines.
5. **Common screening investigations available**
   – mammography, cervical cytology (smear test), and faecal occult blood tests such as haem-occult.
6. **Tumour imaging**
   – using **contrast agents**: barium swallows, barium meals and enemas (barium enema will detect 70–90% of colon cancer lesions, endoscopy is used to identify cancers of the oesophagus and stomach), intravenous urograms, lymphangiograms (used in staging Hodgkin's disease and lymphoma), cholangiograms, and myelograms.
   – **radio-isotope scanning** such as a bone scan.
   – **ultrasound imaging.**

- **computerised tomography (CT)**, a technique whereby serial X-ray exposures are taken of sections of the body, which are then reconstructed into a computer-generated three-dimensional image. CT scanning is commonly used for diagnostic and staging investigations. While the scan is painless, it does require lying on a table while the scanner rotates taking many pictures. Contrast media may be injected intravenously to enhance images.
- **magnetic resonance imaging (MRI)**, which derives similar cross-sectional images as CT scanning, but places a magnetic field around the body, and uses radiofrequency pulses to re-align magnetised hydrogen nuclei throughout the body. These are excited and relaxed between pulses, creating signals of varying frequency depending on different tissue characteristics. These are then used as data by a computer to generate images, which can also be enhanced using various contrast media.

Such scans are particularly valuable for imaging the brain, spinal cord, and musculoskeletal system. An MRI scan, however, is lengthy, taking between 30 minutes and 1 hour. It also requires lying on a table, within the tubular scanner. This can be a very difficult experience, particularly for someone who is anxious, who may experience feelings of claustrophobia, or has pain or breathlessness. The machine can also be noisy, and makes a loud knocking sound. Careful preparation for the experience of the scan is important. Any metal objects that may have been implanted in the body, such as a pacemaker, surgical clips or shrapnel, could be dislodged by the scanner.[4]

Ongoing use of staging investigations allows for the fact that cancer, as a cellular disease, commonly spreads to distant sites but the extent of this spread may be difficult to determine at the time of diagnosis. Ultimately, however, the potential to develop metastatic disease may greatly influence how successful the selected interventions will prove to be. Cancer spreads either by tumour growth, or by the formation of metastases (i.e. the generation of cells within a cancer that have the ability to disseminate to form a new foci of growth at non-contiguous sites).[7] These are the major causes of death due to cancer. Metastatic spread occurs via either the lymphatics or the blood system. Tumours have different patterns of spread, and this will determine approaches to treatment. For example, cancers of the head and neck spread initially to regional lymph nodes and therefore local therapy such as surgery or radiotherapy can be curative. In contrast, in breast cancer, spread to distant sites can occur early, often before cancer is even suspected, via the

lymphatics and blood stream.[7] The formation of metastases is not automatic, and is thought to be a relatively inefficient process. Large numbers of cancer cells are known to circulate in the blood stream, and yet only a tiny proportion, estimated to be less than 1%, will form metastatic growth.[7] The difficulty is that micrometastases are impossible to detect early in the course of cancer, and therefore systemic treatments, such as chemotherapy, in those cancers known to spread widely, are used to reduce the chance of these developing. Figure 9.3 shows the mechanisms by which cancer spreads, and Table 9.1 the typical sites for metastatic cancer to arise from common cancer sites.

Making decisions about treatment

The use of classificatory systems in the diagnosis, staging, and treatment of cancer, although inevitably crude in comparison to the disease and its various manifestations, attempts to represent the particular nature of the cancer in any given individual, and is unquestionably important in the ongoing management of the disease and in making decisions about treatment. Such systems have themselves come under scrutiny. While they are a useful means by which disease can be classified, and then treatment decisions made, these are also inherently constraining and tend to remain for the exclusive use of health professionals.

Sociologists and anthropologists have sought to characterise the diagnosis and treatment of disease in contemporary health care. 'Disease' and the 'biomedical' response to it are seen as socially, historically, and culturally constituted. Bodily functions and malfunctions are seen as constructed ideas, plans, or maps, which are not real in the sense that they are unfailingly accurate representations of the body as a physiological system, but are rather an agreed understanding within Western biomedical science. This means that other understandings of disease and illness may co-exist, such as those seen in other cultures or in lay understandings of illness.[8] Indeed, a clear distinction is made between disease and illness. Disease refers to pathology, with defined signs and symptoms, whereas illness is the person's experience of health or ill-health, and the person's reaction to it.[9]

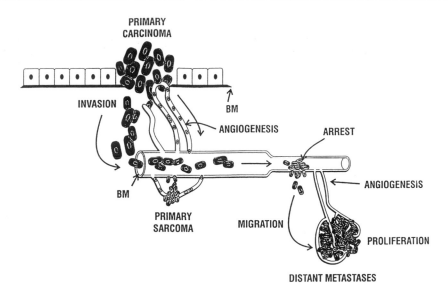

Figure 9.3 A model of the major steps of metastasis. Anchorage-independent growth of epithelial cells results in the formation of a primary carcinoma. The tumour induces the growth of blood vessels into the tumour by angiogenesis. Some cells separate from the primary tumour, invade through the basement membrane, enter the vasculature and eventually arrest in capillaries, where they extravasate out of the blood vessels into the underlying connective tissue at the metastatic site. There, further cell growth and angiogenesis results in the formation of metastatic tumour growth (reproduced with permission from Tannock I. and Hill R.P. (eds.) *The Basic Science of Oncology*, 3rd edition. New York: McGraw Hill).

Michel Foucault,[10] the French historian and philosopher, has traced the origins of modern medicine, identifying the end of the eighteenth century as a critical time in its development. This is where the modern notion of 'the clinic' begins. From this time, developments in science and medicine meant that the body was becoming visible internally. The structure and function of body organs, systems, and cells became known and conceptualised. New understandings emerged; these had a dramatic and important effect on medical thought. Before this time, medicine worked within a classificatory system, where illnesses were understood in terms of their effects, rather than with the malfunctioning body system or part that gives rise to symptoms and can be observed by the 'medical gaze', as in medicine today. As Foucault says:

> This new structure is indicated by the minute but decisive change, whereby the question 'What is the matter with you?', which the eighteenth-century dialogue between doctor and patient and patient began . . . was replaced by that other question: 'Where does it hurt?'

> . . . from then on, the whole relationship of signifier and signified, at every level of medical experience, is redistributed: between the symptoms that signify and the disease that is signified, between the description and what is described, between the event and what it prognosticates, between the lesion and the pain that it indicates. The clinic – constantly praised for its empiricism, the modesty of its attention, and the care with which it silently lets things surface to the observing gaze without disturbing them with discourse – owes its real importance to the fact that it is a reorganisation of depth, not only of medical discourse, but of the very possibility of a discourse about disease [p. xix].

The consequence of this to modern health care is that, while it has given rise to the developments in medicine that have allowed the control and cure of many diseases, it also results in the exclusion of the person from the process of diagnosing and treating or making decisions about disease. What has been created and perpetuated is a system that is professionally dominated, where the doctor holds a different and superior knowledge in relation to disease, and a language that is exclusive and excluding of individuals.

Table 9.1 Pattern of tumour spread for common cancers

Primary site of tumour	Risk of spread	Common sites of spread
Breast	***	Lymph nodes Bone Liver Lung
Lung	***	Lymph nodes Liver Bone, bone marrow Brain
Gastrointestinal tract		
Stomach	***	Local invasion Lymph nodes Liver Lung Bone
Pancreas	***	Local invasion Lymph nodes Liver Lung
Large bowel	**	Local invasion Lymph nodes Liver
Gynaecological		
Ovary	***	Local spread and invasion Lymph nodes Liver
Uterus (womb)	*	Local invasion Lymph nodes Liver
Cervix	**	Local invasion Lymph nodes
Urological		
Kidney	**	Local invasion Lymph nodes Bones Lung
Bladder	**	Local invasion Lymph nodes
Prostate	***	Local invasion Lymph nodes Bone
Melanoma	**	Local invasion and skin Lymph nodes Liver Lung Brain

Table 9.1 (Continued)

Primary site of tumour	Risk of spread	Common sites of spread
Head and neck	* or **	Local invasion Lymph node Lung
Lymphomas Hodgkin's disease	***	Lymph nodes Spleen Liver Lungs Bone/bone marrow
Non-Hodgkin's lymphoma	***	Lymph nodes Liver Bone/bone marrow Brain Lungs

(Reproduced with permission from Williams C. *All About Cancer: A Practical Guide to Cancer Care*. New York: © John Wiley and Sons).

Cancer has its own nomenclature, classifications and graphic representations of disease, as has already been shown. Paradoxically, developments in molecular biology mean that understanding of cancer is advancing beyond any model actually possible to observe in any visual sense. Increasingly, cancer is being modelled and represented in complex subcellular systems as medical science seeks to understand the disease at ever more minute levels.

The effect of the separation of the person from 'disease' is evident in Jackie Stacey's account of her experience leading up to the discovery that she had cancer. While empirical, observable information was acquired so that a definitive diagnosis could be made, she was maintained outside the system into which she was about to be initiated: the system of cancer and cancer treatment.

Unfortunately, changing this situation does not simply mean employing 'patient-centred' care, where greater involvement in decision making is encouraged, and there is more open dialogue between doctor and patient. As Silverman[11] points out:

> . . . the problem is not simply one of a benevolent totalising medicine . . . [there is] a naive view of the human subject. It seems to be assumed that we are carriers of unique experiences and that the role of conversations

(and therefore more patient-centred care) is to discover an authentic language in which these experiences can be truly understood [p. 195].

Even if we were to discover this, there is nothing to say that any new form of dialogue with health carers would necessarily be more 'authentic', nor that there are 'private languages' ready to be revealed in any straightforward way.[11] There is some evidence to suggest that where a different agenda exists and social and family experiences are taken into account during medical encounters, these may also be used as a form of medical surveillance of more intimate and personal areas of life, allowing judgements to be made about appropriate treatment, in a cost-driven health care arena, which may not be just in the interests of the individuals concerned.[11]

A number of studies has been undertaken to explore the desire of people newly diagnosed with cancer to be involved in making decisions about their treatment. In response to the general call for greater consumerism within health care, an important strand of this work has been initiated by Lesley Degner.[12] A series of investigations has been undertaken into decision-making preferences with people diagnosed with cancer, using a series of vignettes, which set out different scenarios surrounding the nature of a relationship with doctors. These can broadly be described as follows.

- *Health provider controlled decision making*: health personnel have final control over the type of treatment, while the person and family are involved to varying degrees in the actual implementation of treatment.
- *Patient controlled decision making*: the person exercises final control over the type of treatment received.
- *Family controlled decision making*: the family has final control over what treatment is given.
- *Jointly controlled decision making*: Control over the design of therapy is shared by one or more participants in decision making.

Degner and Sloan[13] have developed a tool for evaluating such preferences on a continuum from playing an active role in decision making, through a collaborative or shared role, to a passive role, where the physician or other health carer is the primary or sole decision maker. While for a general population, the majority of people would wish to have an active role, there is increasing evidence to suggest that this is not the case when diagnosed with a life-threatening illness such as cancer. In the study by Beaver *et al.*[14] of 150 women newly diagnosed with breast cancer and 200 women with benign breast disease, the majority of women with breast cancer preferred a passive role, with 20% wanting an active role, and 28% a shared role. Women who were older, were from lower socio-economic groups, or had completed less education, were more likely to elect a passive role. This contrasted with the women with benign breast disease, where only 31% wanted a passive role. The work of Beaver *et al.* illuminates an important distinction between participation and a desire to make decisions about care or treatment, and the need for information. Women express a uniformly high desire for information, but not necessarily for active participation. Where medical communications are supplemented by giving people an audiotape of the consultation, this has enhanced the satisfaction with information received, although this does not reduce psychological distress. For a minority of women, however, listening to a tape recording of the consultation is distressing.[15]

Treatment

Treatment may take the form of a clinical trial, a conventional treatment plan, a novel plan recently published in a reputable journal, or a more individualised approach based on the judgement of the clinician (using a combination of their experience and expertise). Approaches involving a combination of therapies are more likely to control cancer and the primary treatment for breast cancer, for example, may firstly involve surgery followed by adjuvant chemotherapy or hormone therapy. Recently, systemic treatments have been given prior to surgery and are known as neo-adjuvant treatment. These are given to reduce the metastatic potential prior to removal of the primary tumour.[16]

Once the options are determined, and a treatment plan is drawn up, a long relationship with the cancer treatment team commences. This involves a large number of different professionals and a long treatment trajectory, frequently over weeks and months, an unreal situation, where side-effects may be minimal, or more often severe. The enormity of this experience and the struggle to endure treatment are expressed in the second account by Jackie Stacey, which this time describes chemotherapy.

Personal account 9.2: Chemotherapy

I arrive at the hospital for the first dose. I am equipped with organic food, dozens of vitamins and minerals and I have a few visual images at the ready. My oncologist has warned me of hair loss and vomiting, so I take extra vitamin C against nausea and a homeopathic remedy against hair loss. I also have a diary to record what drugs I am given and what effects they have on me. I plan to get through the treatment by using these 'regimes of self-management' to structure the days in hospital as I have done my days at home.

. . . I write down the names of the drugs in my diary: Bleomycin, Etoposide, Cisplatinum. I take more vitamin C. The treatment begins. Twenty-four hours into the treatment I am vomiting regularly, I have a high temperature, I am sweating and I ache everywhere with flu-like symptoms. None of the anti-emetic drugs work – instead they produce new unpleasant side-effects (one of them makes you feel as if you have an ants nest in your anus). Had someone offered me carrot juice or organic nut roast (both of which I have brought with me) I'd certainly have thrown it at them. Vitamins are out of the question. Regular vomiting renders such grand plans redundant. This goes on for 3 days. When I finally get home, I develop a burning itchy rash all over my body. I scratch like crazy. I am readmitted for an antihistamine. The scratch marks remain all over my neck, arms, breasts, back and stomach. Traces of my desperation become permanent scars. Bleomycin can do this sometimes I am told.

Back at home the itching has stopped but not the vomiting. We phone the hospital. Just hold on. It will stop eventually. No there's no chance of dehydration, she's had plenty of fluids. But the sickness continues. The next day it's about every hour or so. And I am getting weaker and weaker. That evening, I collapse in the bathroom, my partner in attendance. My eyes roll, my teeth chatter and my throat croaks, my body goes cold and I pour with sweat. I am unconscious and my breathing is uneven. The hospital is 'phoned again. We should call the GP, we are told. Could the seizure be connected with chemotherapy? Could one of the drugs cause potassium deficiency as it says in our book? The doctor laughs at our amateur medical knowledge. I am just dehydrated nothing to worry about.

When I return to hospital and tell the story it generates medical panic. I have to have an EEG to test for brain damage and may even need a lumbar puncture to test the spinal fluid. This is probably caused by potassium deficiency from the drugs and I should come straight into hospital, I am told. Tempers are rising, family appears on the scene and nurses are reprimanded. I should have stayed in hospital longer, I am told;

next time, I am to stay in hospital until the vomiting stops.

Some days after the second treatment I awake with severe chest pains. Is this a heart attack? The GP is called, my usual doctor arrives and is sympathetic. He is perplexed. Everything seems fine. On returning to the hospital I complain of the chest pain. An X-ray is taken but all is clear. I insist that something is wrong. The chemotherapy is thus postponed until I have a lung function test at another hospital. This shows lung damage. One of the three drugs is cut from the treatment, which lessens the overall effectiveness, and this may mean more treatments.

The vomiting continues after the third treatment, and after the fourth, I have a repeat performance of the first and the vomiting is relentless. In addition, I have now developed tinnitus (a loud high-pitched ringing in my ears), neuropathy (numbness and tingling in my hands and feet), infections in my mouth, I have stopped menstruating, and I have intermittent chest pains. I am on steroids for a few months to try and help the lungs repair themselves, and as a result my appetite for starch and sugar has increased tenfold. I put on about two stone in weight and my face is puffy from the steroids. My hair has fallen out.

By the end of the fourth treatment my body has reached a limit, but I still have to have one more dose. I am vomiting, I have diarrhoea, my hands and feet are completely numb and my ears are ringing loudly all the time. My body has been transformed, colonised by the drugs and their side-effects. I can't walk properly in the mornings, as I have no feeling in my feet, which sends me off balance. My hearing is damaged and I find it hard to follow conversations if there is any competing background noise. All my body hair has fallen out and I am completely bald, except for a few stray eyebrow hairs. No eyelashes are left. My skin is marked with what look like whip marks. I am having hot flushes about once an hour because the other ovary has been affected and my periods have stopped. Am I beginning early menopause? No one can be sure. Urination becomes hard because the nerves in the bladder have also become numb.

My dreams focus on pollution and physical disgust: one night I dream I have to eat a huge pile of car tyres which are stacked up in front of me in a pyramid, and I keep protesting that I can't possibly eat them all. Why would one willingly poison oneself?, I keep thinking in my dream.

I write to my consultant and tell him of my fears. Receiving no reply, I go in for my fifth and final treatment. By this time I am without any pretence of self-control. Even the will-power I rely on to get me to the hospital is running out. To have to go for chemotherapy willingly is expecting a lot. When I arrive at the hospital something is odd: nurses smirk and no bed has my name on it. I perch on a spare one. My consultant appears on the ward. This is unprecedented. He thinks I've probably had enough. I can go home. It is over.

(Reproduced with permission from Stacey J. (1997). *Teratologies: A Cultural Study of Cancer*. London: Routledge, pp. 181–183.)

There is evidence to suggest that treatment, while difficult, is accepted. Research has shown that facing the prospect of cancer, the majority of people would opt for treatment offering only a slim chance of cure, and willingly accept toxic treatments because they fear certain death if they do not.[17] Indeed, there may be an association, in the minds of some people undergoing cancer treatment, between side-effects and more effective treatment, a sort of 'nasty medicine being good for you', or a feeling that suffering during treatment is part of fighting the disease, and necessary for survival. Gamble,[18] in an interview study of people undergoing treatment for cancers of the lung and head and neck, found that what most wanted at the end of treatment was someone to acknowledge what they had been through, and to congratulate them for 'getting through it'.

The state of cancer science, however, is such that there has been heavy investment in developing more effective treatments; in many instances this has been at the expense of both short-term and long-term effects on the body. Relative to this there has been a neglect of strategies to reduce or minimise the side-effects of treatment.[19] For example, it has taken 60 years to arrive at the conclusion that mastectomy, a radical and mutilating procedure, is no more effective in early stage breast cancer than more limited surgery, which conserves the breast and is an effective treatment for a large number of women.[20] The most powerful influence on this 'discovery' was not medical science but the pressure of the women's movement, and a determination that the level of disfigurement involved in surgery for breast cancer is unacceptable.

Little attention has been paid to the daily difficulties encountered by people as a result of radiotherapy, which continues for weeks, months or even years after initial treatment. Impotence, incontinence, painful sexual intercourse, bowel problems, lymphoedema, breathing difficulties, limb dysfunction, tiredness, and loss of appetite are just a few difficulties people face. Even less research has been directed towards strategies for preventing or minimising these problems, or for assisting in their management once they arise. Encounters with health professionals frequently do not include discussions about such 'trivial' and perhaps unmentionable problems, alongside the much larger project of life-saving treatment.[21]

Chemotherapy is the mainstay of much cancer treatment; treatment-induced problems such as hair loss, vomiting, sterility, menopause, and fatigue are accepted as a justifiable part of cancer treatment. At times the seductiveness of the 'battle' is such that letting go of treatment becomes very difficult, even when all hope of containing the disease for an individual with advanced cancer has passed. This may frequently be at the request of the person who has cancer, and is not simply a difficulty in health professionals 'letting go'.

These difficulties are central to nurses' roles in cancer care, since in many instances nurses deliver cancer treatment (for example, administering chemotherapy regimes), monitor side-effects, assist people receiving cancer treatment to prepare for anticipated side-effects or difficulties, and work towards alleviating or ameliorating the effects of these. A detailed knowledge of the problems accompanying treatment is needed in order to optimise nursing input.

Increasingly, nursing research effort is being directed towards gathering data about the nature of cancer symptoms and problems that result from treatment, and towards evaluating interventions for these. Much of this work is detailed in the section on managing cancer-related problems. Nursing roles in cancer treatment are changing, so that nurses are taking on more responsibility for the delivery of certain cancer treatments, and for the management of support for people undergoing treatment and their lives beyond this. Accessing insight into the difficulties faced during cancer treatment is central to effective cancer care. These themes recur throughout this section on treatment for cancer.

The treatment trajectory for cancer is frequently long and arduous, and may involve a whole series of treatments. Treatment of breast cancer, for example, involves surgical removal of the tumour and sampling of the axillary lymph nodes as part of determining disease stage, as well as radiotherapy to the chest wall, followed by a course of chemotherapy and/or long-term treatment with tamoxifen, an anti-oestrogen drug. If the disease recurs, there may be more chemotherapy, or radiotherapy for bone metastases. Treatment for cancer of the colon involves surgical removal of part of the bowel; this may be followed by a course of chemotherapy for disease that is more advanced.[22]

Aftercare

After treatment, contact with the cancer centre traditionally continues for many years, since post-treatment surveillance using screening investigations known as 'follow-up' has been routine, and aims to detect any disease recurrence as early as possible. This model of aftercare has meant that people have frequent interactions with the health system. This, on the one hand, may be reassuring if it confirms that there are no signs that the cancer has returned, but also maintains a dependence on the health system, and reinforces cancer as a kind of career from which one never escapes. Follow-up visits are associated with considerable anxiety as tests and investigations are anticipated, and what might be found can be a preoccupation for days or weeks before the hospital appointment. Recently, there has been much questioning of routine follow-up for cancer since it is costly and there is little evidence that it is effective in detecting cancer recurrence. In fact, most recurrence is identified by the person themselves following a new symptom arising or a change in body function.[23]

Studies of alternative models of follow-up have been undertaken. Grunfeld et al.[24] conducted a randomised, controlled trial comparing conventional, hospital-based follow-up of women with breast cancer with follow-up in primary care by the GP. No differences were found in the effectiveness of the two models. Of the 26 out of 269 women who developed a recurrence during the study, nine had experienced delays of more than 28 days in the diagnosis of recurrence. These were largely due to administrative errors, in particular delays in obtaining out-patient appointments when the case was not considered to be urgent. The majority of women with signs of recurrence visited their GP in the first instance regardless of whether they were in the hospital or primary care follow-up system. An important finding was that 36% of women refused to participate in the study, suggesting that at least one-third of women with breast cancer want the reassurance of ongoing care by a specialist. Unfortunately, no information regarding satisfaction with the two models of care was collected by the researchers. An interview study of attitudes to follow-up amongst people with colorectal cancer in The Netherlands[25] found a high level of satisfaction with the system; a similar level of satisfaction was found in a UK study[26] of 252 people attending a general oncology follow-up clinic. Also, a reluctance to accept a system based on follow-up outside the hospital setting was expressed. These studies indicate that it may not be straightforward to transfer this area of care into primary care settings, unless the sources by which people obtain support and reassurance that their cancer has not returned are also available.

It may be that simply replacing a hospital-based system with a less intensive model of care will not address the ongoing need for information and support following cancer treatment. It is likely that in the future specialist nurses may play an increasing role in managing ongoing support and follow-up in partnership with general practitioners and the primary health care team. James et al.[27] evaluated a model of care using telephone support offered by a nurse specialist and surveillance for people with neurological tumours. The Royal Marsden Hospital and Institute of Cancer Research in London have devised a model of nurse-led follow-up care in lung cancer, which has moved away from disease surveillance as its central purpose to a system of nurse-led support. Care is managed over the 'phone, with a telephone screening procedure to assess for signs of illness progression. In addition, an open access nurse-led clinic is available to address any problems, symptoms, or concerns, in a relaxed and informal atmosphere. The system also emphasises close links with GPs and palliative care services so that ongoing care and support needs are addressed as early as possible, in a group whose cancer is frequently progressing and prognosis is poor. This system is being evaluated in a randomised, controlled trial.

Cancer and its treatment are complex, and are increasingly understood as an ongoing journey, with multiple pathways through an increasingly complex treatment and health care environment. There are critical stages in these pathways, where decisions need to be made about an appropriate course of treatment and the care and support that may be required. Stages such as diagnosis, or signs of cancer progressing or returning, require a series of clinical investigations and these events are stressful and difficult.

The role of nursing in relation to cancer treatment is central, and is not simply about being a participant in the team making decisions about treatment, and then taking responsibility for administering and monitoring the effects of treatment. Nurses are central to determining the level of care and support required for individuals, and to establishing a package of care strategies to provide for these. These strategies are distinct from cancer treatment, and since they relate to emotional, practical, and functional problems, it may be more difficult to identify the most appropriate responses required or how these may need to alter as an individual progresses through the treatment journey. This requires the active identification of problems and needs of people undergoing treatment, and the creation of an environment that can acknowledge and address these needs. Often such decisions have to be made in the absence of evidence on which one might draw to support one's decisions. The journey through cancer treatment is difficult and insufficient attention has been given to how to manage problems caused by treatment or how to help people to sustain themselves through it. After treatment, unlike other conditions, fear of cancer returning and the need to be constantly vigilant for this, mean that returning to 'normal' may be difficult to achieve, and ongoing contact with the health care system is common. The following chapters examine these issues in more detail in relation to the major modalities of treatment for cancer, and explore the role of nursing in caring for, and supporting, those receiving them.

References

1. Stacey J. (1997). *Teratologies: A Cultural Study of Cancer.* London: Routledge.
2. O'Mary S. (1997). Diagnostic evaluation, classification and staging. In Groenwald S., Hansen Frogge M. and Henke Yarbro C. (eds.) *Cancer Nursing*, 4th edition. Sudbury, MA: Jones and Bartlett.
3. Maxwell M.B. (1997). Principles of treatment planning. In Groenwald S., Hansen Frogge M. and Henke Yarbro C. (eds.) *Cancer Nursing*, 4th edition. Sudbury, MA: Jones and Bartlett.
4. Hermanek P., Hutter R.V.P., Sobin L.H., Wagner G. and Wittekind C. (eds.) (1997). *UICC TMN Atlas*, 4th edition. Berlin: Springer.
5. Souhami R. and Tobias S. (1995). *Cancer and Its Management.* London: Blackwell Science.
6. Eddy D. (1996). Diagnostic and staging investigations. In Tschudin V. (ed.) *Nursing the Patient with Cancer.* London: Prentice Hall.
7. Chambers A. and Hill R.P. (1998). Tumour progression and metastases. In Tannock I.F. and Hill R.P. (eds.) *The Basic Science of Oncology*, 3rd edition. New York: McGraw Hill.
8. Atkinson P. (1995). *Medical Talk and Medical Work.* London: Sage.
9. Bond J. and Bond S. (1986). *Sociology and Health Care.* Edinburgh: Churchill Livingstone.
10. Foucault M. (1973). *The Birth of the Clinic.* London: Tavistock.
11. Silverman D. (1987). *Communication and Medical Practice: Social Relations in the Clinic.* London: Sage.
12. Degner L. and Russell A. (1988). Preferences for treatment and control among adults with cancer. *Research in Nursing and Health* 11, 367–374.
13. Degner L. and Sloan J.F. (1992). Decision making during serious illness: what part do patients really want to play? *Journal of Clinical Epidemiology* 45, 944–50.
14. Beaver K., Luker K., Glynn Owens R., Leinster S.J. and Degner L. (1996). Treatment decision making in women newly diagnosed with breast cancer. *Cancer Nursing* 19, 8–19.
15. McHugh P., Lewis S., Ford S. *et al.* (1995). The efficacy of audiotapes in promoting well-being in cancer patients: a randomised controlled trial. *British Journal of Cancer* 74, 388–392.
16. Smith I., Walsh G., Jones A. *et al.* (1995). High complete remission rates with primary neoadjuvant infusional chemotherapy for large early breast cancer. *Journal of Clinical Oncology* 13, 424–429.
17. Slevin M.L., Strubbs L., Plant H.J. *et al.* (1990). Attributes to chemotherapy: comparing views of patients with cancer with those of doctors, nurses, and general public. *British Medical Journal* 300, 1458–1460.
18. Gamble K. (1996). *Communication and information: the experience of radiotherapy patients.* Unpublished D.Phil. thesis, Open University, Milton Keynes.
19. Corner J. (1997). Nursing and the counter culture for cancer. *European Journal of Cancer Care* 6, 174–181.
20. Baum M. (1993). Breast cancer 2000 BC to 2000 AD: time for a paradigm shift? *Acta Oncologica* 32, 3–8.
21. Faithfull S. (1995). 'Just grin and bear it and hope it will go away'. Coping with urinary symptoms from pelvic radiotherapy. *European Journal of Cancer Care* 4, 158–165.

22. NHS Executive (1997). *Guidance on Commissioning Cancer Services. Improving Outcomes in Colorectal Cancer.* London: Department of Health.
23. Brada M. (1995). Is there a need to follow up cancer patients? *European Journal of Cancer* **31A**, 655–657.
24. Grunfeld E., Mant D., Yudkin P. *et al.* (1996). Routine follow-up of breast cancer in primary care: randomised trial. *British Medical Journal* **313**, 665–669.
25. Stiggelbout A.M., de Haes J., Van de Velde C., Bruijninck C., van Groningen K. and Kievet J. (1997). Follow-up of colorectal cancer patients with quality of life and attitudes towards follow-up. *British Journal of Cancer* **75**, 914–920.
26. Thomas S., Glynne-Jones R. and Chait I. (1997). Is it worth the wait? Survey of patient's satisfaction with an oncology outpatient clinic. *European Journal of Cancer Care* **6**, 50–58.
27. James N.D., Guerrero D. and Brada M. (1994). Who should follow up cancer patients? Nurse specialist based outpatient care and the introduction of a phone clinic system. *Clinical Oncology* **6**, 283–287.

CHAPTER TEN

Surgery

Julia Downing

Surgery is the oldest form of cancer treatment and is one of the most important treatment modalities in individuals with solid tumours. Over the years there have been many changes in the treatment of cancer and although surgery still remains the treatment of choice for many cancers,[1] our understanding of the biology of cancer, along with the developments of other treatment modalities and those within surgery itself, have necessitated a re-evaluation of the methods and types of surgery used. At the same time, changes in the delivery of cancer services, such as the use of day care facilities and shorter stays in hospital, have had an influence on the treatment given.

Advances in surgery that have had an impact on the treatment given to individuals with cancer are wide-ranging. These include improved technical abilities of surgeons resulting in the possibility of more complex and radical surgery, the use of radiolabelled monoclonal antibodies to facilitate the excision of the whole tumour, a decrease in morbidity from secondary infection due to the use of a wide range of antibiotics, increased survival after radical surgery due to advanced technology in the intensive care unit and improved prosthetics, which help to reduce distress and disfigurement from radical surgery.[2]

The knowledge of the biological basis of cancer has had an impact on the development of different treatment modalities such as radiotherapy, chemotherapy, and biological therapies and how these can be used both independently and in combination with each other. This has resulted in an increase in disease-free intervals and survival rates.[3] Along with this, the extent of surgery has changed and whereas in the past surgery may have been quite radical, it may now be more conservative.[4] For instance, in the past women may have been given a mastectomy for breast cancer, whereas now they may be given a lumpectomy followed by radiotherapy.

Box 10.1: Principles of surgical oncology[3,5]

In order to understand the theory behind treatment decisions one needs to understand the biology and natural history of tumours. Treatment decisions are made according to the growth rate, differentiation, metastatic pattern and metastatic potential of a tumour, along with the status of the individual. Multi-disciplinary teamwork and treatment planning is necessary in order to select the most effective treatment for an individual. For treatment to be effective all cancer cells must be removed; any cancer cell that is left can be a potential hazard, therefore surgery must involve the resection of the entire tumour mass and a safe margin of normal tissue around it.

Factors affecting treatment decisions are:

- Growth rate:
  - the time taken for tumour mass to double in size
  - tumours with a slow growth rate, that is with cells that have a prolonged cell cycle, are best for surgical treatment and are more likely to be contained locally than tumours with a high growth rate.
- Metastatic potential:
  - some tumours metastasise late or not at all and may be cured by surgical treatment

- some tumours metastasise to local or regional sites and a cure may still be achieved through surgery
- other tumours metastasise early to distant sites and do not warrant surgery except as an adjuvant therapy or for loco-regional control.

- Tumour location, histology, and invasiveness:
  - the ability to surgically remove a tumour or not may rest on its position, whether it is near vital structures or not, and its invasiveness
  - superficial and encapsulated tumours are easier to remove than deep or embedded tumours, for example, a basal cell carcinoma of the skin is relatively superficial, whereas a melanoma invades deeply
  - certain histological types are not treated with surgery as they are disseminated at onset, such as leukaemias.

- Individual's physical status:
  - pre-operative assessment is vital
  - the severity of the underlying condition and concurrent conditions must be taken into account when planning surgery.

- Quality of life and individual choice:
  - the individual's desire for treatment must be assessed: they may not want surgery
  - the goal of therapy varies according to the stage of the disease but the benefits and risks must be weighed up in all circumstances and be acceptable to the individual.

The initial treatment plan for an individual with cancer is critical, and a multidisciplinary approach is needed in order to achieve the best results. Although surgery can be curative in localised disease, as many as 70% of individuals will have micrometastases at diagnosis.[6] Hence surgery does not happen in isolation, but in combination with other treatment modalities such as chemotherapy or radiotherapy. Slow-growing tumours are the most amenable to surgical treatment and initial surgery is more successful than secondary operations for recurrence, and as long as it does not result in serious disfigurement, the removal of the tumour and adjacent lymph nodes is preferential to removing only the tumour itself.[2]

In looking at the role of surgery in the care of the individual with cancer it can be helpful to look at what is meant by the term 'surgery' and how this has changed over the years. Surgery has been defined as 'the branch of medicine that treats disease by operative measures'[7] or as 'that branch of medicine which treats disease, injuries, and defor-

mities by manual or operative methods'.[8] While both definitions may have described the use of surgery in the past, more recently the dimensions of surgery have expanded, involving areas such as prevention, diagnosis, and palliation, as well as the actual treatment of disease; hence these definitions of surgery are limited. A more appropriate way of defining surgery is 'the branch of medicine concerned with diseases and trauma requiring operative procedures',[9] thus encompassing other aspects along with the treatment of disease.

Current surgical interventions are not therefore limited to tumour removal but also involve areas such as diagnosis and staging of disease, prevention, reconstruction (rehabilitation), palliation, and supportive surgery.[2,3,10,11] It therefore has a central role to play in the management of an individual with cancer and most individuals with cancer will undergo a surgical procedure at some time in their cancer career, be it a biopsy for diagnosis, the insertion of a central line for chemotherapy or the formation of a colostomy for colorectal cancer.

For each individual having that surgical procedure, the surgery does not happen in isolation, but within the context of that person's social, psychological and illness career and therefore the meaning of that procedure will vary. The meaning that an individual gives to any surgical intervention will depend on the explorative or definitive nature of the surgery, the operable or inoperable status of the tumour and the functional consequence or deficits.[12] The meaning of the surgery will be different for an individual having a biopsy, a mastectomy, or surgery to relieve bowel obstruction in advanced ovarian cancer.

Prophylactic surgery

Surgery has a limited but important role in prophylaxis and in some cases its benefit is not yet known. It is indicated in individuals who have a family history of a specific type of cancer, for example colorectal cancer, and have an underlying condition or congenital predisposition that increases the risk of them getting cancer.[3,6] The surgical removal of non-vital benign tissue or organs can lower this risk and prevent the occurrence of cancer; however, the knowledge that an individual has a genetic defect that can be passed on, along with the removal of parts of the body and changes to their body image, may also decrease an individual's quality of life. Therefore the benefits of avoiding the disease may not be as great as the individual had anticipated.[13]

There are various underlying conditions or genetic dispositions where prophylactic surgery may be used (Table 10.1). The benefits of prophylactic surgery have in some instances been accepted, for example in individuals with familial adenomatous polyposis (FAP) where prophylactic surgery is necessary to prevent cancer.[14] With hereditary non-polyposis colorectal cancer (HNPCC),[15] prophylactic colectomy is generally indicated, although factors such as co-morbidity, age, sphincter function, and compliance with future surveillance must be considered.[14] If prophylactic surgery is not indicated then there is a continual need for screening, which may in itself involve regular colonoscopies.

Controversy exists, however, in other instances, such as the use of prophylactic mastectomy for women at a high risk of getting breast cancer.[16] The mutant predisposing gene for breast cancer was first identified in Utah in 1994,[17] and although influenced by other factors and the environment, germ line genetic mutations are responsible for 5–10% of all cases of breast cancer.[18] Up to 50% of familial breast cancer malignancies occur in individuals with BRCA-1 mutations.[18] Hence individuals who have either the BRCA-1 or BRCA-2 gene are at a higher risk of developing breast cancer than those individuals without them. The identification of these breast cancer genes has had a rapid and significant clinical impact.[19]

So, apart from keeping a close eye on women who have been identified as having the gene, what can be done to reduce their risk of developing breast cancer? The effectiveness of intensive screening in young high-risk women is not known and may cause psychological distress to some and reassurance to others.[18,19] The benefits of taking tamoxifen prophylactically are such that although the incidence may be decreased, it does not remove the risk,[20] hence prophylactic mastectomy, with or without reconstruction, is an option that should be considered and discussed, although reports about its efficacy are conflicting. Burke et al.[16] suggest that the evidence for the subsequent prevention of cancer by prophylactic mastectomy is lacking and that case reports document the occurrence of cancer following prophylactic surgery. However, in their recent study Hartmann et al.[21] found a statistically significant decrease in the incidence of breast cancer and of death from breast cancer after prophylactic mastectomy, compared with the expected incidence in women at high risk of breast cancer on the basis of family history who do not undergo the procedure.

Many of these women have family members who have been diagnosed, treated, and may even have died from breast cancer; they are living not only with the fear of when it may be their turn, but whether they will have to have a mastectomy, radiotherapy, chemotherapy, hormone therapy, whether they will survive or die too, and worries about their partners, children, friends, and how they will cope. For them, the fear of living with the threat of cancer over them is greater than the anticipated fear of losing their breasts, and for many, the option of a prophylactic mastectomy is perceived as the only option.

Table 10.1 Examples of prophylactic surgery for cancer [3,6,14,16]

Predisposing condition	Type of surgery	Cancer
Familial breast cancer	Mastectomy	Breast
Familial ovarian cancer	Oophorectomy	Ovary
Familial prostatic cancer	Prostatectomy (rare)	Prostate
Familial adenomatous polyposis (FAP)	Colectomy	Colon
Hereditary non-polyposis colorectal cancer (HNPCC)	Colectomy	Colon
Ulcerative colitis	Colectomy	Colon
Cryptorchidism	Orchidectomy	Testicular
Multiple endocrine neoplasia types II and III	Thyroidectomy	Thyroid

Women have a difficult decision to make with regard to prophylactic surgery, for it is not without its own cost, for example, surgical complications and its impact on self-image and sexual functioning.[22] It is not an easy decision for individuals to make and nurses have an important role in supporting them through their decision. Accurate information regarding both the benefits and the costs of surgery, along with the option of reconstructive surgery is vital. The individual will also need help in coming to terms with the implications of their decision, whether it be to have surgery or not.

Specific indications for a prophylactic mastectomy in high-risk women have been given by Hartmann *et al.*[21] as:

- family/personal experience of breast cancer
- multiple previous breast biopsies
- unreliable results on physical examination due to nodular breasts
- dense breast tissue on mammography
- cancerphobia.

However, these are medically orientated and do not necessarily take into account the wider context in which individuals find themselves, such as their roles and responsibility within their family and society, their age, occupation, culture, and religion, their own subjective assessment of the risk of developing cancer and their previous experiences with illness, death, and the medical system.

The decision to have a prophylactic mastectomy is not one to be taken lightly or quickly, individuals need to be encouraged to take their time over the decision, and their autonomy in this decision making is important and needs to be recognised.[23] Once the decision has been made to have a prophylactic mastectomy, with or without reconstruction, the procedure will need to be clearly explained.

One woman's thoughts about having a prophylactic mastectomy ran along the following lines:

> The decision to have the operation itself (bilateral mastectomy) was not hard . . . my mum and aunt both died from breast cancer when I was growing up and my eldest sister has already had a mastectomy for breast cancer . . . so . . . I was afraid that I too would get it . . . the operation has meant that I no longer live with that fear

> . . . that fear of getting cancer . . . it was taking over my life . . . it did not feel like 'if' I get it but 'when' I get it . . . The hard part . . . well . . . that is getting used to my new body . . . wondering whether I will still be able to get a boyfriend . . . and . . . feeling guilty that I might pass the gene on to any children I may have . . . but . . . at least I will hopefully be alive to care for them . . . unlike my own mum.

Although the women have chosen to have the mastectomy and the operation may relieve them from the fear of cancer, coming to terms with the effect of the operation may still be hard for them. As well as experiencing physical discomfort from the surgery, their body image may be altered by the surgery; they may fear what their loved ones will think, or fear that they will find it hard to get a partner. The impact on their sexuality may be enormous, not only in terms of sexual function but also in their perception of their femininity, their inability to breast feed in the future, and above all the knowledge that they may never have developed cancer and therefore mastectomy with all its consequences may have been unnecessary.

Prophylactic surgery is, therefore, an option in individuals who are at a high risk of developing a specific type of cancer. The willingness to undergo prophylactic surgery may, however, depend on the ability of current treatments to cure the hereditary cancer,[23] and if treatment outcomes improve then the role of prophylactic surgery may decrease.

Diagnostic surgery

In order to be able to make the correct decisions about treatment, it is important that doctors are able to get as much information as possible about a suspected malignancy, hence the accuracy of the information gained during the diagnostic process is important. The need to gather as much information as possible about the nature of a malignancy necessitates that the individual undergoes numerous investigations, of both a non-surgical and a surgical nature. The major role of surgery at this stage is in the acquisition of tissues in order that a histological diagnosis can be made.[1,6] Numerous surgical investigations may be used in the diagnosis and staging of cancer, ranging from fine needle biopsies to bronchoscopies or even in rare cases a staging laparotomy (see below).[24]

Biopsies

- A tissue biopsy is essential in confirming diagnosis and identifying the histology of the disease.
- It involves removing a piece of living tissue from the patient and examining it under the microscope to determine whether the tissue is malignant or not.
- The principles of surgical biopsies are:[6]
  - the needle tracks and scars should be placed so that they are removed by subsequent definitive surgery, for cosmetic reasons and to prevent tumour cells seeding along the biopsy site
  - new tissue planes should not be contaminated during biopsy
  - the biopsy technique should be carefully selected in order to obtain an adequate sample of tissue
  - the handling of the biopsy specimen by the pathologist is important as bad handling can render the sample useless.

Fine needle aspiration

- It is the aspiration of cells and tissue fragments through a needle that has been guided to a suspected malignant tissue.[2,6]
- It is the procedure of choice if high risk of malignancy.
- It is quick, safe, reliable, and easily repeated.
- It is well tolerated, with little trauma.
- A local anaesthetic may be used.
- It may be guided by CT scan or ultrasound.
- There is a possibility that the tumour might be missed, therefore only a positive test is diagnostically significant.

Needle core biopsy

- This involves obtaining a core of tissue through a specially designed needle introduced into suspected malignant tissue.[2,6]
- A local anaesthetic is used.
- It is adequate for the diagnosis of most tumours.
- There is the possibility that the tumour might be missed, therefore only a positive test is diagnostically significant.

Incisional biopsy

- This is the removal of a small wedge of tissue from a larger tumour mass.
- It is the preferred method for diagnosing soft tissue and bony sarcomas and used for large tumours that will need major surgery.
- The biopsy site is totally excised with major surgery.

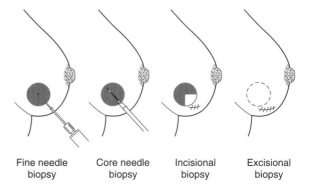

| Fine needle biopsy | Core needle biopsy | Incisional biopsy | Excisional biopsy |

Figure 10.1 Types of biopsy (reproduced with permission from Love Susan M. (1995). *Dr Susan Love's Breast Book*. New York: Perseus Books Publishers).

Excisional biopsy

- This is the excision of the entire suspected tumour mass with no attempt to obtain generous margins of adjacent normal tissue.[1,2,6]
- It is the procedure of choice for small accessible tumours.
- It can sometimes be the definitive treatment; for example, basal cell carcinoma on the nose or ear, although surgery may be needed post-diagnosis to ensure adequate excisional margins.

Endoscopies

- These are used to have a look down accessible lumens and get a biopsy specimen where possible.
- The advent of flexible instruments has made it easier and more tolerable for the individual.
- There are different types of endoscopy, e.g. bronchoscopy, gastroscopy, laryngoscopy, and colonoscopy.
- Depending on the type, they may be carried out with sedation, under anaesthetic or without either.
- The placement of the biopsy site is important, e.g. for cosmesis.

Examination under anaesthetic (EUA)

- Occasionally it is not possible to examine an individual or to take a biopsy without putting them under an anaesthetic, due to the inaccessibility of the tumour, pain, or anxiety, particularly in individuals with nasopharyngeal tumours.

Laparotomy

- This is an exploratory procedure to help diagnose and stage intracavitary tumours.
- It is traditionally used in lymphomas and ovarian cancer.
- This can provide critically important staging information that cannot be ascertained by other methods.
- The use of staging laparotomies has decreased as other non-surgical investigative procedures have been developed.

To the medical staff a needle biopsy or incisional biopsy may be a routine procedure requiring little or no surgical preparation, yet for the individual it is far from routine and the time leading up to and including diagnosis is one filled with great anxiety and fear – fear of the unknown, fear of what the results may or may not show, and the effects that the diagnosis could have on the rest of their lives. Anxieties such as attending hospital, medical staff, or past experiences may all affect an individual's willingness to undergo diagnostic procedures and their willingness to seek medical care in the first place. In his book about his experiences of head and neck cancer, John Diamond[26] writes how, when he thought that his lump was benign, he was prepared to forget about the lump rather than have it removed, due to his fear of anaesthetics:

> The problem was that having it [the lump] removed would have meant a general anaesthetic and I have an irrational fear of general anaesthetics. And not so very irrational, come to that: people, middle-aged male people especially, go under the anaesthetic and don't come round again. I forgot about the lump [p. 26].

It can also be a time of waiting, waiting for referrals to come through, waiting in out-patient department, waiting for X-rays, and waiting for results – results that could turn lives upside down. In other cases, such as one-stop breast clinics, an individual may be seen, have various X-rays, mammograms and needle biopsies in one day, and get the results back a few days later; thus, everything moves very quickly. Both of these situations can affect the way that an individual copes with and comes to terms with a diagnosis – too much waiting can cause an increase in anxiety and fear, and carries with it the feelings of 'Why is it all taking so long? What if it is cancer; will it not still be growing? Don't we need to start treatment now?' The opposite situation, with things moving very quickly, can mean that an individual is having to make decisions about treatment before they can realise the impact of the diagnosis and they do not have time to take stock and think about what is happening – it all passes in a blur and the individual has no sense of control over the situation:

> I had a bone marrow aspirate and the biopsy, which I didn't anticipate. I didn't know anything about it and

I can't remember if it all happened. The next day the doctor confirmed the diagnosis. The next day I was in a blood bank undergoing leucopheresis.[27]

> A week and a half later (since referral), on a Monday, the urologist also thought it was an infection after a physical examination but immediately performed an ultrasound scan and then decided it could possibly be a tumour. He scheduled surgery for the Wednesday and as a result the testicle was removed because of the results of a biopsy. A week later the stitches came out and the full diagnosis (non-seminoma, embryonal cell carcinomas) was given to me and my wife . . . I have been rather shocked by the speed of it all.[28]

The individual having the diagnostic tests does not go through it alone, but is part of a wider family and social context. They may be concerned not only about the tests and their outcome but also about the effect that this might have on their role in the family or their job, and friends and relatives may feel worried and frightened as well, not knowing how best to support their loved one. The fear of cancer is still great, with individuals seeing the word 'cancer' as synonymous with suffering and death:[29]

> We could only try to imagine what Mum must have been feeling during those days of endless tests. We ourselves were extremely worried and frightened. Eventually it was established that it was . . . cancer, that dreaded illness that either meant weeks of horrible treatment or death. Just how far the cancer had spread had not been ascertained and there were more tests. It was then decided to remove the spleen, at the same time giving doctors an opportunity of finding out exactly what was happening. Mum came through the operation well and I spent many hours with her afterwards . . . I wanted her to feel that I was there to comfort her as much as possible . . . Removing the spleen had in fact helped Mum's discomfort but had also proved that the cancer had spread and I was told that Mum had about two months to live [pp. 81–82].

Once an initial diagnosis has been made, this may not be the end of the tests as the exact extent and staging of the disease is needed in order to decide on the most appropriate treatment. The delivery of the news that an individual has cancer may then be compounded by the fact that it may be inoperable or that it has already reached an advanced stage, and this fear that it is already 'too late' may be at the back of peoples' minds throughout the diagnostic process. However, those whose malignancy has been picked up through a routine screening programme may feel relieved that it has been picked up so soon.

Surgical diagnostic techniques include needle aspirations and biopsies, lumbar punctures, bone marrow biopsies, endoscopies, cystoscopies, and occasionally a laparotomy, and they will be undertaken according to the type of malignancy suspected and the 'position' of the area being studied, such as on the surface of the body, whether it is by an orifice/lumen that can be scoped, or whether it is in deep tissue.[11] Sometimes, as in the case of disease in deep tissues, a diagnosis may be suspected but not confirmed until definitive surgery is undertaken. With the exception of a staging laparotomy, most of the other investigative procedures will be undertaken on an out-patient or day care basis,[3] thus preventing any unnecessary hospital admissions. However, this means that the time that nurses have to spend with the individual is short and individual anxiety may be increased due to fear of something going wrong once they get home. It is important that individuals are given as much information as possible about the procedure before they have it and that they are given the opportunity to think about it and ask questions. Information needs to be given to them with regard to how to care for their biopsy site, what they should look out for, and what to do and who to call if any complications should arise. Possible complications from a biopsy, depending on the site, are pain, bleeding, haematoma, and infection. The individual also needs to know when and how they will get the results of the investigations.

For investigations where a general anaesthetic or sedation may be used and individuals are admitted to the day care unit, more extensive preparation is needed. Day care surgery has been defined as 'an investigation or operation where the management intention is planned as non-residential and requires some form of anaesthesia and recovery facilities'.[31] Education and planning for day care surgery, both for the individual and for their family, is an important challenge to nurses and one that can drastically affect the way an individual copes with the experience and future day care treatment. While giving information with regard to investigations and what the patient can expect to happen

will help to allay some of the fears and anxieties of the individual, it is not possible for nurses to relieve all their anxiety and fears. There will always be the fear of the unknown, the fear that it might be cancer, and this is something that one can try and support the individual through, but neither nurses nor anyone else can take it away from the individual or their family, because it might, after all, be cancer:

> The pill is taking hold. I shall go to bed now. A public bed in a public ward, but one with clean sheets and surrounded by nurses who accept that men who are about to go under the knife get angry. And frightened. Because while BUPA covers most contingencies, it doesn't cover fear.[31]

Definitive surgery

The goal of definitive surgery is to remove as much of the tumour as possible, along with a safe margin of normal tissue surrounding it.[11] It can be a simple, safe method to cure patients with solid tumours when the tumour is confined to the anatomical site of origin.[6] The stage of disease is important when trying to identify whether an individual can be cured by surgery alone; examples of such malignancies are basal cell carcinomas, early melanomas, and Dukes A rectal carcinomas.[11] Owing to advances that have been made in surgery, the focus is on both tissue and functional preservation; for example, lumpectomy as opposed to mastectomy (see Figure 10.2). Tumours that are to be surgically removed need to be solid and accessible, with well-

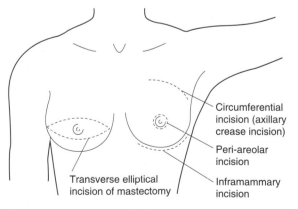

Figure 10.2 Incisions for lumpectomy and mastectomy. (Reproduced with permission from Chapman & Hall Medical, London, Nash and Mokbel.[32])

defined margins and no evidence of spread. The type and extent of the surgical procedure will vary according to the tumour and its stage. Local resections are done for small tumours and the whole tumour is excised along with a margin of tumour-free tissue; more radical resections involve the resection of the tumour along with local and regional tissue, the lymphatics and a margin of tumour-free tissue. The lymphatics are removed to try to prevent spread and to stop local recurrence.[3]

Surgery is, however, a localised treatment and due to the fact that 70% of individuals will have micrometastases at diagnosis, it is often used in combination with other treatment modalities and thus requires careful consideration of all the effective treatment options available. The combination of therapies is used to try and increase cure rates and disease-free survival. Adjuvant therapies may be given at different stages of the treatment process, for example, pre-, intra- or post-operatively. Where possible, safe conservative surgical techniques are used due to multi-modal treatment and the tailoring of treatment to individual needs.[11]

The use of multi-modal treatment does, however, bring with it some difficulties. The timing and extent of the surgery is important and this may change after treatment with radiotherapy or chemotherapy. Wound healing may be a problem if radiotherapy has been given previously. Treatment will not necessarily fit into the treatment plan as the needs of an individual change and surgery may be needed in the middle of chemotherapy treatment, due to obstruction or the need for a vascular access device to be inserted. Some cytotoxic drugs can also be toxic to major organs, causing long-term side-effects, which may then affect an individual's suitability for surgery; for example, bleomycin can have an effect on the lungs, which can cause respiratory problems with surgery leading to acute adult respiratory distress syndrome (AARDS).[3]

The surgical options in the treatment of cancer are great and as well as surgery being aimed at cure, both on its own and in combination with other modalities, it can also be used to reduce the bulk of tumours, for example in Burkitt's lymphoma or ovarian cancer, in an attempt to control any residual gross disease.[6] However, debulking is only of benefit when there are other effective treatments to help to control the residual disease. By decreasing the tumour mass it is possible to increase the effectiveness of radiotherapy or chemotherapy.[2]

There is also a role for surgery in the resection of metastatic disease with a curative intent. Individuals with a single site of metastatic disease in a position where it can be resected without major morbidity, where the primary tumour is believed to have been eradicated, should undergo that resection.[3] Resection of pulmonary metastases in individuals with soft tissue or bony sarcomas can lead to a cure in up to 30% of individuals.[6] Other areas where metastases can be resected are the brain or the liver.

Other types of surgery, such as cryosurgery and laser surgery, may also be used in the treatment of cancer. Cryosurgery is where malignant cells are destroyed by liquid nitrogen and might be used for cancer of the skin, oral cavity, or prostate. Laser surgery may be used for the local excision of laryngeal and cervical cancers.[6]

The person with cancer undergoing surgery will experience many of the same physical effects and complications as a person without cancer, such as pain, infection, bleeding, and poor wound healing. However, some of these will be further complicated by the effect on the individual of their cancer or its treatment.

The control of post-operative pain needs to be discussed prior to surgery in order to allow people to talk about any fears or previous experience they may have, and to inform them of methods of post-operative pain control. Discussion should include information on pain assessment, expectations of pain, methods of pain control, such as patient-controlled analgesia (PCA), analgesics used and other non-pharmacological methods of pain control.

Malnutrition is a common problem in individuals with cancer, especially those with advanced disease, and may be due to the effects of treatment or to the cancer itself. Malnutrition results from:[5]

- decreased oral intake
- increased enteral losses as a result of malabsorption or intestinal fistulae
- increased nutritional requirements due to hypermetabolism or the tumour itself.

The cancer patient who is nutritionally compromised is a poor surgical candidate[3,5] as they are unable to mount the usual defences when faced with major stress such as surgery. Complications of surgery due to malnutrition include:

- poor wound healing
- anaemia
- pneumonia
- sepsis
- further malnutrition
- increased morbidity
- reduced tolerance to further chemotherapy.

An individual's nutritional status therefore needs to be assessed prior to surgery and nutritional support considered where necessary, such as enteral nutrition via a nasogastric tube or total parenteral nutrition (TPN). The nutritional plan is as important as the treatment plan in order to minimise some of the adverse effects of the surgery.

Anaemia is common amongst cancer patients,[5] along with platelet dysfunction and alterations in white blood cells. They are also more susceptible to minor changes in the haemostatic process and are more likely to develop post-operative thrombosis than an individual without cancer.[3,5] Anaemia and any alterations in haemostasis should therefore be corrected prior to surgery.

Surgery specific complications may also occur and efforts need to be made to try and reduce these, such as the need for arm exercise post-operatively after breast surgery to prevent restricted mobility due to the development of a 'frozen shoulder'. Mobility after surgery is important and concerns about restriction of mobility have been expressed due to the presence of drains, a delay in their removal, the formation of post-drain seroma, and the potential for poor wound healing.[33]

Complications of surgery include:

- shock
- haemorrhage
- thrombophlebitis
- pulmonary complications – pneumonia, atelectasis, bronchitis, pleurisy, acute adult respiratory distress syndrome, embolism
- urinary retention or incontinence
- intestinal obstruction
- wound complications – haemorrhage, haematoma
- sepsis
- oncological emergencies.

As can be seen, the options for surgery in the active treatment of cancer are great, as are the impacts of that surgery on the individual. For many, surgery will come at the start of their overall cancer treatment, for others it may come after months of chemotherapy or radiotherapy treatment. Some individuals may have had a recurrence of their disease and surgery will be a last attempt to try to find that cure; still others might be on their fourth or fifth operation, desperately hoping that this will be the last. So what does that surgery mean to those individuals; how will they react?

The fears and anxieties associated with having surgery for cancer represent those of having surgery in general; however, there is also the added meaning of the cancer itself and its threat to life.[10] Cancer is a disease, but it also carries with it a series of experiences that will profoundly affect the individual and those who share the experience of the disease and its treatment, along with society's beliefs and fears surrounding the disease.

Despite the advances in treatment, cure, and disease-free survival rates for some cancers, the diagnosis of cancer still brings with it feelings of dread, fear of horrible treatment and ultimately of death.[31,34] It is one of the most feared diseases in our society.[29] A diagnosis of cancer causes significant emotional distress, family upheaval, and psychosocial disruption, shatters one's illusions of immortality and invulnerability and causes one to lose the view of the world as being safe. Individuals feel vulnerable and fearful, have a sense of loss of control and a need to re-evaluate their priorities, and all this may lead to a spiritual crisis.[34] Unfortunately, the fears and anxieties of society can be confirmed by our reactions and attitudes as nurses. This can be illustrated by the following quote from Jackie Stacey[35] when the nurse's attitude and behaviour change towards her once she has a diagnosis of cancer, and no one on the surgical ward where she is will actually say the word 'cancer'.

> Whatever you do, don't say cancer. The unspoken word, written on everyone's lips, must not be voiced . . . Even after my diagnosis no one on the surgical ward says the word cancer to me. The nurses' rounds, which previously involved introducing the patients to the new shift by explaining the nature of their illness or surgery, suddenly have a different format; in my case, the C word, is whispered about in the office before the round, and not men-

tioned when they pass my bed twice a day. Instead of pausing to introduce me as they had done previously, by name and then by medical problem, 'This is Jackie and she's had a right laparotomy', they introduce me by name, 'This is Jackie . . .' followed by an awkward smile which fills the place of the second half of the naming ritual. In my imagination, and I am sure in theirs too, an anonymous voice whispers 'and she has cancer'. This non-naming ritual is repeated twice a day at every shift change until I leave the ward and come under the treatment of an oncologist who feels more relaxed about naming his specialism more openly [p. 65].[35]

In a study looking into the lived experience of having cancer, Halldorsdottir and Hamrin[36] found five themes that ran through the experience of having cancer:

- uncertainty
- vulnerability
- isolation
- discomfort
- redefinition.

The first two of these – uncertainty and vulnerability – were very evident during the treatment phase of the illness. The search for meaning is a significant part of the cancer experience[37] and nurses can assist the individual in their efforts to find meaning in and make sense of the cancer experience as a whole.[27] However, at the time of initial diagnosis and treatment, while the individual is trying to come to terms with the diagnosis, they are also expected to make decisions regarding their treatment options. An individual's concerns about treatment – what are the options? How will it effect my daily life? What are the chances of cure? – may be an effort to make sense of their situation and derive some meaning from their experience.[27] The diagnosis of cancer challenges an individual's sense of control and this may be evident in the extent to which they want to be involved in the decision-making process with regard to treatment options.

Individuals will have different needs or wishes with regards to medical care: some will want to have an active role in decision making, others will want to be passive and hand the decisions completely over to the medical staff.[29,38] In reality, the uncertainty of treatment outcomes for the newly diagnosed oncology patient and the stress caused by the

diagnosis itself, make the decision-making process hard and many individuals may prefer the doctor to take the lead.[39] Allowing choice in treatment decisions may help with long-term psychological adjustment to the disease and the effects of treatment[40] and in order for patients to do this, effective communication is important so that they are fully aware of the treatment options open to them.

Factors influencing an individual's decisions regarding treatment include:[41]

- superstitious beliefs about doctors, treatment and prognosis
- spiritual beliefs
- disbelief in medical technology
- commitment and belief in 'alternative' healing culture
- impact of previous exposure to cancer treatment as a patient, carer, or observer
- memories of the death of a loved one from cancer
- a lack of understanding of information or consent
- time pressures for decision making
- emotional reactions.

The provision of information is an important factor in helping an individual participate in the decision-making process and in pre-operative care, and is an important intervention strategy for nurses.[42] Information needs to be given in a clear and concise manner in ways that are understandable to the individual, avoiding where possible the use of medical jargon. Often individuals will retain very little of what is said to them initially about treatment and so it is important that where possible information is reinforced and an individual's understanding is checked out. There are many different ways of giving and explaining information, examples of which could be written information, drawings, or tape recording the conversation so that it can be played back at a later date. It is important to remember that everyone will retain information in different ways and so what is appropriate for one person may not be so for another:

. . . we met the second surgeon who examined me and then drew some sketches of what he was going to do to remove the cancer and repair the bowel (an anterior resection). The sketches made the procedure seem quite simple but of course it's not . . . this approach (drawing sketches) is in my opinion the very best way to put people at their ease and remove any mystery from treatment . . .[43]

In supporting someone through the decision-making process and the pre-operative process, one must be aware of the meaning of the treatment to that person, their need for control, the history of their illness, their personality, social position in life and coping abilities,[27] and the factors that will influence their decision making. They need to weigh up the personal consequences of cancer surgery, recognising both the benefits and risks of having surgery, the chances of cure, effects on their body image and sexuality, and the effects on their roles in the family and society. Psychological preparation for surgery is important and can aid post-operative recovery, adjustment, and adaptation.[10] However, nurses must also be aware that as they support the individual through the process of decision making and pre-operative care, the individual may make decisions that the nurse may not agree with, and though the nurse may find this hard, the individual needs to feel supported in whatever decision they make, whether it be to go through with surgery or not.

The place of surgery within the individual's cancer experience is important. Each part of their cancer treatment is set within a unique set of life experiences.[27] An individual may feel optimistic towards surgery – 'They have found it early and once it has been cut out I will be OK' – or they may be having surgery for local recurrence after the failure of chemotherapy or radiotherapy, and fear further side-effects from treatment. It could be that they have had many years of treatment and it seems to be continuous, never ending – taking a bit more of the individual away every time:

> We all sat quietly for a few moments while I took in the offer of this new operation. I couldn't think properly. This was worse, somehow, than even the original diagnosis. I felt the oppressive weight of the interminable surgical process suddenly, slicing me inch-by-inch, sucking me into even more drastic remedies, even more unbearable disabilities.

'What happens' I said, 'if I don't have the operation? [p. 249]'[26]

The following are a ward sister's comments on her experience with a 48-year-old man with a tumour of the upper jaw:[44]

> The strain of five years of illness was beginning to tell on the family when . . . John was due to have his left eye removed, the fourth operation to his face. The family was stunned by the shock and unable to do anything but close ranks and try not to think of the implications . . . When John came out of hospital . . . they still presented a united and optimistic front . . . but . . . they shared with me some of the difficulties they were experiencing in dealing with his wound and I was able to make practical suggestions. It was almost as if we could talk about the wound or the discharge as though they were entities separate from John himself, and therefore safe to talk about [p. 36].

The type of cancer that an individual has will affect their response to surgery. Surgery to some areas of the body may cause more distress to an individual than in other areas.[45] Surgery to the head and neck may alter an individual's appearance and fundamental functions and interactions such as eating, breathing and talking. Nowhere else is the site of surgery so exposed to society's view and so intertwined with who we are.[46] Fears about the concerns of others are natural, along with fears of isolation and rejection. Not only that, but the loss of functions such as speech will affect most areas of life, including family and social roles.[10]

The formation of a colostomy due to colorectal cancer so that normal bowel function is lost and faecal elimination is carried out through a surgically constructed stoma can give rise to thoughts of disgust, anger, embarrassment, and shame. For some individuals, their sense of cleanliness is violated and some may refuse to look at or have anything to do with their stoma.[10] Along with the change in their body image the formation of a stoma has implications on how they dress, their sexual functioning and their whole self-identity and confidence.

For individuals with gynaecological cancer, their identity as a woman is at stake, along with temporary or permanent loss of sexual functioning. This loss of sexual functioning along with loss of sexual desire and a decreased sense of femininity can greatly affect self-esteem and a lot of emotional care and support may be needed.[50] Similarly, breast surgery

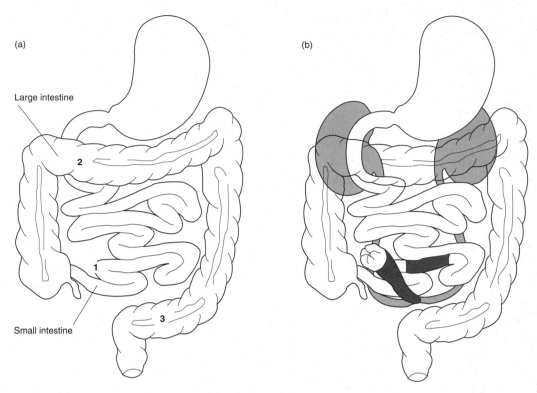

Figure 10.3 (a) Position of bowel stomas. (1) Ileostomy; (2) transverse colostomy; (3) sigmoid colostomy. (b) Ileal conduit (reproduced with permission from Salter M. (1997). *Altered Body Image: The Nursing Role*, 2nd edition. London: Ballière Tindall, p. 181).[49]

Box 10.3: Colorectal surgery

The goal of surgery for colorectal cancers is resection of the disease, leaving a disease-free margin. Surgical resection includes resection of associated vascular and lymphatic structures along with the tumour, in order to prevent seeding of the malignant cells.[47] Extensive procedures may therefore be needed. The type and extent of the surgery is determined by:

- tumour size
- tumour location
- presence/absence of metastases
- age
- nutritional status
- complications such as perforation or obstruction.

Surgery may be site specific for small localised tumours, though radical surgery is usually preferred[47] and may involve one of three types of major surgery:

- resection of the tumour with re-anastomosis

- resection of the tumour with the formation of a colostomy, either temporary or permanent
- abdomino-perineal resection.

Extensive metastases may require more radical surgery such as pelvic exenteration, where the bladder, rectum, and other structures are removed and an ileal conduit and sigmoid colostomy are created. However, sphincter-preserving surgery is now performed on over 50% of surgically resectable rectal tumours.[47]

If a colostomy is to be performed, the individual should be seen by a stoma care nurse as soon as possible. The siting of the stoma is very important and it should be away from the waistline, scars, skin folds or where the abdominal incision will occur. It should also be in a position where the individual can see and reach it. Post-operatively, the stoma site should be observed for colour and size, it should appear pink and moist; if it looks blue, black, or dusky in appearance it is showing signs of necrosis and ischaemia.

Post-operative complications can occur and include infection, paralytic ileus, pulmonary complications, anastomatic leaks leading to fistula formation, urinary problems, stoma retraction, and prolapse.[49]

can lead to feelings of a loss of femininity, sexuality, and self-esteem, and this varies according to the point of the surgery in the patient's lifetime.[10]

Research study 10.1

Corney R., Everett H., Howells A. and Crowther M. (1992). The care of patients undergoing surgery for gynaecological cancer: the need for information, emotional support and counselling. *Journal of Advanced Nursing* 17, 667–671.[50]

Aim of study
To investigate the psychosocial and psychosexual adjustment of women following major gynaecological surgery for cancer.

Method
Out of 177 women who underwent surgery for gynaecological malignancy in a London teaching hospital, 138 were contacted 6 months after their operation and invited to participate in a semi-structured interview. In total 105 women were interviewed, 28 of whom had had a radical vulvectomy, 69 a Wertheims' hysterectomy and eight a pelvic exenteration.

Results
Sixty-eight per cent of respondents said that they had been markedly or severely distressed at some stage in their illness, with the periods of most distress corresponding to the periods of most uncertainty. At the time of the interview (a minimum of 6 months post-surgery) 31% of the women were depressed and 41% anxious as classified by the Hospital Anxiety and Depression (HAD) Scale.

A high proportion of the women would have liked more information pre-operatively with regards to the after-effects of the surgery. Of the 40 partners that responded to the questionnaire, 25% would have liked more information on the illness and its treatment. 29% of the women would have liked information on the effects of the surgery on sexual function, with over 50% of the under 40-year-old women wanting their partners to be more involved in this.

Conclusions
The women indicated a need for more information with regards to all aspects of their surgery, covering physical, sexual, and emotional issues, and also indicated a need for emotional support, discussion, and counselling.

Limitations
The study was limited to women seen by one consultant in one hospital and will have reflected information/support networks within that one hospital, thus limiting the generalisability of the findings. However, the need for information pre-operatively is known to be important. With a time period of a minimum of 6 months, experiences of the treatment process, such as feelings and fears, may have diminished and other life events may have affected the womens' responses to the interview and HAD scale other than their surgery, as the individual does not go through treatment in isolation but amongst the intricacies of their daily lives. It was also noted that a greater proportion of women was prepared to discuss sexual issues post-surgery compared with pre-surgery. This reflects the lack of ease with which such subjects are discussed and may not therefore show the true picture among the sample.

The effects of surgery are felt not only by the individual undergoing that surgery but by their family and loved ones. Cancer is a family illness, affecting everyone that it touches. Partners will be affected by the change in body image of their loved ones along with the change in sexual desire and functioning. They too will need the care and support of health care professionals in coming to terms with what is happening to them and their loved ones. Some people may feel guilty and ungrateful in voicing their concerns about how things have affected them, for example in their sexual functioning, when their loved one has been saved from a perceived death sentence,[51] but they need to be encouraged to talk about this and explore how they feel. To others, the effects of the disease and disfigurement of surgery can be all too much, as described in the experiences of a ward sister looking after a man with head and neck cancer:

> . . . I had a frantic phone call to say that Pam, the 18-year-old daughter, had taken an overdose and was unconscious. Pam was a shy, highly strung girl who adored her father. His illness had distressed her deeply and his disfigurement was past enduring. She had refused to talk about this illness and tried to keep away from the house as much as possible [p. 38].[44]

It tends to be thought that individuals will be prepared to endure any type of disfigurement or change in functional ability in an effort to increase the probability of a cure.[29] However, an individual's willingness to tolerate any form of surgery merely to survive may become secondary once they are cured and have to face the psychosocial adaptation to the results of their surgery.[45] The amount of disfigurement or functional disability that an individual is prepared to take may vary at different times of their illness; what is or is not acceptable at one point of treatment may later change and become acceptable at a later date, when the life experiences and expectations of that individual have changed and moved on. This can be seen in the following illustration from John Diamond's book.[26] To him, the possible removal of his tongue was inconceivable at the time of his first surgery, when he was still hoping for a cure and could not imagine life without a tongue and the effect that this would have on his family and work life. However, further down the line, his feelings have changed and he is prepared to go through the operation and have his tongue removed in order that he might live for longer.

> Before the operation in 1997 I'd been handed the standard it's-not-our-fault-guv disclaimer to sign on which was detailed the nature of the procedure I was to undergo. I wrote in above the description the rider that however bad the tumour appeared to be they should not perform a total glossectomy – which is to say remove the whole of my tongue. Looking back on it now this seems a futile sort of gesture. If the only cure was removing my whole tongue then what point was there leaving it there? I wrote at the time that there would have been serious competition between living without a tongue and dying with one, but looking back now, I'm not so sure. Then again, at the time I still had no idea how long this road could run or how far down it I was prepared to go . . . The truth is that when I wrote that rider it wasn't because I didn't want them to remove my tongue but that I couldn't conceive of a state of tonguelessness and that denying it on the consent form was my acknowledgement of that. Now here we are again . . . listening to details of the next operation which was, of course, to remove the rest of my tongue [pp. 246–247].[26]

The delivery of surgical care in the UK has changed over the past decade due to both central government initiatives and medical advances.[52] The result of this has been the growth of day surgery and shorter in-patient admissions. Hospitalisation is expensive and stressful for the individual, with surgical patients experiencing more stress than medical patients.[53] Changes in the delivery of cancer services with shorter hospital stays for patients have meant an increased input from specialist and community nurses and more responsibility given to family and friends.

With shorter hospital stays, planning, and pre- and post-operative information becomes even more important, along with adequate assessment of the individual and family's needs and abilities to care for the individual after discharge. Information needs to be given on discharge about possible complications, what to do if these are experienced, and who to contact. While shorter hospital stays can reduce anxiety and allow individuals to recover in their own home, it can also increase anxiety if the appropriate resources are not available or in place.

The experience of surgery for the treatment of cancer is different for each individual and while information should be given to individuals before surgery about what to expect, we can never prepare them fully for how they will be and feel. Individuals can be told how many drains they will have *in situ*, where the scar will be, how much movement they will have, what pain control regime they will be on, or how to communicate if they are unable to talk, but we can never tell them what they will feel – how it will feel for them:

> The problem with major surgery – any surgery – is that there is no real way of anyone telling you how it will be when you come round. I'd had conversations with various of the medical people and . . . I had some idea of the wreckage that my physical form would suffer – that I'd be cut, and bandaged, and scarred. And I'd guessed that I'd feel pretty miserable, although misery wasn't really the term to describe the mixture of drug-dampened pain, irritation and physical constraint. But nobody can tell you how it feels to be that post-operative person, the person who is lying there waiting for the new chapter to start and with no idea how that chapter will read. I knew that everything that had been done to me would have a permanent effect, but I couldn't say what the effect – on my constitution, my looks, my voice, my career, my persona would be. I lay there and contemplated the new me and was frustrated by the shallowness of contemplation which was possible [pp. 188–189].[26]

Reconstructive surgery

Reconstructive surgery is 'surgery concerned with the restoration, reconstruction, correction or improvement in the shape and appearance of body structures that are defective, damaged or misshapen by injury, disease or growth and development'.[8] With the developments in surgery that have occurred over recent years, it has become more and more common for surgeons to repair anatomical defects and improve both function and cosmesis in order to restore an individual to as near a normal life as possible following cancer surgery;[3] for example, breast reconstruction, head and neck surgery, artificial joints for sarcoma patients, skin grafting, and penile implants.

Radical cancer surgery often leaves significant deformity and loss of function, causing major psychological morbidity and social isolation and reconstructive surgery has done much to restore or preserve function, self-image, and quality of life.[1] Reconstructive surgery should be considered at the initial stage of treatment as well as later in the course of the disease and can be carried out at the time of the initial operation where possible, even if an individual's life-expectancy is limited, as people should not have to face the added burden of physical and functional disability.[11]

Research study 10.2

Neill K.M., Armstrong N. and Burnett C.B. (1998). Choosing reconstruction after mastectomy: a qualitative analysis. *Oncology Nursing Forum* 25(4), 743–749.[54]

Aim of study
To describe the perspectives of women with breast cancer who chose to have a reconstruction, on the factors that influenced their decision.

Method
A descriptive qualitative design was used. Eleven women with a diagnosis of breast cancer who had undergone breast reconstruction were interviewed. They were all under the care of a plastic surgeon from an academic health centre in America. Inclusion criteria were a primary diagnosis of breast cancer, and admission to the centre for treatment and reconstruction. Subjects also had to speak English. Out of the 11 subjects, six had TRAM flap reconstruction, four saline implants, and one had a silicone implant. All reconstructions were undertaken immediately following surgery for breast cancer.

Intensive in-depth interviews were carried out either at the subject's home or at the health centre; these lasted for 45–90 minutes and were tape-recorded. Information was obtained about demographic information, their breast cancer diagnosis, and the decision-making process for having a reconstruction, such as their thoughts and behaviours when seeking information, personal reasons, and the feelings about the decision post-reconstruction. The information given at interview was

analysed at several different levels and sorted into different categories. Eight of the subjects were able to confirm the interpretation of the data at a later interview.

Results
The main theme that came out of the interviews was that of 'Getting one's life back' and this goal guided the decision-making process. The decision-making process was split into three themes: information seeking, talking it over, and seeking normality and these themes were interactive.

Conclusions
Getting one's life back was seen as a sense of normality in appearance, a social self with no need to explain one's physical self, and a return to work and physical activities. Breast reconstruction was seen to offer the best opportunity for achieving this and retaining a positive sense of self. Thus, reconstruction minimised the negative consequences of breast cancer and its treatment for the women in the study.

Limitations
A small sample was used for the study and all participants were all under the same surgeon. Subjects were mainly white (*n* = 8) and were well educated with regard to the health care resources available. The study only looked at women who had chosen to have a reconstruction and did not consider the decision-making process of those who had not. The women were also having to make lots of decisions at the same time on top of being given a cancer diagnosis, such as local disease control, adjuvant cancer therapy and decisions about reconstruction and it may be hard to separate out thoughts and feelings for each of these decisions. Hence the results of this study, although interesting, are not easily transferable to other women with breast cancer.

Some individuals, for example those having a mastectomy for breast cancer, will be given the option as to whether they would like breast reconstruction surgery or not. This option should be given to them at the time of their initial surgery. Hence, not only will they be trying to come to terms with the diagnosis of cancer and the fact that they need to have a mastectomy but also whether they would like reconstructive surgery as well, resulting in lots of decisions having to be made at once.[54] A variety of reconstructive options will be available to them; they may be offered an implant that goes under either the muscle or the skin that covers their chest, or muscle may be taken from another part of the body to form a new breast [*latissimus dorsi* flap or transverse *rectus abdominis* musculocutaneous (TRAM) flap], or they may be able to have a mixture of the two. The aim of the surgery is to cre-

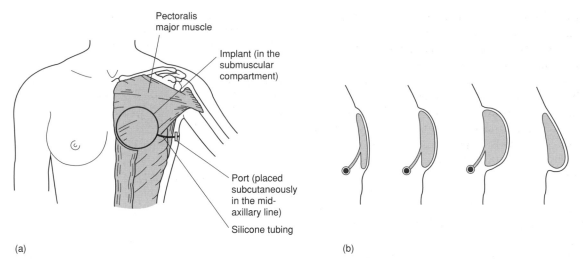

Pectoralis
major muscle

Implant (in the
submuscular
compartment)

Port (placed
subcutaneously
in the mid-
axillary line)

Silicone tubing

(a)

(b)

Reconstruction by expansion using a Becker's prosthesis.

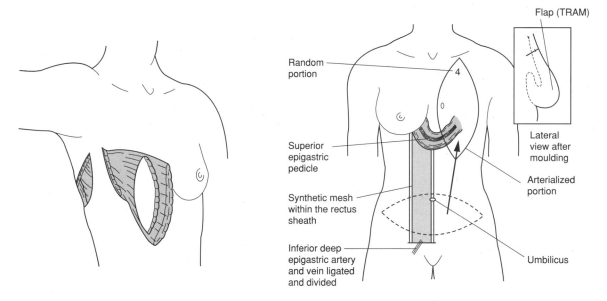

Flap (TRAM)

Random
portion

Lateral
view after
moulding

Superior
epigastric
pedicle

Arterialized
portion

Synthetic mesh
within the rectus
sheath

Inferior deep
epigastric artery
and vein ligated
and divided

Umbilicus

(c) Latissimus dorsi flap reconstruction. The myocutaneous
flap is delivered through the mastectomy wound.

(d) Conventional (pedicled) TRAM reconstruction.

Figure 10.4   Types of breast reconstruction surgery. ((a), (c) and (d) Reproduced with permission from Chapman & Hall Medical, London, Nash and Mokbel.[32] (b) Reproduced with permission from Baum M., Saunders C. and Meredith S. (1995). *Breast Cancer: A Guide for Every Woman*. Oxford: Oxford University Press, p. 70).[55]

ate a breast that is similar in size and shape to their own, but it will not be identical. While breast reconstruction is available at the time of the initial excision of the disease, and this is often seen to be in the individual's best interests,[11] it can also be performed at a later date if an individual would prefer or cannot decide whether to have it done or not.[3]

In other cases, for example those with head and neck cancer, there may be no choice as to whether reconstructive surgery is desired or not: it is a necessary part of the surgery to excise the tumour. Surgery of the head and neck is more complex than in other regions due to the essential and social functions that challenge the surgeons and also the importance of the individual's appearance. As well as the distress caused to the individual by having cancer, people who have had head and neck surgery see themselves as having changed; they are different to what they were, physically, emotionally, and in their self-identity, and this may have a negative impact on their relationships and sexuality.[45] Disfigurement acts as a physical barrier between the individual and their partner and some individuals will do all they can to hide any evidence of their surgery. Therefore in head and neck surgery, all attempts are made to reduce physical disfigurement and loss of function, and optimise cosmesis.

When performing surgery for cancers of the head and neck, a balance has to be made between surgical excision, reconstruction, and the prospect of early local recurrence in relation to morbidity and quality of life.[46] The loss of the ability to eat and talk is a high price to pay if one's expectation of life is limited.[11]

A diagnosis of cancer brings physiological, psychological, and social challenges and the decision or the ability to have reconstructive surgery will affect lifestyle and sense of self.[54] Reconstruction can facilitate self-esteem and return to a normal lifestyle, and helps the individual to cope with their diagnosis and treatment.[54] Careful emotional and physical planning is needed and people need to be given all the options, and information about those options, so that they can make an informed decision. It is important that they understand that while reconstructive surgery will give them 'a breast' or 'a tongue', it will not be the same as the real thing. A reconstructed breast will not feel or move in the same way or have the same sensual feeling. Likewise, the replacement of a tongue with a platform of tissue (a *latissimus dorsi* myocutaneous flap) can help to restore some of the ability to swallow and maintain intelligible speech, but it will not be the same. A balance therefore needs to be given between optimism and realism, and between quality of life and length of life:

> . . . This time plastic surgery would be needed: a lump of muscle in my back would be cut out and used to replace the tongue. For a while I thought this meant the recreation of a new tongue, of something which would have some of the function of the old one. But no: the flap would be no more than a platform, filling in the empty space in my lower jaw [p. 247].[26]

Some people with cancer have a strong desire to 'be normal again' and getting their life back to near what it was before is an overriding goal, to be a social individual with no need for explanations about their physical self, and to be able to return to work and physical activities.[54] These people and their families will need support not only in coming to terms with their diagnosis and decisions with regard to surgery but also in coming to terms with their new self, their new identity. Uncertainties will still exist about the outcome of treatment and the future but reconstructive surgery may play a vital role in allowing the individual to face that uncertain future:[11]

> Everybody was uncomfortable to some degree over the 'phone, but when they saw me and when I looked and acted so normal, I think they acted normal which normalised the whole situation . . . A body is supposed to be symmetrical. It's terribly lopsided the other way.

> All I wanted to do was to get back to normal as soon as possible, and I wanted to be cured . . . There was never any consideration of not having [reconstruction]. I don't know why any woman wouldn't have it . . . there's just no point in not looking normal and feeling normal when you've got those options in today's world [p. 748].[54]

Palliative surgery

Surgery can be effective in relieving symptoms in the advanced stages of cancer. In those people receiving palliative care there is usually no indication for further treatment of the underlying main diagnosis,[56] although in some instances, for example in head and neck cancer, there is often no distinction between what comprises 'palliative' or 'curative' surgery and palliative treatment may be so effective that a cure becomes possible.[57] The goal of palliative surgery is to relieve suffering and to minimise the symptoms of the disease.[3] The experience of the surgery will be different for each person, as a cure is no longer possible.

If quality of life will not be improved or if there is an unnecessary risk of morbidity or mortality, then surgery should not be undertaken. It is important that individuals are aware of the goals and aims of the surgery so that they can be realistic in their expectations of the surgery and are able to make informed decisions as to whether to go ahead with the surgery or not. For some, the thought of another operation or more time spent in hospital is too much and they would rather enjoy the time that they have left. Others will continue treatment right up to the last minute and will take whatever is offered to them in the hope that it might, after all, cure them or at least prolong their life that much more.

The role of surgery in the palliation of advanced disease includes:[57]

- the initial evaluation of disease when an individual presents with advanced disease
- local control of disease
- control of discharge or haemorrhage
- control of pain
- reconstruction or rehabilitation.

Surgery is essential in the control of local disease, whether that be for a fungating breast wound in an individual who is not yet dying from metastases[57] or to relieve bowel obstruction in an individual with cancer of the ovary. Removing or debulking the primary tumour in the presence of metastases may control discharge or the formation of fistulae or haemorrhage. Haemorrhage may occur from any ulcerated surface or from any tumour pressing onto a vital blood vessel, for example a 'carotid blowout'. In such instances, surgery may be considered as a preventive measure. Attempts to control the cancer may be taken before infiltration of the nerves occurs, which causes pain that is hard to control. Prophylactic or therapeutic pinning of metastases in long bones to prevent fracture may also be considered.[57] Surgery may also be required in the treatment of acute events in cancer care, such as spinal cord compression.

Box 10.4: Surgical treatment of bowel obstruction due to gynaecological malignancy

Bowel obstruction is a common complication of advanced ovarian cancer; it is hard to treat and often causes great distress. It is caused by occlusion to the lumen or a lack of normal propulsion, preventing or delaying intestinal contents from moving along the gastrointestinal tract.[58] Usually the tumour is scattered diffusely on the bowel surface, infiltrating the mesentery, resulting in a stiff, immobile bowel in areas that are encircled and compressed.[48] Presenting symptoms are nausea and vomiting, abdominal distension, spasmodic cramp-type pain and constipation.[59]

Treatment can be divided into conservative techniques, such as nasogastric intubation, fluids and resting the gut, sympto-

matic treatment such as octreotide, and surgery. Surgery is the primary treatment but not all individuals will be fit for surgery, so conservative or symptomatic treatment will be given. The decision to operate will depend on the following factors:[58]

- age, general medical condition and nutritional status
- presence of ascites or palpable abdominal masses
- previous radiotherapy to the abdomen or pelvis, or combination chemotherapy
- degree of abdominal distension
- patients' wishes.

The type of surgery given will depend on the area of the obstruction and, if present at more than one site, a combination of approaches may be taken. Surgical approaches include:[58]

- resection and re-anastomosis
- decompression, either colostomy or ileostomy
- bypass, such as gastroenterostomy
- lysis of adhesions.

Survival is greater in those having surgery; however, there is a high level of morbidity and mortality connected to it.[58,60] The mortality and morbidity rates are partly due to poor wound healing or infection due to a poor nutritional status.

Palliative care surgery needs to be carefully considered on an individual basis by the multi-disciplinary team. It should be considered in relation to each person's symptoms and their quality of life, and only if this can be improved should it be undertaken. Within the palliative care context it is the individual that should be treated first and the cancer second and not the other way round.[57] Surgery may be offered at a time when individuals are trying to come to terms with the fact that their cancer is no longer curable and that they have a shortened life expectancy, that they may not see their children or grandchildren grow up, when they may be mourning the loss of their future. The thought of surgery may interrupt this process and they may think that there is hope, only to have it destroyed again; however, the prospect of further surgery, which might improve their quality of life, may mean that they can be involved in important family events.

One man's comments on his wife's cancer run as follows:

We had been told that there was no further treatment for my wife's cancer . . . that they did not expect her to live for very long . . . well um . . . we were devastated . . . especially as our eldest daughter was due to get married in a couple of months . . . Jean so wanted to be there, but she was getting weaker and weaker and the tumour in her abdomen was getting bigger and bigger so she was very uncomfortable and could not eat . . . They said that they could operate and make the tumour smaller so that she would be more comfortable and may be able to eat more . . . she did not really want any more surgery but she thought that if she had it then she might just make our daughter's wedding after all . . . so she had the surgery and her appetite did get better for a bit and she was a lot more comfortable . . . and yes . . . she did manage to see our daughter married before she died and that was so special for all of us.

The control of pain is important in advanced cancer as 65–85% of individuals with advanced cancer have pain.[61] Pain assessment and evaluation of management strategies is vital in the control of pain and nurses have an important part to play in this. Surgical interventions for pain relief are required for some, though the majority will get adequate relief through oral analgesics and adjuvant medications. Less than 10% of those with cancer pain will require spinal opioids or neurolytic blocks.[62] The use of spinal opioids or neurolytic blocks necessitates the surgical insertion of access devices, such as intra-epidural and intrathecal catheters, intraspinal ports, or intraventricular reservoirs (Ommaya reservoirs).[63] These may be inserted under general or local anaesthetics and are normally well tolerated by the individual (see Chapter 17 for further information on pain control).

It is important that the appropriate considerations are taken before inserting access devices for pain control, such as individual and social factors, the availability of nursing care, who is going to look after the device, and whether the individual or their family will be able to cope with it. Issues around change in body image should also be considered, though for many the sheer relief of having their pain controlled will outweigh any potential implications and complications.

Supportive surgery

The surgical team may be required to undertake supportive surgery for the individual with cancer, such as providing venous and arterial access for the safe and reliable delivery of cytotoxics or for nutritional support or additional adjuvant therapies, such as the removal of the ovaries in women under 50 years old with early breast cancer. The ablation

of functioning ovaries in pre-menopausal women with early breast cancer significantly improves long-term survival in the absence of chemotherapy.[64] Ablation can be undertaken therapeutically through the use of hormones such as goserelin acetate, or by using radiotherapy or surgery.

The provision of venous access is very important in the treatment of cancer, both for the administration of chemotherapy and for supportive care during treatment. Vascular access can be achieved through short-term peripheral lines or longer-term central catheters (see Figure 10.5). The use of indwelling catheters has meant a marked improvement not only in safety but also in quality of life for people with cancer.[65] The decision of whether to insert an indwelling catheter will depend on the nature and duration of the anticipated intravenous therapy, the need for blood supply, and individual preference; for example, in those having a bone marrow transplant, or those with a needle phobia.

Box 10.5: Insertion of a central venous catheter

The catheter is inserted under the skin of the chest wall and into a large vein that leads to the heart. It may be inserted directly into the vein or tunnelled subcutaneously for a short distance before entering the vein. Catheters that are tunnelled subcutaneously have a Dacron cuff around the catheter, which anchors the catheter under the skin so that it does not slip out. Two incisions will be made, an 'insertion site' and an 'exit site'. The insertion site will heal once the sutures have been removed. The exit site of the catheter will need to have special care in order to prevent infection. The hazards associated with the insertion of a central catheter are numerous and include sepsis, air embolism, pneumothorax, haemorrhage, brachial plexus injury, catheter embolism, and thrombosis.

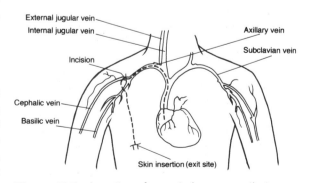

Figure 10.5   Insertion of a central venous catheter.

Careful assessment of the individual is needed when having a catheter inserted. Individuals and their families need to be taught about all aspects of care, function, and maintenance before the line is inserted, to ensure that they understand the implications and are able to care for it safely. Failure to do this can result in an indwelling catheter needing to be removed if the individual or family is unable to care for it properly. Catheters can usually be inserted on an out-patient or day care basis and may be inserted under either local or general anaesthetic, depending on both doctor and personal preferences.

For the health care professional, the use of indwelling catheters such as Hickman or Groshong lines may be routine, and thought may not be given as to how it could affect an individual and the implications of this. The reason why the line is being inserted also needs to be considered. Is it going to be used for intensive treatment such as a bone marrow transplantation, where the goal of that treatment is cure, or is it being used for palliative treatment where the goal is to control symptoms and maybe to prolong life? The following examples show how this difference may be perceived. In the first example, the individual is having intensive treatment with the hope of a cure, and can see the benefits of having a Hickman line and the freedom and control that it gives him. In the second example, a woman with advanced ovarian cancer is being offered palliative chemotherapy in an attempt to prolong her life; instead of seeing the benefits, she sees it as a threat to her body image and to her femininity, which is particularly important to her as she struggles to come to terms with what is happening.

> The oncologist who is in charge of my chemotherapy suggested . . . with the aid of diagrams that I should have a Hickman line put in and the chemicals administered by an infusion system. So, instead of having to go into hospital for two or three days every two weeks to have the chemo put in and the lines flushed through, my wife and I could 'do it ourselves at home'. I went into hospital to have the Hickman line fitted and for the first chemo to be put in, so that we could learn sterile procedures . . . Being responsible for administering the chemical at home has given us the feeling that we are making a positive contribution towards my recovery . . . so in conclusion – if you are given the chance to have a Hickman line fitted and if you are given the chance to have the chemicals at home – go for it and live life to the full![43]

Care strategy 10.1: Principles of care for a central venous catheter

Careful attention to the maintenance of the patency of the line and care of the insertion site will prolong the life of the catheter.

1. **Prevention of infection**
- Prevention of infection is very important, as many patients with cancer who have an indwelling central catheter will have periods of immunosuppression due to disease or its treatment and infection can be life-threatening.[65,66]
- There are three types of catheter-related infections: exit site infections, tunnel infections, and line sepsis.[65,66]
- An aseptic technique should be used when cleaning around the insertion and exit sites until the sutures have been removed.
- Once the sutures have been removed a dressing is not necessary over the catheter unless the person would like one, and a clean technique should be used to clean around the exit site.
- The exit and insertion sites should be observed for inflammation and/or discharge.

2. **Maintenance of a closed system**
- If equipment becomes disconnected, profuse blood loss or air embolism may occur.
- When a catheter that has a clamp is used, this should remain closed except when the catheter is in use.
- All connections should be carefully checked to ensure that they are air tight.

3. **Maintenance of a patent catheter**
- Occlusion of the catheter can occur due to the administration set being turned off for long periods, insufficient flushing or precipitate formation between incompatible medications.[66]
- The catheter should be flushed before and after it is used.
- Regular flushing of the catheter is needed, though there is considerable variation as to the solution and the frequency of flushing required (see guidelines for individual institutions).[65]

4. **Preventing damage to the catheter**
- Catheters may split if handled incorrectly.
- Catheters should be secured to the body by tape to prevent dislodgment.
- The catheter should be kept away from sharp objects such as scissors, shears or knives and other objects that could cause damage to the catheter.
- If damage does occur, the catheter should be clamped proximal to the damage and professional guidance sought.

If complications do occur then these should be dealt with by a health care professional.

The view of a woman with advanced cancer on having a Hickman line inserted is different:

> . . . they told me that I needed to have a 'line' put in so that I could have chemotherapy at home. They said they would put the line in under general anaesthetic, well it's . . . not the anaesthetic that I fear . . . no it's . . . the fact that the line goes in my chest . . . Well . . . I don't want a scar . . . my chest . . . well it's . . . it's the only part of my womanhood that they haven't touched . . . you see . . . my hair's gone . . . my womb has gone . . . and well . . . I don't want a scar on my chest as well . . .[43]

Indwelling catheters may be inserted for reasons other than for intravenous chemotherapy, such as a gastrostomy tube for nutrition, or intra-arterial, intraperitoneal, or intraventricular catheters for regional delivery of chemotherapy.[11,67] Whatever the reason, adequate planning is needed and the context surrounding the experience for the individual should be explored, enabling the right decision to be taken for that person.

Conclusion

It is clear that surgery has a major role and can be used in many different ways and contexts within the care and management of the person with cancer, whether it be on its own or alongside other treatment modalities, such as chemotherapy or radiotherapy. The meaning of surgery to the individual is important and in order to give the care that is needed we must be able to see the surgery within the context and experience of the individual.

The different types of surgery (definitive, reconstructive, and supportive) have been examined individually and in terms of what they might mean to the individuals experiencing them. In reality, however, it might not be as clear cut as that, with individuals not receiving a definite diagnosis until after definitive surgery. Surgery to excise a tumour may include definitive surgery to remove the tumour, diagnostic surgery through removal and subsequent testing of tissue and lymph glands, reconstructive surgery to repair the functional or cosmetic deformity made by the definitive surgery, and supportive surgery through the use of central lines or a gastrostomy; and after all that it may be that the surgery was palliative, if the disease had spread further than originally thought. Hence, what might start off in the eyes of the individual as a fairly

simple operation may turn out to be a lot more complex:

> But I felt pretty sanguine about the whole thing. I imagined a fairly routine operation to cut a bit out of me, stitch me up and kick me out on to the street again . . . Suddenly the single operation to cut out the cancer had become five operations – the cancer removal, two neck dissections, a tracheostomy and a gastrostomy. But there was more. He wasn't sure how much of my tongue he'd have to remove . . . it might be a job for the plastic surgeon . . . seven ops in one. Whoopee. I was scared again. Well of course I was . . . [pp. 135–137].[26]

The impact of surgery on the individual with cancer, whether it be major reconstructive surgery or the insertion of a Hickman line, should not be underestimated, and as nurses we need to focus our care on the individual and not on the cancer itself.

References

1. Moffat F.L. and Ketcham A.S. (1994). Surgery for malignant neoplasia: the evolution of oncologic surgery and its role on the management of cancer patients. In McKenna R.J. and Murphey G.P. (eds.) *Cancer Surgery*. Philadelphia, PA: Lippincott, pp. 1–20.
2. Buhle E.L. (1999). Introduction to surgical oncology. *Oncolink: University of Pennsylvania*. http://www.oncolink. upenn.edu/cgi-bin/print.pl
3. Frogge M.H. and Kalinowski B.H. (1997). Surgical therapy. In Groenwald S.L., Frogge M.H., Goodman M. and Yarbro C.H. (eds.) *Cancer Nursing: Principles and Practice*, 4th edition. London: Jones and Bartlett, pp. 229–246.
4. Thompson J.F. (1999). Principles of surgical oncology. In Bishops J.F. (ed.) *Cancer Facts: A Concise Oncology Text*. Singapore: Harwood, pp. 72–75.
5. Pfeifer K.A. (1994). Surgery. In Otto S.E. (ed.) *Oncology Nursing*, 2nd edition. St Louis, MO: Mosby, pp. 443–466.
6. Rosenberg S.A. (1997). Principles of cancer management: surgical oncology. In DeVita V.T., Hellman S. and Rosenberg S.A. (eds.) *Cancer: Principles and Practice of Oncology*, Vol. 1, 5th edition. Philadelphia, PA: Lippincott-Raven, pp. 295–306.
7. Cape B.F. and Dobson P. (eds.) (1974). *Baillière's Nurses' Dictionary*, 18th edition. London: Baillière Tindall.
8. *Doland's Illustrated Medical Dictionary* (1985). 26th edition. Philadelphia, PA: W.B. Saunders.
9. Anderson K.N. (1996). *Mosby's Medical, Nursing and Allied Health Dictionary*, 4th edition. St Louis, MO: Mosby.
10. Jacobsen P.B., Roth A.J. and Holland J.C. (1998). Surgery. In Holland J.C. (ed.) *Psycho-oncology*. New York: Oxford University Press, pp. 257–268.

11. Davidson T. and Sacks N.P.M. (1995). Principles of surgical oncology. In Horwich A. (ed.) *Oncology: A Multidisciplinary Textbook.* London: Chapman and Hall, pp. 101–115.
12. Holland J.C. (1989). Clinical course of cancer. In Holland J.C. and Rowland J.H. (eds.) *Handbook of Psycho-oncology: Psychological Care of the Patient with Cancer.* New York: Oxford University Press, pp. 75–100.
13. Grann V.R., Panageas K.S., Whang W., Antman K.H. and Neugut A.I. (1998). Decision analysis of prophylactic mastectomy and oophorectomy in BRCA1-positive or BRCA2-positive patients. *Journal of Clinical Oncology* 16, 979–985.
14. Church J.M. (1996). Prophylactic colectomy in patients with hereditary nonpolyposis colorectal cancer. *Annals of Medicine* 28, 479–482.
15. Lynch J. (1997). The genetics and natural history of hereditary colon cancer. *Seminars in Oncology Nursing* 13, 91–98.
16. Burke W., Daly M., Garber J., Botkin J., Kahn M.J.E., Lynch P. *et al.* (1997). Recommendations for follow-up care of individuals with an inherited predisposition to cancer. *Journal of the American Medical Association* 277, 997–1003.
17. Miki Y., Swensen J., Shattuck-Eiders D. *et al.* (1994). A strong candidate for the breast and ovarian cancer susceptibility gene BRCA-1. *Science* 266, 66–71.
18. Fentiman I.S. (1998). Prophylactic mastectomy: deliverance or delusion? *British Medical Journal* 317, 1402–1403.
19. Klijn J.G.M., Janin N., Cortes-Funes H. and Colomer R. (1997). Current controversies in cancer: should prophylactic surgery be used in women with a high risk of breast cancer? *European Journal of Cancer* 33, 2149–2159.
20. Powles T.J., Hardy J.R., Ashley S.E. *et al.* (1989). A pilot study to evaluate the acute toxicity and feasibility of tamoxifen for prevention of breast cancer. *British Journal of Cancer* 60, 126–133.
21. Hartmann L.C., Schaid D.J., Woods J.E. *et al.* (1999). Efficacy of bilateral prophylactic mastectomy in women with a family history of breast cancer. *New England Journal of Medicine* 340, 77–84.
22. Schrag D., Kuntz K.M., Garber J.E. and Weeks J.C. (1997). Decision analysis – effects of prophylactic mastectomy and oophorectomy on life expectancy among women with BRCA1 or BRCA2 mutations. *New England Journal of Medicine* 336, 1465–1471.
23. Eisinger F., Julian-Reynier C., Stoppa-Lyonnet *et al.* (1998) Correspondence: breast and ovarian cancer prone women and prophylactic surgery temptation. *Journal of Clinical Oncology* 16, 2573–2575.
24. Eddy D. (1996). Diagnostic and staging investigations. In Tschudin V. (ed.) *Nursing the Patient with Cancer.* London: Prentice Hall, pp. 43–60.
25. Love S. (1990). *Dr Susan Love's Breast Book.* Reading, MA: Addison-Wesley.
26. Diamond J. (1999). *C: Because Cowards Get Cancer Too . . .* London: Vermilion.
27. Haberman M. (1995). The meaning of cancer therapy: bone marrow transplantation as an exemplar of therapy. *Seminars in Oncology Nursing* 11, 23–31.
28. Askew N. (1998). *Your Contributions. CancerHelp UK.* http://medweb.bham.ac.uk/cancerhelp/public/forum/askew/index.html
29. Sanson-Fisher R.W. (1999). Patients' expectations of cancer. In Bishop J.F. (ed.) *Cancer Facts: A Concise Oncology Text.* Singapore: Harwood, pp. 372–376.
30. Murley A. (1990). A quality of dying. In Saunders C. (ed.) *St Christopher's in Celebration.* London: Hodder and Stoughton, pp. 80–83.
31. Otte D.I. (1996). Patients' perspectives and experiences of day case surgery. *Journal of Advanced Nursing* 23, 1228–1237.
32. Nash A.G. and Mokbel K. (1996). Techniques for local excision and reconstruction. In Allen-Mersh T.G. (ed.) *Surgical Oncology.* London: Chapman and Hall, pp. 373–382.
33. Crane R. (1994). Breast cancer. In Otto S.E. (ed.) *Oncology Nursing*, 2nd edition. St Louis, MO: Mosby, pp. 90–129.
34. Sherman A.C. and Simonton-Atchley S. (1996). Psychological aspects of treating oncology patients. In Myers E.N. and Suen J.Y. (eds.) *Cancer of the Head and Neck.* Philadelphia, PA: W.B. Saunders, pp. 917–925.
35. Stacey J. (1997). *Teratologies: A Cultural Study of Cancer.* London: Routledge.
36. Halldorsdottir S. and Hamrin E. (1996). Experiencing existential changes: the lived experience of having cancer. *Cancer Nursing* 19, 29–36.
37. Taylor E.J. (1995). Whys and wherefores: adult patient perspectives of the meaning of cancer. *Seminars in Oncology Nursing* 11, 32–30.
38. Davison B.J. and Degner L.F. (1998). Promoting patient decision making in life-and-death situations. *Seminars in Oncology Nursing* 14, 129–136.
39. Barry B. and Henderson A. (1996). Nature of decision-making in the terminally ill patient. *Cancer Nursing* 19, 384–391.
40. Beaver K., Luker K., Glynn Owens R., Leinster S.J. and Degner L. (1996). Treatment decision making in women newly diagnosed with breast cancer. *Cancer Nursing* 19, 8–19.
41. Szendroe A. (1999). Working with and managing cancer patients. In Bishop J.F. (ed.) *Cancer Facts: A Concise Oncology Text.* Singapore: Harwood, pp. 377–380.
42. Griffiths M. and Leek C. (1995). Patient education needs: opinions of oncology nurses and their patients. *Oncology Nursing Forum* 22, 139–144.

43. Adkin T. (1999). *Your contributions. CancerHelp UK.* http://medweb.bham.ac.uk/cancerhelp/public/forum/adkin/index.html.

44. McNulty B. (1990). A holding role. In Saunders C. (ed.) *St Christopher's in Celebration.* London: Hodder and Stoughton, pp. 35–44.

45. Gamba A., Romano M., Grosso I.M., Tamburini M., Cantu G., Molinari R. *et al.* (1992). Psychosocial adjustment of patients surgically treated for head and neck cancer. *Head and Neck* 14, 218–223.

46. Rhys-Evans F. (1996). Tumours of the head and neck. In Saunders C. (ed.) *Nursing the Patient with Cancer.* London: Prentice Hall, pp. 178–201.

47. Murphy M.E. (1994). Colorectal cancer. In Otto S.E. (ed.) *Oncology Nursing,* 2nd edition. St Louis, MO: Mosby, pp. 130–144.

48. Souhami R. and Tobias J. (1998). *Cancer and Its Management,* 3rd edition. Oxford: Blackwell.

49. Salter M. (1997). Stoma care and its effects on body image. In Salter M. (ed.) *Altered Body Image: The Nurse's Role,* 2nd edition. London: Baillière Tindall, pp. 180–208.

50. Corney R., Everett H., Howells A. and Crowther M. (1992). The care of patients undergoing surgery for gynaecological cancer: the need for information, emotional support and counselling. *Journal of Advanced Nursing* 17, 667–671.

51. Jones B. (1994). Drop-in centre for cancer care. *Nursing Standard* 9, 23–25.

52. Mitchell M. (1997). Patients' perceptions of pre-operative preparation for day surgery. *Journal of Advanced Nursing* 26, 356–363.

53. Fallowfield L. (1998). Editorial: early discharge after surgery for breast cancer: might not be applicable to most patients. *British Medical Journal* 317, 1264–1265.

54. Neill K.M., Armstrong N. and Burnett C.B. (1998). Choosing reconstruction after mastectomy: a qualitative analysis. *Oncology Nursing Forum* 25, 743–750.

55. Baum M., Saunders C. and Meredith S. (1995). *Breast Cancer: A Guide for Every Woman.* Oxford: Oxford University Press.

56. Bruera E. and Lawlor P. (1998). Defining palliative care interventions. *Journal of Palliative Care* 14, 23–24.

57. Baum M., Breach N.M., Shepherd J.H., Shearer R.J., Merion Thomas J. and Ball A. (1995). Surgical palliation. In Doyle D., Hanks G.W.C. and MacDonald N. (eds.) *Oxford Textbook of Palliative Medicine.* Oxford: Oxford University Press, pp. 129–140.

58. Baines M. (1995). The pathophysiology and management of malignant intestinal obstruction. In Doyle D., Hanks G.W.C. and MacDonald N. (eds.) *Oxford Textbook of Palliative Medicine.* Oxford: Oxford University Press, pp. 311–316.

59. Dennison S. and Dawson T. (1996). Gynaecological cancers. In Tschudin V. (ed.) *Nursing the Patient with Cancer.* London: Prentice Hall, pp. 279–300.

60. Chan A. and Woodruff R.K. (1992). Intestinal obstruction in patients with widespread intra-abdominal malignancy. *Journal of Pain and Symptom Management* 7, 339–342.

61. Grond S., Zech D., Diefenbach C. and Bischoff A. (1995). Prevalence and pattern of symptoms in patients with cancer pain: a prospective evaluation of 1,635 cancer patients referred to a pain clinic. *Journal of Pain and Symptom Management* 9, 372–382.

62. Swarm R.A. and Cousins M.J. (1995). Anaesthetic techniques for pain control. In Doyle D., Hanks G.W.C. and MacDonald N. (eds.) *Oxford Textbook of Palliative Medicine.* Oxford: Oxford University Press, pp. 204–221.

63. Brant J.M. (1995). The use of access devices in cancer pain control. *Seminars in Oncology Nursing* 11, 203–212.

64. Early Breast Cancer Trialists' Collaborative Group (EBCTG) (1999). Ovarian ablation in early breast cancer: overview of the randomised trials (Cochrane Review). In *The Cochrane Library,* Issue 1. Oxford: Update Software.

65. Alexander H.R. (1997). Vascular access and specialized techniques of drugs delivery. In DeVita V.T., Hellman S. and Rosenberg S.A. (eds.) *Cancer: Principles and Practice of Oncology,* Vol. 1, 5th edition. Philadelphia, PA: Lippincott-Raven, pp. 725–734.

66. Mallett J. and Bailey C. (1996). *The Royal Marsden Hospital Manual of Clinical Nursing Procedures,* 4th edition. Oxford: Blackwell.

67. Almadrones L., Campana P. and Dantis E.C. (1995). Arterial, peritoneal, and intraventricular access devices. *Seminars in Oncology Nursing* 11, 194–202.

CHAPTER ELEVEN

Chemotherapy

Lisa Dougherty and Christopher Bailey

The term 'chemotherapy' was originally coined at the beginning of the twentieth century to refer to the theoretical possibility of utilising substances with specific toxicity towards micro-organisms such as bacteria.[1] Cancer chemotherapy – the administration of antineoplastic agents either alone or in combination – frequently makes use of drugs that disrupt cellular replication by inhibiting the synthesis of new genetic material or causing irreparable damage to DNA itself.[2]

Cyto- (or *-cyte*) = cells or a cell

chemo- = chemical

neoplasm = new or abnormal growth of tissue in some part of the body, especially a tumour.

Chemotherapy in cancer may be used in the expectation of achieving a cure, when all cancer cells are destroyed and life expectancy is similar to the life expectancy of a person who does not have cancer. It may be used to achieve control over the disease by preventing or slowing down the growth of a malignant tumour, and thus prolonging survival, and it may be used palliatively in the management of symptoms such as pain or breathlessness. Chemotherapy used for the palliation of symptoms is not expected to achieve either cure or control.

Definitive chemotherapy is chemotherapy given as the sole treatment of a disease; the term *salvage chemotherapy* is sometimes used to denote treatment given to patients who have relapsed following initially successful treatment with another modality (such as surgery or radiotherapy). Experimental chemotherapy is given to investigate the usefulness of a new drug whose role is not proven at the time of treatment.

Adjuvant chemotherapy refers to the use of antineoplastic drugs after removal of the primary tumour to eliminate as many remaining cancerous cells or micrometastases as possible.

Neoadjuvant chemotherapy refers to the use of chemotherapy or radiotherapy before surgery to 'debulk' or reduce the size of the primary tumour and to maximise the effectiveness of subsequent therapies. In the treatment of rectal cancer, for example, neoadjuvant radiotherapy may be given to patients with resectable tumours to destroy microscopic tumour cells that could not be surgically removed without increasing the risk of major post-operative complications. If the tumour is not resectable (which may be the case if it has become attached to adjacent organs such as the bladder), pre-operative radiotherapy may be given to shrink the tumour and 'downstage' the disease.[3]

When evaluating the response to chemotherapy, it remains remarkably difficult to define 'cure' reliably in cancer care. One definition is that cure is achieved when the life expectancy of a person with cancer is the same as for a person of the same age and sex who has not been affected by cancer.[4] Many research trials use duration of survival as a measure of the success of treatment. In general, survival is likely to be longer with treatment than if treatment had not been given, but shorter than it would have been had the person not developed cancer.[5] Objective criteria are needed, based on the immediate response of the tumour and a patient's physiological status, to evaluate the effects of treatment. Tumour regression often occurs early and can be expressed in terms of tumour size. To summarise some key definitions of response:

- complete reponse (CR) – disappearance of all known disease
- partial response (PR) – a decrease in total tumour of 50% or more
- no change (NC) – neither a 50% decrease nor a 25% increase in tumour size can be demonstrated
- progressive disease (PD) – increase in tumour size of 25% of more.

(Adapted from Horwich A. (ed.) (1995). *Oncology: A Multidisciplinary Textbook*. London: Chapman and Hall, p. 136.)[6]

Patients' own accounts and reflections are also extremely valuable to clinicians, and often help the patient to understand and make sense of their illness and treatment. Measures of performance status are sometimes used to assess response to treatment (e.g. Karnofsky Performance Status Scale,[7] visual rating scales, verbal rating scales, and patient diaries). Measurement tools such as this reflect one aspect of function rather than multi-dimensional function[8] and may not give a comprehensive picture of the effects of illness or treatment.

The cell cycle

The sequence of phases through which cells must pass as they replicate (the *cell cycle*) is the fundamental biological context for many of the anti-cancer drugs.

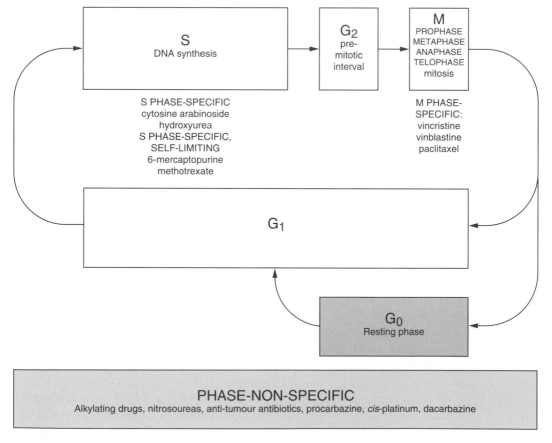

Figure 11.1 The cell cycle and the relationship of anti-tumour drug action to the cycle (reproduced with permission from Hardman J.G. *et al.* (eds.) (1996). Goodman and Gilman's *The Pharmacological Basis of Therapeutics*, 9th edition. McGraw Hill, New York, p. 1231).[2]

The term 'cell cycle' refers to the process through which cells, both normal and malignant, grow and replicate (see Figure 11.1). The cycle is comprised of five phases: G_0, G_1, S, G_2, and M. The 'G' phases are gap phases, in which cells are preparing for active DNA (deoxyribonucleic acid) synthesis and mitosis (division), or are resting.

G_1 is the first gap or growth phase (also known as the intermitotic phase), in which cells prepare for DNA synthesis by producing RNA (ribonucleic acid) and protein. Cells in G_0 are resting (that is, not preparing for cell division), though they remain viable and are capable of division if suitably stimulated. G_0 is considered a sub-phase of G_1.

S is the synthesis phase, in which cells double their DNA content (DNA is the coded genetic information required for the growth, repair, and reproduction of cells). Many cytotoxic drugs work by disrupting genetic codes during DNA synthesis.

G_2 is the second gap or growth phase (premitotic phase). Synthesis of RNA and proteins continues in preparation for mitosis.

M is the mitotic phase, in which cell division (mitosis) takes place. The cell divides into two daughter cells, each containing the same number and type of chromosomes as the parent cell. At the end of the M phase, cells either rejoin the cell cycle at G_1, or enter the resting sub-phase G_0.

Cytotoxic drugs affect both normal and malignant cells by altering activity during one or more phases of the cell cycle. Though both types of cells are destroyed by chemotherapy, normal cells have a greater ability to repair minor damage and remain viable than malignant cells. The susceptibility of malignant cells to irreparable damage is utilised to achieve the therapeutic effects of cytotoxic chemotherapy.

Yarbro (in Perry[1]) describes the delicate balancing act that is the goal of cytotoxic chemotherapy in this way:

> The metabolism of the cancer cell is so similar to that of the normal cell that we have been forced to utilise rather minute differences through which drugs might exert a differential effect. The most important such difference is the rapid rate of division of the cancer cell relative to most other body tissues . . . this small difference allowed chemotherapeutic cures in rapidly proliferating animal tumours such as the L1210 mouse leukaemia . . . Human tumours, however, are more com-plex. They . . . follow . . . the more complex Gompertzian growth curve in which there are resting, non-proliferating cells resistant to chemotherapy . . . [p. 2].

Tumour growth

Tumour growth is affected by *cell cycling time* and *growth fraction*.

Cell cycling time

Originally tumours were thought to grow because they consisted of cells that multiplied more rapidly than cells in the surrounding tissue. In fact, the average cell cycle of 48 hours for human tumour cells is slightly longer than the cycle of non-malignant cells. If the rate of cell division were the only factor to determine tumour growth, cancers would grow at the same rate as or more slowly than normal tissue and cause no problems.

When a normal cell divides, it does so only to replace a cell that has been lost and in this way a constant cell population is maintained. In tumour cells the control mechanism appears to have been lost: as the cell divides it adds to existing numbers of cells and increases the total population. The cause of this phenomenon remains unclear.

A measure of the rate of tumour growth is the time taken for a given population of malignant cells to double in size (*doubling time*). If the cell cycle takes between 15 and 120 hours, the doubling time can be between 96 hours and 500 days, depending on the histological type of the tumour, its age, and whether it is a primary or metastatic growth. A shorter doubling time (less than 30 days) is seen with teratomas, non-Hodgkin's lymphomas, and acute leukaemias; common solid tumours such as squamous cell carcinoma of the bronchus and adenocarcinoma of the breast and bowel have doubling times in excess of 70 days. In any patient the growth of a cancer is only detectable and observable during the last 10–14 of its 35–40 doubling times.

Growth fraction

In the early stages of development tumour volume is low, but the proportion of viable cells in the active division cycle at any one time (the *growth fraction*)[9] is high. However, most malignant neoplasms are only detected at a later stage. By this time, poor tumour vascularity and consequent hypoxia, or poor nutrient supply together with other factors, mean that the rate of growth is decelerating, and the tumour contains a high fraction of slowly dividing or resting (G_0) cells (i.e. the growth fraction is low).[10] Studies of adenocarcinoma in mice have shown that as the tumour increases in size, the mass doubling time (time taken for the tumour mass to double) increases many-fold, while the growth fraction is drastically reduced[11] (that is, the mass doubling time is inversely proportional to the growth fraction). This pattern of growth is close to what is known as a *Gompertzian* growth curve: cells accumulate slowly at first, then more rapidly, achieving a maximum growth rate at about one-third of maximum tumour volume.[1] The rate of growth then slows gradually and almost levels out (the 'plateau phase') (see Figure 11.2).

Most chemotherapeutic agents are most effective against rapidly dividing cells, i.e. when tumours are still in the proliferating stage. Some are phase specific, and are most effective against cells in a particular phase of the cell cycle. Therefore, at the point at which most tumours are detected clinically, the situation is not immediately best suited for intervention with cytotoxic therapy. However, reducing the number of malignant cells with surgery, radiotherapy or non-cycle-specific drugs may lead to an increase in the rate of cell division and may induce (or 'recruit') resting cells to re-enter the cell cycle, where they are more vulnerable to cycle-specific agents. The proportion of malignant cells destroyed may therefore increase over repeated courses of treatment.

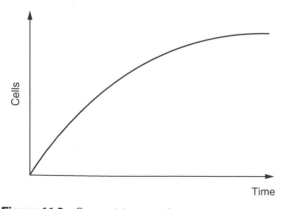

Figure 11.2 Gompertzian growth.

First-order kinetics

Cancer cells appear to be destroyed by chemotherapy according to first-order kinetics, that is, a certain dose of drug will destroy a constant proportion of malignant cells, rather than a constant number. Pratt *et al.*[12] explain some of the implications of 'first-order kinetics':

> . . . it will take just as much drug to lower the tumour cell number from 10^6 to 10^3 (a loss of less than 1 mg of tissue) as to lower the tumour cell number from 10^9 to 10^6 (a loss of 1 g of tissue) . . . at the time of diagnosis of a number of disseminated malignant diseases, as many as 10^{12} tumour cells may be present. This may be close to the fatal number for certain tumours. Successful chemotherapy may kill 99.9% of the cells . . . and still leave 10^9 cells in the patient. This number is barely detectable, and clinically, the patient may appear to be 'in remission'. But it is necessary to continue therapy even in the face of an apparent remission to eliminate the many malignant cells that are still present . . . to produce a cure, therapy must be continued until the last tumour cell is killed. There is ample experimental evidence that one viable tumour cell can produce a tumour that will kill a susceptible host animal [pp. 29–30].

Pharmacology

The way that cancer chemotherapy is selected, calculated, and administered depends on a variety of pharmacological factors. Knowledge of the *pharmacodynamic* properties of a drug ('what drugs do and how they do it') is 'essential to the choice of drug therapy' and 'the basis of intelligent use of medicines'.[13] Doses have to be set to achieve neither too much nor too little of the right effect. Too much may cause unwanted and dangerous toxic effects; too little may not achieve any therapeutic goals.

Pharmacokinetics is about achieving:

> . . . the right effect at the right intensity, at the right time, for the right duration, with minimum risk of unpleasantness or harm . . . [and] . . . is concerned with the rate at which drug molecules cross cell membranes to enter the body, to distribute within it and to leave the body, as well as with the structural changes [metabolism] to which they are subject within it [p. 83].[13]

The therapeutic effect of a drug thus rests on achieving a balance between what the drug does, its action or its pharmacodynamic properties, and its behaviour within the body, or its pharmacokinetic properties, to achieve the right kind of effect with the right intensity and duration.

Route of administration

The route of administration is dictated by the characteristics of individual drugs and is chosen to optimise drug availability. Careful selection of an appropriate route of administration can improve the anticancer effect of a drug by enabling a higher concentration to reach the tumour.

Drug distribution

The distribution and transport of drugs within the body can significantly influence the effects of chemotherapy. After they have been administered drugs can bind to serum albumin, which affects the proportion of free or pharmacologically active drug in the blood stream. When free drug leaves the blood stream (for example, when it is metabolised or excreted), it is replaced by drug that was previously protein bound. Drugs sometimes compete for binding sites: one drug can displace another from a binding site, which can lead to toxic levels of the drug that is displaced. Methotrexate is displaced by aspirin and probenecid and possibly by other non-steroidal anti-inflammatories in this way, causing severe toxicity.[13]

Biotransformation

Cytotoxic drugs undergo a wide range of metabolic transformations, including oxidation, reduction, hydrolysis, or configuration, most of which take place in the liver.

Excretion

Drugs are commonly excreted via the kidneys or the liver. The function of these organs is crucial to successful treatment, as impaired clearance may cause increased toxicity.

Drug interactions

Interactions between drugs are not uncommon. One drug may either inhibit or potentiate the action of another, thus modifying its therapeutic or toxic effects, or its enzyme inhibition or induction.

Drug resistance

The value of any cytotoxic agent can be severely limited by tumour resistance. There are two main types of tumour resistance. *Primary resistance*

occurs when tumours show no response when drugs are administered; it is thought to be a major factor in the failure of chemotherapy drugs. *Secondary resistance* is said to occur when tumour regression is initially seen following administration of a drug, but is temporary, with the tumour reappearing and the patient relapsing. Factors contributing to secondary resistance include:

- variations in drug bioavailability
- drug metabolism or elimination
- tumours possibly located in 'sanctuary sites'
- changes in cell kinetics
- drug-related toxicity in the recipient
- reduced blood supply to the tumour.

There are four main categories of drug resistance.

1. *Kinetic resistance.* Anti-cancer drugs may be cell cycle or cell cycle phase specific, so cells can be less sensitive to particular agents by virtue of their position in the cell cycle.
2. *Biochemical resistance* will occur if drugs are not transported across the cell membrane, if they are not activated within the cell, if they are confronted with an excess of their target substance within the cell, or if cells possess an enhanced ability to repair their DNA.[1]
3. *Pharmacological resistance.* Tumour cells may be located in areas where it is difficult to achieve the required drug concentration, and may therefore in effect be less sensitive. The central nervous system is one such area. Changes in the way a drug is metabolised in an individual patient may also make it more difficult to achieve adequate concentration of a drug.[1]
4. *Selected/induced resistance.* One possible explanation of the biological reasons for drug resistance (or reduced sensitivity) in tumours is that it is due to genetic factors. This type of resistance is known as *selected resistance.* However, it is also possible that resistance is a direct result of exposure to an anti-cancer drug. This type of resistance is known as *induced resistance.* It is argued[1] that the most likely explanation is that acquired resistance has a genetic and therefore a selective basis. Resistance may also be *intrinsic*, as opposed to *acquired*: that is to say, it is present in cells that have not previously been exposed to a particular drug.

Multi-drug resistance (MDR) is now a well-recognised phenomenon: exposure to a single drug is followed by cross-resistance to other apparently unrelated drugs. Impaired drug transport appears to be a critical factor in MDR, resulting in reduced or altered drug accumulation in the cell. Two mechanisms have been proposed to account for this: (a) drug enters the cell at the normal rate but is removed by a biochemical 'pump'; (b) a biochemical barrier controls entry to the cell. Evidence suggests that a cell surface glycoprotein (P-glycoprotein) acts as a pump, removing toxins from the cell. Drugs are thought to become bound to P-glycoprotein, and are subsequently moved across the cell membrane and out of the cell. Tumour cells appear to be able to increase the amount of P-glycoprotein on their surface membrane.

Effects of cytotoxic drugs

All cytotoxic drugs share two properties: an ability to inhibit the process of cell division and an inability to distinguish between normal and malignant cells. The effects of cytotoxic drugs are most obvious in normal tissues where cells are dividing most rapidly, and it is the appearance of toxicity in these tissues that limits their usefulness as anticancer agents.

Tissues that are rapidly and continuously proliferating include the following:

- *Bone marrow.* Here there is continuous cellular repair and replacement of two types of cell: *stem cells* (progenitor cells from which all other cells are derived) and *differentiated* (mature) cells.
- *Gastrointestinal tract.* The mucosal epithelium that lines the gastrointestinal tract is composed of cells that frequently divide to repair the day-to-day damage caused by nutrients and waste on their way through the gut.
- *Hair follicles.* Between 60% and 90% of hair follicles are actively dividing at any one time. Cytotoxic drugs can damage the epithelial cells of the hair follicle: stem cells at the base of the shaft atrophy, hairs become thinner and more fragile, and can break off or fall away.[14]
- *Testicular germ cells.* The germinal epithelium of the seminiferous tubules of the male testicles replicates continuously throughout adult life and is therefore highly sensitive to the effects of anticancer agents.[4]

Some tissues proliferate slowly and continuously (e.g. tracheobronchial and vascular epithelium), some proliferate in a cyclical fashion (e.g. glandular female breast cells and the endometrial lining of the uterus), some possess the capacity to proliferate after injury (e.g. liver and bone tissue), and some do not proliferate at all (e.g. skeletal and cardiac muscle, cartilage, and neurones).

Care strategy 11.1: Managing hair loss

Our hair plays an important part in the way we see or think of ourselves, and hair loss (alopecia) can badly damage our body image and self-concept,[15] particularly in view of current stereotypes of physical beauty.[16] Freedman[17] explains that:

> Embodied in the symbolism of hair is a concept of the whole self, a completed person, who has the possibility of expressing individualism through the design of her hair. If hair is seen as being associated with the person's identity, then the meaning of the loss of hair can be understood as symbolic of the devastating sense of the diminishing and eventual loss of the self. The loss of hair is an extremely traumatic experience precisely because it is the symbolic precursor to the loss of the self. This raises the psychological terror and consequent fear that the known self will no longer exist [p. 336].

Sudden changes in body image or alterations of body structure or function are perceived as threats and invariably cause anxiety. The hair loss caused by anti-cancer chemotherapy represents such a threat.[18] It has been suggested that of all the side-effects of chemotherapy, hair loss is the most distressing, and it may be the reason that some patients decline treatment.[16,19,20] A patient's own account[21] of hair loss expresses how distressing an experience it is:

> Mentally I had prepared myself for the likelihood of losing my hair and having to wear a wig; but the physical reality of the hair falling out posed emotional and practical problems which I had not anticipated. For two weeks I was in tears every morning, plucking the clumps of hair from all over the bedclothes . . . intellectually I understood what was happening, but emotionally it reinforced my feelings that I was losing part of myself.[20]

In her research, Tierney[22] described three broad categories of feelings that emerge when people discover that they will lose their hair. There are those who are upset and worried:

> Yes, it worries me because it would be an outward sign of my incapacity and that is upsetting when one is trying to be normal, even with cancer . . . actually I realise that hair loss worries me a lot, even though I was told

it might not happen . . . I think it's been worse to come to terms with than having my mastectomy. I can live with the fact that I've lost a breast, but no, I couldn't do with hair loss.

There are those who appear to have gone through the stage of feeling upset and have become resigned to hair loss, simply accepting it as the price of treatment:

Well, if it happens, it happens . . . you just have to accept it. I console myself with the knowledge that it is only temporary and it can be hidden.

Other patients are clearly not bothered by the prospect of hair loss:

No, I'm not really bothered . . . I can wear a wig and that will be alright.

A small group of patients, though, was very distressed, to the point of considering whether to have treatment at all:

I was heartbroken about it . . . it really upset me to the point of wondering if I could accept chemotherapy. I couldn't think how I'd cope with it. For me, the possibility of losing my hair is much, much worse than losing a breast.

Freedman[17] discusses the meaning or symbolism of hair loss:

For many . . . the meaning of the shaved head can be symbolic of a state of disgrace, which becomes a stigmata of sin or wrongdoing. This symbolic meaning . . . may be part of the reason that women describe themselves as being in a state of shame when they lose their hair . . . 'Losing my hair was the most traumatic part of the cancer/chemo process for me. It makes it so obvious that you are sick. Under the wig I knew there was a shiny bald head. It really takes some getting used to. It's really hard to express how you feel when your hair is coming out in handfuls. Some words are panic, fear, hurt, and even shame for how you look, even though you know it is not your fault.' [p. 337]

While the prospect of hair loss is a source of distress and anxiety for some (particularly if it occurs a second time),[23] not every patient will share this experience. It cannot be assumed that every patient will be distressed, and some may find that there are positive aspects to the situation.[22,24] An opportunity to talk about how you are feeling can be very helpful, and for nurses, developing an understanding of the meaning and importance of hair loss for different patients can lead to important insights into the caring process.[17] Nurses are well placed to provide support and information, and to highlight choices. They can offer realistic information about hair loss, details about what actually happens and when, and advice and assistance with practical problems (if and when to cut hair or choose a wig, for instance).[25,26] Scalp cooling, although it is not effective in all cases, can be offered in appropriate

circumstances to prevent or reduce hair loss, though it may be a lengthy and uncomfortable procedure.[27–29] It should be carefully explained in advance, measures should be taken to minimise discomfort and anxiety, and patients' reactions should be carefully monitored.[30–32]

Giving anti-cancer chemotherapy

Single agent continuous cytotoxic therapy
Priestman[4] notes that in the early period of anti-cancer chemotherapy the principles of anti-microbial chemotherapy were used as the basis for single agent continuous therapy, the object being to produce and maintain a constant level of cytotoxic agent in the patient until:

. . . unacceptable toxicity, drug resistance, or cure resulted. Toxicity determined the amount of drug that could be given. As it was considered that the blood level of the drug should be as high as possible, the dose was adjusted upwards until toxicity was apparent and then maintained at a level which caused minimal side-effects (such as slight nausea or a small depression in the white cell count) [p. 55].

Continuous infusional chemotherapy
Anti-cancer chemotherapy is often most effective when tumour cells are cycling, or when they are in a specific phase of the cell cycle. When chemotherapy is given by continuous infusion, the anti-cancer agent is present when a sensitive phase of the cycle is reached, irrespective of the length of the cell cycle. The transport of the agent across the tumour cell membrane may depend not only on drug concentration but also on the length of time the drug is available to the cell membrane. Most chemotherapeutic agents have a short pharmacological half-life and may be more effective if tumour cells are exposed to them for prolonged periods, which cannot be achieved if they are given by intermittent bolus injection. When given continuously the concentration of drug in the plasma may be lower than levels reached immediately following bolus injection or intermittent bolus infusion, and many of the toxicities associated with a drug may thus be avoided. Perry[1] notes that:

. . . the potential enhancement of antitumour activity by continuous infusion may not be accompanied by commensurate enhancement of toxicity . . . Because of diminished toxicity, some chemotherapeutic agents, such as 5-fluorouracil, may be given in more dose-intense schedules if delivered by continuous infusion. However, measured dose intensity between differing schedules of administration may not relate to antitumour activity [p. 232].

Intermittent chemotherapy

Populations of normal cells are diminished by treatment with anti-cancer chemotherapy, but initially recover far more rapidly than malignant cells. Because restoration is achieved more quickly in normal tissue than in malignant tissue, if a series of treatments is given with intervals to allow normal tissue to recover, it may be possible to eradicate a tumour without jeopardising the population of normal cells. Timing of the treatments is very important. If the interval between treatments is too short, normal stem cells will not have recovered sufficiently and cumulative toxicity will result, preventing adequate treatment. If the interval between treatments is too long, tumour cell recovery will be complete, and tumour size will remain static or increase between treatments. Dividing chemotherapy regimens into short, intensive treatments followed by intervals is known as intermittent chemotherapy. Intermittent chemotherapy has enabled combinations of drugs to be used to increase response rates without irreversible toxicity.

Combination chemotherapy

Chemotherapeutic agents have a variety of actions on the dividing cell. A tumour cell that is resistant to one drug with a particular mode of action may well be sensitive to a different agent with an alternative form of cytotoxicity. Combining drugs with different mechanisms of action should reduce the likelihood of resistance, increase the fractional cell kill, and improve response rates. All drugs used in combination chemotherapy should be of proven value in the disease they are intended to treat; they should have different modes of cytotoxic action and, if possible, the dose-limiting toxicities of the chosen agents should be different, so that the additive toxicity does not limit the dose intensity of the treatment.

High-dose chemotherapy

A few drugs (those that principally cause toxicity to the bone marrow) may be used in very high doses if bone marrow is taken from the patient prior to treatment and returned later (autologous bone marrow transplantation or 'autografting'). In this way doses of a drug that are very toxic to the bone marrow may be given, as the autograft of bone marrow or stem cells is not exposed to the chemotherapeutic agent. Following reinfusion of the autograft, the patient's blood count will gradually return to normal. Autografting of bone marrow does not, however, reduce the toxicities of high-dose chemotherapy that affect tissues other than the bone marrow.

Drug dosage and scheduling

There is a definite relationship between drug dose and response in sensitive tumour cell populations. Therapeutic effect may be compromised by an inadequate dose of chemotherapy, and commonly results from a reduction of the prescribed dose. Three parameters are used to define the dose component of treatment: size, total amount delivered, and rate.

Treatment protocols

Decisions about whether to administer anti-cancer chemotherapy on an in-patient or an out-patient basis depend on numerous considerations, including:

- the age and general health of the patient
- the planned drug regimen and the recommended method of administration
- the necessity for additional therapy (e.g. intravenous hydration)
- the need to correct deficits prior to commencing treatment (e.g. blood transfusion, nutritional support)
- the anticipated severity of side-effects and/or toxicity and the necessity for anti-emetics or other medication
- the wishes of the patient, family, or friends.[33]

The initial decision is not absolute. Therapy that starts on the ward may continue in the clinic or vice versa. The same course of treatment may include both periods as an in-patient and a series of out-patient attendances. However, increasingly standardised regimens and more effective anti-emetics and other supportive therapies have enabled greater accuracy in the prediction and treatment of side-effects and toxicities. As a result, out-patient, day care, and home chemotherapy have become increasingly common.

Development and assessment of new anti-cancer chemotherapy

Clinical evaluation of new drugs has developed into a standard pattern of three clearly defined phases:

- *Phase I*: assessment of the maximum tolerated dose of drug with a given schedule and route of administration, and definition of the toxicity profile of the compound. This involves identifying the side-effects and whether they are predictable, tolerable, and reversible in patients who would potentially benefit from the drug.
- *Phase II*: assessment of the efficacy of a drug in a group of patients with a single tumour type. The number of patients depends on the expected response rate. Often patients have not received previous treatment or they have malignancies that have shown little or no benefit from chemotherapy. Information is collected about tumour activity, techniques for administering the drug, precautions to be taken, possible dose modifications, acute toxicities, and necessary supportive care.
- *Phase III*: the drug is tested in clinical trials against existing agents or other forms of treatment known to be of value. Measures of efficacy involve demonstrating one or more of the following: improved cure rates, improved survival times, improved response rates, improved palliation, and improved quality of life.

Informed consent

The principle of informed consent recognises an individual's autonomy and right to self-determination.[33] In health care, informed consent has been defined as giving patients sufficient information to allow them to make the decision to undertake, or not, the proposed procedure or treatment, and to give or withhold consent.[34] Informed consent is intended to ensure that patients are in possession of comprehensive information about the treatment or research process they are about to undergo. Legally it is a doctor's responsibility to obtain informed consent, but nurses have an ethical obligation to ensure that such consent is obtained before chemotherapy is administered. Nurses have an obligation to ensure that patients truly understand what chemotherapy is, and what the possible side-effects are, before it is administered.

Although there is a great deal of literature on the ethical principle of informed consent, there are only a few examples of work that discusses informed consent in the context of anticancer chemotherapy. It is possible that too little information is given about the risks and difficulties of the side-effects of chemotherapy. Nurses may infer from this that they have an ethical and a professional responsibility to engage in a caring way in the process of informed choice. There are real and valid reasons why patients may want to decline, and do decline, to be treated.

Routes of administration

Intra-arterial

Intra-arterial chemotherapy allows high concentrations of drugs to be delivered directly into the tumour, and has the advantage of decreasing systemic drug concentration and side-effects. This method of treatment delivery can be used to treat a number of cancers, including cancer of the liver, colon and rectum, head and neck, as well as sarcomas and melanomas of the upper and lower limbs ('isolated limb perfusion'). The tumour site determines which artery is used to deliver the chemotherapy: the artery providing the blood supply to the tumour is cannulated. The anti-tumour drug is delivered directly through the arterial catheter to the tumour bed. 5-Fluorouracil (5-FU), doxorubicin, mitomycin C, and methotrexate are the agents most commonly delivered intra-arterially. Drugs can be administered either by slow push (bolus) injection, large or small volume infusion, or through an implanted pump.[36–38]

The two methods of administering intra-arterial infusional chemotherapy are termed *external* or *internal*. The external method involves X-ray placement of an arterial catheter and attachment to an external infusion pump for 3–7 days. Therapy is given intermittently for several courses. In the long term (6 months or longer) this method of administration is uncomfortable, inconvenient, and costly. Use of an arterial port has benefits in terms of patient comfort and freedom. The internal or implantable method involves surgical placement of a totally implantable pump. A catheter is inserted into the appropriate artery and attached to the pump; the pump chamber is filled with the prescribed anti-cancer drug. This method offers patients a greater level of freedom and has a lower complication rate than the external method.[36,39,40]

It is important that nurses caring for people receiving intra-arterial chemotherapy are able to recognise and act to minimise drug side-effects, infection, extravasation, or malfunction. Patients require careful teaching to enable them to maintain an implantable pump, and to recognise complications or malfunctions.

Intrapleural

Pleural effusions are a frequent complication of a number of cancers, including lung cancer, breast cancer, lymphoma, and cancer of the ovary, and cause severe breathlessness. Chemotherapeutic agents such as bleomycin or mustine, and other agents (such as tetracycline) can be administered into the pleural cavity following aspiration of fluid to prevent or delay recurrence of an effusion. After aspiration alone, some 60% of pleural effusions will recur.

The prescribed agent is administered into the pleural space through the chest wall using a catheter, causing the two pleural surfaces to sclerose and adhere. This procedure can be repeated daily for several days if required. Local pleural pain for 24–48 hours after instillation is the most common side-effect. Alternative methods for treating pleural effusions may be used, including insertion of a percutaneous small-bore catheter or port, or insertion of a pleuroperitoneal shunt, which may be effective in the management of recurrent effusions.[38,41-43]

Intravesical

Direct instillation of anti-cancer chemotherapy into the bladder can be a simple and effective means to treat or control multiple or diffuse superficial papillary tumours. Agents such as thiotepa, doxorubicin, mitomycin C, and bacillus, Calmette-Guérin (BCG) have all been shown to be effective. Instillation is usually carried out weekly for 4–12 weeks, and involves insertion of a urinary catheter, drainage of the bladder, and instillation of the drug, which is retained for 1–2 hours and dispersed throughout the bladder by frequent changes of position. The bladder is emptied of the chemotherapeutic agent by either unclamping the urinary catheter, or voiding. Systemic toxicity can be a problem when thiotepa is used, and most agents can cause irritation of the bladder. It is important that patients practise careful personal hygiene, including hand washing and cleansing of the genitalia after voiding, and the toilet should be flushed at least twice after use. Following treatment patients may experience urinary frequency, dysuria, and occasional haematuria. Increased intake of fluids after the 'dwell time' of the chemotherapy in the bladder will dilute the drug and can reduce side-effects.[39,41]

Intrathecal/intraventricular

Most chemotherapeutic agents are unable to cross the blood–brain barrier. In an attempt to reach tumour deposits within the central nervous system, drugs can be administered into the cerebrospinal fluid by means of a lumbar puncture.[36,38,43] This is known as the intrathecal route. Involvement of the central nervous system is most commonly seen in leukaemia, and to a lesser extent in breast cancer and lymphoma. Anti-cancer agents are injected directly into the intrathecal or intraventricular space (e.g. through a catheter placed in the ventricle of the brain), either to provide prophylaxis or to manage existing disease. Methotrexate, cytarabine, thiotepa, and interferon are the drugs most commonly used in this way. Drug preparations must be preservative free to reduce neurotoxicity and should be prepared aseptically to reduce the risk of infection. Care must be taken to ensure that the volume of cerebrospinal fluid removed is equivalent to the volume of drug instilled. When administered by the intrathecal or intraventricular route, chemotherapy is usually given on a daily or weekly basis. The intrathecal route is quick and easy but the drug may only reach the epidural or subdural spaces, and concentrations in the ventricles may only be one-tenth of those in the spinal cord.[4] To ensure better drug distribution, Ommaya reservoirs have been used. Ommaya reservoirs are surgically implanted re-usable silicone ports placed subcutaneously and connected by a catheter to a lateral ventricle in the brain. Placement of such reservoirs involves a greater risk than a lumbar puncture. However, they provide permanent access. Neurotoxic side-effects of drugs administered intrathecally or intraventricularly include headache, nausea, vomiting, drowsiness, fever, stiff neck, ataxia, blurred vision, and (rarely) meningitis.[36,38,43]

Intraperitoneal

Direct instillation of drugs such as cisplatin, 5-FU, methotrexate, mitomycin C, and doxorubicin into the peritoneal cavity has been performed with two different objectives: control of ascites following aspiration, and control of tumour growth. Positive results have been observed with intraperitoneal cisplatin in the treatment of small or microscopic tumours in ovarian cancer, and 5-FU has been shown to reduce peritoneal cavity recurrences in colon cancer, but without conferring a survival advantage over intravenous 5-FU.[1] The intraperitoneal route allows high doses of chemotherapeutic agents to be delivered directly into the abdominal cavity, exposing patients to higher concentrations of drugs for prolonged periods, but with minimal systemic side-effects. For intraperitoneal chemotherapy to be effective, tumours must be confined to the abdominal cavity and the tumour burden must be small.[38]

Prior to delivery by the intraperitoneal route, anti-cancer agents are mixed with large volumes of fluid to maximise distribution within the peritoneal cavity, exposing as much of this area as possible to the effects of the drug. Lower concentrations enter the blood stream, and consequently systemic side-effects are mild or delayed. There are three methods of accessing the peritoneal space:

1. Intermittent placement of a temporary indwelling catheter for short-term use; for example, in symptom relief or palliative care.
2. Placement of a Tenckhoff external catheter. An external catheter requires care and maintenance by the patient and there is a greater likelihood of infection and leakage around the catheter, but very rapid flow rates can be achieved. Fluids should be warmed to body temperature prior to instillation.
3. Placement of an implantable peritoneal port. The port is internal and requires no care when not in use. It therefore carries a lower risk of infection, and may be more acceptable to patients, although flow rates may be relatively low.[36,39]

Side-effects of intraperitoneal chemotherapy include respiratory distress, abdominal pain, pyrexia and diarrhoea, and may result from increased intra-abdominal pressure, mechanical difficulties with the catheter, infection, or electrolyte imbalance. Intraperitoneal chemotherapy is usually well tolerated, without severe disruption of lifestyle.

Topical

A number of anti-cancer agents has been incorporated into creams and ointments for treatment of cutaneous malignant lesions such as cutaneous T-cell lymphomas, basal cell carcinomas, and squamous cell carcinomas. The most widely used preparation is 5% 5-FU cream, which is usually applied once or twice a day in the treatment of actinic or solar keratoses. Applications may continue for up to 4 weeks until local erythema, blistering, or ulceration occurs. Once a slough is formed on the affected area, regranulation of normal tissues begins and continues for approximately 8 weeks. This method of application is only suitable for superficial lesions, but positive results have been demonstrated. Unaffected skin must be protected when applying the cream. Adverse reactions such as pain, pruritis, and hyperpigmentation may occur, making it necessary to discontinue therapy before recommencing with a reduced dose.[38,39]

Oral

A variety of anti-cancer agents is administered orally. The oral route is convenient, economical, non-invasive, and sometimes less toxic.[39] Most oral drugs are well absorbed if the gastrointestinal tract is functioning normally. However, the oral route may be unreliable for the following reasons.

- Rarely, patients may not be willing to comply with therapy.
- Doses may be accidentally omitted.
- Tablets may cause intolerable nausea.
- Patients experiencing difficulty swallowing tablets or capsules may crush them, reducing their effectiveness.[37]

It is therefore important for patients to understand the need for careful dosing and scheduling, and the importance of following the regimen correctly. Equally important is effective prophylaxis of side-effects such as nausea.

Intramuscular/subcutaneous

Only a few chemotherapies can be administered by the intramuscular or subcutaneous route, owing to the irritant nature of the drugs involved, the risk of tissue damage, bleeding caused by thrombocytopenia, and pain or discomfort. Drugs may also be incompletely absorbed. When drugs used in the treatment of cancer can be administered by one of these routes, there may be advantages for patients receiving maintenance treatment at home or at the GP's surgery, or if venous access is limited. The amount and type of diluent may differ from those recommended for IV administration. Specific guidelines for the administration of drugs intramuscularly or subcutaneously should be followed, including rotation of sites, and use of large muscles and the 'Z-track' technique to prevent leakage into the skin. The smallest needle that will allow passage of the solution should be selected to minimise discomfort and scarring.[38,39]

Intravenous

Of all the routes of administration, intravenous delivery is most frequently used for anticancer agents and ancillary drugs (e.g. anti-emetics) and supportive therapy (e.g. antibiotics, blood transfusions). Absorption is more reliable than by the intramuscular or subcutaneous route, and may reduce the need for repeated injections. The means of gaining venous access should be considered before treatment starts: nursing assessment of the patient's physical status and needs plays an important part in this process. Venous access is either peripheral, using a winged infusion device or intravenous cannula; or central, involving the insertion of an indwelling catheter or implanted port.

The veins of the upper limbs are the preferred site for peripheral venous access as they are more numerous, cause fewer complications, and are more convenient to use than the peripheral veins of the lower limbs, for example. Using specific criteria in the selection of veins for peripheral access helps to ensure that the best vessel is chosen for the given purpose on each occasion. This is important as vein status may change in accordance with the patient's clinical condition: for example, anaemia or dehydration may reduce the circulating volume and cause veins to become flaccid. Choice of a vein for peripheral access is influenced by the type of medication to be used (e.g. vesicant or non-vesicant), the volume to be injected or infused, and the rate of administration desired and the duration of

therapy (e.g. minutes, hours, or days).[44] Even with guidelines such as these, there remain areas of controversy involving the administration of chemotherapy (see Table 11.1).

Factors to consider when choosing a means of venous access include the following.

- *The condition and accessibility of the peripheral veins.* There are many reasons why the choice of vein may be limited. In children and obese patients veins may be obscured by subcutaneous fat. In the elderly they may be fragile and inelastic. Previous surgical procedures (for example, amputation or axillary node dissection) may restrict the available vessels or compromise venous return. Lymphoedema may be present and other clinical conditions such as arthritis may reduce the number of available sites. The most common cause of reduced venous access is previous intravenous therapy, resulting in scarred or thrombosed veins.

- *The nature and duration of therapy.* The length and nature of treatment may be difficult to predict but with most cancers a fairly reliable estimate is possible. Differences in the nature and duration of therapy can make different demands upon patients and their veins. Regimens vary from the injection of a single agent twice a month, to continuous infusion of large volumes for 5 days every 3 weeks, a combination of three or more drugs given cyclically and requiring weekly venepuncture, or high-dose single-agent regimens delivered over a few hours but producing acute toxicity lasting several weeks and during which intensive supportive therapy is required.

- *The type of chemotherapy prescribed.* Some anticancer drugs are thrombo-irritants, and cause chemical phlebitis; some are vesicants with the potential to cause tissue necrosis. Diluents with which the drugs are mixed may be alkaline (pH > 7) or acidic (pH < 7) and cause extra irritation and scarring of the venous pathway. Supportive therapy, involving intensive use of antibiotics or other drugs, may limit the availability of veins for future intravenous therapy.

- *Patients' feelings about repeated venepuncture.* This is perhaps the single most important factor to be considered. Repeated venepuncture for blood sampling and administration of chemotherapy is

Table 11.1 Some controversial issues in the administration of IV chemotherapy

Issue		
Using veins in the antecubital fossa	• *For*: larger veins permit more rapid administration of drugs; increased blood flow dilutes irritant agents and reduced the likelihood of phlebitis.	• *Against*: extravasation of drugs is difficult to detect due to subcutaneous tissues; risk may be increased if the patient coughs or vomits; important arteries or veins may be damaged by extravasation, and skin grafting to repair tissue damage may greatly reduce the function of the whole limb.
Needle size	• *Large gauge*: irritant drugs reach the central veins more rapidly, so reducing contact time with small vessels; more rapid administration means that patients are under stress for shorter periods.	• *Small gauge*: smaller needles are less likely to cause a through-puncture and cause less pain and scar tissue; increased blood flow around the small needle dilutes the irritant drugs, buffers the vein wall, and reduces phlebitis.
Vesicants first or last?	• *First*: vascular integrity decreases with time – the vein is healthiest at the beginning of treatment; patients' and nurses' assessment of vein patency and problems is most accurate at the outset of administration.	• *Last*: these drugs are irritant and may increase vein fragility and prevent delivery of prescribed therapy if given first; venepuncture and initial injection of the drug may cause spasm, making extravasation more likely – it can be difficult to distinguish between vein spasm and extravasation.

at best uncomfortable, but may be the cause of considerable anxiety as treatment progresses and peripheral venous access diminishes. This anxiety may be influenced by the relationship between intravenous therapy and underlying illness. Fear of needles may develop and occasionally become phobic in nature. This additional stress compounds the problem. Veins disappear and each venepuncture becomes an ordeal for all concerned. Ways to minimise this include: establishing and maintaining a relationship of trust; explanation of procedures and involvement of patients in decision making; careful preparation to achieve maximum dilation of veins, together with skilful technique when placing or accessing the device; reducing discomfort by careful maintenance of the intravenous device once established and consideration of patients' thoughts, fears, and previous experiences.[44]

Venous access deteriorates over time, and it is important that technically proficient staff are avail-

able to reduce the likelihood of both physical and psychological trauma for patients, and the incidence of local toxicity and complications such as infection. Nurses are well placed to extend their caring role into this field of practice.

Central venous access
The advantage of central venous access is the absence of repeated venepuncture and reduction of the risk of local toxicities such as extravasation or phlebitis. Careful discussion of the management of central venous access devices with a patient is essential, as they are often asked to take on aspects of the maintenance of the device themselves. Infection is a major hazard, and home circumstances and personal hygiene are of prime importance. Dexterity and quality of eyesight also have to be taken into consideration when assessing someone's ability to manage a central venous device. Family members or friends may need to be taught the basic skills and principles involved in caring for the catheter at home. Written information should be provided to guide procedures,

though these must be performed successfully both with and without supervision before a patient leaves hospital. Nurses have a responsibility to educate patients and others in the care of their device, and whenever possible should allow them to continue to manage the device when readmitted to hospital.[45]

Current technology and materials make it possible to maintain long-term central venous access effectively. There is a number of different methods and devices, including the following.

- *PICCs (peripherally inserted central catheters)* are inserted in the cephalic, median cubital or basilic veins at the antecubital fossa, and are threaded along the veins in the upper arm until the tip rests in the superior vena cava. PICCs do not require a surgical procedure to place them and are ideal for short-term central venous access over periods of 1 week to several months. They have been associated with decreased rates of infection. A PICC can be inserted quite simply at the bedside by an experienced nurse, provided that the patient has suitable veins in the antecubital fossa. This is an advantage for patients, but they must be able to care for the catheter effectively themselves.[41,46,47]

- A *skin-tunnelled catheter* provides safe and reliable long-term access with a low rate of infection. The catheter is made of an inert material such as silicone or polyurethane, which enables it to remain in position for months or even years. The most well-known catheter of this type is the Hickman catheter, developed by Robert Hickman in the mid-1970s. It incorporates a Dacron cuff, which lies under the skin. Granulation tissue forms around the cuff, keeping it in place and reducing bacterial tracking along the outside of the catheter.[48]

  Skin-tunnelled catheters are available with a single, double, or triple lumen, and are either open or closed (e.g. Groshong type with a slit valve) at the tip. Pneumothorax can occur during insertion, and once in place catheters can become occluded or infected, or provide a site for thrombus formation. There is a risk of infection at the exit site of the catheter, but the site of the catheter coming out from the skin is also a constant reminder to patients of their illness and need for treatment. Surgical procedures, weight loss, and hair loss from chemotherapy may add to the effect on body image and self-esteem. The presence of the catheter may be seen as another insult and can affect sexual function. Although the catheter may not be in use at home it may still be regarded as an intrusion in intimate situations. In one study,[49] patients felt that long-term central venous access adversely affected their body image, affected their partner, and reminded them of their disease.

- *Implantable port.* A silicone catheter leading to a central vein is attached to a port implanted under the skin of the chest wall. Access to the port is gained through the skin using a special needle. The port is only visible as a bump under the skin. The skin acts as a barrier to infection and has been shown to reduce the risk of bacterial contamination. The advantage of an implanted port over a skin-tunnelled catheter is that when not in use, the port requires almost no care or maintenance. Access is provided by inserting a non-coring needle through the skin into a silicone septum in the port. Implantable ports are expensive to insert, but the cost of routine maintenance is low. They are ideal for intermittent therapies and for patients who are unable or unwilling to care for an external device, who are concerned about altered body image, and who are particularly active physically (for example, patients who swim frequently). The disadvantage of an implanted port is that it involves using a needle, although local anaesthetic cream can reduce the discomfort of inserting the needle. Needles can be left in place for up to 7 days, after which time they must be replaced if treatment is to continue. After a course of therapy, the port is heparinised and the needle removed. When not in use, it is recommended that a port is heparinised every month.[50–52]

Infusional ambulatory chemotherapy

Cancer chemotherapy has traditionally been administered using a schedule of intermittent doses, requiring patients to be admitted to hospital or to attend as day cases, and separating them from home, family, and work.[53] The trend towards ambulatory chemotherapy being administered as a continuous infusion has dramatically changed the administration of cancer treatment. The development of improved venous access devices, together with the availability of portable infusion pumps, has made it possible for patients to receive chemotherapy at home, for conditions such as myeloma and cancers of the breast, colon, and rectum.

A number of anti-cancer agents has been found to maintain prolonged concentrations in the plasma when given by continuous infusion. Drugs such as doxorubicin and bleomycin, which have relatively short half-lives, are more effective when administered in this way because they remain present at effective levels when malignant cells replicate. Cells of solid tumours must be exposed to chemotherapeutic agents for prolonged periods because the length of cell cycles varies and is generally measured in days rather than hours.[54] Continuous infusion has been shown to reduce the toxicity of some agents (for example, the cardiotoxicity of doxorubicin) when given over several days in low doses, reducing peak plasma levels; conversely, some cytotoxics given in this way may cause greater toxicity than single-bolus infusions (for example, cytarabine and methotrexate).[1] The cost-effectiveness of home chemotherapy has been demonstrated in the USA, where this system has been in use for almost 20 years. A properly managed programme of home chemotherapy can reduce the costs associated with hospitalisation and increase treatment availability.[55]

Home chemotherapy is thought to enhance patients' independence and sense of control, particularly if it is self-administered.[55,56] The opportunity for patients to be actively involved in their treatment can encourage a positive attitude, and patients receiving treatment at home have reported psychological benefits because they are among people and possessions that are important to them.[57] Patients also appear to be more able to tolerate drug-related side-effects in this setting.[49] While the families of people with cancer can feel helpless and inadequate, home chemotherapy may enable them to become more involved and to give greater assistance and support. Chemotherapy at home reduces the risk of exposing immunocompromised individuals to the harmful pathogens found in hospitals.[49]

Overall, the benefits of home chemotherapy, including convenience, the opportunity for active participation, and cost-effectiveness, may well outweigh the disadvantages, though these must be considered carefully. In hospital staff are always available to assist and support patients when needed, whereas this may not always be the case at home. In spite of recent increases in the number of community nurses who have the skills and knowledge to manage IV therapy in the home, it is not possible for them to be present round the clock. For this reason, it is vital to make careful decisions with patients about whether home chemotherapy is suitable and likely to be successful. Some patients may not be able to undertake the procedures necessary for maintaining treatment at home, either because they are confused by the instructions, because they are fearful, or because there is a physical reason why some part of the care of their drugs and infusion device may not be possible. Some people may prefer the feeling of security that being in hospital can give, and may not wish to take on a programme of treatment at home. Complications do occur, and can cause severe anxiety or stress for some patients.

Catheter-related complications include extravasation of drugs and clotting within the catheter, which may lead to occlusion. Loss of patency often occurs after failure to switch the pump on, during periods of malfunction, or if the catheter is not flushed using the correct solution or the recommended technique.[56] Patency can usually be restored with a fibrinolytic agent.[58]

Drug-related complications can be caused by precipitation of a drug,[53] or by toxicities such as bone marrow suppression, mucositis, diarrhoea, or palmar-plantar erythrodysesthesia syndrome (i.e. 'hand–foot syndrome', where high-dose continuous infusion of 5-FU causes pain, tenderness, and erythema of the palms and soles). Such toxicities may necessitate a break in treatment.

Infusion device-related complications can occur as a result of leakage or rupture of the drug reservoir,[56] pump malfunction,[56,57] or incorrect infusion rate. Depletion or failure of the pump battery can also be a problem.[53,59]

Consideration must also be given to the changes in body image caused by the location of the central venous catheter, which may be connected to an infusion pump for days or weeks at a time. Some patients find even a portable pump cumbersome, and day-to-day and sporting activities and holidays may become difficult or intolerable. Chemotherapy, which takes a considerable time to complete, may be difficult to tolerate for patients who prefer to get their treatment over and done with as quickly as possible.

Finally, it is possible to argue that the economic case for home chemotherapy is open to question. While this method of providing treatment may release hospital beds, costs could be said to increase, as the beds made available in this way are subsequently occupied by additional patients.[49]

When considering whether to begin a programme of home chemotherapy, a number of factors must be carefully weighed. Careful discussion with patients about the implications and comprehensive teaching are essential. Patients must be willing participants in their own care and either they or their family and/or friends must be comfortable with and skilled in the operation of the infusion pump and venous access device, as well as able to respond to the effects of the chemotherapeutic agent in use.[56] From a medical point of view, disease stage and the patient's general health status must be such that home chemotherapy is appropriate and feasible.[60] Thought must be given to the choice of infusion device: given the effect of central venous catheters on lifestyle and activities, it is important to meet each individual's needs as closely as possible. A wide variety of ambulatory infusion pumps is now available, from external syringe drivers to totally implantable systems, including disposable pumps. One type may be more appropriate than another, given a person's particular circumstances.[45]

Fernsler and Cannon[61] point out that the objectives of a learning programme for patients include adherence to a therapeutic regimen, increased satisfaction, enhanced self-determination, increased ability to manage symptoms, and enhanced recovery from surgical procedures. However, increased knowledge is possibly the outcome that is most often seen in nursing documentation. Before conducting a programme of learning it is important to consider the process of learning and the factors that affect a person's ability to learn, both in everyday situations, and in potentially more stressful health care-related situations.

Patients facing the possibility of a central venous catheter, continuously or intermittently infused medications, the need to become familiar with and operate infusion equipment, as well as the likelihood of drug-related side-effects, are not in an easy situation for learning. Initially they may find it difficult to become motivated, as it is likely that they are feeling frightened and anxious, powerless and out of control. Sometimes the amount of information to be absorbed about their illness and their treatment can be overwhelming. They may also be anxious about personal issues, and the environment in hospital is often intimidating and stressful.[45] Patients may not share a common language with hospital staff, there may be an organic obstacle to communication such as dysphasia, and literacy may be limited. Culturally, patients may feel ill at ease with the organisation of Western hospitals and treatment, and may be suffering from the effects of their illness and/or its treatment.

Studies conducted with patients receiving chemotherapy, pain management, and stoma care indicate that learning can enhance self-care.[62] The goals of chemotherapy-related learning include:

- adjusting to the demands of treatment
- exploring the effects of treatment on cancer
- understanding the scheduling of treatment
- recognising and reporting side-effects
- identifying ways of minimising side-effects.

Anxiety makes it more difficult for patients to absorb and retain the information they need, but an added obstacle may be their existing beliefs and perceptions about cancer and chemotherapy.[62] Initial assessment of patients' needs should include information about their response to their diagnosis, their communication style, and their ability to read and understand written information. It may be useful for nurses to ask patients to explain their understanding of their situation in their own words, to provide a basis for further explanations. Supporting written information should be provided so that patients and their families are able to refer back to relevant points about the illness and treatment when they are at home. It may be necessary to begin with simple information or instructions, and to move towards more complex information gradually, as a relationship is established between nurse and patient.[45,63] Patients must feel able to ask for further instructions if they feel worried or unsure, and a contact number should be provided for this purpose. Listening and observing a patient's demeanour to become familiar with characteristic mannerisms and anxieties is always as important as giving explanations.

A successful learning programme depends on individualised and mutually identified goals and objectives. Verbal information ought be supported by clear and effective written information. Learning can be formal or informal, and can include videos, booklets, or audio tapes, or a combination of these. Learning about treatment can help to reduce fear, increase feelings of being in control, make treatment regimens more manageable, and make taking responsibility for one's own care a more positive experience.

The nurse's role in administration of anti-cancer chemotherapy

Aims of care
The aims of care encompass both physical and psychological preparation of patients to receive chemotherapy, and can be summarised as follows.

1. To provide information about chemotherapy and its effects at the level requested by patients and their families and friends; to repeat, expand, or reinforce this as necessary, answering questions and resolving misconceptions.
2. To allow time for patients to adjust to the idea of chemotherapy and its significance; to share any thoughts or anxieties.
3. To deliver therapy effectively to patients without discomfort or injury.
4. To anticipate possible side-effects and toxicities and plan nursing interventions to minimise or alleviate these.
5. To involve patients in the planning, execution, and evaluation of these interventions; to encourage discussion of unusual occurrences and feelings.
6. To encourage family and friends to participate in the provision of care at home and in hospital; to support them in their search for solutions to side-effects and dilemmas.
7. To identify actual and potential problems for patients that cannot be resolved by nursing measures, and initiate referral to the appropriate member of the multi-disciplinary team.
8. To enable patients to live as normal a life as possible during therapy, taking account of what constitutes each individual's chosen lifestyle.[33]

Handling cytotoxic drugs and disposal of waste
The actual or potential hazards of exposure to cytotoxic drugs are such that careful attention must be paid to safe handling and disposal of waste. Cytotoxic drugs are known to be potentially mutagenic (i.e. induce genetic mutations), teratogenic (i.e. produce physical defects in the foetus), and carcinogenic (i.e. induce tumours), and some studies of hospital staff have demonstrated an incidence of chromosomal abnormalities and excretion of mutagenic products.[1,39,64] Abnormalities have been found to disappear when staff are no longer exposed to these substances, and the total amount of drug absorbed is likely to be small. Nevertheless, these drugs are hazardous, and may be inhaled when powder or liquid is 'aerosolised' or emitted in a fine airborne powder or spray during reconstitution, or if spillage occurs during preparation or administration. They may also be ingested or come into contact with the skin.[38] They therefore represent a health risk for staff regularly involved in their preparation and administration. The safest way of working with cytotoxic drugs is to develop and apply policies and guidelines to reduce the possibility of direct exposure to them.

Cytotoxic chemotherapy presents two levels of health risk: first, a definite risk arises from the fact that a number of chemotherapeutic agents is known to be extremely irritant and to produce harmful local effects after contact with the skin or eyes; second, a potential risk exists because such substances have been shown to cause changes in humans on the cellular or genetic level. Local effects of exposure to cytotoxic drugs include dermatitis, inflammation of the mucous membranes, excessive lacrimation (production of tears), pigmentation, blistering, and a range of other allergic reactions. Systemic effects include dizziness, hair loss, headaches, blurred vision, light-headedness, cough, pruritis, and general malaise.

The Health and Safety at Work Act (1974)[65] and control of substances hazardous to health (COSHH) regulations[66] make it mandatory to assess occupational health risks and hazards, and guidelines for preparation, handling, and management of spillage must be in place before nurses handle chemotherapeutic agents.

In ideal conditions, safety cabinets provide a balance between protection for the operator and the necessity to handle equipment and products. Adequate levels of safety must be provided for both patients and staff preparing and administering drugs, using, for example, vertical laminar flow cabinets or isolators.[38] Some form of protective clothing must be worn at all times when handling cytotoxic agents, though the degree of protection required depends on the type of preparation facility available, the nature of the agents being handled, and the extent of the exposure. The minimum requirement is for an overall and gloves of suitable quality; additional protection can be provided by non-absorbent armlets, plastic apron, eye protection, and face mask. Disposable gloves should be worn throughout preparation and checking of cytotoxic chemotherapy. Recommendations about the best type of glove material vary, but when selecting gloves the user must be certain that the material is of a suitable thickness and integrity to maximise protection.[67] Double gloving is recommended for dealing with spillages.[38]

The key to reducing the risk of exposure is good technique. The Health and Safety at Work Act[65] and COSHH regulations[66] provide important additional guidelines on safe working environments and handling hazardous substances, including management of spillage and disposal of waste. All possible precautions should be taken to avoid accidental spillage, though staff should be aware of the approved written procedure for managing spillage should it occur. Staff must receive education and training in procedures and guidelines to a level appropriate to their level of involvement with the handling, preparation, or administration of cytotoxic drugs.[68,69]

A Dutch survey[70] highlighted a number of issues related to the handling of cytotoxic chemotherapy. Out of a total of 824 respondents in 10 hospitals, 750 (91%) wore gloves when administering drugs, but only 173 (21%) wore a gown or an apron; 634 (77%) were aware of the risk posed by 'aerosolisation', but 157 (19%) did not believe that opening a glass ampoule was accompanied by any risk; 775 (94%) felt that protective measures were adequate, though 280 (34%) attached bags or bottles to IV administration sets with the bag or bottle on the stand. Researchers concluded that nurses do not always follow safety guidelines or use recommended protective measures because they may be perceived as inconvenient or unnecessary. Nurses may take their own safety less seriously than that of their patients.

Extravasation

A number of cytotoxic anti-cancer drugs is known to cause venous irritation; others, known as *vesicants*, can cause intense local tissue inflammation and pain, progressing to necrosis and ulceration if they leak from the vein during administration. This leakage of drugs into the tissues surrounding the vein is termed *extravasation*.[71] Tissue damage can be severe and long term. It is essential that nurses know which of the drugs they are administering are vesicants, as well as how to recognise and manage extravasation should it occur. Extravasation can normally be avoided by using good administration techniques, but even with the greatest care and skill accidents can occasionally occur. The incidence of extravasation is low amongst experienced cancer nurses in specialised settings, but higher in general hospital settings.

A number of factors can increase the risk of extravasation:

- additional difficulties present during cannulation or administration of drugs (for example, if a patient is very young)
- the IV cannula may be placed in an awkward position where monitoring of administration is more difficult (e.g. over a bony prominence or joint)
- some equipment (such as steel needles) is unsuitable; plastic cannulae are safer
- poor standard of practice (for example, incorrect amount or type of diluent, failure to observe IV site correctly while drugs are administered, or use of inappropriate peripheral vein as opposed to central vein).[44,48,71,72]

Early recognition of extravasation is imperative to minimise potential tissue damage. The following signs and symptoms of extravasation can occur singly or in combination:

- swelling (most common)
- stinging, burning, or pain (not always present)
- redness (not seen initially)
- lack of blood return into the syringe (though this is not always indicative of extravasation)
- pressure or resistance to syringe plunger or infusion.[37,48]

Implanted ports and skin-tunnelled catheters are considered to be safe and reliable means of drug delivery, but extravasation can also occur with these devices. The consequences in these circumstances are very serious, and careful note should be taken of any complaints of pain or change in sensation around the port or catheter during administration. If extravasation from a central venous catheter is suspected, the infusion or injection must be stopped immediately and medical staff notified.

While there is agreement about the signs and symptoms of extravasation, its management remains controversial. However, if there is reason to believe that extravasation of a vesicant agent has occurred, it is essential that immediate action is taken to minimise tissue damage and prevent further serious consequences. Nurses must ensure that all appropriate antidotes and diluents are readily available and accessible. Management of extravasation often includes the following steps.

1. Stop administration of drug.
2. Attempt to aspirate any residual drug.
3. Remove the IV access device (if peripheral).
4. Apply heat with vinca alkaloids, or cold with anthracyclines, as recommended.
5. Prepare antidote and inject subcutaneously around the site of the extravasation using a 25 G needle.
6. Elevate the affected limb.
7. Notify medical staff.
8. Document the incident and if necessary photograph affected area.
9. Request advice from a plastic surgeon if necessary.
10. Instruct the patient in care of the affected area, ensure adequate systemic analgesia, and plan follow-up.[37,38,44,48]

Care strategy 11.2: Patients receiving intravenous therapy

Cancer patients undergo numerous blood tests and are often required to have an intravenous cannula sited for chemotherapy or supportive therapy (for example, blood products or antibiotics). They are also subjected to a variety of diagnostic tests including bone scans, CT scans, lumbar punctures, and bone marrow aspirates, all of which require the insertion of a needle. Coates et al.[73] found that patients ranked having a needle inserted sixth out of the 15 most difficult cancer-related

experiences, which gives an indication of how important this event is for many patients. Cohn[74] writes:

> As my veins become increasingly scarce, mobile and collapsible, I sometimes had to be needled as many as five times, because laboratory technicians would not listen when I said that Vacutainers did not work any more.

Technical skill is not the only requirement when inserting a peripheral venous access device. It is just as important to understand the fears and anxieties that surround the cannulation procedure, and the implications of the presence of the device during hospital admission. The intrusion and restriction caused by the siting of an intravenous cannula can affect a patient's body image, and the cannula can be a constant source of anxiety while it is in place.[75] Kaplan[76] suggests that once an intravenous infusion is in progress, anxieties may change, but do not necessarily diminish: questions such as 'Will the drip stop or run dry?', 'Will the pump alarm and if so why?', and 'What if the cannula is dislodged or becomes occluded?' can still persist. Concerns over a cannula being dislodged may not always relate to fear of having another device put in place; it is sometimes a matter of wanting to avoid inconvenience and delays in being treated.[77]

Patients also worry about the security of intravenous devices. One report describes how a patient needed a family member present during every infusion because a previous infusion had leaked into subcutaneous tissues.[78] Anxieties may focus on the contents of injections or infusions, in particular possible side-effects, or the fear that blood may be incompatible or infected.[77,79] Patients may be disturbed by changes in routine, for example if chemotherapy is administered in a way with which they are not familiar.[76]

Nursing interventions play an important part in allaying patients' fears and in ensuring that treatment is correctly and efficiently given. The manner in which nurses undertake the care of IV sites, and the way in which drugs are administered has an important influence on whether patients feel safe or anxious. Patients like to feel that IV devices are secure and will remain in position:[77] a nurse may 'know' what should be done, but a patient knows what feels best, making it important that the two discuss the care involved in intravenous therapy.[80] Fear and anxiety stirred up by a painful experience can persist for some time: measures taken to comfort and reassure a frightened person (holding hands, for example) may need to continue after the end of the procedure that caused the distress. Nurses often leave once a procedure has been completed, and do not realise the impact of post-event stress. Skill and familiarity on the part of nurses handling and using equipment, and regular checks to make sure that equipment is functioning correctly and that infusions are running properly and safely, can be emotionally supportive for patients and their relatives and reduce levels of anxiety.

Mobilising patients' strengths and coping strategies, using relaxation or distraction techniques, being able to listen and talk, paying attention to detail, and experience and confidence[77,78] have been found to be highly valued approaches. Inexperienced nurses:

> . . . can produce fear in patients . . . sensitive nurses who feel unsure of a particular procedure will ask someone with experience to assist them.[76]

Patients may feel more in control of their IV therapy if they are given the opportunity to become active participants, for example by choosing the site for their IV access device. One study suggested that patients who were able to choose the arm from which to donate blood experienced less discomfort and pain when compared with patients who were not given a choice.[81] Being able to care for oneself even in a small way is an important dimension of health care,[82] even when patients are faced with the emotionally difficult experience of being confined to bed with an IV infusion. Providing patients with options and choices may have an important influence on behavioural and physiological stress reactions.[81] Patients may feel a greater degree of control over their situation if they have a say in the scheduling of treatment. (For example, they may want to have treatment overnight to give them more freedom during the day.) Having a choice about where an IV device is placed may ensure that it remains effective and in place longer and that treatment is completed with fewer interruptions.[83] It is important to have the opportunity to participate and to foster a sense of independence and control in a potentially difficult situation.

Caring for patients receiving chemotherapy

Nurses are constantly involved in helping patients to meet the challenges of daily living. Interventions focused on physical care are likely to be evaluated frequently, providing a means of monitoring the quality of this aspect of care. It is as important to understand the role of other non-physical factors in maintaining quality of life.

Loss of control
Control has been described as the belief that one has at one's disposal a response that can influence awareness of an event. Loss of control, a feeling that chemotherapy is 'done for you or done to you', is a frequent experience for cancer patients; having a blood sample taken can feel like 'relinquishing control over access to personal space'.[84] Feelings of loss of control, together with possible lack of understanding about the rationale and procedures related to chemotherapy, contribute greatly to anxiety.

Greater knowledge and understanding can help to restore part of the feeling of being in control. As one researcher with personal experience of treatment for Hodgkin's disease[85] puts it:

> I decided before being hospitalised . . . that my best chance of staying sane lay in using my skills as a researcher and ethnographer to demystify my disease and its treatment, and thereby to restore some sense of control. Treatments of indefinite length and uncertain outcome invariably inspire fear and rage, and rob the cancer patient of much of his personal autonomy. In such circumstances knowledge is the only kind of power available. It imposed order, pattern and meaning to a life that had suddenly taken on a frighteningly random character, and so made it possible to manage the fear [p. 316].

'Behaviour control', the belief that behaving in a particular way can affect awareness of an event, has been said to reduce anticipatory anxiety and increase tolerance of difficult or painful experiences,[86,87] as has 'cognitive control', the belief that knowing things or thinking in a particular way can exert a positive influence. Involvement in decision making and taking personal responsibility for aspects of health care can be constructive:

> . . . my relationship with my oncologist continued to change, involving more and more negotiation and compromise . . . as my understanding of the treatment processes expanded and my physical condition deteriorated. I brought all my capacities for identifying and analysing pattern to bear on my body's increasingly violent response to chemotherapy, using every treatment as an opportunity to try out my theories on my oncologist. He came to respect my ability to observe and report sensitively and accurately . . . as I began to negotiate more aggressively (and more successfully) for lower doses. This was no fiction of participation; it was based on a mutual understanding of chemotherapy . . . [p. 333].[85]

Patients may choose to adopt a lifestyle that helps them to foster the sense that they are 'fighting' their illness, the side-effects of treatment, or both.

Feelings associated with chemotherapy
Receiving chemotherapy has been likened to riding a 'physiological roller coaster' of alternating sickness and health.[74] A wide range of emotions is associated with chemotherapy, from feeling 'weepy' or on edge, to frustration, annoyance, and rage, all com-

pounded by accumulating tiredness as treatment progresses.[33] Events that may seem trivial to health care professionals can assume major proportions for patients, from the frustration of waiting for blood results to indicate whether treatment can go ahead, to the exasperation and rage experienced when an injection has to be postponed. Events that have not been anticipated and prepared for are often traumatic, as are changes in routine:

> Any event that occurs unpredictably, regardless of the cause, should be expected to produce feelings of helplessness and outrage.[74]

Fear and anxiety are felt both before and after chemotherapy treatments, and have numerous causes, including the possibility of side-effects, venepuncture, feelings of isolation or loss of independence, just being in hospital, or conversely having to manage treatment and equipment at home. Conflicting emotions often arise when patients relapse after treatment, when either further chemotherapy is recommended, or treatment is halted. The end of chemotherapy can be viewed with both delight and fear. The feelings of security and opportunities to discuss worries that come with regular hospital visits can be lost. Patients sometimes experience the fear that without chemotherapy their illness will recur, and relapse can provoke intense feelings of vulnerability and mortality. It is also possible that some patients will feel better able to cope with chemotherapy the second time around.

Nurses need to be aware that chemotherapy evokes strong and varied emotions that need to be expressed and received with understanding and compassion. Buckalew[78] proposes three broad approaches to psychosocial care:

1. Helping patients to identify and utilise sources of support to alleviate anxiety (for example, support from the family or from relaxation exercises or guided imagery).
2. Providing the opportunity to ventilate or express feelings about treatment and side-effects freely and without judgement being passed: anxiety is a normal reaction to the stress and trauma of chemotherapy.
3. Referral to appropriate members of the multi-disciplinary team (for example, stoma therapists, breast care specialists, the palliative care team, cognitive therapists) or support groups.

Isolation

Physical weakness, an inability to write or concentrate, and forgetfulness can reduce a patient's ability to take part in social and recreational activities. Many of the most valued parts of people's lives, including their social life, careers, relationships, outward appearance, and self-respect can be 'stripped away' by chemotherapy. Patients may be apprehensive about the ability of family and friends to adjust to their illness and treatment, and sometimes initial attentiveness by families and others is followed by withdrawal at what is a crucial time.

Johns[88] describes the process of guided reflection, a means of facilitating learning through reflection on lived experiences, through which:

> The practitioner must expose, confront, and understand the contradictions between what is practised and what is desirable . . . the conflict of contradiction and the commitment to achieve desirable work . . . empowers the practitioner to take action to appropriately resolve these contradictions.

Johns[89] gives an account of how guided reflection may be used to develop practice by describing how a nurse, Caitlin, moves towards a better understanding of how a patient, Ray, who is dying, can be helped to feel closer to his wife, Lucy, and how eventually they can find a way to say goodbye. Caitlin recounts how Lucy:

> . . . was there with him by herself. She was crying. I went in there and sat down with the two of them. Lucy said she was sorry, wiping her tears away. I said 'No, it's okay to cry. I am sure you have had some very good times together.' Ray knew what we were talking about. He opened his eyes but seemed sad. There was that air about him.

A sense of isolation can be linked with a feeling of being unable to communicate with nursing staff, or that nurses are too busy to 'waste time' talking to them.[90] However, nurses are well placed to help patients to manage feelings of isolation. A willingness to listen, to identify needs and worries, and to collaborate to maintain physical and emotional well-being will contribute to feelings of being part of a joint effort, as opposed to being something of an outcast, or not belonging.

Personal growth

> The opportunity for personal growth during chemo-therapy can and should be conveyed to patients because the heightened self-esteem which results from that growth will increase patients' stamina during treatment and diminish the likelihood of their discontinuing ther-apy prematurely.[74]

Accounts by patients of their experience of chemotherapy refer to positive aspects, such as per-sonal growth. It may be true to say that strength comes from within, but nurses can offer guidance to patients searching for a way of regaining their self-esteem. One approach is jointly to set goals that are achievable and consistent with realistic expec-tations. Goals are sometimes therefore necessarily short term and based on a 'take each day as it comes' philosophy. It is often important to provide patients with encouragement to maintain their commitment, and achieving goals may not always become easier as time goes on. Side-effects may get worse, or new ones might appear, and if patients experience a deterioration in their overall situation, some goals may have to be reassessed. Steps taken and strategies agreed during an initial course of chemotherapy may positively influence a patient's ability to manage subsequent courses, and could explain why some people are better equipped and more assertive the second time around. Psycho-logical well-being is often related to physical well-being, so efforts to prevent, minimise, or treat the physical effects of illness and treatment can play an important part in sustaining feelings of integrity and help patients to adjust in periods of personal upheaval and disturbance.

Sexuality and body image

Sharing intimacy and giving pleasure to a partner is a major source of personal value. When diag-nosed with cancer, some people do not experience any changes to their sexuality or sex lives, while oth-ers may choose this point to cease sexual activity. However, cancer and cancer treatment do some-times affect frequency of sexual activity, sexual satisfaction, and sexual confidence and body image.[91] Young-McCaughan[92] found that:

> While short-term effects of [adjuvant] therapy on sex-ual functioning, such as nausea, hair loss, and fatigue resolve shortly after treatment is completed and no longer require adaptive responses, long-term effects of therapy on sexual functioning, such as body image changes and premature ovarian failure, can affect women for years . . .

Indirect effects of illness such as anorexia, nau-sea, and vomiting can cause significant changes in appearance, body image, and feelings of well-being. Hair loss, pallor, malaise, and lethargy may exac-erbate these effects. Emotional and psychological reactions to illness can potentiate fatigue. Under-standably, sexual activity may be difficult to sustain, for both partners in a relationship. This in itself may further reinforce disruptions to an already threatened body image.[93] Society remains uncom-fortable with overt expressions of concern about sexual function, but nurses need to be able to dis-cuss this aspect of our lives without being dismis-sive or getting embarrassed. It helps to be comfortable with the idea of your own sexuality and attitudes towards sex, and counselling skills may help.[94] If nurses lack the confidence to participate in discussions about sexuality or the possibility of modifying sex to take account of health care needs, referral to a counsellor or specialist with the appropriate skills should be considered.

Worries related to sexual function (for example, the effects of chemotherapy on future pregnancies) also need to be addressed. Advice on contraception during and for some time after chemotherapy should always be given to women of childbearing age to avoid the possibility of teratogenic effects; the need for sperm banking should be considered for men before the start of chemotherapy. Treat-ment with chemotherapy does not preclude expressions of physical affection, though familiar activities like kissing can be difficult if, for exam-ple, someone is suffering badly with stomatitis. Chemotherapy can cause hot flushes, vaginal dry-ness, amenorrhoea, and painful intercourse (dys-pareunia), and may induce an early menopause. It is difficult to predict whether patients will become sterile or not as a result of chemotherapy, though in women the risk appears to be related to age. Men may experience temporary sterility as a result of the effects of chemotherapy on the seminiferous tubules of the testicles; if the damage is not per-manent, normal function should return within 2 years.[14]

Side-effects, toxicities, and nursing implications

Chemotherapy is a systemic treatment, which can produce a great number and variety of side-effects throughout the body. These effects depend upon the drug or the combination of drugs used, the dose, the schedule of administration, and the route of administration. Perhaps the greatest variable of all, however, is the reaction of individuals given their physical and/or emotional circumstances when they are given chemotherapy.

Medical and nursing assessment of patients, and the investigations carried out before starting chemotherapy, have three main objectives:

1. To assess each person's physical condition, including nutritional status, renal, liver, and cardiac function, bone marrow reserve, and performance status; to resolve problems where possible and to identify anyone at risk of specific short- or long-term toxicities.
2. To determine the extent of a person's cancer to provide a baseline against which to measure response to therapy, for example, using X-rays, scans, or measurement of tumour markers.
3. To calculate the correct dose of drug or drugs, avoiding unnecessary risk of toxicity; dosage is often based on body surface area in m^2, calculated from height and weight.

Assessment and investigations may be repeated at regular intervals to detect at an early stage toxicities that could lead to irreversible damage if not reversed. The information gathered, together with patients' descriptions of their usual level of function and activity, will assist medical and nursing staff to plan a safer course of chemotherapy, either preventing or minimising physical discomfort and distress. Anticipation of toxicities makes it possible to provide effective prophylaxis in some cases. It is essential to be familiar with protocols in use when taking responsibility for patients receiving chemotherapy or for administering the drugs; in addition to giving details of chemotherapy, protocols contain vital information about prophylactic medications such as anti-emetics and antidotes given as part of a particular course of treatment.

Assessing the toxicities of anticancer chemotherapy in practice requires knowledge of the effect of cytotoxic drugs on the body in general, and familiarity with the effects of the specific drugs or combinations of drugs in use. It is important to observe the onset, severity, and duration of toxicities, to recognise any risk to patients, and to initiate interventions and make prompt referrals to ensure that chemotherapy-related problems are dealt with effectively. The World Health Organisation has developed a detailed system of common toxicity criteria, both to facilitate the reporting of toxicities in clinical practice and clinical trials, and to provide a framework for acceptable practice.[1]

The side-effects of chemotherapy can be divided into three categories according to their time of onset.[33,44] Immediate side-effects (Table 11.2) can be said to occur within 30 minutes of the start of treatment; short-term side-effects (Table 11.3) can be said to occur between 3 and 7 days after therapy begins; and long-term side-effects (Table 11.4), which are often cumulative, can be said to occur after 7 days.

Table 11.2 Immediate side-effects of chemotherapy

- Pain at insertion site
- Venous pain
- Cold sensation along the vein
- Red flush along the vein
- 'Nettle' rash along and adjacent to the vein
- Facial flushing
- Bodily flushing
- Hypotension
- Hypersensitivity reactions
- Anaphylaxis
- Abnormal tastes or smells

Table 11.3 Short-term side-effects of chemotherapy

- Anorexia
- Nausea
- Vomiting
- Stomatitis
- Possible recall of radiation skin reactions
- Pain at tumour site or jaw area
- Malaise
- Flu-like syndrome, including fever
- Chemical cystitis
- Haematuria
- Red urine/green urine
- Constipation
- Diarrhoea

Table 11.4 Long-term and cumulative side-effects of chemotherapy

- Bone marrow depression
- Alopecia
- Skin reactions, including rashes, inflammation, pigmentation, photosensitivity
- Nail ridging
- Pulmonary fibrosis
- Thrombophlebitis
- Pulmonary fibrosis
- Congestive cardiac failure
- Liver dysfunction
- Renal toxicity
- Sexual dysfunction, including amenorrhoea, sterility, possible chromosomal damage.
- Neurological problems, including peripheral neuropathy, muscle weakness, high-frequency hearing loss, paralytic ileus, bladder atony
- CNS toxicity, including lethargy, fatigue, depression, headaches

Immediate side-effects

Local effects of chemotherapy, which are related to the venepuncture site and the venous pathway, are often transient. It is important to inform patients of what to expect so that they can provide the information nurses and clinicians need to help them to distinguish between events such as local allergic reaction, and extravasation.

Short-term effects

Anorexia

Anorexia can be described as a decrease in appetite, and is frequently experienced by people with cancer and patients receiving chemotherapy. It can contribute to a reduced intake of calories and subsequent weight loss, and can have a significant impact on both physical and emotional well-being.[95] Anorexia can be secondary to a number of factors, including fatigue, nausea and vomiting, dry mouth, stomatitis, constipation, and alterations in taste and smell. Taste alterations, which can vary in degree, type, and duration, are thought to be caused by the direct effect of chemotherapeutic agents on the taste buds of the tongue, which are replaced every 5–7 days.[14] Patients may experience a metallic or bitter taste, and there may be an increased threshold or aversion to sweet food. Within the family, a disinclination to eat or participate in meal times can be seen as a rejec-

tion of caring feelings and actions, and may lead to uncomfortable pressures and tensions.[95] It is important that patients and their families understand this, and that they are given help to set realistic goals in terms of meeting nutritional requirements.

The first step is often nutritional assessment, which includes physical assessment, dietary history, what may have caused the loss of appetite, and specific measures such as weight, intake and expenditure of calories, or skin-fold thickness. It may be necessary to refer patients to a dietician for advice on nutritional supplements and on whether enteral or parenteral feeding is required. Patients and their families and friends should be assisted to maintain an interest in nutrition and the dietary choices available to them, and an awareness of the role of a well-planned diet in sustaining energy levels and physical and emotional well-being. It can be helpful to experiment with flavours, and strongly flavoured sweets to mask tastes or smells may make it easier to tolerate the administration of some drugs. Factors that contribute to the enjoyment of food, such as presentation, odour, texture, timing, social setting, and alcoholic drinks, can be discussed and taken into account when planning meals. Measures can be taken to prevent or minimise some of the conditions that impair sensation or perception and affect the intake of food and fluids, including scrupulous oral hygiene, and treatment of dry mouth, stomatitis, nausea, vomiting, and constipation. Alterations in taste are likely to be temporary, and it may help to reassure patients that their liking for favourite foods will return. In the meantime, regular, small meals can be offered, or alternatively, a good meal served at a time when a patient feels particularly able to eat.

Diarrhoea

Diarrhoea can be defined as an increase in stool volume and liquidity resulting in three or more bowel movements a day, and may be accompanied by abdominal cramps and/or flatus. By inhibiting normal cell replication, chemotherapy can disrupt the process of cell replacement and disturb the integrity of the epithelial lining of the bowel, which becomes inflamed and oedematous. The overall size of the absorptive surface becomes smaller as villi and microvilli are flattened and become atrophic;[95] intestinal contents pass rapidly through the gut, with a consequent lessening in the absorption of nutrients. The degree and duration of diarrhoea depends on the chemotherapeutic agent in use, the dose, the timing of the nadir (lowest point in the peripheral blood count after chemotherapy), and the frequency of administration.[52] 5-FU is known to cause diarrhoea, as are actinomycin-D, doxorubicin, cisplatin, hydroxyurea, and the nitrosureas. While diarrhoea is a less common complication with methotrexate, therapy must be halted if it occurs, to prevent serious gastrointestinal problems.[14]

Patients should be assessed to establish their normal bowel habit, ways of managing elimination, and nutritional status. Nutritional status, fluid balance, the frequency and characteristics of the diarrhoea, and the effectiveness of anti-diarrhoeal drugs (e.g. loperamide) in relieving diarrhoea and/or cramps should be frequently monitored. High-calorie, high-protein, low-residue, soft, bland, easily digested foods (e.g. fish, chicken, pasta, boiled or steamed vegetables) should be provided, and milk, milk products, high-fibre foods, and others that exacerbate diarrhoea avoided. Adequate fluid replacement is essential, as is careful perianal care.

Constipation

Constipation has been defined as infrequent, excessively hard and dry bowel movements resulting from a decrease in rectal filling or emptying.[52] The vinca alkaloids (e.g. vincristine and vinblastine) most commonly cause constipation, secondary to autonomic nerve dysfunction that is manifested as colicky abdominal pain and adynamic ileus.[14] Symptoms occur within 3–7 days after drug administration. Constipation is an uncomfortable and distressing side-effect, which can create nutritional problems and result in anal tears, bleeding, and infection.

The emphasis should be on prevention rather than treatment. The risk of constipation can be reduced through good knowledge of dietary measures such as adequate fibre and fluid intake, and through regular physical activity. Stool softeners and laxatives can be prescribed in conjunction with chemotherapeutic agents known to cause constipation; early notification of medical staff when problems are developing, and appropriate use of prescribed medication can help to prevent the more serious and distressing consequences of this condition. The use of laxatives and/or stool softeners such as lactulose is especially recommended for patients with a history of constipation. Choosing an appropriate medication from the range of enemas, suppositories, stimulants, and softeners available depends on what effect is required.

Stomatitis

Stomatitis is an acute inflammation of the oral and oropharyngeal mucous membranes, including the lips, tongue, gingiva (gums), buccal mucosa, palate, or floor of the mouth. Many chemotherapeutic drugs can disrupt or destroy the tissues of the mouth, by either direct or indirect mechanisms. Direct mechanisms are those that interfere with intracellular metabolic processes and disrupt growth, maturation, or replication of cells; indirect mechanisms include suppression of the bone marrow, which increases the risk of bleeding and infection in areas such as the mouth and gastrointestinal tract.[96] Studies have shown that 40% of adults and 90% of children receiving chemotherapy experience some form of oral complication.[97–99] Many drugs, including 5-FU, methotrexate, doxorubicin, bleomycin, cytosine arabinoside, daunorubicin, and mitomycin C, are known to induce stomatitis. The mucosal lining of the mouth consists of non-keratinised squamous epithelium that regenerates every 10–14 days; the first symptoms of stomatitis, including pale, dry mucous membranes, can be seen as early as the third day after administration of the chemotherapeutic agent, and may be accompanied by a burning sensation. Diffuse ulceration may not appear for up to 7 days after treatment is given. A number of factors can influence the frequency and severity of oral complications, including drug type, dosage, nutritional status, oral health prior to treatment, and quality of oral care given during treatment.

Younger patients experience stomatitis more frequently than older patients, and the incidence of oral complications is two to three times higher in haematological malignancies than in solid tumours, possibly due to the immunosuppression that characterises haematological cancers. Patients whose oral hygiene is poor, or who have poor dentition, are also more likely to experience oral problems with chemotherapy. However, a decrease in oral complications can be achieved if dental problems are corrected and mouth care is scrupulously attended to. Both the more minor effects of chemotherapy on the mouth (for example, a burning sensation, intolerance to hot, spicy, or acidic foods, inflammation, and changes to saliva production) and the major effects, including sloughing, ulceration, bleeding, and bacterial, fungal, or viral infections, have profound effects on quality of life, and can undermine an individual's ability and willingness to tolerate further chemotherapy. Stomatitis can indeed be so severe and painful that eating and drinking become extremely difficult, and it may be necessary to reduce the dose of chemotherapy or to delay subsequent courses.

Before the start of chemotherapy a baseline oral assessment is recommended, including a review of the patient's daily oral care routine. Effective oral hygiene, with a soft toothbrush to prevent damage to delicate tissues, is essential to reduce the potential for infection. Specific nursing interventions depend on the extent of stomatitis, which may range from a potential problem to bleeding, ulceration, and an inability to take food or fluids (sometimes described as grade 4 stomatitis).[14] Measures include use of anti-bacterial mouthwashes, and sodium bicarbonate solution or dilute hydrogen peroxide to remove thick secretions or debris.[14] The mouth should be rinsed with water after using hydrogen peroxide. Soft foods with a smooth consistency are recommended; spicy or acidic foods should be avoided. Application of emollients or medicated topical applications are often required to prevent cracking and drying of lips and to treat infections. Anti-bacterial and anti-fungal oral suspensions are often required to treat oral infections. In the most severe cases patients will require intravenous hydration, measures to control pain (which may include a morphine infusion), and on occasions enteral or parenteral feeding.

With some drugs (such as 5-FU) cryotherapy may be helpful in preventing stomatitis: patients start sucking ice chips 5 minutes before chemotherapy is given, and continue for 30 minutes afterwards.[40]

Nausea and vomiting

While clinicians often regard suppression of the bone marrow as being the major dose-limiting toxicity of chemotherapy, patients are likely to see nausea and vomiting as the most distressing side-effect:[72,100]

> After the second course, I found that thinking about going there made me vomit, in fact it was almost as bad as when I was actually having treatment. Even now [2 years later] I start feeling sick when I pass the hospital.[101]

Nausea is often experienced as the need to vomit, a dreadful sensation of impending sickness focused on the stomach. Patients suffering from nausea often appear pale and sweaty; they may have a rapid pulse and feel cold and clammy. *Retching* is a rhythmic, often forceful, movement of the respiratory muscles, which moves stomach contents in and out of the oesophagus. *Vomiting* occurs when the contents of the stomach are expelled forcefully through the mouth. This is achieved by sudden powerful contractions of the respiratory muscles at the same time as relaxation of the upper oesophageal sphincter. Vomiting is often followed by lethargy and pronounced weakness of the muscles.

Chemotherapy-induced nausea and vomiting occurs at a variety of time points relative to the time that treatment was given. Nausea and vomiting occurring within 2 hours of treatment (and lasting up to 24 hours) is referred to as *acute*; *delayed* nausea and vomiting can last for 3–5 days or more; *anticipatory* nausea and vomiting occurs before or during the administration of chemotherapy, at a time when this symptom would not normally be expected.[102] Younger patients tend to experience more nausea and vomiting than older patients.[103] Chemotherapeutic agents can be described as having *mild*, *moderate*, or *severe* emetogenic potential, according to the severity of nausea and vomiting with which they are associated (see Table 11.5). Poor prophylaxis or control of nausea and vomiting has the potential to affect quality of life badly by initiating a number of undesirable consequences, including anticipatory nausea and vomiting, unwillingness to continue with treatment, delays in treatment, dose reduction, dehydration, electrolyte imbalance, anorexia and aversion to food, oesophageal tears, dental erosion, muscular strain, and fatigue.

Mechanism of nausea and vomiting

The vomiting reflex in chemotherapy-induced nausea and vomiting is co-ordinated by the vomiting centre in the medullary reticular formation in

Table 11.5 Emetogenicity of common chemotherapeutic agents

Mildly emetogenic	Moderately emetogenic	Highly emetogenic
Etoposide (oral)	Carboplatin	Cisplatin
Mitomycin C	Daunorubicin	Mustine
Methotrexate	Carmustine	Dacarbazine
Bleomycin	Lomustine	Cyclophosphamide (IV >1000 mg/m^2)
Chlorambucil	Doxorubicin	Melphalan (IV >100 mg/m^2)
5-FU (continuous infusion)	Dactinomycin	
Melphalan (oral)	Cytarabine	
Vincristine	Procarbazine	
Vinblastine	Mitoxantrone	
	5-FU (IV bolus)	
	Etoposide (IV)	

the brain; the vomiting centre is located close to the chemoreceptor trigger zone (CTZ), which is sensitive to chemicals, drugs, and toxins, including chemotherapeutic agents, and radiation. The vomiting centre is sensitive to stimulation from the CTZ, afferent nerve fibres in the gastrointestinal tract, cerebral cortex, vestibular apparatus, and heart.[96] Vomiting occurs when the vomiting centre is stimulated from the CTZ or other areas. Histamine (H_1 and H_2), dopamine, acetylcholine, and opiate receptors are known to be located in the CTZ, but the mechanism of chemotherapy-induced nausea and vomiting has yet to be fully explicated. Damage to the mucosa of the small intestine caused by chemotherapy releases serotonin ($5\text{-}HT_3$), which stimulates receptors on afferent nerve fibres, which in turn stimulate the vomiting centre. $5\text{-}HT_3$ antagonists (e.g. ondansetron and granisetron) have shown considerable success in preventing and controlling acute nausea and vomiting in patients receiving chemotherapy, but have been less successful in treating delayed nausea and vomiting.[14]

Assessment of nausea and vomiting

Nausea and vomiting are distinctive experiences, which are usefully assessed separately, though some studies appear not to distinguish between the two. The experience of nausea affects individuals in different ways, and assessment relies on eliciting patients' accounts. The word 'nausea' is not always understood: 'feeling sick' or 'feeling queasy' are more commonly used. It is possible to interpret the experience of nausea in terms of dimensions such as frequency, intensity, and duration, which can then be recorded by means of visual analogue scales (10 cm lines marked with a cross to indicate severity) or descriptive ordinal scales (where a choice is given between descriptors such as 'never', 'sometimes', or 'frequently', each of which is allocated a sequential score). However, patients' own accounts remain a fundamental source of information about nausea and/or vomiting, recorded in specially designed diaries or journals. Using a scale in conjunction with a diary or journal provides a simple means of comparing scores and assessments, though a scale necessarily omits much of the complexity of the experience.

Anticipatory nausea and vomiting

Although it occurs less frequently than post-treatment nausea and vomiting, anticipatory nausea and vomiting (ANV) can be just as distressing, and anti-emetic drugs do not appear to control it once it has developed. Improvements in the management of chemotherapy-induced emesis have led to a reduction in the severity but not the incidence of ANV. Estimates of the incidence of ANV vary from 14%[104] to 65%,[105] though it would appear that post-treatment nausea and vomiting has to occur before ANV can develop.

ANV has been described as a conditioned response:[106] in other words, neutral stimuli such as the odour or appearance of the treatment room or the sight of the nurse become strongly associated with the chemotherapy. They therefore lose their 'neutrality' and become 'conditioned stimuli'. Responses elicited by conditioned stimuli are known as conditioned responses. Conditioned responses (such as nausea and vomiting) may occur in the presence of conditioned stimuli (for example, the room, smell, or nurse) without the presence of the unconditioned stimulus (the chemotherapy itself).

Factors influencing ANV include age (younger patients are more susceptible), anxiety, susceptibility to nausea and/or motion sickness, abnormal taste associated with chemotherapy drugs, fear of venepuncture, and poorly controlled or prolonged nausea and vomiting after treatment.

Preventing ANV

It has been suggested that the development of anticipatory side-effects could be avoided or at least significantly reduced by better management of post-treatment nausea and vomiting. Allowing nausea and vomiting to develop before prescribing anti-emetics is a poor strategy in the management of the problem in general, and in the management of ANV in particular.

Hypnosis has been used in the control of nausea and vomiting and may be effective in reducing ANV in children and adolescents. Progressive muscle relaxation, which involves a series of muscle-tensing and relaxing exercises often accompanied by guided imagery (soothing imaginary scenes), is considered by some to have an influence on patients' responses to anxiety and nausea. The emphasis of this technique is on gaining self-control and combating feelings of helplessness. It has the advantage of being non-invasive and easy to learn. 'Systematic desensitisation' is a method of disconnecting learned associations used in the management of phobias. Although it is time consuming, it has been shown to have a positive role in the management of ANV.[107] Biofeedback, stress inoculation, and distraction techniques have also been shown to have a positive effect.[108]

Choice of anti-emetic drugs

A number of factors may be relevant in determining the susceptibility of an individual to emesis following chemotherapy, including previous emesis during chemotherapy, a history of motion sickness, the emetic potential of chemotherapeutic agents (both singly and in combination), and the dose and schedule of anti-emetics. In practice, though, these factors do not usually influence the choice of anti-emetic drug, which is based on the emetic potential of the type of chemotherapy in use.

Anti-emetic agents

A variety of anti-emetic agents is in common use. No single drug has proven ideal, giving complete control of emesis and no toxicity. Combinations of different anti-emetics are frequently used to provide the most effective management. Phenothiazines (e.g. chlorpromazine and prochlorperazine) are useful in the treatment of motion sickness and other forms of emesis not related to chemotherapy; chlorpromazine has also been shown to give anti-emetic control in some 50% of non-platinum-containing chemotherapy regimens.[109] Corticosteroids (e.g. dexamethasone) are widely used to provide control of emesis with moderately emetogenic chemotherapy, usually in high concentrations and in combination with metaclopramide or serotonin ($5\text{-}HT_3$) antagonists. Cannabinoids such as nabilone have an anti-emetic effect but also cause dysphoria, hypotension, and dizziness in up to 30% of patients. They are absorbed unpredictably when taken orally, and are not widely used in current anti-emetic practice. Butyrophenones (doperidol and haloperidol) have short plasma half-lives but are effective when given by intravenous or subcutaneous infusion. Their anti-emetic effect is dose dependent, and toxicity at therapeutic levels, including dystonia, dry mouth, and sedation, limits their use. Use of benzodiazepines such as lorazepam is also limited by their sedative effect, which precludes use in out-patients' departments for instance. However, their amnesic and anxiolytic properties may be useful in the treatment of anticipatory nausea and vomiting if given at least 24 hours before chemotherapy.[110]

Of the class of drugs known as substituted benzamides, metaclopramide is the most commonly used. Given by the oral route, it has little anti-emetic effect, but given over 15 minutes in higher doses by short intravenous infusion it is very effective in the treatment of acute emesis in moderately and highly emetogenic regimes, including platinum-based chemotherapy. Side-effects may occur, including akathesia and dystonic reactions; the overall incidence of extrapyramidal side-effects is between 10 and 15%.

The development of selective serotonin receptor antagonists has provided a class of drug that is very effective in controlling emesis without causing sedation or extrapyramidal effects. Side-effects of 5-HT$_3$ antagonists do include mild or moderate headache, flushing, fatigue, diarrhoea (1%), and constipation (3%). A number of 5-HT$_3$ antagonists has been tested in clinical trials, including ondansetron, granisetron, and tropisetron. Ondansetron and granisetron have been shown to be effective in the prophylaxis of emesis caused be platinum compounds, with complete or major control of side-effects in around two-thirds of patients. They have been shown to be effective in the control of emesis caused by moderately emetogenic drugs, and in controlling emesis that has not responded to treatment with conventional agents such as dexamethasone or metaclopramide. Despite their role in the control of acute emesis, 5-HT$_3$ antagonists are less effective in the management of delayed emesis.

Nursing interventions

> The worst time was after the first chemotherapy. I was so frightened probably because I didn't know what to expect. It didn't seem so difficult after that, even though it was as bad, once I knew I'd survive it.[111]

Supporting patients who are coping with vomiting presents a challenge for nurses. Honesty and realism about the likelihood and duration of the problem must be combined with an explanation of why it is happening and a sensitive approach to the fears provoked. One survey suggests that the decision about when anti-emetic therapy is required rests with the nurse in about 80% of cases,[112] which indicates the magnitude of nurses' responsibilities in this area, but also perhaps the scope for recognising the opportunity to involve patients fully in decisions affecting their well-being.

Patients are likely to benefit from opportunities to learn about the nature of the side-effects of chemotherapy and when they are likely to happen; exploring patients' expectations and previous experiences of vomiting with a particular chemotherapy regimen can help to identify care priorities. Knowledge and effective use of the range of pharmacological options for managing nausea and vomiting is essential and written information on what to expect and how best to deal with it is often useful. Non-pharmacological measures are equally important. Advice

on adjusting eating habits can help, including assessment of the most suitable timing, size, and content of meals. Small, frequent, low-fat meals, eaten cold to avoid cooking odours and accompanied by fizzy drinks are often more easily tolerated. Sipping nourishing fluids regularly can assist in achieving the desired fluid and dietary intake. Nibbling on dry toast, crackers, or biscuits may help to settle a nauseous stomach. Relaxation and distraction exercises (guidelines can be found in *Pain: A Clinical Manual for Nursing Practice*[113]), therapeutic touch, massage, and aromatherapy can also have a positive effect.

It is important to pay careful attention to the patient's environment by using restful colours, and providing music, television, comfortable furniture including reclining chairs, and access to fresh air. It has been suggested that patients experience less severe nausea and vomiting when they are seated during administration of chemotherapy, rather than lying down.

Acupressure bands, which are commercially available, have been found to reduce feelings of nausea. Acupressure is a non-invasive technique, which involves applying pressure to the P6 acupressure point located on the inner aspect of the wrist three fingers' width above the distal skin crease of the wrist joint. It is easy to administer and safe to use. Patients can put the bands in place as soon as chemotherapy has been administered, pressing the stud incorporated in the band at regular intervals. Studies have shown that acupressure and acupuncture provide benefits for the majority of patients, though the numbers involved in research have been small.[114]

Other side-effects

In one study[111] of patients receiving chemotherapy, 25% of those involved reported suffering from *impaired concentration*. One woman described it as 'constant mental cloudiness', while another wrote:

> The loss of concentration I suffered had a devastating effect on me. I was unprepared for this and kept trying to do things which required concentration and became very anxious about it. Once I discovered this was due to the drugs and would pass, I became more philosophical about it and accepting of it.

It is important for patients to be able to distinguish between this kind of short-term drug-related effect on their concentration, and effects of disease on mental functioning or signs of dementia, which they may fear are affecting them. Forewarning them that they may experience some 'mental cloudiness' can help to avoid unnecessary distress.

The less well publicised side-effects of chemotherapy (for example, vaginal dryness and joint laxity), that may not be seen as priorities by nursing or medical staff, can trouble patients greatly. Patients may experience a great number and variety of effects which, without preparation and explanation, can seem to indicate a general deterioration in well-being that is not necessarily seen as relating to chemotherapy at all. Therefore, it is always important to take an inclusive approach to the subject of side-effects and to work together with patients so that as little as possible is unexpected, and a broad range of management strategies is made available.

Fatigue

This is a multi-dimensional concept including feelings of tiredness, lack of energy, and inability to continue, and is a common and distressing effect of both cancer and chemotherapy,[115] with research suggesting that between 60 and 90% of patients receiving chemotherapy experience it:[116]

> I'm exhausted all the time, both physically and mentally. I go to bed after lunch while my daughter sleeps and I just can't manage without that and then going to bed at night when she does. I'm doing nothing except existing.[111]

Acute fatigue can be seen as protective, in that it is an intermittent response to such things as overwork or a hectic timetable, and provides an opportunity to restore energy levels and preparedness. Chronic fatigue, in contrast, has been described as generalised, with extreme tiredness and very low energy, and is perceived as abnormal and excessive.[117] It affects the whole body, and is constant and difficult to resolve.

A number of theories has been put forward to explain chronic fatigue, though no conclusive explanation exists as yet. One theory is that fatigue is caused by an accumulation of waste products and metabolites; another is that muscular activity is impaired when the necessary 'materials' are not available. It has been suggested that increased energy expenditure, and changes in the production, utilisation, and distribution of hormones may influence feelings of fatigue, as well as having a functional effect. The neurophysiological model of fatigue[118] suggests that fatigue is due to alterations in the central nervous system, and it has also been suggested that each of us has a specific amount of energy to aid adaptation to stressful situations and that once this is depleted, fatigue is inevitable.[119] Other factors, including the extent of tumour burden, physical symptoms, psychological stress, psychosocial changes such as isolation and boredom, and drugs such as anti-emetics have also been put forward as possible explanations.

The time of onset, duration, pattern, and severity of chemotherapy-related fatigue may vary and appear to be related to the drug in use. In one study,[116] patients receiving 3–4-week cycles of chemotherapy experienced high levels of fatigue in the 4–5 days after treatment. Fatigue then decreased until the low point of the blood count (nadir) at around 15 days, when it increased again temporarily. Patients who received weekly injections, however, were found to experience moderate, cyclically fluctuating fatigue. It has been suggested that fatigue may be associated with disruption of neurotransmitters, and that drugs that cross the blood–brain barrier or cause neurotoxicities (for example, vinca alkaloids, 5FU[120] or adjuvant chemotherapy for breast cancer[121,122]) are therefore more likely to cause it.

Rhodes[123] has described how patients were able to care for themselves after chemotherapy, but still found tiredness and weakness to be the symptoms that interfered most with self-care activities:

> I could not get out of bed and walk to the bathroom and would have to sit down and rest, then go to the shower . . . I would have to rest between each activity . . . because I had no energy left.

Objective assessment of fatigue is possible, but may be of less relevance practically than the patient's own assessment.[117]

Interventions

Little attention has been paid to assessing the value of specific interventions for managing fatigue. Tierney et al.[111] found that patients felt that tiredness was one of the few side-effects of chemotherapy that they had any control over themselves, and most reported using specific measures to alleviate it.

In particular, coping with tiredness involved actions directed at conserving energy. Rhodes[123] has described how patients planned their activities to this end:

> . . . scheduling activities, stuff like that – became the most important thing for me . . . I had to figure out how far I could walk.

The aim is to alternate periods of activity with periods of rest, to build up or maintain levels of function:

> In the afternoon, I would be tired, so usually I would rest and then we would have to do any socialising we did in the evening.

Rest or sleep, in the form of naps or periods of inactivity, is frequently recommended to allow recuperation or conservation of energy, but extended periods of sleep do not always alleviate tiredness. Minimising boredom, and involving friends and relatives in household chores and food preparation, can prevent loss of focus and reduce the burden of unwanted activities. Exercise has been reported to have an influence on both perceptions and the experience of fatigue.

Long-term effects

Bone marrow suppression

Bone marrow suppression (myelosuppression) is the most frequent dose-limiting side-effect of cancer chemotherapy and is potentially life-threatening: when death occurs in the myelosuppressed patient it is most often due to infection or haemorrhage. Many of the agents used in cancer chemotherapy affect the rapidly dividing stem cells in the bone marrow: the red blood cells (erythrocytes), the white blood cells (leucocytes), and the platelets (thrombocytes). The onset of myelosuppression can be rapid: white blood cells divide every 6–8 hours, platelets every 7–10 days, and because chemotherapy interferes with dividing cells, these cells are most quickly affected by myelosuppressive drugs. Loss of white blood cells (neutropenia) is seen before loss of platelets (thrombocytopenia); and, generally speaking, neutropenia is more severe.[96] Red blood cells are replaced every 120 days or so and anaemia develops more slowly.

The lowest point to which the peripheral blood count of red and white cells and platelets falls is known as the 'nadir' (opposite of 'zenith'), which usually occurs 7–14 days after chemotherapy has been administered. As cells are replaced the nadir resolves; with high-dose chemotherapy, however, populations of stem cells may be unable to regenerate quickly, leading to a prolonged nadir period. Some of the alkylating agents, including nitrogen mustard (mechlorethamine), dacarbazine, busulfan, and the nitrosureas (e.g. carmustine and lomustine) are regarded as particularly myelosuppressive.[96] Steroids do not cause myelosuppression, with the exception of tamoxifen, which affects the white cell and platelet count. Several factors are cited as contributing to the degree of bone marrow suppression, including age (though some older people tolerate normal doses),[124] class of drug, combination of drugs, poor nutrition, reduced bone marrow reserve, poor renal or liver function, and previous treatment (for example, radiotherapy to sites of bone marrow production).[14]

Bone marrow suppression leading to loss of white cells, particularly neutrophils, increases the risk of patients experiencing severe bacterial infection. Neutrophils, which are one of three types of white cells known as granulocytes, are the largest group of white cells and act as phagocytes, playing a vital role in the body's inflammatory response and defence against micro-organisms. The normal neutrophil count is 2500–7000/mm^3; neutropenia is defined as an absolute neutrophil count of <2500/mm^3; risk of infection increases in proportion to a decreasing neutrophil count. Fever is often the first sign of infection, though when infection occurs in the neutropenic patient, signs such as inflammation or formation of pus at infected sites may be absent or less conspicuous. Infection with organisms such as *Pseudomonas aeruginosa*, *Staphylococcus aureus* and the fungus *Candida albicans* are common; common sites include the blood, respiratory tract, and oral mucosa.

Thrombocytopenia, reduction of platelet counts below the normal level of 150 000–350 000/mm^3, increases the risk of bruising, bleeding from the gums or nose, petechiae, and haemorrhage in the central nervous system or gastrointestinal tract. Risk of bleeding increases in proportion to the decrease in numbers of platelets; the risk is regarded as moderate when counts fall below 50 000/mm^3, and severe below 20 000/mm.^{3}[3,14]

Severe anaemia is less often seen with cancer chemotherapy; when it occurs it develops later than chemotherapy-induced neutropenia or thrombocytopenia, because of the long half-life of red blood cells. Signs of anaemia include pallor of the skin, mucous membranes, conjunctiva, and nail beds, and increased heart rate, breathlessness, headaches, and fatigue.

Patients should be asked to report any of the signs and symptoms associated with bone marrow suppression, and measures taken to reduce the risk of bleeding and infection. It is important to maintain the integrity of the skin and mucous membranes to provide a barrier against infection. Care should be taken to maintain personal hygiene, and to avoid cuts and bruises, for example by using a soft toothbrush for oral care and an electric shaver in preference to a wet razor. The risk of constipation and straining can be reduced with the use of stool softeners, and adequate intake of fluids and dietary fibre.

Invasive procedures like injections and catheterisation, which breach the integrity of the skin and increase the risk of infection, should be kept to a minimum, and medications that interfere with clotting (such as aspirin) treated with caution. Patients may be asked to avoid crowded places or people with known infections; in severe cases of neutropenia, protective isolation and antibiotic and/or anti-fungal therapy are often required.

Anaemia may not prevent continuation of chemotherapy but has a significant effect on how patients feel about and cope with their treatment; blood transfusions may be required, especially if patients are symptomatic. Both anaemia and thrombocytopenia can be corrected by transfusions of blood or platelets.

In recent years the use of haematopoietic growth factors has had an impact on the management of chemotherapy-induced neutropenia. Granulocyte colony stimulating factor (G-CSF) and granulocyte-macrophage colony stimulating factor (GM-CSF) increase the number of neutrophils (G-CSF) and neutrophils, eosinophils, and basophils (GM-CSF). Haematopoietic growth factors have been found to limit the duration of neutropenia, reduce antibiotic use, decrease the incidence of mucositis, and facilitate the administration of chemotherapy according to schedule.[1]

Gonadal toxicity

In women, chemotherapeutic agents are known to affect ovarian function. Busulfan has been shown to cause ovarian failure; nitrogen mustard (in combination therapy), chlorambucil, melphalan, procarbazine, and cyclophosphamide are also known to affect ovarian function adversely. Gonadal toxicity has been reported with bleomycin, mitomycin C, vinblastine, etoposide, and cisplatin (in combination therapy). 5-FU, methotrexate, bleomycin, and vincristine are not known to be gonadotoxic.[1] Women can experience amenorrhoea with hot flushes, insomnia, and vaginal dryness, as well as decreased fertility or permanent infertility. They may also experience decreased sexual interest and disruptions in self-confidence and close relationships. Menstruation sometimes recommences months or even years after treatment has finished. Damage to ovarian function appears to be age related, with women aged over 30 less likely to regain ovarian function:

> I went to my GP because my period was so late and also with these hot flushes I thought something might be up. He told me that chemotherapy can sometimes bring on the menopause. Well, I was really devastated. I could remember, after the mastectomy, that my period came and I thought to myself, well, that's good, at least I'm still a woman. I'd really be depressed if this treatment now finishes it off for me. I wouldn't be so upset maybe if I'd known this was possible . . . but no-one mentioned it.[111]

Clearly, it is important to work with women sensitively and supportively to enable them to discuss and consider the implications of chemotherapy on ovarian function, and to review and if necessary adapt themselves sexually, with their partner, to changed sexual feelings. New approaches to sexual activity, including different positions for intercourse, alternatives to intercourse, and recognition that sex may be easier before rather than after a tiring day, may be helpful if previous approaches are now difficult or painful. Help from a specialised therapist or counsellor should be sought if necessary. Birth control measures should be continued for about 2 years after chemotherapy to avoid the potentially teratogenic or mutagenic effects of cytotoxic drugs (that is, their capacity to cause physical defects or genetic mutations in the foetus); few teratogenic complications have been reported with chemotherapy given in the second or third trimester, but have been reported with antimetabolites and alkylating agents given in the first trimester;[52] mutagenic effects are probably unlikely, though theoretically possible.[1]

Cardiotoxicity

A number of chemotherapeutic agents has toxic effects on the heart, the most prominent of which are doxorubicin and daunomycin. Doxorubicin can cause acute changes to heart rate and rhythm during or shortly after administration, including tachycardia, and ectopic ventricular and atrial contractions. These effects are rarely fatal,[1] and often resolve quickly without complications. Doxorubicin can also lead in the longer term (weeks and months) to chronic damage of the myocardial cells (cardiomyopathy) with heart failure. Up to 9% of patients receiving doxorubicin experience drug-induced cardiomyopathy; the condition is thought to be fatal in over 60% of these cases.[96] Chronic cardiotoxicity can be difficult to detect, as patients may be asymptomatic before presenting with the signs and symptoms of congestive cardiac failure, including tachycardia, breathlessness, non-productive cough, distension of the neck veins, and ankle oedema. Sub-acute toxicities such as myocarditis and pericarditis are also seen in the days and weeks after administration (primarily with daunorubicin), though they are infrequent. Daunorubicin is also known to cause cardiac dysrhythmias and congestive cardiac failure, which is associated with high mortality and morbidity, as with doxorubicin. Clearly, the chronic cardiotoxic effects of doxorubicin and daunorubicin are such that administration is discontinued as soon as signs and symptoms are detected. Epirubicin, a drug in the same class of anthracycline antibiotics as doxorubicin and daunorubicin, was developed to provide a drug with reduced cardiotoxicity; mitoxantrone, while similar in structure to doxorubicin and daunomycin, is also less cardiotoxic. Other chemotherapeutic agents with reported cardiotoxic effects include amsacrine, bleomycin, cyclophosphamide (high dose), cisplatin, diethylstilbestrol, paclitaxel (Taxol), and 5-FU, which has been associated with angina, and with myocardial infarction, which is fatal in a proportion of cases.

Neurotoxicity

Neurological effects related to chemotherapy are not uncommon, but can be difficult to distinguish from the effects of cancer itself. In the majority of cases, neurotoxicity is temporary, although permanent neurological damage can occur. Severe neurotoxicity may lead to discontinuation of the drug involved or make it necessary to interrupt treatment to allow symptoms to resolve before dose modification or replacement of the drug.

When used in high doses, methotrexate can affect the central nervous system, leading to stiff neck, headache, nausea and vomiting, fever, and lethargy (arachnoiditis); occasionally, paraplegia is seen following intrathecal administration of methotrexate or cytosine arabinoside. Methotrexate is also associated with encephalopathy, especially when administered intrathecally or intraventricularly, and in combination with cranial irradiation.[96] 5-FU can cause a number of reversible central nervous system effects, including acute ataxias, loss of muscle control, and speech and occulomotor disturbances when given as a bolus in high doses. Vincristine is known to cause peripheral neuropathy, which can be dose-limiting. Its effects include loss of the Achilles tendon reflex, sensory loss in the hands and feet and weakness or atrophy of the muscles; vincristine can also affect the autonomic nervous system, with effects such as constipation, urinary retention, and impotence.[1] Neurotoxicity is common with cisplatin, and includes such effects as hearing loss and peripheral sensory disturbances, which may be experienced in the first instance as tingling and numbness, followed by proprioceptive disturbances. Barton Burke *et al.*[14] note that proprioceptive losses, which involve 'the loss of the ability to determine the position of body parts without visual cues' can be devastating. Effects may be dose-limiting and may not be reversible. Neurotoxicity has been reported with BCNU, and neurological effects, including difficulty with walking and standing, and mood and sleep disturbances, are common with corticosteroids. Some of the neurological effects of steroid therapy can be avoided or minimised by gradual dose reduction before discontinuation.

Pulmonary toxicity

Pulmonary toxicity, often in the form of pneumonitis or fibrosis, is a result of damage to the endothelial cells of the lungs. A large number of chemotherapeutic agents is known to cause pulmonary toxicity,[1] including bleomycin, BCNU and CCNU, methotrexate, cyclophosphamide, mitomycin C, chlorambucil, cytosine arabinoside, melphalan, fludarabine, and busulfan.

Bleomycin is known to cause widespread interstitial fibrosis and damage to the alveoli, resulting in impaired respiratory function and in some cases death. Patients may present with breathlessness on exertion and an unproductive cough, progressing to breathlessness at rest. The toxic effects of bleomycin on the lungs are increased when it is combined with irradiation of the lungs, and patients of 70 years and over are at increased risk. Treatment often involves withdrawing the drug and administering steroids, though 'bleomycin lung' may not be reversible. A known toxicity of the biological response modifier interleukin-2 is severe respiratory distress, which may necessitate mechanical ventilation.

Hepatotoxicity

Liver damage as a result of cancer chemotherapy may become apparent through (sometimes transient) elevations in hepatic enzymes detected in liver function tests, or when the liver is found to be enlarged, or when a patient becomes jaundiced or experiences abdominal pain. Drugs known to be hepatotoxic include chlorambucil, streptozotocin, methotrexate, cytosine arabinoside, 6-mercaptopurine, mithramycin, cisplatin, L-asparaginase, amsacrine, and dacarbazine. Because many chemotherapeutic agents are metabolised by the liver, dose modification may be necessary with impaired liver function. Hepatotoxicity is an uncommon but serious complication of chemotherapy, and it is important to monitor liver function through liver function tests throughout a course of treatment.

Haemorrhagic cystitis

This toxicity is associated only with cyclophosphamide and ifosfamide; with these agents toxic metabolites are excreted in the urine. The complication varies in severity from transient cystitis to major damage to the bladder and life-threatening haemorrhage. MESNA (2-mercaptoethane sulfonate) is administered with ifosfamide and high-dose cyclophosphamide as prophylaxis against cystitis; adequate hydration, together with frequent voiding of the bladder, have an important role in protecting the bladder. Urine should be monitored for traces of blood.

Nephrotoxicity

Many chemotherapeutic agents are known to be nephrotoxic, including cisplatin, streptozotocin, BCNU, CCNU, mitomycin C, mithramycin, ifosfamide, methotrexate, cyclophosphamide, and vincristine. With cisplatin, nephrotoxicity is dose-limiting. Its effects on renal function range from mild and reversible to acute renal failure. Reductions in glomerular filtration are seen following administration, though they are often temporary. Pre- and post-hydration and intravenous mannitol is used when administering cisplatin to prevent or minimise impairment of renal function; diuretics may also be used in high-dose regimes. Streptozotocin causes nephritis and tubular atrophy, and nephrotoxicity is again dose-limiting. Toxicity can take the form of a reversible proteinuria but may be severe, necessitating dialysis, and can be fatal. BCNU and CCNU sometimes give rise to delayed renal failure. Mitomycin C is associated with a syndrome comprising renal failure and microangiopathic haemolytic anaemia (MAHA)[1] with hypertension; and mithramycin is known to cause necrosis of the renal tubules. High-dose methotrexate can precipitate in the renal tubules, leading to impairment of the glomerular filtration rate; the nephrotoxicity of methotrexate can be minimised by simultaneous administration of sodium bicarbonate to maintain the alkalinity (pH > 7) of the urine. Hyponatraemia occurs in some patients receiving vincristine, and is associated with the peripheral and autonomic neuropathy occurring with this drug. The effect is clinically similar to inappropriate secretion of antidiuretic hormone.[1]

Common anti-cancer agents

Anti-cancer agents can be classified according to their mechanism of action.[1]

The anti-metabolites

The anti-metabolites inhibit enzymes necessary for the DNA synthesis part of the cell cycle, and are most active during this phase (S phase). Examples of anti-metabolites include 5-FU, methotrexate, cytosine arabinoside (araC), hydroxyurea, 6-mercaptopurine, 6-thioguanine, deoxycoformycin and fludarabine.

Fluorouracil (5-FU) acts through a metabolic pathway in which it is enzymatically converted to delete thymidine triphosphate (TTP), an important constituent of DNA. 5-FU is useful in the management of cancers of the breast, head and neck, and gastrointestinal tract. Further reported usages include hepatoma, carcinoma of the ovary, cervix, bladder, prostate, pancreas, and oropharynx.

Methotrexate is an anti-folate/folate antagonist, which inhibits the enzyme dihydrofolate reductase, depleting the folates (derived from dietary folic acid) necessary for the synthesis of precursors of DNA (thymidylate and purines) and RNA (purines). Methotrexate is used in the treatment of acute lymphoblastic leukaemia in children, in choriocarcinoma, and osteosarcoma. It is used in combination with other agents in the management of non-Hodgkin's lymphoma, and carcinoma of the breast, head and neck, ovary, and bladder. High-dose methotrexate is given in conjunction with folinic acid rescue to prevent excessive toxicity.

When activated, the anti-metabolite *cytosine arabinoside (araC)* is a potent inhibitor of DNA synthesis. To enable this sequence of events to take place, it is likely that cells must be exposed to araC during the 'S' phase of the cell cycle (i.e. inhibition of DNA must continue for at least one complete cell cycle).[2] Administration schedules must be tailored to achieve this result: typically, araC is given in bolus doses every 12 hours for 5–7 days, or by continuous infusion for 7 days.[2] AraC is used in the treatment of acute myelocytic leukaemia, and is a particularly important factor in the induction of remission.

Hydroxyurea acts upon an enzyme (ribonucleoside diphosphate reductase) essential to the synthesis of DNA. Hydroxyurea acts upon cells in the 'S' phase of the cell cycle at the G_1–S interface when they are sensitive to irradiation. *In vitro* studies indicate that combinations of hydroxyurea and irradiation cause synergistic toxicity.[2] Uses include treatment for chronic granulocytic leukaemia.

The anti-metabolites *mercaptopurine and thioguanine* inhibit the action of enzymes required for the synthesis of DNA, and cause critical alterations in the synthesis of RNA.[2] Mercaptopurine is a particularly important agent in the treatment of acute childhood leukaemias, and is also used in the adult form of the disease. Thioguanine is an important agent in the treatment of acute leukaemias (in combination with cytarabine for acute granulocytic leukaemia).

Deoxycoformycin inhibits DNA synthesis and impairs replication in the G_1 and S phases of the cell cycle. It is used in the treatment of chronic lym-

phoid malignancies such as hairy cell leukaemia.[10]

Fludarabine inhibits DNA and RNA synthesis. It is active against tumours with a low growth fraction (e.g. indolent lymphomas);[10] other uses include treatment of chronic lymphocytic leukaemia and hairy cell leukaemia.

The spindle poisons
The spindle poisons are most active during the synthetic (S) phase of the cell cycle, but also arrest cells in mitosis (M). Examples include *vincristine, vinblastine*, and *vindesine*.

Together with another vinca alkaloid, vinblastine, vincristine is derived from the pink periwinkle plant (*Catharanthus roseus* or *Vinca rosea*). Vindesine, a semisynthetic derivative of vinblastine, has primarily investigational rather than therapeutic applications. The vinca alkaloids have an anti-mitotic effect, blocking cells in mitosis. The microtubules of the mitotic apparatus (which are essential to the formation of the 'mitotic spindle') are disrupted and cell division is arrested; chromosomes are free to disperse ('exploded mitosis') or clump within the cytoplasm.[2] Vincristine is used in the treatment of childhood leukaemias and solid tumours, as well as lymphomas in adults. Vinblastine is most frequently used in the treatment of testicular teratomas. *Vinorelbine*, a further vinca alkaloid, is active against non-small cell lung cancer and breast cancer, though its applications are still the subject of clinical trials.

The alkylating agents
The alkylating agents damage the DNA template and appear to act throughout the cell cycle. Alkylating agents include cyclophosphamide, melphalan, ifosfamide, and chlorambucil (nitrogen mustards); carmustine (BCNU), lomustine (CCNU), semustine (methyl/CCNU), streptozocin and chlorozotocin (nitrosureas); thiotepa, busulphan, dacarbazine, mitomycin C, and procarbazine.

Cyclophosphamide is the most widely used of the alkylating agents. Following metabolic activation after administration, cyclophosphamide severely disrupts DNA molecules during the synthesis phase of the cell cycle. It is used in the management of lymphomas, chronic leukaemias and carcinomas (e.g. in combination with methotrexate or doxorubicin and 5-FU as adjuvant therapy for carcinoma of the breast).

Chlorambucil and melphalan, two nitrogen mustards used in the early 1940s, were the first drugs shown to have anti-tumour activity. Teicher[125] writes that researchers at the Chester Beatty Research Institute in London (now part of the Institute of Cancer Research) produced two now familiar derivatives of nitrogen mustards: chlorambucil and melphalan. Chlorambucil and melphalan induce alkylation of DNA and thus inhibit DNA replication. Priestman[4] explains alkylation as follows:

> The alkylating agents used in cancer chemotherapy form covalent bonds with a number of biologically active molecules including nucleic acids, proteins, amino acids and nucleotides and have the potential to damage cell membranes, deplete amino acid stores and inactivate enzymes. It has been shown that these drugs attack both a number of enzymes taking part in protein synthesis and also the linking enzymes which are needed for the construction of new DNA strands on their parent templates. Alkylation prevents these enzymes from carrying out their biological role within the cell and so stops the formation of new DNA which . . . inhibits mitosis . . . a more important action of these drugs in arresting cell division, is the formation of cross-linkages between DNA chains [pp. 28–29].

Clamon[126] adds:

> Depending upon the alkylating agent, a reactive intermediate such as a carbonium ion is formed which binds to DNA and causes single- or double-stranded DNA breaks and may cross-link the chains of DNA. The cytotoxic effect of alkylating agents correlates with their capacity to form cross-strand covalent linkages. Bifunctional alkylating agents, which have two reactive sites on the drug, are often more effective in inducing such links [p. 286; see also Hardman *et al.,*[2] pp. 1233–1236].

Ifosfamide is an analogue of cyclophosphamide. When metabolised, both agents produce alkylating compounds that destroy DNA. Ifosfamide is used as salvage therapy in testicular cancer or lymphoma. Because ifosfamide causes urotoxicity, a 'uroprotector' (MESNA) is administered concurrently during therapy.

Carmustine (BCNU, bischloroethylnitrosurea) is a nitrosurea, which alkylates DNA and produces DNA–DNA and DNA–protein cross-links.[10] BCNU has been used in the palliation of Hodgkin's disease, non-Hodgkin's lymphoma, multiple myeloma, and melanoma, but most significantly in primary brain tumours.[1] Chabner and

Longo[10] note that:

> . . . the nitrosureas are used singly and in combination in the therapy of lymphomas, lung cancer, colon cancer, and drug resistant multiple myelomas . . . When used as an adjuvant to radiation therapy, they enhance survival in patients with grade III and IV astrocytomas. The severe haematopoietic depression (especially thrombocytopenia) produced by these agents is a significant limiting factor in their use [p. 303].

Lomustine (CCNU, cyclohexylchloroethylnitrosurea) is an alkylating agent that inhibits RNA and DNA synthesis.

Streptozotocin is an alkylating agent that is a naturally occurring antibiotic methylnitrosurea derived from *Streptomyces*. Uses include treatment for carcinomas of islet cells in the pancreas.

Thiotepa is one of a group of drugs thought to produce alkylation in a similar way to the nitrogen mustards. It has been used in the treatment of carcinoma of the bladder, breast, and ovary.

Busulphan is an alkylating agent that disrupts DNA synthesis and cell division. While alkylating agents may act on cells at any stage of the cell cycle, toxicity is usually more apparent at the end of the G_1 phase and the beginning of the S phase. The primary use of busulphan is in chronic granulocytic leukaemia; it is also used in high-dose regimens with cyclophosphamide prior to bone marrow transplantation.

Dacarbazine is referred to as a 'non-classical' alkylating agent. It inhibits synthesis of DNA and RNA. Dacarbazine is metabolically activated following administration, and is active in several phases of the cell cycle. It has been used in the treatment of malignant melanoma, soft tissue sarcomas, and Hodgkin's disease.

Procarbazine is also referred to as a non-classical alkylating agent. Procarbazine has been used in combination with other agents in the treatment of Hodgkin's disease (mechlorethamine, vincristine, procarbazine, and prednisolone – MOPP) and non-Hodgkin's lymphoma. It has been shown to inhibit DNA, RNA, and protein synthesis. Cells in the premitotic G_2 phase may be most susceptible.[3]

Mitomycin C is an antitumour antibiotic derived from *Streptomyces*. It acts as an alkylating agent[14] and inhibits DNA synthesis by cross-linking of strands. Mitomycin C has been used in the treatment of carcinoma of the anus, bladder, breast, head and neck, lung, stomach, pancreas, and colon and rectum.

Other agents

Other agents that damage the DNA template through a variety of mechanisms include cisplatin and carboplatin (platinum analogues); doxorubicin, daunorubicin, mitoxantrone, idarubicin, epirubicin, and bleomycin (anti-tumour antibiotics); etoposide and teniposide (podophyllotoxins); dactinomycin and mithramycin (block RNA synthesis).

The anti-neoplastic properties of the platinum compounds:

... were discovered as the result of fortuitous observation ... during a study of the effects of electric current on growing bacteria. When alternating current was delivered through platinum electrodes to a growing bacterial culture, the bacterial cells stopped dividing and grew into long filaments ... filamentous growth was known to occur in bacteria subjected to alkylating agents or radiation ... It was found that platinum was released by electrolysis as hexachloroplatinate, which, in the presence of ammonium salts and light, generated the platinum complex ... now known as the anticancer drug cisplatin.[9]

Cisplatin binds covalently to DNA bases in a similar way to bifunctional alkylating agents, inhibiting DNA synthesis. It has been used in the treatment of carcinoma of the ovary and cervix, testicular cancer, head and neck cancer, bladder cancer, and small cell cancer of the lung.

Carboplatin is an analogue of cisplatin with a similar mode of action, but causes less nausea, neurotoxicity, ototoxicity, and nephrotoxicity than cisplatin.[2] Its dose-limiting toxicity is thrombocytopenia. Carboplatin is most often used in the treatment of carcinoma of the ovary.

Doxorubicin is an anti-tumour antibiotic derived from the fungus *Streptomyces*. Its cytotoxic activity may result from an ability to cause breaks in strands of DNA. Perry[1] summarises the mechanisms of action of various anti-tumour antibiotics as follows:

The focal point for the cytotoxicities of antitumour antibiotics is DNA ... antibiotics can intercalate [i.e. bind] in between base pairs of DNA (doxorubicin, daunorubicin, dactinomycin, bleomycin), bind to DNA (mitomycin C, plicamycin) and generate toxic oxygen free radicals, which cause single- or double-stranded DNA breaks (doxorubicin, daunorubicin, bleomycin, mitomycin C). From this ... DNA damage come some

of the ... cytotoxic actions of these agents, such as inhibition of DNA-directed RNA synthesis, protein synthesis ... [pp. 320–321].

Doxorubicin, which is most toxic during the S phase of the cell cycle, is used in treatment of acute lymphocytic and non-lymphocytic leukaemia, chronic lymphocytic leukaemia, Hodgkin's and non-Hodgkin's lymphoma, carcinoma of the breast and ovary, small cell carcinoma of the lung, osteogenic and soft tissue sarcomas, and metastatic carcinoma of the thyroid.[2] *Daunorubicin,* also S-phase specific, is used in the treatment of acute non-lymphocytic (with cytarabine) and acute lymphocytic leukaemia (with vincristine and prednisolone). *Bleomycin,* an antitumour antibiotic originally produced by fermentation of *Streptomyces verticullus,* is used in the treatment of germ cell tumours of the testis (in combination with cisplatin/vinblastine or cisplatin/etoposide) or ovary. Other usages include treatment for squamous cell carcinomas of the head and neck, oesophagus, and genito-urinary tract (e.g. in combination with cisplatin) and in combination therapy for Hodgkin's and non-Hodgkin's lymphoma. Bleomycin causes accumulation of cells in G_2 phase and fragmentation of DNA.

Mitoxantrone is an anti-tumour antibiotic, which inhibits DNA and RNA synthesis. It has been used in the treatment of advanced carcinoma of the breast and in initial treatment of acute non-lymphocytic leukaemia.

Epirubicin is an analogue of the anti-tumour antibiotic doxorubicin. Uses include carcinoma of the breast, biliary tract and oesophagus, and advanced gastric cancer.[127]

Together with *teniposide, etoposide* is derived from podophyllotoxin taken from the mandrake plant (*Podophyllum peltatum*). Etoposide and teniposide are most active against cells in the S and G_2 phases of the cell cycle, causing irreparable DNA breaks, which lead to cell death. In combination with bleomycin and cisplatin, etoposide is used in the management of testicular cancer; in combination with cisplatin, it is given in the treatment of small cell carcinoma of the lung. Other uses include treatment of non-Hodgkin's lymphomas, acute non-lymphocytic leukaemia, carcinoma of the breast, and Kaposi's sarcoma in AIDS. Teniposide is used in the management of acute lymphoblastic leukaemia in children and acute monocytic leukaemia in infants.

Dactinomycin (actinomycin D) is an anti-tumour antibiotic. It is used in the management of gestational choriocarcinoma in combination with etoposide, methotrexate, folinic acid, vincristine and cyclophosphamide (EMA/CO) and in the treatment of childhood rhabdomyosarcoma. Dactinomycin inhibits RNA and protein synthesis.

Mithramycin (plicamycin) is an anti-tumour antibiotic derived from *Streptomyces plicatus*. It inhibits RNA synthesis. Mithramycin reduces calcium and phosphorus resorption from the bones[127] and has been used in the management of malignant hypercalcaemia.

Taxanes: paclitaxel (taxol) and docetaxel (taxotere)

Taxol was produced from the bark of the Western yew tree in 1971 and has both anti-tumour and anti-leukemic effects. It disrupts many cellular activities by inducing abnormal stability in cell microtubules and causes cells to arrest in the G and M phases of the cell cycle. Taxotere is a semi-synthetic analogue of taxol. Taxol in conjunction with a platinum compound is now a widely accepted standard therapy for ovarian cancer. It has also been used in metastatic breast cancer when patients have not responded to previous therapy, as has taxotere. Nabholtz *et al.*[128] note that:

> Docetaxel [taxotere] represents a clear treatment option for patients with MBC [metastatic breast cancer] progressing despite previous anthracycline-containing chemotherapy.

Hormones and hormone antagonists

These include oestrogens, progestational agents, and corticosteroids (hormones); also anti-oestrogens, and aminoglutethamide, leuprolide, goserelin, and flutamide (hormone antagonists).

High doses of *oestrogens* (e.g. *diethylstilbestrol*) have been used in the treatment of metastatic breast cancer, though the mechanism of action of oestrogens in this role is not fully understood. (Paradoxically, oestrogens are known to stimulate tumour cell growth.[127]) When a tumour is oestrogen-receptor positive, a response rate of about 60% can be achieved in metastatic breast cancer.[13] The *anti-oestrogen* tamoxifen is used in the treatment of oestrogen-dependent breast cancer and has been the subject of clinical trials as a means of primary prevention of breast cancer in high-risk groups.[13] *Progestogens* (e.g. *megestrol* and *medroxyproges-*

terone) are used in the treatment of metastatic breast cancer and have also been used in renal cell carcinoma and cancer of the endometrium. In advanced prostate cancer, hormonal therapy with oestrogens or luteinising hormone-releasing hormone (LHRH) agonists is palliative in as much as 80% of patients.[127] Anti-androgens (e.g. *leuprolide*, *goserelin* and *flutamide*) are used in total androgen blockade (TAB) for advanced carcinoma of the prostate. *Aminoglutethamide* is an aromatase inhibitor, which causes suppression of the adrenal gland and inhibits production of oestrogens and androgens. It has been used in the treatment of metastatic cancer of the prostate and breast. Patients receiving aminoglutethamide require corticosteroid supplements to avoid the symptoms of adrenal suppression.

Corticosteroids (or *adrenocorticoids*) 'modulate DNA synthesis, mitosis, cell growth, differentiation, and . . . metabolism in normal and neoplastic target tissues'.[1] They are used in combination with other agents in the primary treatment of acute and chronic lymphocytic leukaemia, multiple myeloma, and Hodgkin's and non-Hodgkin's lymphoma. Barton Burke *et al.*[14] note that corticosteroids 'may recruit malignant cells out of G_0 phase, making them vulnerable to damage caused by cell cycle phase-specific agents'. Corticosteroids are also frequently used as anti-emetics, as well as in the management of hypercalcaemia associated with breast cancer, in the palliation of bone pain, to reduce cerebral oedema due to primary or metastatic tumours, and to alleviate breathlessness (e.g. in lymphangitis carcinomatosa).

Biological response modifiers

Biological response modifiers include interferons, interleukins, BCG, and levamisole.

The *interferons*, α- (alpha-), β- (beta-), and γ- (gamma-), were originally derived from leucocytes, fibroblasts, and T-cell lymphocytes, respectively; they cause inhibition of protein, DNA, and RNA synthesis. Perry[1] notes that interferons augment cell-specific T-cell cytotoxic and natural killer-cell activities. Interferon is an important treatment for metastatic renal cell carcinoma, hairy cell leukaemia, and chronic myeloid (or myelogenous) leukaemia. It has also been used in the treatment of follicle centre lymphomas and adult T-cell lymphomas, islet cell tumours of the gastrointestinal tract, malignant melanoma, and multiple myeloma.

Interleukin-2 has been most widely tested as a potential anti-tumour agent. Interleukins are, like interferons, produced by leucocytes. Interleukin-2 is derived from peripheral T-helper lymphocytes. Interleukin-2 stimulates immune responses, including cytotoxic T-cells, natural killer cells, other interleukins, and γ-interferon. Interleukin-2 has been used in the treatment of metastatic renal cell carcinoma. Trials have been conducted with interleukin-2 combined with lymphokine activated killer cells, though no significant differences in response rate or survival have been demonstrated.

BCG is derived from the live bacterium *Mycobacterium bovis*. BCG is administered intravesically to delay tumour progression and death in patients who present with superficial bladder cancer.

ʟ-Asparaginase

Asparaginase is an enzyme that can be isolated from many animal tissues, bacteria (including *Escherichia coli*), plants and the serum of some rodents. Asparaginase deprives leukaemia cells of asparagine, causing destruction of DNA and cell death; the cell cycle is arrested in G_1 phase.[129] It is used in combination with other agents in the treatment of acute lymphoblastic leukaemia and in some types of non-Hodgkin's lymphoma.

Research study 11.1: On the receiving end – patients' perceptions of the side-effects of cancer chemotherapy

Coates A., Abraham S., Kaye S.B. *et al.* (1993). *European Journal of Cancer and Clinical Oncology* **19**, 203–208.[73]

This study was conducted at a time when most chemotherapy was given with palliative rather than curative intent, and the decision to use chemotherapy involved weighing the benefits (i.e. anti-tumour effects) against the costs (i.e. side-effects). Assessment, particularly of the psychological side-effects of anti-cancer chemotherapy, had not received a great deal of attention up to this point. This study represents a first step towards developing quantitative measures to assist in the evaluation of chemotherapy side-effects.

Method

Ninety-nine patients (39 men/60 women aged 18–78 years, median 52 years) attending an out-patient clinic in Sydney took part. All had advanced cancer, and had received chemotherapy in the 4 weeks before the study. Patients were asked to select any number of cards from two groups (group A: 45 physical side-effects, group B: 28 non-physical side-effects) describing a potential side-effect of chemotherapy. They were then asked to rank the symptoms in order of importance. The top five ranked cards from each group were combined and the patients asked to select the five most severe symptoms regardless of group, in order from most to least severe. Patients were interviewed about general physical status and opinions about chemotherapy and were asked to complete a personality questionnaire. Chemotherapy regimens were divided into: (a) those containing cisplatinum; (b) those containing doxorubicin but no cisplatinum; and (c) those containing neither cisplatinum nor doxorubicin. Responses were analysed according to age, sex, diagnosis, treatment, opinions about progress, and marital and domestic status.

Results

The median number of non-physical symptoms selected was seven, compared with 12 for physical symptoms. Certain subgroups of the study group showed differences from the overall ranking of symptoms. For example, 'length of time treatment takes' was ranked fifth overall, but third by men, and 14th by women; 'having to have a needle' was ranked sixth overall, but 16th by men, and fifth by women.

Patients aged <45 years indicated that anxiety was more severe than sleeping difficulties and tiredness; 45–60-year-old patients emphasised sleeping difficulties but expressed less concern about having a needle and length of treatment time. Patients aged over 60 years mentioned fewer effects on the family and sleep, but included 'sore throat' in their list of symptoms.

A small number of patients with progressive disease ranked constant tiredness, trouble swallowing, loss of appetite, and sore throat highly, in contrast to patients with stable disease.

Although in total there was a smaller number of non-physical symptoms to choose from, 37 out of the 99 patients identified more non-physical effects in their list of the five most serious symptoms. Patients with high 'neuroticism' scores according to the personality questionnaire selected more non-physical symptoms; patients with high 'extraversion' scores selected fewer physical and non-physical symptoms. Older patients selected fewer non-physical symptoms.

Discussion

Of the 15 side-effects identified as most severe overall, 54% were non-physical, which suggests that this type of side-effect is at least as important as physical side-effects. The researchers cite the relative importance of 'fear of coming for treatment' and 'having to have a needle' as justification for the use of amnesic agents (lorazepam, for example). They conclude:

> Our findings highlight the importance of considering factors such as age and sex and the marital and domestic status of the patient when assessing the impact of

chemotherapy. The importance of loss of sexual feeling or ability suggests the need for helping patients cope with age-related problems which may be exacerbated by disease or treatment . . . The identification of patient subgroups and their particular potential problems with treatment contributes to the more accurate evaluation of the balance between morbidity and therapeutic benefit inherent in every decision to use cancer chemotherapy [pp. 206, 208].

References

1. Perry M.C. (ed.) (1992). *The Chemotherapy Source Book.* Baltimore, CT: Williams & Wilkins.
2. Hardman J.G., Limbird L.E., Molinoff P.B., Ruddon R.W. and Gilman A.G. (eds.) (1996). *Goodman & Gilman's The Pharmacological Basis of Therapeutics*, 9th edition. New York: McGraw Hill.
3. Bleiberg H., Rougier P. and Wilke H.-J. (1998). *Management of Colorectal Cancer.* London: Martin Dunitz.
4. Priestman (1987). *Cancer Chemotherapy: An Introduction*, 3rd edition. London: Springer.
5. Skeel R.T. (1987). *Handbook of Cancer Chemotherapy.* Boston, MA: Little Brown.
6. Horwich A. (ed.) (1995). *Oncology: A Multidisciplinary Textbook.* London: Chapman and Hall Medical.
7. Karnofsky D.A. and Burchenal J.H. (1949). The clinical evaluation of chemotherapeutic agents in cancer. In McLeod C.M. (ed.) *Evaluation of Chemotherapeutic Agents.* New York: Columbia University Press.
8. Fretwell D.F. (1990). Comprehensive functional assessment (CFA) in everyday practice. In Hazzard W.R., Andres R., Bierman E.L. and Blass J.P. (eds.) *Principles of Geriatric Medicine and Gerontology.* New York: McGraw Hill.
9. Mendelsohn M.L. (1960). The growth fraction: a new concept applied to tumors. *Science* 132, 1496.
10. Chabner B.A. and Longo D.L. (1995). *Cancer Chemotherapy and Biotherapy: Principles and Practice.* Philadelphia, PA: Lippincott-Raven.
11. Schabel F.M. Jr (1969). The use of tumor growth kinetics in planning 'curative' chemotherapy of advanced solid tumours. *Cancer Research* 29, 2384.
12. Pratt W.B., Ruddon R.W., Ensminger W.D. and Maybaum J. (1994). *The Anticancer Drugs.* New York: Oxford University Press.
13. Laurence D.R., Bennett P.N. and Brown M.J. (1997). *Clinical Pharmacology.* New York: Churchill Livingstone, p. 560.
14. Barton Burke M., Wilkes G.M. and Ingwersen K. (1996). *Cancer Chemotherapy: A Nursing Process Approach.* Sudbury, MA: Jones and Bartlett.
15. Baird S.B. (1988). *Decision Making in Oncology Nursing.* Philadelphia, PA: B.C. Decker.
16. Baxley K.O., Erdman L.K., Henry E.B. and Roof B.J. (1984). Alopecia: effect on cancer patients' body image. *Cancer Nursing* 7, 499–503.
17. Freedman T.G. (1994). Social and cultural dimensions of hair loss in women treated for breast cancer. *Cancer Nursing* 17, 334–341.
18. Wagner L. and Bye M.G. (1979). Body image and patients experiencing alopecia as a result of cancer chemotherapy. *Cancer Nursing* 2, 365–369.
19. Dean J., Salmon S.E. and Griffiths K.S. (1979). Prevention of doxorubicin-induced alopecia with scalp hypothermia. *New England Journal of Medicine* 301, 1427–1429.
20. Love R.R., Leventhal H., Easterling D.V. and Nerenz D.R. (1989). Side-effects and emotional distress during cancer chemotherapy. *Cancer* 63, 604–612.
21. Clement-Jones V. (1985). Cancer and beyond: the formation of BACUP. *British Medical Journal* 291, 1021–1023.
22. Tierney A.J. (1987). Preventing chemotherapy-induced alopecia in women treated for breast cancer: is scalp cooling worthwhile? *Journal of Advanced Nursing* 12, 303–310.
23. Gallagher J. (1996). Women's experiences of hair loss associated with chemotherapy: longitudinal perspective. *Proceedings of 9th International Conference on Cancer Nursing*, Brighton, UK, 1996.
24. Munstedt K., Manthey N., Sacchse S. and Vahrson H. (1997). Changes in self-concept and body image during cancer chemotherapy-induced alopecia. *Supportive Care in Cancer* 5, 139–143.
25. David J.A. and Speechley V. (1987). Scalp cooling to prevent alopecia. *Nursing Times* 83, 36–37.
26. Keller J.F. and Blausey L.A. (1988). Nursing issues and management in chemotherapy-induced alopecia. *Oncology Nursing Forum* 15, 603–607.
27. Tierney A.J. (1991). Chemotherapy-induced hair loss. *Nursing Standard* 5, 29–31.
28. Lemenager-Blondel, M. *et al.* (1998). Chemotherapy-induced alopecia: a controllable side-effect. *Oncology Nurses Today* 3, 18–20.
29. Ron I.G., Kalmus Y., Kalmus Z., Inbar M. and Chaitchik S. (1997). Scalp cooling in the prevention of alopecia in patients receiving depilating chemotherapy. *Supportive Care in Cancer* 5, 136–138.
30. Cavalli F., Hansen H.H. and Kaye S.B. (1997). *Textbook of Medical Oncology.* London: Martin Dunitz.
31. Crowe M., Kendrick M. and Woods S. (1998). Is scalp cooling a procedure that should be offered to patients receiving chemotherapy-induced alopecia for solid tumours? *Proceedings of the 10th International Conference on Cancer Nursing*, Jerusalem, 1998.

32. Dougherty L. (1996). Scalp cooling to prevent hair loss in chemotherapy. *Professional Nurse* 11, 507–509.

33. Speechley V. (1987). Nursing patients having chemotherapy. In Tiffany R. and Borley D. (eds.). *Oncology for Nurses and Health Care Professionals*, Vol. 3 (*Cancer Nursing*). London: Harper and Row, Chapter 13, 74–121.

34. Gillon R. (1986). *Philosophical Medical Ethics*. Chichester: John Wiley.

35. McGrath P. (1995). It's OK to say no! A discussion of ethical issues arising from informed consent to chemotherapy. *Cancer Nursing* 18, 97–103.

36. Otto S.E. (1995). Advanced concepts in chemotherapy drug delivery: regional therapy. *Journal of Intravenous Nursing* 18, 170–176.

37. Mallett J. and Bailey C. (1996). Cytotoxic drugs: handling and administration. *The Royal Marsden Hospital Manual of Clinical Nursing Procedures*. Oxford: Blackwells, Chapter 13, 191–212.

38. Allwood M., Stanley A. and Wright P. (1997). *The Cytotoxics Handbook*. Oxford: Radcliffe Medical Press.

39. Goodman M. and Riley M.B. (1997). Chemotherapy: principles of administration. In Groenwald S.K., Frogge S.H., Goodman M. and Yarbro C.H. (eds.) *Cancer Nursing: Principles and Practice*. Boston, MA: Jones & Bartlett.

40. Doyle M.A. (1995). Oncologic therapy. In Terry J., Boranowski L., Lonsway R.A. and Hedrick C. (eds.) *Intravenous Therapy: Clinical Practice and Principles*. Philadelphia, PA: W.B. Saunders.

41. Reymann P.E. (1993). Chemotherapy: principles of administration. In Groenwald S.K., Frogge S.H., Goodman M. and Yarbro C.H. (eds.) *Cancer Nursing: Principles and Practice*. Boston, MA: Jones and Bartlett.

42. Tsang V., Fernando H.C. and Goldstraw P. (1990). Pleuroperitoneal shunt for recurrent malignant pleural effusions. *Thorax* 45, 369–372.

43. Chisholm L.G., Berman A.R., de Carvalho M. and Gorrell C.R. (1993). Cancer chemotherapy: alternative administration routes. *Cancer Nursing* 16, 237–246.

44. Dougherty L. and Lamb J. (1999). *Intravenous Therapy in Nursing Practice*. Edinburgh: Churchill Livingstone.

45. Dougherty L., Viner C. and Young J. (1998). Establishing ambulatory chemotherapy at home. *Professional Nurse* 13, 356–358.

46. Gabriel J. (1996). Peripherally inserted central catheters: expanding UK nurses' practice. *British Journal of Nursing* 5, 71–74.

47. Macrae K. (1998). Hand-held dopplers in central catheter insertion. *Professional Nurse* 14, 99–102.

48. Weinstein S.M. and Plumer A.L. (1996). *Plumer's Principles and Practice of Intravenous Therapy*. Philadelphia, PA: Lippincott, Williams & Wilkins.

49. Thompson A.M., Kidd E., McKenzie M., Parker A.C. and Nixon S.J. (1989). Long term central venous access: the patient's view. *Intensive Therapy and Clinical Monitoring* 10, 142–145.

50. Speechley V. and Davidson T. (1989). Managing an implantable drug delivery system. *Professional Nurse* 4, 284–288.

51. Alexander H.R. (1994). *Vascular Access in the Cancer Patient: Devices, Insertion Techniques, Maintenance, and Prevention and Management of Complications*. Philadelphia, PA: Lippincott-Raven.

52. Camp Sorrell D. (1993). Toxicity management in cancer nursing. In Groenwald S.K., Frogge S.H., Goodman M. and Yarbro C.H. (eds.) *Cancer Nursing: Principles and Practice*. Boston, MA: Jones and Bartlett.

53. Lokich J., Bothe A. Jr, Fine N. and Perri J. (1982). The delivery of cancer chemotherapy by constant venous infusion: ambulatory management of venous access and portable pump. *Cancer* 50, 2731–2735.

54. Garvey E.C. (1987). Current and future nursing issues in the home administration of chemotherapy. *Seminars in Oncology Nursing* 3, 142–147.

55. Sewell G.J. and Summerhayes M. (1993). Home-based cytotoxic chemotherapy. In Allwood M. and Wright A. (eds.) *The Cytotoxics Handbook*. Oxford: Radcliffe Medical Press.

56. Schulmeister L. (1992). An overview of continuous infusion chemotherapy. *Journal of Intravenous Nursing* 15, 315–321.

57. Teich C.J. and Raia K. (1984). Teaching strategies for an ambulatory chemotherapy program. *Oncology Nursing Forum* 11, 24–28.

58. Nanninga A.G., de Vries E.G., Willemse P.H. *et al.* (1991). Continuous infusion of chemotherapy on an outpatient basis via a totally implanted venous access port. *European Journal of Cancer* 27, 147–149.

59. Koeppen M.A. and Caspars S.M. (1994). Problems identified with home infusion pumps. *Journal of Intravenous Nursing* 17, 151–156.

60. Garvey E. and Kramer R. (1983). Improving cancer patients' adjustment to infusion chemotherapy: evaluation of a patient education program. *Cancer Nursing* 6, 373–378.

61. Fernsler J.I. and Cannon C.A. (1991). The whys of patient education. *Seminars in Oncology Nursing* 7, 79–86.

62. Dodd M.J. (1982). Assessing patient self-care for side-effects of chemotherapy, part 1. *Cancer Nursing* 5, 447–451.

63. Butler M.C. (1984). Families' response to chemotherapy by an ambulatory infusion pump. *Nursing Clinics of North America* 19, 139–143.

64. Valanis B.G., Vollmer W.M., Labuhn K.T. and Glass A.G. (1993). Acute symptoms associated with antineoplastic drug handling among nurses. *Cancer Nursing* 16, 288–295.

65. HMSO (1974). *Health and Safety at Work Act (1974).* London: HMSO.

66. Health and Safety Executive (1988*). Control of Substances Hazardous to Health (COSHH) (1988).* London: HMSO.

67. Laidlaw J.L., Connor T.H., Theiss J.C., Anderson R.W. and Matney T.S. (1984). Permeability of latex and polyvinyl chloride gloves to 20 antineoplastic drugs. *American Journal of Hospital Pharmacy* **41**, 2618–2623.

68. Goodman I. (1998). Development of national, evidence-based clinical guidelines for the administration of cytotoxic chemotherapy. *European Journal of Oncology Nursing* **2**, 43–50.

69. Baker E.S. and Connor T.H. (1996). Monitoring occupational exposure to cancer chemotherapy drugs. *American Journal of Health Systems and Pharmacy* **53**, 2713–2723.

70. Nieweg R.M., de Boer M., Dubbleman R.C. *et al.* (1994). Safe handling of neoplastic drugs: results of a survey. *Cancer Nursing* **17**, 501–511.

71. How C. and Brown J. (1998). Extravasation of cytotoxic chemotherapy from peripheral veins. *European Journal of Oncology Nursing* **2**, 51–58.

72. Boyle, D.M. and Engelking C. (1995). Vesicant extravasation: myths and realities. *Oncology Nursing Forum* **22**, 57–67.

73. Coates A., Abraham S., Kaye S.B. *et al.* (1983). On the receiving end – patient perception of the side-effects of chemotherapy. *European Journal of Cancer and Clinical Oncology* **19**, 203–208.

74. Cohn K.H. (1982). Chemotherapy from an insider's perspective. *Lancet* **i**, 1006–1009.

75. Price B. (1992). Living with altered body image: the cancer experience. *British Journal of Nursing* **1**, 641–642, 644–645.

76. Kaplan M. (1983). Viewpoint: the cancer patient . . . being hospitalised on a cancer floor. *Cancer Nursing* **6**, 103–107.

77. Dougherty L. (1994). *A study to discover how cancer patients perceive the intravenous cannulation experience.* Unpublished M.Sc. thesis, University of Surrey.

78. Buckalew P.G. (1982). On the opposite side of the bed: a nurse clinician's experiences with anxiety during chemotherapy. *Cancer Nursing* **5**, 435–439.

79. Kaberry S. (1991). Blood simple? *Nursing Times* **87**, 56.

80. Messina S.M. (1989). The nurse with a central line: when the patient is you. *Journal of Intravenous Nursing* **12**, 29–30.

81. Mills R.T. and Krantz D.S. (1979). Information, choice, and reactions to stress: a field experiment in a blood bank with laboratory analogue. *Journal of Personality and Social Psychology* **37**, 608–620.

82. Richardson, A. (1992). Studies exploring self-care for the person coping with cancer treatment: an overview. *International Journal of Nursing Studies* **29**, 191–204.

83. Hudek J. (1986). Compliance in intravenous therapy. *CINA: Official Journal of the Canadian Intravenous Nurses Association* **2**, 7–8.

84. Kelly M.P. (1985). Loss and grief reactions as responses to surgery. *Journal of Advanced Nursing* **10**, 517–525.

85. DiGiacomo S.M. (1987). Biomedicine as a cultural system: an anthropologist in the kingdom of the sick. In Baer H.A. (ed.) *Encounters with Biomedicine.* New York: Gordon & Breach.

86. Thompson S.C. (1981). Will it hurt less if I can control it? A complex answer to a simple question. *Psychological Bulletin* **90**, 89–101.

87. Gill K.M. (1984). Coping effectively with invasive medical procedures: a descriptive model. *Clinical Psychology Review* **4**, 339–362.

88. Johns C. (1996). Visualizing and realizing caring in practice through guided reflection. *Journal of Advanced Nursing* **24**, 1135–1143.

89. Johns C. (1997). Caitlin's story – realizing caring within everyday practice through guided reflections. *International Journal of Human Caring* **1**, 33–39.

90. Holmes S. and Dickerson J. (1987). The quality of life: design and evaluation of a self-assessment instrument for use with cancer patients. *International Journal of Nursing Studies* **24**, 15–24.

91. Lamb M.A. (1985). Sexual dysfunction in the gynaecologic oncology patient. *Seminars in Oncology Nursing* **1**, 9–17.

92. Young-McCaughan S. (1996). Sexual functioning in women with breast cancer after treatment with adjuvant therapy. *Cancer Nursing* **19**, 308–319.

93. Holmes S. (1990). *Cancer Chemotherapy.* London: Austen Cornish.

94. Yates A. (1987). Sexual healing. *Nursing Times* **83**, 20–30.

95. Holmes S. (1987). Nutritional problems in the cancer patient. *Nursing* **3**, 733–735, 737–738.

96. Perry M.C. and Yarbro J.W. (eds.) (1984). *Toxicity of Chemotherapy.* Orlando: Grune and Stratton.

97. Sonis S.T., Sonis A.L. and Lieberman A. (1978). Oral complications for patients receiving treatment for malignancies other than head and neck. *Journal of the American Dental Association* **97**, 468–472.

98. Chemotherapy in paediatric patients. *Journal of Pedodentics* **3**(2), 122–128.

99. Graham K.M., Pecadoro D.A., Ventura M. and Meyer C.C. (1993). Reducing the incidence of stomatitis using a quality assessment and improvement approach. *Cancer Nursing* **16**, 117–122.

100. Colbourne L. (1995). Patients' experiences of chemotherapy treatment. *Professional Nurse* **10**, 439–442.

101. Fallowfield L. and Clark A. (1991). *Breast Cancer*. London: Routledge.

102. Jenns K. (1994). Importance of nausea. *Cancer Nursing* 17, 488–493.

103. Dodd M.J., Onishi K., Dibble S.L. and Larson P. (1996). Differences in nausea, vomiting and retching between younger and older outpatients receiving cancer chemotherapy. *Cancer Nursing* 19, 155–161.

104. Love R.R., Nerenz D.R. and Leventhal H. (1983). Anticipatory nausea with cancer patients: developments through two mechanisms. *Proceedings of the American Society of Clinical Oncology*, C-242.

105. Coons H.L., Leventhal H., Nerenz D.R., Love R.R. and Larson S. (1987). Anticipatory nausea and emotional distress in patients receiving cisplatin-based chemotherapy. *Oncology Nursing Forum* 14, 31–35.

106. Pratt A., Lazar R.M., Penman D. and Holland J.C. (1984). Psychological parameters of chemotherapy-induced conditioned nausea and vomiting: a review. *Cancer Nursing* 7, 483–490.

107. Morrow G.R. and Morrell C. (1982). Behavioural treatment for the anticipatory nausea and vomiting induced by cancer chemotherapy. *New England Journal of Medicine* 307, 1476–1480.

108. Andrews P.L.R. and Sanger G.J. (1993). *Emesis in Anti-Cancer Therapy: Mechanisms and Treatment*. London: Chapman and Hall.

109. Cunningham D., Evans C., Gazet J.C. *et al.* (1987). Comparison of antiemetic efficacy of domperidone, metoclopramide, and dexamethasone in patients receiving outpatient chemotherapy regimens. *British Medical Journal* 295, 250.

110. Lazlo J., Clark R.A., Hanson D.C., Tyson L., Crumpler L. and Gralla R. (1985). Lorazepam in cancer patients treated with cisplatin: a drug having antiemetic, amnesic, and anxiolytic effects. *Journal of Clinical Oncology* 3, 864–869.

111. Tierney A.J., Taylor J. and Closs S.J. (1992). Knowledge, expectations and experiences of patients receiving chemotherapy for breast cancer. *Scandinavian Journal of Caring Sciences* 6, 75–80.

112. Pritchard A.P. and Speechley V. (1989). What do nurses know about emesis? *International Cancer Nursing News* 1, 68.

113. McCaffery M. and Beebe A. (1989). *Pain: Clinical Manual for Nursing Practice*. St Louis, MO: CV Mosby.

114. Dundee J.W. and Yang J. (1990). Prolongation of the antiemetic action of P6 acupuncture by acupressure in patients having cancer chemotherapy. *Journal of the Royal Society of Medicine* 83, 360–362.

115. Tanghe A., Evers G. and Paridaens R. (1998). Nurses' assessment of symptom occurrence and symptom distress in chemotherapy patients. *European Journal of Oncology Nursing* 2, 14–26.

116. Richardson A., Ream E. and Wilson-Barnett J. (1998). Fatigue in patients receiving chemotherapy: patterns of change. *Cancer Nursing* 21, 17–30.

117. Piper B., Lindsey A. and Dodd M. (1987). Fatigue mechanisms in cancer patients: developing a nursing theory. *Oncology Nursing Forum* 14, 17–23.

118. Grandjean E.P. (1970). Fatigue. *American Industrial Hygiene Association Journal* 31, 401–411.

119. Selye H. (1974). *Stress without Distress*. Philadelphia, PA: J.B. Lippincott.

120. Nerenz D.R., Leventhal H. and Love R.R. (1982). Factors contributing to emotional distress during cancer chemotherapy. *Cancer* 50, 1020–1027.

121. Knopf M.T. (1986). Physical and psychologic distress associated with adjuvant chemotherapy in women with breast cancer. *Journal of Clinical Oncology* 4, 678–684.

122. Ehlke G. (1988). Symptom distress in breast cancer patients receiving chemotherapy in the outpatient setting. *Oncology Nursing Forum* 15, 344–346.

123. Rhodes V.A. (1988). Patients' descriptions of the influence of tiredness and weakness on self-care abilities. *Cancer Nursing* 11, 186–194.

124. Blesch K.S. (1988). The normal physiological changes of ageing and their impact on the response to cancer treatment. *Seminars in Oncology Nursing* 4, 178–188.

125. Teicher B.A. (1997). *Cancer Therapeutics: Experimental and Clinical Agents*. Totowa, NJ: Humana Press.

126. Clamon H.G. In Perry M.C. (ed.) (1992). *The Chemotherapy Source Book*. Baltimore, MD: Williams & Wilkins.

127. Cavalli F., Hansen H. and Kaye S.B. (1997). *Textbook of Medical Oncology*. London: Martin Dunitz.

128. Nabholz J.M., Senn H.J., Bezwoda W.R. *et al.* (1999). Prospective randomized trial of docetaxel versus mitomycin plus vinblastine in patients with metastatic breast cancer progressing despite previous anthracycline-containing chemotherapy, 304 Study Group. *Journal of Clinical Oncology* 17, 1413–1424.

129. Ueno T., Ohtawa K., Mitsui K. *et al.* (1997). Cell cycle arrest and apoptosis of leukaemia cells induced by L-asparaginase. *Leukaemia* 11, 1858–1861.

CHAPTER TWELVE

Radiotherapy

Sara Faithfull

Radiotherapy plays a central role in the treatment of cancer. Over 50% of people with cancer will receive radiation therapy at some time. In the context of cancer therapy, its value lies in the local management of disease. Radiotherapy may be aimed at cure, may be palliative, or given as an adjunct to existing treatment. Its success depends on tumour bulk and the tumour's sensitivity to radiation, as well as the tolerance of surrounding tissues to radiotherapy.

. Radiotherapy is the use of ionising radiation. The ionisation damages DNA and consequently causes cell death, especially when the cell attempts to replicate. Radiation affects both normal and malignant cells; however, the goal of radiotherapy is to preserve normal tissue function, while damaging the tumour. This is possible owing to various factors. For example, more damage is caused to cancer cells than to normal cells. The kinetics of the cell usually favours the recovery of normal tissue over that of the tumour, and this is exploited by giving radiation in small daily doses (fractionated radiotherapy), over several weeks. Side-effects from treatment are a result of normal tissue damage and may continue long after radiotherapy has finished. Radiotherapy treatment is often seen as an acute event from which recovery is rapid. However, when side-effects of radiation therapy are superimposed on existing functional difficulties, morbidity can be significant.

Nurses are often unaware of the effects of radiotherapy or of how treatment works; the severity of side-effects and their implications for resuming normal life are also underestimated. Radiotherapy is mainly organised as an out-patient treatment and as a result nursing support may not be available routinely to people undergoing treatment.

The invisible and highly technical nature of radiotherapy contributes to the fact that 'few therapeutic modalities in medicine induce more misunderstanding, confusion and apprehension'.[1] Radiation therapy has been in existence since the 1900s. In the past the hazards and biological basis of it were little understood, but there is now a growing body of knowledge that provides new and exciting prospects for how the treatment is used, and in developments for the future.

Radiation is given in the form of X-rays, gamma-rays or electrons. Particles such as neutrons or protons are seldom used. Ionising radiation by definition is those types of radiation that produce ionisation of atoms and molecules with which they come into contact.[2] A simple understanding of atomic structure can help to explain the nature of these changes.

Atoms are essentially electric in nature. Ionising radiation has sufficient energy to cause atoms of cells in its path to lose orbiting electrons. When an electron is dislodged from its orbit the atom fragments acquire a positive electrical charge. These

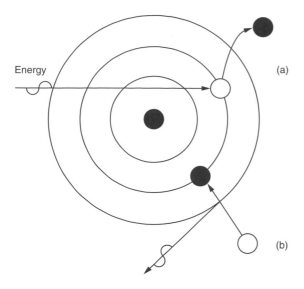

Figure 12.1 Ionisation and excitation of atoms. When an atom or molecule has too many electrons, it is called a negative ion. An atom with fewer electrons is called positive. The atom is said to be ionised when an electron is (a) completely removed, but (b) only excited when it moves from one orbit to another. This movement produces the emission of electromagnetic radiation or X-rays (based on Bomford *et al.*[75]).

'free' electrons interact with neighbouring atoms and hence these atom fragments acquire a negative electrical charge. When electrons are released from their orbit, energy in the form of free electrons is released at high speed and dislodges more electrons from neighbouring atoms, which in turn release energy, and continue further ionisations until all energy is dissipated (see Figure 12.1).[3]

Although this process is hard to visualise, it is almost like playing marbles, where one marble may knock others in its path causing them to scatter, creating more movement in a cascade. The electrically charged particles are called ions and the process of their development is called ionisation. This ionisation is responsible for the chemical and biological changes that occur to tissues in the form of radiotherapy.

Ionising beams used in radiotherapy fall into two main types: (1) those that are electrically produced X-rays from a filament; and (2) through the decay of radioactive isotopes, either naturally occurring or those manufactured specifically in reactors.

Where do the rays come from?

The rays produced by radiotherapy machines are electromagnetic beams such as X-rays. These are similar to light but of a higher energy and shorter wavelength, consisting of photons (see Figure 12.2). The rays occur when speeding electrons hit high atomic weight targets such as tantalum. The early kilovoltage machines produced electrons from heated filaments. Modern megavoltage machines, known as linear accelerators, use a radiowave guide to accelerate further electrons produced in this way. These electrons bombard the target at high energy producing X-rays in the range of 4–24 MeV (million electron volts). This form of radiotherapy is termed 'external beam' and is used for a variety of different treatments outlined in Table 12.1.

At low energies the X-rays produced are absorbed to varying degrees by different tissues and result in a clear distinction between bone, soft tissue, and air interface, which is visible on diagnostic radiographs (X-ray films). Superficial irradiation occurs with photon energies of 150 keV and orthovoltage at 300 keV. At megavoltage energies (4–25 MeV) photons penetrate the deeper tissues. These differences in energy levels are important, as increased energy of radiation produces a greater penetration of tissues. The different energy levels are often used for differing sites of radiotherapy treatments. Electrons created by removing the target travel only short distances so are limited in their therapeutic use, but are very good for superficial treatments such as basal cell skin cancers.

Radiation dose is defined as the amount of energy absorbed per unit mass of tissue. This is measured in gray (Gy): 1 gray = 1 joule/kg. For a conventional curative course of external beam radiotherapy the dose ranges from 55 to 65 Gy and is given in daily treatments of 1.6–2.5 Gy over 4–6 weeks. This is termed fractionation. External beam radiotherapy utilises a beam from which the patient is placed at a defined distance (usually 100 mm). The isodose is the distribution of absorption of radiation in the tissues and varies at any point within the tissue, depending on the distance from the X-ray source. These distributions often look like contours on a map and reflect changes in radiation dose (Figure 12.3). High-energy X-rays produced by the linear accelerator deposit most of their

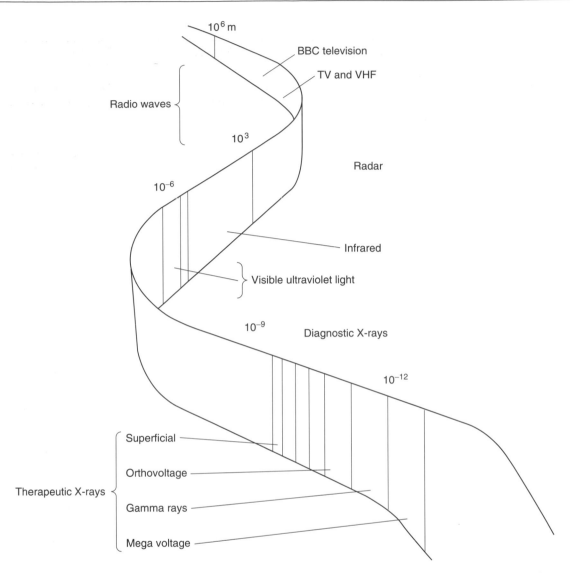

Figure 12.2   The electromagnetic spectrum. The electromagnetic spectrum extends from wavelengths of many kilometres (10^3) to less than 1 picometre (10^{-12}). These invisible waves are called X-rays and gamma (γ)-rays.

energy at some distance from the skin surface. This is known as the 'skin sparing' effect and can diminish skin damage, which was often seen in the early days of radiotherapy treatment, when lower energies were used.

Alternative radiation sources are those from naturally occurring radionucleotides; these elements have unstable nuclei, which release energy in the process of spontaneous disintegration. This may be in the form of gamma-rays, high-speed electrons, or other particles. A variety of isotopes is also used (see Table 12.1). These have a range of therapeutic uses that are continually being developed.

Brachytherapy involves the delivery of radiation by placing sources close to the tumour. The dose of radiotherapy decreases equal to the square of the distance from the source. Therefore the tumour receives a higher dose, with little radiation reaching the surrounding normal tissues. The most

Table 12.1 Types of radiation

Type	Energy	Source	Clinical use
Oral or parenteral radiotherapy Radioactive isotopes administered orally or parentarally; their effect is targeted to tissues where they concentrate.		Iodine-131 Strontium-89	Thyroid tumours Multiple bone metastases
Brachytherapy Placing of radiation sources close to the tumour. A high dose is received by the tumour and less by surrounding normal tissues.		Iridium-192 (seeds or wires) Iodine-125 seeds Caesium-137	Sources can be implanted directly into small tumours such as the tongue, lip or breast. Intracavity sources for cervical and uterine cancers.
External beam (teletherapy) Superficial Orthovoltage Low energy X-rays do not possess skin-sparing properties.	50–150 keV 250–500 keV	X-ray tube X-ray tube	Skin tumours Superficial sites, e.g. breast, rib, sacrum.
Megavoltage High energy and have skin-sparing effects.	>1 MeV (usually 4–16 MeV)	Linear accelerator	Main source of therapeutic beams for sites other than skin.
Gamma rays	2.5 MeV 4–30 MeV	Cobalt Linear accelerator	Superficial sites, e.g. skin, lymph nodes; (depth depends upon electron energy).

common example of brachytherapy is the insertion of interactive sources (see Table 12.1); for example, uterine or cervical carcinomas. Techniques of placing the source in small catheters that can then be safely inserted and withdrawn, termed 'afterloading', are designed to provide maximum radiation protection for staff.[4]

Radioactive isotopes for systemic treatments are administered orally. Localisation of the isotopes around tumours occurs when the chemical that is radioactive is metabolised. An example of this is iodine-131, which is used to treat cancer of the thyroid. Research into tagging of radioactive nucleotides to monoclonal antibodies has been progressing; however, this so-called 'magic bullet' has not lived up to its promise because of technical difficulties in making it work.

Cells in action: radiobiology

Radiation interacts either directly or indirectly with tissue to produce short-lived ion radicals. These are associated with damage to deoxyribonucleic acid (DNA) and result in single- or double-strand breaks in its structure. This damage may subsequently be repaired by the cell. Normal tissues have a greater ability to repair themselves than cancer cells.[5] Differences in how cells respond to irradiation are some of the reasons for the differences seen in the radiosensitivity of different cancers. The response to radiation is also affected by oxygenation, the number of cells actively dividing, and the rate at which cells grow within the tumour. These parameters are often termed the 4 Rs and are important in understanding the rationale behind radiotherapy treatment, since they are used to max-imise damage to cancer cells while minimising normal tissue damage.

The scattering 'marbles' effect described earlier has two modes of action. They interact directly or indirectly with the tissues. The direct damage is in the nucleus of the cell and affects the DNA, rather like chopping up spaghetti, and the cell is either unable to repair itself or does so inaccurately, result-ing in cell death after several cell divisions. The indirect effects involve interaction of free radicals within the cells. These free radicals are OH ions and

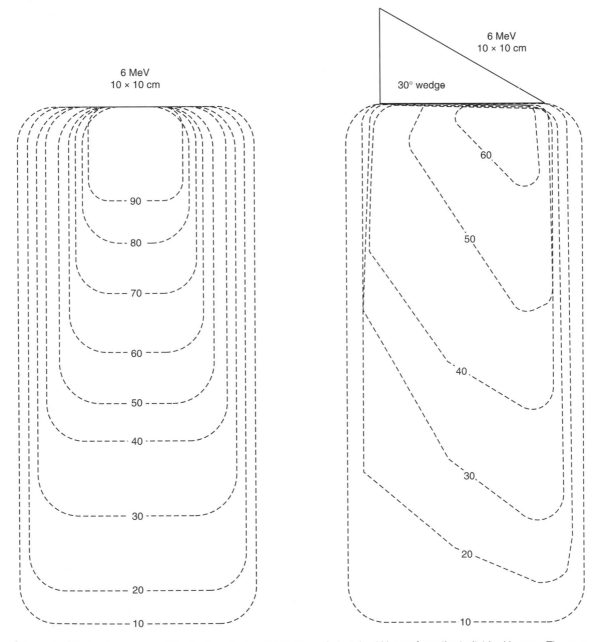

Figure 12.3 Isodose curves. The isodose is the distribution of absorbed X-rays from the individual beams. The max-imum value is labelled 100% and lower dose values are drawn at 10% intervals. The isodose curve can be altered by insertion of 30° edge into the beam.

are oxidising agents. The mechanism is poorly understood but the result is a disruption in cellular and tissue function.[3] The direct effects are thought to be most damaging to cells (see Figure 12.4). This disturbance of DNA synthesis leads to abnormal mitosis. Cells that have a short mitosis (for example, mucosa and skin) will show signs of radiation damage more quickly than those whose cycle is long and explains why some of the symp-

toms experienced appear many months to years following treatment.

The considerable variation in radiosensitivity of different tissues is not fully understood. In experiments in the laboratory it is possible to analyse these differences and it is clear that cell survival after irradiation shows an initial curve of cell multiplication followed by rapidly declining cell numbers (see Figure 12.5). This curve represents the ability

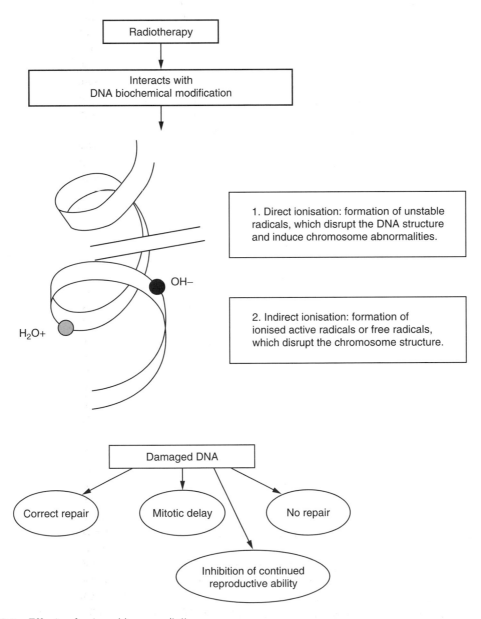

Figure 12.4 Effects of external beam radiation.

of cells in some way to repair themselves and this is termed 'sub-lethal damage'. Differences in this repair capacity between cancers may be part of the explanation for the different responses of tumours to fractionation regimes, especially when using low doses of radiation.[6]

A series of fractionated doses increases the difference in repair ability between normal tissue and

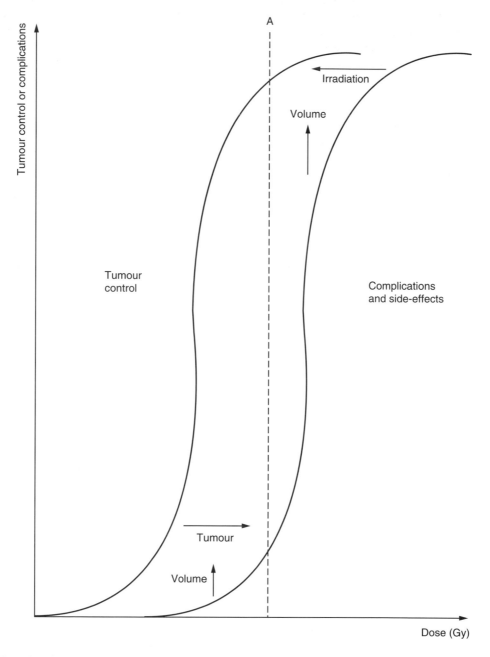

Figure 12.5 Dose–response curves for tumour control and complications. Small changes in radiation dose have major effects on the possible complications. A — the optimal dose giving high tumour control with a low complication rate. If you move this to the right, it significantly increases the number of side-effects. To the left, this reduces the tumour control.

tumour for several reasons. These are termed the 4 Rs: (1) repair of injury; (2) redistribution of cells within the cell cycle; (3) repopulation; and (4) re-oxygenation.[7] Normal tissues surrounding the cancer also show different degrees of sensitivity in the extent of damage and the timing of the effect of this damage. These mechanisms are linked to the side-effects experienced: 'acute' reactions occur within 3 months of treatment, while 'late' reactions may occur up to several years after treatment. Tissues having a fast multiplication, such as skin and mucosal surfaces, show damage more quickly, whereas damage to slow-dividing cells may be responsible for many of the late complications of radiation.[8]

The dose of radiotherapy can have major implications for the response of tissues to irradiation. The dose–response curves both for normal tissues and cancer cells are similar. A relatively small change in the dose can have major implications both for tumour control and in the side-effects of treatment. The optimum dose is often balanced against the possible complications; however, some individuals appear to be more sensitive than others.[9,10] Certain tissues are very sensitive to radiotherapy (for example, eyes, lung, ovaries, and testes) and the dose that can safely be given to these areas is very limited. This tolerance to treatment is often the factor that limits the dose of radiation.[8] The relationship between dose and the probability of curing the cancer is shown in Figure 12.5. There is a threshold dose below which tumours are not controlled but above which control increases steeply. This also applies to normal tissue damage, but with fractionation it is displaced to the right. The greater the difference between the two curves, tumour control and complications, the greater the therapeutic ratio.[7] The link between acute and late effects of radiation is often disassociated in that a severe late reaction does not necessarily follow acute toxicity. Late tissue damage seems to be more related to fraction size than acutely reacting tissues.[2]

Fractionation is a technique that reduces the damage to normal tissues by giving the radiotherapy in smaller parts. Using smaller fraction sizes spares the normal tissue rather than the tumour, since small, frequent, sub-lethal damage allows normal cells to be repaired between the daily treat-

ments. Many tumours have a poor blood supply and have regions of hypoxia that are relatively resistant to radiotherapy. Increasing the treatment time using a fractionated schedule allows hypoxic cells to re-oxygenate and redistribute themselves within the tumour so that more are in the radiosensitive phases of the cell cycle (Figure 12.6).

Box 12.1: The 4 'Rs' of radiotherapy

It is possible to think of the 4 Rs as being similar to the effects of a journey on a tube train in rush hour. The cancer cells are a group of people huddled together in the carriage. The train is packed, people are unable to move, you feel like a sardine if you are standing, but relieved if you have a seat. This is like the hypoxic cells in the tumour squashed together, with the surrounding cells having more space and being well oxygenated. The train pulls into a station and the train empties, those near the door now have more space so people spread out. This is rather like repopulation; the cells grow with the additional space and those that are hypoxic become better oxygenated. The train continues until at the end of the rush hour few standing people remain. The stops at the stations represent the fractions of radiation until there are no more viable cancer cells remaining.

Conventional fractionation is in 2 Gy treatment doses; however, there is very little consensus on optimal radiotherapy regimens.[4] Recent developments in radiotherapy have explored improving fractionation schedules and there are several regimens that are currently used. Accelerated treatment aims to overcome the problem of tumour cells repopulating as rapidly as the normal tissues, as this is a type of radioresistance.[11] Treatments are given twice per day to reduce the overall treatment time. Hyperfractionated treatment aims to improve the therapeutic ratio, reducing the dose given in each fraction.[12] This is to reduce late side-effects while also permitting an increased total dose to the tumour. Hypofractionated treatment, in contrast, gives a smaller number of radiation fractions, but the dose per fraction is increased. The total dose is lower than conventional treatments because of enhanced late side-effects. Hypofractionated regimens are often used for palliative treatments so that the course of treatment can be shorter.[13]

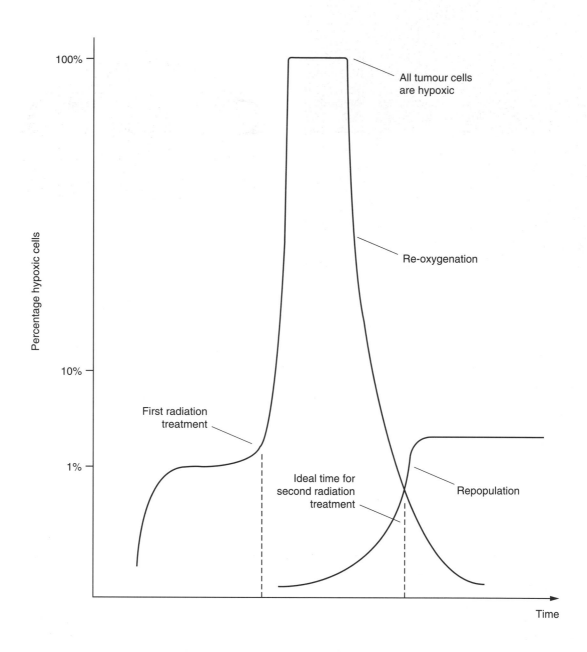

Figure 12.6 The pattern of oxygenated and hypoxic cells during radiotherapy. Radiotherapy is commonly given as a series of equal doses. Each daily dose or 'fraction' kills the same proportion of cells. When solid tumours grow, they often outstrip their blood supply and have areas of hypoxia. Hypoxic cells are two to three times as radioresistant. When multiple small doses of radiation are given, the oxygenated cells, being more sensitive, are killed first. During the interval between dose fractions, killed cells are eliminated and the previously hypoxic cells gain better access to oxygen. This process of re-oxygenation is utilised by giving the total radiation dose in many smaller doses.

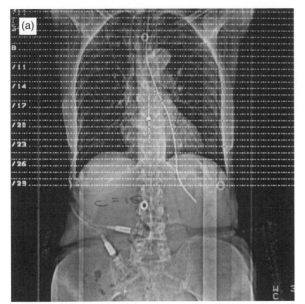

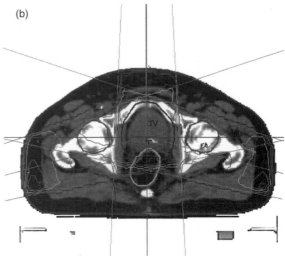

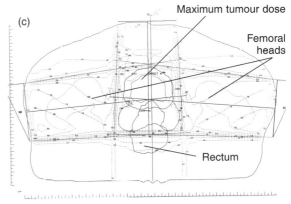

Figure 12.7 Principles of treatment planning. (a) CT topogram of chest to show levels of CT images. (b) CT image through the centre of the target volume. The target volume is drawn with a 1 cm margin. This example shows that of a pelvic treatment for carcinoma of the prostate. Sensitive normal tissues such as femoral heads and rectum are also outlined. TV – target volume; T – tumour; SC – spinal cord; FA – femoral heads; R – rectum. (c) The isodose distribution is outlined. This example is of a pelvic treatment for carcinoma of the prostate. Maximum tumour dose = 100%, minimum tumour dose = 95%. The femoral heads and rectum are identified to help avoid sensitive tissue as much as possible.

Maximum tumour dose

Femoral heads

Rectum

The homogeneity and accuracy of the radiotherapy are important as the dose received by the target determines the outcome of the therapy and the probability of treatment side-effects.[7] Accuracy is achieved by using two or more radiation fields.[14] A composite isodose plan is drawn showing the isodose distributions from the individual beams. These beam characteristics may be altered with wedges or compensators when angled fields are used, or when there are changes in the patient's contour (see Figure 12.3). Most rectangular fields of radiotherapy are determined by thick collimators that are on the radiotherapy machine head, which, once set, determine the size of each field being given. Further shaping of the beams can be achieved by using shaped lead or alloy blocks, placed on trays in the path of the planned irradiation volume.

The volume of the tissue to be treated is determined by findings from diagnostic computed tomographic (CT) or magnetic resonance imaging (MRI) scans and knowledge of the usual patterns of spread of the cancer (see Figure 12.7). The target volume includes a margin of surrounding tissues, which might contain microscopic disease, but also allows for any inaccuracy of the treatment techniques; for example, patient movement or machine positioning.[7,14] The reproducibility of daily treatment is an important factor in delivering accurate radiotherapy.

Most radiotherapy is planned in two dimensions but more sophisticated computer programs are used for shaping complex field arrangements for three-dimensional planned treatment. This type of planning requires reconstruction of tumour and target volumes from CT or MRI images so that the treatment volume can be localised and defined accurately for deep internal structures (see Figure 12.7). During these procedures, localisation of the target volume is achieved with reference to the person's contours, as well as indelible skin markers such as tattoos or ink. Structures that may be at risk from toxicity of treatment can be identified and the field sizes and beam arrangements modified if appropriate. When sensitive tissues are adjacent to the treatment fields, fixation devices such as moulds or plastic casts are used to keep the person as still as possible (see Figure 12.10). The radiotherapy dose prescription and fractionation regime is then defined, detailing the dose to be delivered to target volume from each beam during radiotherapy. The standard dose is defined at the isocentre where the beams intersect. Once this plan of therapy has been devised, simulation of therapy is performed to verify the size, shape, and placing of the proposed beams (Figure 12.8).[14]

A simulator machine is identical to a therapy machine in its geometric specification and movements but differs in that it emits diagnostic X-rays that produce an image of the tissue structures to be irradiated. At this time, the positioning of radiation beams can be checked and the reference markers on the skin used to set up the treatment (see Figure 12.9).

The treatment trajectory

The start of radiotherapy can be a lengthy affair, beginning with the planning of treatment, visits to the simulator and possibly a mould before starting radiotherapy. Although radiotherapy is given daily there are different stages of treatment, which can produce differing anxieties and fears. Anxieties at the start of treatment may not necessarily become less as familiarity with treatment is gained. Studies have shown that emotional distress may be exacerbated by the completion of treatment and unexpected physical side-effects may continue for many months after treatment is completed. This trajectory of radiotherapy treatment can be thought of in three parts: the initial planning and preparation before starting treatment; the lengthy time of undergoing radiotherapy; and completion of treatment when visits to the treatment machine end.

Planning

The prospect of radiotherapy adds considerably to the fear and anxiety that may already be present following a diagnosis of cancer. Fear and misunderstandings of the use of radiation treatment and negative attitudes regarding its effectiveness are known to be common.[15–17] In a study of women who were deciding whether to have either a mastectomy, or a lumpectomy with radiotherapy, concerns about the efficiency of radiation and its side-effects significantly influenced decisions.[18] Fear of being 'burned', becoming radioactive, or of terrible side-effects is common.[19]

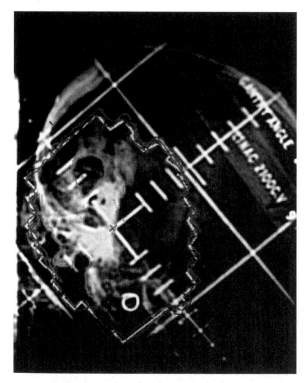

Figure 12.8   A simulator film shows the localisation of the target volume. The simulator is identical to a therapy machine but differs in that it emits diagnostic X-rays. The positioning of the radiation beams can be checked in relation to the tattoos used to set up treatment.

Radiation therapy machines are frequently situated in hospital basements and are therefore isolated. This may serve to create a mystique about the treatment and add to the apprehensions about having radiotherapy. The planning stage of radiotherapy is often perceived as taking a long time; this may be misconstrued as being on a waiting list for treatment, or having an indolent cancer as there appears to be no rush to provide therapy. People are often unaware that much of the preparation before treatment is essential for the accuracy and reproducibility of their radiotherapy. Planning and preparation for radiotherapy is 'behind the scenes' so that the extent of work required before treatment can proceed is not obvious. Once treatment has started it may take only a few seconds to deliver the therapy; however, checking the accuracy and reproducibility of that radiotherapy is just as important. The feeling of delay, and CT or MRI tests can raise anxieties over the extent of disease or suggest that full information about the radiotherapy has not been given. Research study 12.1 revealed these to be central concerns of people undergoing radiotherapy.

Research study 12.1

A study by Eardley[15] highlighted the general apprehension about treatment and misconceptions surrounding it. Thirty-nine patients were interviewed 1 week into their radiotherapy treatment and asked about how they felt about radiotherapy. One man described his wife's anxieties:

> She's not very happy because she's just hanging around – she thought she'd start straight away. She worried because she had those X-rays and no one's explained what they're for . . . it's not knowing what's going to happen . . . she was upset today after this X-ray, two doctors walked away from her whispering to each other, not saying a word to her. She got it into her head now that she's got something else.

Another had a fear that he would be crushed by the machine:

> I have a fear of machines, a fear of something coming on top of me.

It was clear from the interviews that the amount of knowledge and understanding of radiotherapy varied considerably:

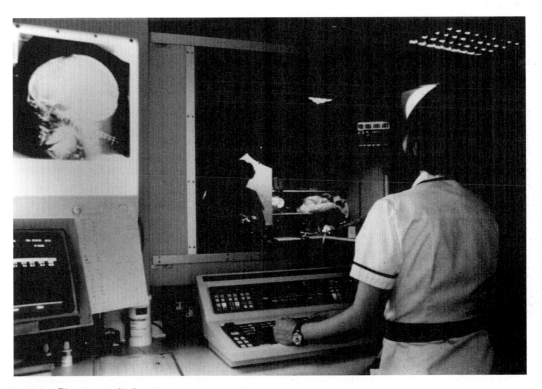

Figure 12.9 Planning radiotherapy.

Even now, I don't know anything about the treatment – I just know I'm having preparation (mould room), not what the preparation is for.

Over half of those interviewed had worries about some aspect of treatment. Eighty-two per cent knew about their treatment and how long it would take; those remaining had little knowledge of what to expect. Thirty-six per cent were unaware that they might experience side-effects from the radiotherapy. Worries were expressed concerning cancer symptoms that had increased or arisen since radiotherapy referral.

This can be a very lonely time; lots of investigations have to be undergone, but there is little contact with health professionals. Studies have identified the extent of fear and psychological morbidity associated with this stage of therapy. A controlled study[20] using mock radiotherapy showed that 75% of people developed symptoms of nausea and fatigue following what they thought was therapy. High levels of anxiety were found prior to treatment in a similar study.[21] Although these studies are now considered unethical, they do indicate the level of anxiety associated with radiotherapy generally.

Restlessness, anxiety, apprehension, social isolation, unfounded pessimism over the likely outcome of treatment, and feeling withdrawn have been reported.[16,17,22] This misapprehension about radiotherapy may be due to the lack of information given prior to the planning of treatment. Peck and Boland[17] found that 60% of people were unprepared for the frequency, number of sessions, and prolonged course of therapy. Most had received little information about the nature of radiotherapy and instead had gathered information from relatives and friends. Another study found that 52% of patients referred for radiotherapy felt that their referring physician had been no help in preparing them for radiation treatment, and neither the referring doctor nor the radiotherapist was considered by patients as an individual to whom they would bring their fears or emotional problems. Eardley,[23] in a survey of 227 radiographers, found that the most common questions patients asked prior to treatment were about side-effects of the radiotherapy, whether they would feel ill after the treatment, and practicalities about how long the treatment would take. Providing an orientation to

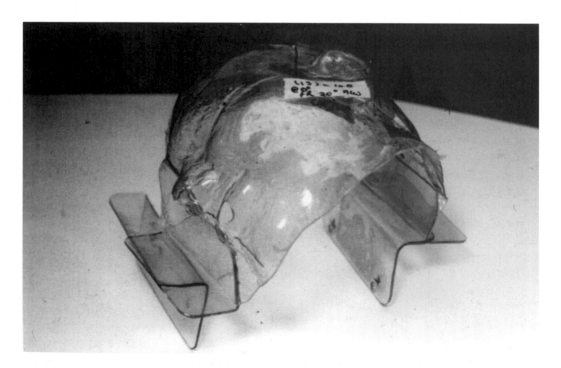

Figure 12.10 Mould for immobilisation for treatment of head and neck cancer.

the radiotherapy machines and an initial interview prior to radiotherapy is known to reduce anxieties, and enhance compliance with therapy, which in turn contributes to better treatment.[25,26]

Preparation for radiotherapy should include:

- provision of information about the treatment and the process of planning
- provision of information about practicalities such as car parking, driving and length of time of treatment
- prior to starting therapy, orientation to the machines and radiotherapy unit
- offering clear guidance on what to do prior to planning, such as to have a full bladder and on how to care for radiotherapy skin marks
- assessment of levels of anxiety and depression prior to starting therapy.

During treatment

A course of radiotherapy may last for several weeks, during which time daily visits to the hospital become routine. Radiotherapy is a difficult treatment modality to comprehend: 'being alone in a room and exposed to an invisible force that can destroy cells is an abstract experience that takes time and repeated information to become clear'.[27] The daily routine and practicalities of travel to the hospital can be an additional burden for those who may be feeling unwell or frail due to their disease. The experience of radiotherapy is emotionally and physically demanding, and distress or anxiety may change during treatment. A study[28] of 45 patients treated with external beam radiotherapy found significant changes in anxiety during the course of treatment. Those who had an initially high level of anxiety reported a significant reduction as treatment progressed. Those with moderate anxiety reported no change, and those with low levels of anxiety reported significant increases as treatment progressed. It appeared that fear at the outset of treatment was predictive of adaptation to treatment. Radiotherapy side-effects, which may appear near the end of treatment, could have caused the increases in anxiety, particularly if these were interpreted as a sign of recurrent disease.

After treatment

The completion of radiotherapy treatment can be an extremely difficult time. The day-to-day contact with radiotherapy staff and fellow patients may have provided informal support and reassurance. This is a time when nursing and medical support is to some extent withdrawn. Community care professionals may provide help, but they do not always have an expert knowledge of radiotherapy or its side-effects. Readjusting to 'normal life' at the end of treatment may not be easy. Loss of hope or confidence about the effectiveness of treatment, and depression, have been shown to feature at this time.[22] Ward's[18] study of women's reactions to completion of treatment identified that the end of treatment did not always bring relief. Out of the 38 women interviewed, 30% found termination of treatment upsetting, and that this was frequently connected to a worsening of side-effects, not just a withdrawal of treatment. Women who were most anxious or depressed at the beginning of treatment were those who were most upset at treatment completion. Other studies suggest that emotional distress at the beginning of treatment is predictive of post-treatment functioning. Eardley's[15] longitudinal study of radiotherapy for head and neck cancer revealed that two-thirds of people felt that they had been inadequately prepared for discharge and were surprised at the length of time they took to recover from radiotherapy.

There is an assumption on the part of health carers that the end of treatment will come as a relief. The loss of stability resulting from a cancer diagnosis may find temporary resolution in the routine of treatment but this can be shattered when it is completed.[18] 'Separation anxiety' may be seen at the end of treatment. Personal account 12.1 illustrates the extent of one person's anxiety.

Personal account 12.1: One woman's experience of radiotherapy

This account concerns a 65-year-old women with cancer of the right breast who, following surgery and wide axillary node clearance, was treated with 15 fractions of adjuvant radiotherapy. At interview prior to completing treatment, she was obviously well informed about her treatment and had supportive relationships with her family. She was keen to talk and had very mixed feelings about finishing her treatment.

> One part of me is pleased because I've begun to feel a bit unwell (on treatment) but . . . I also feel vulnerable . . . coming here, there are people I can talk to, people looking after me.

She wanted to regain control of her life, feeling that she had somehow 'lost her way'. She seemed unsure and fearful of both treatment and its cessation. She had found radiotherapy 'frightening' and 'alien'. Many of her fears had been fuelled by media publicity about damage caused by radiotherapy. At a subsequent interview, when she was beginning to feel better, most of the physical symptoms identified at the end of treatment were no longer a problem.

She felt that she had been keeping up appearances for her family and friends, who expected her to be relieved that treatment was over. Friends kept saying 'you must be so pleased it's all over':

> I was saying yes I am, it's great, but it was all lies really . . . the day after I finished my treatment, I felt quite awful . . . not well . . . and abandoned really . . . It seemed as though there is nothing. You get all this intensive treatment and then it's shut off . . . after the radiotherapy's finished, you shouldn't need to have any more contact but you do . . . I felt that everything had been taken away from me, although coming here had been a tiring routine I felt safe, I knew I could ask . . . what you need is a daily contact and a gradual weaning away from your dependency. I can't be isolated in feeling like this . . . a gradual weaning off and I wouldn't have felt so bereft.[29]

Since completing treatment can be very difficult, it may be helpful to ask about feelings surrounding this, so that the insecurity over losing a 'safety net' can be acknowledged and discussed;[18] these feelings can be complex and may affect adjustment to cancer more generally. The feeling of needing to gain control after treatment and 'get back to normal' may be pressing, while for others the end of treatment is experienced as an anticlimax.

Side-effects of radiotherapy

Radiotherapy treatment is limited by the severity and frequency of its side-effects. Adverse effects of treatment can be very debilitating and have a substantial impact on quality of life. Although radiobiological data have revealed the mechanisms that cause side-effects, there is relatively little knowledge on how best to manage these. In the past, unlike when administering cytoxic drugs, where there are clear regulatory mechanisms, there was no requirement to register radiotherapy treatments or to monitor toxicity. The result of this is that toxicity data from patients who have received radio-

therapy are often unreliable and difficult to compare between differing treatments. Dosages and field sizes vary between countries and even clinicians, with conflicting data as to the best methods of treatment. As clinical trials are becoming more extensive and radiotherapy treatments are revised, the adverse effects are becoming clearer.

One major problem is that unlike many anti-cancer agents the side-effects of radiotherapy develop in several stages. Late radiotherapy side-effects may take many years to develop and are often progressive and chronic, whereas acute side-effects resolve in time. Assessing and monitoring the toxicity of radiotherapy treatments is therefore difficult.[10] It is thought that there is no link between acute and late radiotherapy side-effects, and it is hard to predict who is at risk or when problems might occur. This reflects the radiosensitivity of differing tissues, as well as longer term damage resulting from ionising radiation.

The link between total dose of radiation and its biological effect is well known, with the higher doses causing more adverse effects. The sensitivity of particular tissues to radiation also determines the side-effects of treatment. Those tissues with a high cell turnover often show more acute toxicity than tissues with a slow cell turnover.

Table 12.2 shows some of the treatment and biological characteristics that contribute to acute and late radiation reactions.

Often clear distinctions are made as to how different tissues respond to radiation; however, this is more complex than such simple classifications suggest. There are many exceptions and tissues or organs proceed through several phases. For example, the urothelium is very sensitive to radiation. Symptoms are often described as acute, but injury can also become apparent after a long latent period because of the low cell turnover in the urothelium. Another example is that of lung tissue, where two waves of damage may be recognised, the first occurring 3–8 months after irradiation, and lung fibrosis, which develops after about 1 year.[10]

The extent and occurrence of symptoms is linked not only to the susceptibility of the tissue, but also to the innate susceptibility that the individual has to radiotherapy. Clinical and experimental studies are beginning to show that there is a genetic predisposition to hypersensitivity to radiation in nor-

Table 12.2   Characteristics of early and late radiotherapy reactions in normal tissue

Property	Early responding tissue	Late responding tissue
Occurrence	Weeks to months, the latent time is independent of dose, but time for healing to occur is dose dependent.	6 months to 5 years. This is dose dependent.
Sensitivity for dose per fraction	Low	High
Fractionation timing	High	Low
Tissue characteristics	Rapidly self-renewing, stem cells or functional cells.	Slowly self-renewing.
Examples of tissues	Mucosa, skin, intestinal epithelia, urinary epithelia, bone marrow, lung alveolar, testes, and ovaries.	Muscle, liver, kidney, brain, spinal cord, nerves, and cartilage.
Response to radiation injury	Regeneration, resulting in stem cell depletion and functional breakdown.	Repair of sublethal damage, loss of parenchymal cells, fibrosis, and vascular damage.
Symptoms	Transient and usually reversible, but may continue into a late reaction.	Irreversible, progressive changes, but functional compensation may occur.

Reprinted from Bentzen S., Overgaard M., and Overgaard J. (1993). *European Journal of Cancer*, **29A,** 1373–6[10] with permission from Elsevier Science.

mal tissues.[9] This would explain the range of side-effects occurring amongst those who receive similar radiotherapy treatments. Concurrent disease, age, and adjuvant therapy add to the predisposition to side-effects; however, these factors are not as yet clearly defined.

Symptoms occur as a result of tissue damage through the effects of radiation. In acutely responding cells, cell division may fail at some stage during mitosis. Non-proliferating cells may suffer apoptosis or cell death, or remain alive but be unable to perform their function. These biological effects result in tissue breakdown and inflammation. At the end of treatment the remaining cells repopulate and recover.

Late reactions in tissues, which are seen after a long time period, often result from vascular changes. This is seen in telangiectasia, where dilated capillaries appear on the skin surface. The endothelial cells lining the capillaries are damaged, leading to irregular proliferation of surviving cells, changes in thickness, distortion, and thrombosis in the smaller vessels. This affects the blood supply to the tissue leading to secondary damage.

Radiotherapy side-effects can have enormous consequences if poorly managed, and can cause debilitating chronic problems, with a subsequent diminished quality of life. This has led to litigation and claims for compensation by people who have been badly affected, and may not have been warned of the possibility of late effects occurring. An example of this is the late nerve damage experienced by women treated for breast cancer in the 1960s. Changes in cancer therapy to avoid mastectomy led to the prescription of higher total doses of radiation therapy. Late toxicity resulted in brachial plexus injury, leaving some women with the loss of the use of an arm or hand, and substantial pain.[30]

The management of radiotherapy-induced side-effects is an important part of care; symptoms may be experienced during therapy but also many months to years after treatment.

Fatigue

Fatigue is recognised as a common symptom of radiotherapy, which not only occurs during treatment but also continues after the radiotherapy has ended. It is a problem that little is known about, leaving the clinician with few strategies to help to relieve fatigue. The incidence of fatigue following radiotherapy ranges from 65% to 100% of those undergoing treatment, and it is known to fluctuate over the treatment trajectory. Although radiotherapy is a localised treatment with toxicity related to the specific site of the body being treated, fatigue can also be a systemic effect of radiotherapy and can cause considerable distress. Despite this distress, it is not generally considered serious since it is transient, and does not limit the dose of radiotherapy that can be given safely.

Possible causes of fatigue

Little is known about the mechanisms of radiation-induced fatigue. Metabolites from cell destruction caused by ionisation and normal tissue damage accumulate, giving rise to fatigue. Other suggestions are that the increasing requirements for molecular and cellular repair may precipitate fatigue by increasing the body's need for resources for this process. The aetiology of fatigue may also be linked to certain sites of treatment. For example, in radiotherapy to the chest, such as in the treatment of breast cancer, the inclusion of sensitive lung tissue within the radiotherapy field may be linked to fatigue. The occurrence of radiation-induced pneumonitis or later fibrosis may exacerbate fatigue. The difference in incidence according to the site of treatment may be linked to the cell kinetics and ability of the tissues to repair themselves.

The pattern of fatigue

The pattern of fatigue following radiotherapy varies depending on site and the stage of therapy. Haylock and Hart[31] first highlighted the changing pattern of fatigue symptoms during radiotherapy. In a study of 30 adults receiving treatment to different sites, they reported that fatigue increased over the course of radiotherapy treatment. Fatigue declined at weekends when patients were not undergoing therapy (see Figure 12.11). In a more detailed study of women with breast cancer, this weekly variation did not occur but fatigue decreased over the 3 weeks following completion of radiotherapy.[32] Fatigue has been shown to continue after completion of therapy; in one study up to 39% of patients were still experiencing fatigue at 3 months following radiotherapy treatment.[33] In a prospective interview study of the onset, frequency, and severity of side-effects of radiation in 96 patients undergoing radiotherapy, a high incidence of fatigue was found. Specific information was gathered by using a symptom profile checklist, marked on a Likert scale. Patients were interviewed weekly during treatment and monthly for 3 months following completion of therapy. Table 12.3 highlights the differences between site-specific treatments.

The descriptions also give insight into the changing nature of the fatigue. Following radiotherapy to the chest, fatigue was described as intermittent at the start of treatment, but this became more continuous as treatment progressed. Other studies have found that fatigue and skin problems were the most frequently reported side-effects of patients undergoing radiation for lung cancer, although levels of fatigue were higher at the start of treatment compared to women being treated with radiotherapy for breast cancer.[34,35] In head and neck cancer, the pattern of fatigue was at first periodic, but during the last 2 weeks of treatment became more continuous. An interview study ($n = 30$) of the experience of radiotherapy to the head and neck found that two-thirds said they still felt tired and weak 6–8 weeks after radiotherapy had been completed.[15] Men and women experienced different patterns of symptoms following radiotherapy to the pelvic area, men experiencing a lower incidence of fatigue. Women experienced increasing levels of fatigue over the course of the treatment and it was worse in the afternoons. Intracavitary treatment for gynaecological disease has been found to add to the extent of fatigue symptoms.[36] Fatigue is also a very debilitating symptom of cranial irradiation for brain tumours.

A longitudinal study of patients ($n = 19$) having cranial radiotherapy for primary brain tumours found that a specific pattern of incidence was experienced.[37] A daily diary was completed for 6 weeks after treatment and patients were interviewed 1 month and 3 months after treatment. The pattern of symptoms showed a peak of symptoms 2 weeks after therapy; patients complained of feeling fatigued, drowsy, and lethargic. This improved after several weeks but occurred again at 5–6 weeks and was exacerbated by feelings of lack of concentration, drowsiness and lethargy (see Figure 12.12). This pattern of symptoms had not previously been identified, which may be because previous studies

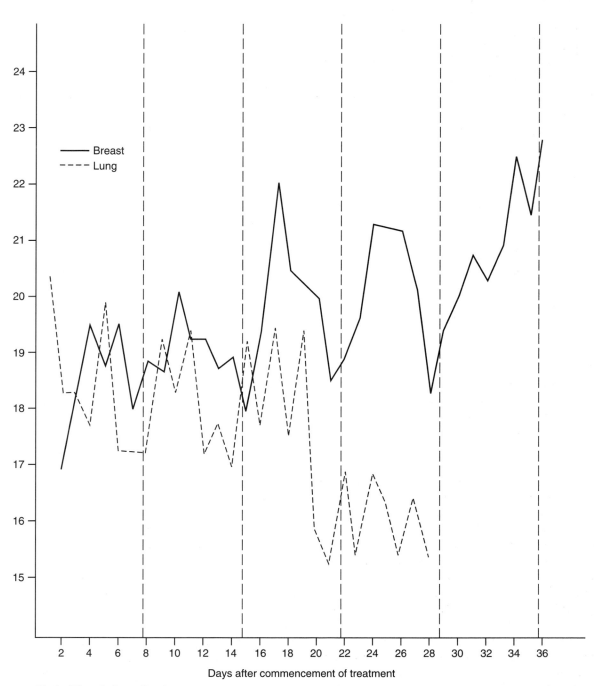

Vertical lines indicate Sundays.

Figure 12.11 Mean fatigue scores during radiotherapy treatment (reproduced with permission from Haycock P. and Hart L. (1979). Fatigue in patients receiving localised radiation. *Cancer Nursing* **2,** 461–467).[31]

had used cross-sectional and retrospective research designs. The daily diary enabled fluctuations in fatigue to be recorded. This pattern of symptoms appears distinct to those patients undergoing cranial irradiation and its aetiology may be due to the specific cells affected by the irradiation. The fluctuations demonstrated in these various studies may not be generalisable, as other researchers have not found similar patterns, but they highlight the need to look at sub-groups in radiotherapy research.[32]

Factors that might influence the occurrence of fatigue
While fatigue is expected to accompany radiotherapy treatment, no specific predictive factors have been identified in the literature. The physical complications of radiotherapy are linked not only to the cell types within the treatment field, but also to the volume and dose. The site of treatment is predictive, in that incidence of fatigue varies by site. Other factors that have been suggested are adjuvant therapy, chemotherapy, or surgery at the time of,

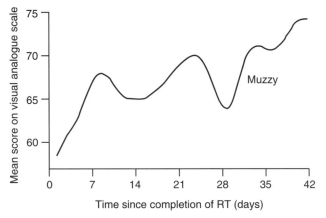

(a) Time series plot of scores from self-completed daily diary. Time trends were recorded only on complete data sets (n = 11). The graph shows smoothed means using resistant smoothers for the symptom termed 'muzzy'. Higher scores indicate alertness.

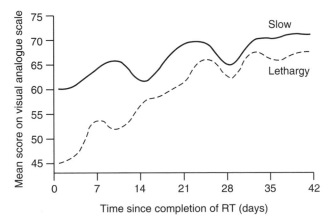

(b) Smoothed mean scores for the sensation of mental slowness and lethargy. Higher scores indicate more vigour and lower scores increased lethargy.

Figure 12.12 Fatigue after cranial radiotherapy (reproduced with permission from Faithfull S. and Brada M. (1998). Somnolence syndrome in adults following cranial irradiation for primary brain tumours. *Clinical Oncology* **10,** 250–254).[40]

Table 12.3 The incidence of fatigue during and after radiotherapy[33]

Treatment site	1st week of treatment	3rd week	Final week	3 months after treatment
Chest ($n = 12$)	60%	93%	80%	46%
Head and neck ($n = 25$)	30%	60%	68%	39%
Male pelvis ($n = 26$)	35%	40%	65%	14%
Female pelvis ($n = 30$)	20%	75%	72%	32%

or before, radiotherapy treatment. There is evidence for increased levels of fatigue with combined modality treatment. In a survey of 403 patients who were receiving a variety of adjuvant treatments, chemotherapy and radiotherapy (58%), radiotherapy (38%), and chemotherapy alone (5%), 90% reported that treatment had an effect on their energy levels.[38] For 37% this did not improve once treatment was completed. The younger patients (<34 years) fared best and felt that they had recovered within 12 months of finishing treatment, while older patients took longer to recover. Factors such as advanced disease, combined treatment modalities, and increased age were significant, although other studies have not shown fatigue and age to be related.[39] Fatigue may be more closely linked to frailty rather than chronological age as such; few studies make this distinction. Differing fractionation regimens may be a factor in the severity of fatigue experienced. In the study of somnolence syndrome, those patients having accelerated fractionation with twice-daily cranial radiotherapy had more fatigue than those patients having once-daily treatments.[40]

Factors influencing the occurrence of fatigue include:

- adjuvant therapy
  - chemotherapy
  - recent surgery
- age
- frailty
- site of radiotherapy
- dosage of treatment
- fractionation regimen
- advanced disease.

Some individuals are more susceptible to the effects of radiation than others, although this is poorly researched and those most at risk are not as yet possible to identify.[9] Stress and anxiety may make fatigue symptoms worse.

The experience of fatigue can cause great distress. Munro explored the distress associated with radiotherapy by asking 72 patients to prioritise which symptoms or feelings were most distressing to them.[41] Fatigue was ranked second to worries about the success of therapy, but above other physical symptoms such as pain. The high levels of distress caused by fatigue could have been a somatic expression of anxiety, and not simply a physical effect of radiotherapy. It is clear that psychological distress is an important variable in fatigue, being linked with depression and anxiety, but it has also been linked to physical symptoms, such as pain.[42] Following radiotherapy, the experience of fatigue is so common that it is unlikely to be wholly a psychological manifestation. The distress of fatigue may be experienced in several ways, including the physical limitations of feeling exhausted and the social isolation that may result. Patients' accounts of what the fatigue is like give a clear picture of the lack of concentration, mental fogginess, and physical effects of experiencing fatigue as a result of radiotherapy treatment.

Personal account 12.2: The experience of fatigue following cranial radiotherapy

The accounts of 12 patients undergoing cranial radiotherapy interviewed for a qualitative study illustrate the pervasive nature of fatigue symptoms.[37]

The feeling of fatigue was described by one individual as 'I have felt like I had lead boots'. When asked to explain about how the fatigue affected them, they had difficulty in articulating what it was like:

I just didn't want to do anything! I didn't feel I could do anything which was the worst thing.

Some described this feeling as lethargy.

> I felt lethargic. There were things which I had to think of doing, wanted to do and I just couldn't muster myself to do them you know.

Most described the effects of fatigue as influencing mental abilities but for those patients who experienced severe fatigue it had repercussions on physical activity:

> I mean physically. I knew I could walk across the kitchen and get myself a biscuit! But to get a biscuit! I would rather sit in a chair and think about it.

Others described how lack of mental concentration affected their lives:

> It felt like every day was a great effort and that just moving and doing anything was exceedingly hard, but not physically. It was more mentally than physically hard.

Feelings of fatigue during radiotherapy for many are an expected result of having cancer therapy, but not following treatment, where the expectation is to recover quickly. The long duration and severity of fatigue symptoms experienced after radiotherapy has been completed can be frightening and may not be understood to be a side-effect of radiotherapy treatment. It may be interpreted as a sign of the cancer progressing, as one man commented:

> I get worried that I'm not recovering. The whole time you think, 'Is it the tumour or is it the side-effect?'

What helps fatigue symptoms is an area where research is still limited. There are no clear ideas as to the aetiology and mechanism of radiotherapy-induced fatigue and consequently interventions are mainly based on anecdotal evidence. Fatigue is often an unexpected side-effect of treatment, and the severity and effects of fatigue symptoms can be a surprise.[37] By warning patients of the likelihood of fatigue occurring and by providing information on strategies that may be helpful, the anxiety of unexpected symptoms can be prevented. However, there is little research evidence because at present fatigue interventions have not been adequately tested in cancer.[42] Exercise, stress management techniques and interventions aimed at reducing emotional distress may be effective ways to decrease feelings of fatigue (see Table 12.4).[42-44]

When experiencing fatigue, most people tend to rest, nap or sleep; however, this may not be the most appropriate strategy to reduce fatigue symptoms.[44]

Table 12.4 Strategies for relieving fatigue

Assessment	Intervention strategy	Suggestions
Check for possible physical and psychological causes of fatigue, e.g. electrolyte imbalance or anaemia.	Reducing activity	Lie down, have a nap, sit and rest. Educate about the bad effects of too much rest.
Evaluate patterns of fatigue: encourage patients to maintain a diary.	Increasing activity	Encourage activity, walking programmes, exercise.
Forewarn patients of the occurrence of fatigue.	Distraction	Listen to music, read, socialise.
Differentiate fatigue from depression.	Schedule	Try different strategies, schedule important activities during times of least fatigue, and eliminate inessential activities.

In a study exploring which strategies were most effective in relieving fatigue associated with cancer treatment (chemotherapy: $n = 45$, radiotherapy: $n = 54$), sleep and exercise were found to be the most effective strategies.[45] The wide range of scores found between individuals for the different interventions suggests that fatigue management needs to be tailored to what works for each individual.

Appropriate assessment is important in managing fatigue. Radiotherapy sites often involve bone tissue and this may affect the production of red cells in the bone marrow. Anaemia, however, may cause fatigue symptoms and should be excluded in someone complaining of fatigue. Assessment of fatigue symptoms should be subjective: asking someone to rate their fatigue on a scale of 0 to 10 may be very useful.[43] There has been much criticism of how fatigue is assessed in the research literature, as a multitude of tools exists and there is a need to explore not only the physical but also cognitive aspects of fatigue symptoms.[42,43] In practice, a more simplistic approach is necessary. Simply asking the person to express in their own words how they would describe their fatigue may be very valuable.

Knowledge about fatigue is insubstantial and does not offer much in the way of intervention support following radiotherapy. Much of the literature in this area is nursing based and highlights the distress experienced. The symptom does not appear to be taken seriously as it is considered subjective and transient. Clinical trials have often focused on observer ratings scores, which do not include fatigue. Quality of life issues in radiotherapy practice are only now beginning to be addressed with tools that reflect the extent of fatigue symptoms. What is clear is that by taking the symptom seriously and offering support, information, and advice, the distressing nature of this symptom should be reduced.

Radiation enteritis

Radiation enteritis is a common side-effect of radiotherapy with fields that involve the pelvis or abdomen. Symptoms include nausea, diarrhoea, abdominal cramps, and proctitis. There may be acute as well as long-lasting late effects, occurring in up to 70% of those whose treatment involves the gastrointestinal tract, while more than 80% of women being treated for gynaecological cancers suffer from diarrhoea during radiotherapy.[33,46] If symptoms are severe, they may interrupt or prolong the course of radiotherapy.

Modern techniques of radiotherapy using bowel-sparing techniques such as conformal treatment and computerised planning have reduced toxicity. There are distinct differences between acute and late side-effects with differing pathophysiology, symptoms, and management. The pathogenesis can mainly be attributed to the inherent sensitivity of the epithelial cells in the intestinal mucosa caused by rapid cell division. Acute damage results in symptoms of nausea, diarrhoea, and abdominal cramps, which are often transient, and return to normal after completion of treatment. Secondary damage is more serious and may occur many months to years after the initial treatment with signs of fibrosis, malabsorption, bleeding, and obstruction, which can be very debilitating (see Table 12.5). The assessment and management of radiation enteritis is an important clinical consideration when trying to balance the therapeutic benefit of treatment with potentially distressing side-effects.

Mechanisms causing radiation enteritis
Acute symptoms may start within the first 2 weeks of radiotherapy treatment. Damage is manifested in the stem cells, and the intestinal villi become shortened, reducing the tissue surface available for absorption.[46,47] The extent of mucosal abnormalities often correlates poorly with symptoms, and may persist after cells are seen to recover.[48] The exact mechanism by which acute symptoms such as diarrhoea and discomfort arise, and what factors contribute to these, are still not known.[49] Several causes have been suggested, such as malabsorption or neuroendocrine stimulation.

1. **Bile acid malabsorption** is considered a major factor contributing to the cause of diarrhoea. Bile salts in the normal gut are nearly totally reabsorbed; this is reduced in radiation enteritis.[50] The unabsorbed bile salts inhibit water reabsorption and stimulate peristalsis distally in the colon.[51] Normal bile salt absorption is thought to take place in the small intestine. Pelvic radiotherapy may include areas of terminal ileum, and may explain the differing

incidence of bowel problems. Evidence for bile salt malabsorption comes from studies that have measured intraluminal fat content and abnormalities in bile salt metabolism. Fat absorption can be measured by faecal fat analysis but more easily by breath tests using a labelled triglyceride.[52] Forty-five per cent of women undergoing pelvic radiotherapy for gynaecological malignancies had abnormal breath tests during radiation treatment; abnormalities were still detected in 21% of these women 3 months following therapy, but returned to normal by 1 year.[53]

2. **Malabsorption of carbohydrate products** has also been suggested as a causative mechanism for enteritis symptoms. Carbohydrate, if not absorbed, also causes raised osmolarity, thereby increasing peristalsis. In the colon, bacterial fermentation of carbohydrate produces gas and results in diarrhoea and discomfort. Few patients show demonstrable signs of malabsorption (for example, weight loss during treatment), but this may be a problem if they already have a pre-existing absorption or carbohydrate deficiency.[54] Malabsorption syndromes may be more of a problem in chronic radiation enteritis.[50]

3. **Neuroendocrine changes** have also been suggested as a causative mechanism for radiation enteritis symptoms. Prostaglandins are released as a response to radiation cell damage. These are known to be stimulators of smooth muscle and have been shown to cause diarrhoea in animal experiments. A double-blind clinical trial using aspirin (a prostaglandin inhibitor) was able to reduce diarrhoea in women receiving treatment for uterine cancer.[55] However, contrary results from a study using olsalazine, a similar drug with minimal systemic absorption, increased symptoms rather than reduced them.[56]

There is evidence that all these mechanisms may play some part in radiation enteritis, but which mechanism is most prominent is not clear. Bile salt malabsorption has been shown to be a feature in most patients with diarrhoea following radiotherapy treatment. Differing sites of treatment may also influence the radiation enteritis.[57] Neuroendocrine changes may also contribute to symptoms but evidence is lacking as to the exact mechanism of action.

Late effects of radiation may occur from 6 to 18 months following completion of treatment and are considered among the most serious complications of radiation therapy.[46] Symptoms can be insidious in onset, such as colicky abdominal pain, weight loss, or bleeding from the rectum or diarrhoea.[47] Late effects have been reported to occur in 5–21% of people and this variation may in part be due to the different doses of radiation used to treat different tumours, but may also relate to the way intestinal symptoms are defined and assessed.[47–49] These late effects include proctitis, colitis, enteritis, ulceration, fistula formation, and obstruction. Chronic changes are often insidious, with progressive symptoms linked to vascular changes. Minor symptoms are often not well reported in the literature on toxicity following radiotherapy. Changes in bowel habit are often under-reported. Many women who have received pelvic radiotherapy for

Table 12.5 Side-effects of radiotherapy

Site	Acute (occurs from 18–22 Gy)	Late (many months to years)
Small intestine	Nausea, peptic ulcers Diarrhoea Cramps Distension	Peptic ulcers, stricture Diarrhoea Malabsorption, Vitamin B_{12} deficiency, lactose intolerance Abdominal obstruction
Rectum and large intestine	Faecal incontinence Bleeding from rectum Anal pain Tenesmus	Fistula formation Bleeding from rectum Ulceration

gynaecological malignancies report that they experience some bowel changes. Danielsson et al.[48] (n = 173) found that 13% of women had diarrhoea 3–35 years (mean 9 years) after pelvic radiotherapy for gynaecological malignancies. Intensive investigations showed that bile acid malabsorption was a common problem. Most studies have focused on gynaecological malignancies and the higher doses of intracavity treatment. These may over-represent the level and degree of late side-effects experienced more generally.

Although acute intestinal effects of radiation are well recognised and are usually transient, chronic enteritis may occur over a long time period and limit the effectiveness of radiation treatment by reducing the dose that can subsequently be delivered.

Factors that might influence the occurrence of radiation enteritis

Factors that influence the occurrence of radiation enteritis symptoms have been studied in relation to the incidence of late effects. These factors can be divided into two types: patient characteristics and treatment factors.

Patient characteristics

- Age and gender are not considered an important factor but in studies, older women are considered to have a higher incidence of radiation enteritis, possibly due to intracavitary therapy.
- Those who are underweight or have a thin physique are more at risk. This is linked to the anterior posterior diameter, and organs which may be included within the field.
- Previous pelvic surgery gives higher risk, although there are contradictory studies.
- Comorbid disease such as diabetes and hypertension give higher risk.
- Hypersensitivity syndromes, e.g. ataxia telangectasia, give higher risk.
- Pre-existing vascular changes, e.g. haemorrhoids, can lead to higher incidence.

Co-existing disease or other characteristics may add to the chance of radiation enteritis occurring.[58] A history of pelvic inflammatory disease may increase the risk of radiotherapy symptoms by 15%.[59] Although pre-existing vascular changes may add to the risk attached to abdominal or pelvic radiotherapy, since these factors are present in older age groups it is difficult to distinguish their importance from age per se as a risk factor.

Treatment factors

- Extended field of radiation treatment is more likely to include small bowel within the field. Acute symptoms have been correlated with the volume of the field.[60]
- Dose of irradiation – it has been shown in laboratory studies that with a lower dose the cells along the villus more rapidly return to normal.
- Fractionation schedule – smaller individual doses given over an extended period are less likely to cause toxicity.

Attempts to minimise the risk may include reducing the volume of small bowel within the treatment field. In pelvic radiotherapy this is achieved with a full bladder, so that the small bowel is pushed out of the field, which reduces radiation enteritis.[61] The precision of planning and conformal techniques can also minimise toxicity.

What does it mean for the person having radiotherapy?

Few studies have explored how enteritis symptoms are experienced. Most have focused on the extent of symptoms rather than the distress or impact for the individual. Padilla,[62] in a study of 101 patients from four radiation oncology clinics, tried to describe the impact of gastrointestinal side-effects, on psychological and physical well-being. Data were collected using a variety of quality of life and quantitative assessments. Few had problems with gastrointestinal symptoms. Psychological distress was linked with gastrointestinal symptoms in 21.5% of patients, whereas anxiety linked to distress was 11.8% and other side-effects 5.5%. The most distressing of physical symptoms was fatigue. Padilla concludes that where side-effects were perceived to be a problem they also had an important impact on psychological and physical well-being. Although this study highlights some of the psychological issues related to radiation enteritis, the quantitative design precludes exploration of what impact the symptoms had on the individual or exploration of what aspect of gastrointestinal symptoms was of greatest concern to those experiencing it.

Diarrhoea from acute radiation enteritis is often considered to be an inevitable consequence of radiation therapy, something that is to be suffered. This is described in one patient's account of his diarrhoea during pelvic radiotherapy (see Personal account 12.3).

Personal account 12.3

Basically I had diarrhoea . . . it was bad news because no sooner had you put a clean pair of underpants on, then I would need to go again and, you know, unfortunately you missed and they were messed again. That was very difficult to take . . . The thing is because I was told, I knew it was going to be okay, if I hadn't been told that's the upsetting thing . . . I think if you know it's a limited time, it's a bit easier . . . needed to be near a toilet and to be perfectly honest some of the times that I would go would be quite unusual I mean it would be 2am, 5am. I found that was difficult.[63]

Diarrhoea disrupts sleep, journeys, or social activities. Medication for diarrhoea can cause side-effects. One man described how he was left feeling remote and dizzy with codeine phosphate tablets:

The diarrhoea hasn't really gone it's a little naughty but the tablets cause a stalling they certainly help. The tablets leave me with a funny feeling I don't know what it is erhm . . . a bit woozy it's a bit hard to explain I mean I can walk and get in or drive the car but at the same time they make you feel a bit woozy.

Others complained of getting constipated:

The tablets they are giving me are blocking me up backwise now and you know they've given me some other medicine to take for that and if I take too much of it I get terrible diarrhoea which I've got at the moment so you know you're doing one thing to stop one thing and you're taking something else and causing other problems.[63]

These accounts have focused on the acute side of radiation enteritis and highlight that patients have numerous problems and feel that there is little that can be done. A low-residue diet and anti-diarrhoea medication have been reported as helpful in managing diarrhoea,[33] although the effectiveness of this approach is open to question since there remains a high incidence of enteritis, despite the use of medication.

Personal experience of symptoms is important in understanding how people interpret their symptoms. Padilla,[62] in observing the impact of acute radiation enteritis, may have found that this was not the most distressing of symptoms, but evidence suggests that if bowel problems persist and become chronic they impact greatly on quality of life.

Personal account 12.4

A man who had received pelvic radiotherapy for prostate cancer 6 months previously was well throughout treatment but had experienced proctitis at the end of it. Months went by with severe pain when opening his bowels. At clinic appointments he had been told he was constipated and he had received differing laxatives. During this time he had periods of diarrhoea and then constipation, the severe pain continued and he found that it was difficult to eat and was losing weight. After many months his cancer was 'cured' but he had despaired of all help; he described how desperate he felt, that 'life wasn't worth living like this'. Finally, with surgical investigations it was found that he had a stricture and required a colostomy to treat this late side-effect. Several months later he told how relieved he was to have someone take his symptoms seriously, and that if someone had listened before to how he was feeling things might not have been as bad.[63]

Bowel symptoms, whether acute or chronic, can profoundly influence social and sexual life.[64] Although most people experience transient and minor symptoms, those who do have uncontrolled diarrhoea or enteritis can find that they become socially isolated, with the symptoms making them feel unclean and not sexually desirable. There is abundant information on the effects of radiation on morphology and intestinal tissue but little on the time course of enteritis symptoms, or how individuals can cope with these symptoms.

Management
A number of management approaches to radiation enteritis has been reported. There is a distinction between acute and late enteritis and each is controlled differently. A key to the management of the problem is to assess accurately the extent of an individual's symptoms and possible causative mechanisms. Breath tests and faecal fat monitoring are not realis-

tic in a clinical setting but asking patients to complete a diary or log of their bowel habit can give valuable information as to the extent of the problem, and the pattern of symptoms. There are three approaches to management: diets, drugs that influence the aetiology, and anti-diarrhoeal agents.

Diet

A low-fat diet has been shown in studies to be beneficial in reducing diarrhoea. Experimental research has shown that specific and elemental diets are useful in protecting cell function during radio-therapy.[60] These alter the fat and lipid content of the diet, but are unpalatable and unlikely to be acceptable. Fat content in the diet has also been associated with bile acid malabsorption and studies suggest that a 40 g low-fat diet can significantly reduce diarrhoea.[49,65] In practice, low-fat diets are rarely used and it is low fibre that patients are recommended with the presumption that reducing bowel bulk will reduce symptoms. There is no clinical evidence that would suggest that this advice is of value and indeed it may cause constipation. One problem with a low-fat diet is that some fat in the diet is inevitable, and therefore dietary control is unlikely to control all symptoms completely.

Drugs influencing aetiology

To combat bile acid malabsorption bile acid sequestrants (colestipol hydrochloride, cholestyramine) have been used in clinical trials. These drugs act to bind with bile acids in the intestine. Although successful in reducing diarrhoea, the side-effects outweigh benefits.[53] Further studies have used the bile acid sequestrant in combination with a 40 g low-fat diet, which resulted in significantly less diarrhoea compared to a low-fat diet without sequestrant.[66]

Anti-diarrhoeal agents

Anti-diarrhoeal agents such as codeine phosphate or Lomotil are often used for symptom management, but these are costly, may cause problems of constipation or dizziness, and may only produce short-term relief.

The management of chronic radiation enteritis is often difficult and is based on the cause of the problem. Strictures, fibrosis, haemorrhage, or ulceration require surgical investigations. Assess-

Table 12.6   Management of acute and late radiation enteritis

Acute	Late
Low-fat diet	Antibiotics
Anti-diarrhoea medication	Low-fat diet
Cholestyramine	Steroids
Sucraflate granules	

ment is clearly very important and in the case of diarrhoea this may be a result of fat malabsorption or bacterial contamination. Studies suggest several strategies, that of a low-fat diet, bile acid sequestrants, antibiotics, or fermented milk, which may be useful in reducing diarrhoea symptoms, while non-steroidal anti-inflammatory agents, steroids and sulfasalazine have been suggested for proctitis (see Table 12.6).

Many of the treatments mentioned in controlling symptoms of radiation enteritis have not been effectively tested and there is a need to improve the clinical assessment and diagnostic tests for radiation enteritis. The possible link between acute and chronic symptoms has been suggested; one study indicates that effective control of acute symptoms may reduce the incidence of chronic radiation enteritis.[66] The question 'Does effective acute symptom management have an impact on later side-effects?' is an important issue for future research to address.

Radiation skin reactions

Skin reactions from radiotherapy are considered a relatively infrequent complication to radiation therapy. Modern megavoltage equipment, with its skin-sparing ability, has reduced the incidence of severe radiation reactions. Although not considered a major problem, skin reactions are still one of the largest issues with which nurses in radiotherapy are asked to deal. Skin changes occur following treatment. Erythema and moist desquamation are often seen as bad signs and may induce fears of having had too much treatment – 'I've been burnt by the therapy'. Symptoms produce discomfort and may take many weeks or months to heal, with a poor cosmetic result.

Little is known about the best way to manage radiotherapy skin problems. In the past, skin reactions were used as a way of monitoring radio-therapy dose. With improved technology some skin reactions have reduced, but have been replaced by wounds in difficult areas, such as skin folds or creases, that are troublesome to manage. The primary aim of modern management is to aid comfort and prevent infection until the skin has regrown. With the increasing prevalence of concomitant therapy, such as chemotherapy and surgery, and new techniques such as escalating radiotherapy dosage and accelerated regimes, it is clear that skin reactions will remain a problem.

Incidence of skin toxicity is unclear, with skin inflammation ranging from 66 to 83%.[67,68] Prevalence studies are rare and few cancer centres use assessments to monitor skin problems. What is known is that acute skin reactions are cumulative with radiotherapy treatment and have a latent healing time after treatment has completed. This highlights the differing aetiology of radiation skin damage compared with conventional wounds.[69] Skin management varies considerably between cancer centres.[70,71] There is a need for studies to evaluate modern wound-care products in the context of radiotherapy skin reactions and a need for innovation to improve this neglected area of radiotherapy side-effects.

Mechanisms

The underlying cause of skin reactions relates to the radiobiological damage to the dermis and epidermis. In normal tissue the epidermis has a renewing cell population in which cell production is balanced by cell loss. Superficial cells are shed and replaced by new cells formed by mitosis in the basal layer.[72-74] The average time for repopulation of cells is approximately 4 weeks. In radiation skin damage, this repopulation is impaired by radiobiological damage to the radiosensitive basal and suprabasal layer and hence this affects the integrity of the upper epidermis layer.[75] The associated erythema represents the secondary inflammation. Skin changes vary and are commonly classified as erythema, dry desquamation, moist desquamation, and necrosis.

These reactions may occur in isolation or in combination over a radiation field. Erythema is a dry, red, warm skin reaction that may feel sensitive and tight.[76] This often starts to occur 2–3 weeks into treatment and subsides 2–3 weeks after therapy. If repopulation of the cells does not keep pace with those being lost, then dry desquamation occurs. This is associated with dry peeling skin that itches. The discomfort of this reaction is compounded by the decreased ability of the sweat and sebaceous glands to produce sweat. This reaction can occur as early as 2–3 weeks into treatment. If new cell proliferation is inadequate and the epidermis layer becomes broken, then moist desquamation may occur. This has distinctive signs in that the skin blisters and sloughs, leaving the denuded areas of dermis exposed. These areas then exude serum, which is associated with pain and discomfort. Necrosis is an infrequent skin reaction caused by a combination of ischaemia and vascular occlusion and is a result of cell death (see Table 12.7).

As in many radiation reactions, the link between acute and late effects is not known. The severity of an acute reaction may have a link to the cosmetic and functional impact on the area that was treated. Scarring from skin breakdown has an affect on body image, as well as on functional morbidity.

Table 12.7 Radiation-induced skin reactions

Early or acute radiation-induced effects	Late or chronic radiation-induced effects
Erythema	Atrophy
Dry desquamation	Thinning
Moist desquamation	Telangiectasia
Alopecia	Altered pigmentation
Reduced sweating	Fibrosis
Itching	Ulcerations
Changes in pigmentation	Necrosis
	Carcinogenesis

Incidence

The incidence of radiation-induced skin problems is relatively unknown. Barkham,[68] in a survey of radiotherapy units in the UK, found that skin reactions are relatively common: 83% of centres reported frequently seeing skin inflammation, dry desquamation was reported in 52% of centres, and moist desquamation in 12%. Acute necrosis was rarely seen. King[33] investigated the timing, onset, frequency, and duration of symptoms among a group of patients receiving radiotherapy. Skin irritation was reported in the last week of radiotherapy in 87% of patients having treatment to the chest, and in the third week of treatment in 80% of patients receiving head and neck radiotherapy. Skin reactions continued to be troublesome in 9% of those treated with radiotherapy to the head and neck, 3 months post-treatment.

The degree of different reactions has been described in work by Dini *et al.*[67] A sample of 42 patients with acute skin reactions was monitored for response to pharmacological management. Erythema and dry desquamation lesions were found in 28% of patients, and moist desquamation lesions in 14%. Skin reactions caused pain, burning, and impairment to normal activity.

Like many of the radiation induced side-effects, factors that influence the occurrence of toxicity are not certain. Clear treatment-related factors such as dose, volume, and fractionation are known to be influencing factors, but other skin variables are not clear.

Treatment factors adversely affecting skin include:

- higher doses of radiation per fraction
- large treatment fields
- tangential fields
- raising the skin surface by wax or moulds
- electron beams – these have a shorter wavelength of radiotherapy and this may result in the skin receiving a larger dose compared to photon treatments.

Factors influencing skin vulnerability include:

- concurrent chemotherapy
- site of radiotherapy – skin folds are more susceptible to damage, e.g. axilla, groin, intra-mammary fold, peri-anal area, and head and neck

- skin areas susceptible to friction
- recent surgery to the skin area
- diabetes or vascular disease
- use of irritant skin-care products.

As with many radiotherapy toxicities, it is difficult to predict those patients most at risk of developing radiation skin damage. Late toxicity is seen in less than 5% of patients and is considered a rare and unexpected complication of curative radiotherapy. Turesson[77] measured early and late radiation skin damage following radiotherapy to the breast. All patients had standard therapy; however, it was clear that the variation in tolerance to radiation was related to an individual's radiosensitivity.

The impact of skin reactions

The discomfort and distress of radiation-induced skin reactions is frequently under-represented as a toxicity, and often goes unnoticed as the physical appearance of the skin does not always correspond with the discomfort experienced by the patient. Pain is often associated with radiation-damaged skin, and can be exacerbated by incorrect wound management.[78] In a small study of women ($n = 20$) having radiotherapy for breast cancer, skin reactions were found to have an adverse affect on home life.[79] Some form of skin reaction occurred in every woman after radiotherapy, with moist desquamation occurring in 45%. The women complained of symptoms of itching and tenderness, a feeling of tightness and throbbing of the skin. However, few complained of marked pain. The skin changes resulted in functional and body image changes: skin damage limited household activities, the discomfort restricted what clothes could be worn, sleep disturbances were reported, and 10% said that the radiotherapy had affected sexual relationships. Few research studies have used qualitative accounts to explore the impact radiation skin reactions have on the individual. One patient with head and neck cancer in Wells' study[80] reported being fearful of people observing him: 'I didn't want people looking surreptitiously at my burns'. Skin was described as feeling 'raw' and as looking like 'crocodile skin', and was painful and itchy. The lack of qualitative research in this area shows how little we know about the impact of skin reactions. Patient accounts and subjective information are necessary to provide insights into how best to assess and support patients through these symptoms.

The management of radiation-induced skin reactions

There are serious gaps in our knowledge of how best to manage skin reactions. Much of the published material is based on anecdotal accounts or tradition.[71] Modern wound-care products are expensive and add to the costs of therapy. In the past, moist wound healing principles have not been applied in the context of radiotherapy-induced skin damage. The latent healing period after therapy is completed means that wound healing is not the same as in conventional cases. Assessment is fundamental in recognising the right approach for skin problems, but preventing skin damage and mediating skin problems is also an essential part of nursing care.

Assessment

The literature is full of descriptions of radiation-induced skin reactions, with scoring for toxicity based on observer reports. Most reflect only the observable reaction and not the subjective symptoms that patients experience. Many of the research assessments have focused on recognition of late toxicity rather than acute effects. Conventional skin assessment tools are often not applicable as the skin damage differs from conventional wounds.

The main aims for caring for impaired skin arising during the course of radiotherapy are to:

- prevent infection
- maximise patient comfort
- minimise trauma and prevent further skin damage.

Following completion of radiotherapy, healing is the priority.

One problem is that there are many assumptions made about how to care for the skin. Research demonstrates little evidence that washing the skin during radiotherapy is harmful or that it contributes to radiation damage.[81] The use of creams and ointments is considered to alleviate some of the discomfort of a dry skin.[71] Creams should not be allowed to build up on the skin and therefore washing should be encouraged. Some creams are contraindicated (for example, petroleum jellies such as Vaseline) as these are poorly soluble and stay on the skin's surface. Lanolin-based creams such as E45 are also not recommended, as the lanolin content increases sensitivity. Topical steroid-based creams are often prescribed for the itching experienced with the dry desquamation; however, prolonged use of steroids is known to delay healing and has no beneficial effects if the skin is broken.[76] The routine use of moisturising creams may prevent the need for steroids. Talcum powder can also be soothing for dry desquamation, although there is little evidence of its efficacy. Clothes should be loose and made of cotton. Irradiated skin is more vulnerable to damage from sun exposure, therefore covering up irradiated skin and using sun blocks after completion of treatment is important.

The routine use of antiseptics such as proflavine in radiation wound management is not considered to confer any advantage over normal saline.[71] Morgan[82] suggests that some products may also have toxic effects on healing tissue such as fibroblasts and therefore normal saline is recommended for wound cleansing. Dressings such as melonin and paraffin gauze were traditionally used for skin reactions; however, they stick to wounds and cause pain and trauma when removed. New dressings have since been developed, such as the alginates and hydrogels. Hydrogels are non-adhesive, absorb wound fluid slowly, have cooling properties and provide a moist environment to enhance re-epithelialisation.[73,74,83,84] Alginate sheets are recommended for wounds with moderate to high exudate during radiotherapy; for example, Sorbsan, which converts to a hydrophilic gel on contact with exudate or saline.[70,78] One of the benefits of alginates is their haemostatic properties, which are useful for areas of bleeding. During radiotherapy, treatment dressings within the radiation field usually need to be removed to prevent changes in dosimetry. In some palliative treatments dressings may be left in place; it is therefore worth checking with the therapeutic radiographer. The use of adhesives such as tape or semi-permeable film dressings within the treatment field may add to skin damage. Occlusive dressings are ideal post-treatment; hydrocolloid sheets can be placed over an area of moist desquamation and left in place for up to 7 days. This minimises cost and friction and maintains comfort. It should be noted that for those who perspire heavily, the dressing may not be suitable. Continuing assessment is advisable once radiotherapy is completed.

Case example 12.1: Managing skin reactions

After having a wide local excision for breast cancer and radiotherapy Hannah started to develop a skin reaction. On assessment, the skin in the treatment field was covered in erythema with an area of moist desquamation in her intra-mammary fold. The overall skin reaction appeared minimal yet she was experiencing sharp burning pain in her breast and puritis around her nipple. Sleep was difficult and the pain caused her to worry about tumour progression. Hannah was anxious about her treatment and the skin reaction very visibly reinforced the nature of her disease.

Nursing intervention not only addressed her anxiety but focused on the physical symptoms. Aqueous cream was applied to the erythema and a hydrocortisone cream applied to her nipple area. The moist desquamation was covered with a hydrogel sheet (Geliperm), which Hannah found soothing and which reduced the pain. Over the next 5 days, the area of moist desquamation enlarged; this was expected, as there is latent healing following radiotherapy. Subsequent to the deterioration the moist desquamation healed within 2 days.

Another example of the use of occlusive dressings can be shown by the case of Joe, who was 8 years old and having radiotherapy to his spine. Near the completion of his treatment he developed an area of moist desquamation on the anterior of his neck. He found it hard not to scratch and peel the dry skin. To prevent him damaging the skin further, Granuflex was applied to his neck. The thin wafer was used as it is more pliable and easier to mould onto the skin folds. A large border was left to enclose any exudate and within 4 days Joe's skin had successfully healed.

The management of skin reactions is a neglected area of practice. There are few research studies to guide practitioners on how best to manage skin problems and research is needed to evaluate modern skin-care products. Innovations such as the use of aloe vera creams, and evening primrose and lavender oils have positive anecdotal reports but clinical trials need to be established to evaluate these formally. Skin reactions, not only those that are acute but also longer term, potentially cause pain and anxiety and should be taken seriously.

Sexual issues and radiotherapy

Sexuality and fertility are an important component of management in radiotherapy practice that is often overlooked by clinicians. Symptoms and side-effects during and following radiotherapy (for example, fatigue, pain, or diarrhoea) may have implications for sexual desire but can also affect sexual function. Talking about sexual issues prior to treatment is difficult, with the consequence that they are often ignored, avoided, or dismissed by staff, despite numerous reports that for many, concerns over fertility or sexuality are common and affect physical and psychological well-being. Symptom management and support should include information on how radiotherapy impacts on fertility, libido, and sexual functioning.

Radiotherapy may affect sexual functioning both physically and psychologically and these effects may be difficult to distinguish from cancer-related ones. Vaginal fibrosis, post-coital bleeding, sterility, and early menopause occur as a result of radiotherapy treatment. Much of the literature focuses on the effects of radiotherapy on women with gynaecological malignancies, but men also have problems with radiotherapy treatment affecting libido and potency. The incidence of sexual problems varies considerably in studies. For example, in one study 50% of women treated for cervical cancer reported reduced sexual activity.[85] In genito-urinary cancer, impotence has been reported in about 35–40% of men following radiotherapy.[86] One problem is that the physical effects of the radiotherapy for genito-urinary and gynaecological cancer are often difficult to distinguish from the sexual dysfunction and impotence that results from the initial disease or adjuvant therapies.

Abbitol and Davenport[87] suggest that it is the physical effects of treatment that result in poor sexual function. This has been disputed following studies where no positive correlation between patients with severe physical changes and those with the greatest decrease in sexual functioning were found.[88,89] Many studies highlight that the physical changes following radiotherapy do not necessarily inhibit sexual desire, but that changes in body image, misconceptions or fears about spreading cancer, or hastening recurrence may all have an impact on sexual function.[90] As with many symptoms, the cause of the problem may be multifactorial, with social, cultural and other symptoms affecting the complexity of sexual desire and function.

Physiological changes

In women treated with radiotherapy for gynaecological cancer, the vaginal canal and ovaries are the areas most sensitive to radiation therapy, and combined modality treatments have a more profound effect.[91,92] If the radiation field includes vaginal tissue, a decrease in vaginal lubrication and sensation may result. The cells in the vagina have rapid cell renewal, which makes the epithelium very sensitive to radiation damage. Depletion of cell supply, slow occlusion of blood vessels, and gradual laying down of fibrosis result in narrowing and lack of elasticity in the vaginal canal.[90] Stenosis and/or shortening of the vagina are late effects that occur progressively over time, with a consequent reduction in size and diameter. In women, radiation to the ovaries causes premature menopause with loss of germinal epithelium and follicles. Very low doses of radiation (4–10 Gy) are required to stop ovulation and permanent loss of menses is inevitable in women over the age of 40.[93] Younger women are more likely to remain functional, but with larger therapeutic doses, cessation of ovulation occurs in any age group (see Table 12.8).

Table 12.8 Possible effects of radiotherapy on the sexual organs

Women	Men
Pelvic fibrosis	Pelvic fibrosis
Atrophy of the vaginal wall	Decreased testosterone
Inelasticity of tissue	Pudendal or sympathetic nerve injury
Scarring	Decreased semen levels
Obliteration of small blood vessels	Aspermia
Thinning of epithelium	Fibrosis of arteries
Loss of lubrication	Reduction in penile blood pressure
Ulceration	

In men radiation to the genital regions as in treatment for prostate or bladder cancer, seminoma, or testicular cancer, can have consequences for sexual functioning. Impotence following external beam radiation therapy for prostate cancer can have physiological affects, causing fibrosis of the pelvic vasculature and damage to the pudendal or sympathetic pelvic nerves.[86,94] Vascular changes result in reduced penile blood pressures, which can contribute to arteriosclerotic changes in the pelvic arteries.[95] Radiotherapy may therefore accelerate changes that were already taking place through other diseases such as diabetes or hypertension. Decreased levels of testosterone may produce a reduction in libido. The testes are also highly radiosensitive. Radiotherapy to the retroperitoneum and pelvis (for example, for seminoma) may compromise gonadal function even at low doses and erectile dysfunction is seen in 10% of cases.[96] Cessation of sperm production (aspermia) may be temporary in those men having lower doses of radiation, but can take 3–5 years to recover.

The common problem from these physiological changes is that they lead to pain on intercourse (dypareunia). Researchers report that 30–50% of women interviewed said that pain on intercourse was the main reason for their decreased enjoyment of sexual activity.[97] Women were also frightened that sex would be painful and this reduced sexual pleasure. Post-coital bleeding has also been found to be a problem.[87,91,97,98]

In men the result of physical changes may be absolute as in the physical inability to have an erection, but men also complain of symptoms of pain on ejaculation and a permanent decrease in semen volume (see Table 12.9).[94]

Table 12.9 Sexual dysfunction following radiotherapy

Women	Men
Pain on intercourse	Impotence
Post-coital bleeding	Pain on ejaculation
Early menopause	Decrease in semen volume
Decreased libido	Male menopause
Feelings of burning with semen	Decreased libido
Pelvic pain	

Loss of reproductive function

The ovaries are very sensitive to radiation therapy and if included within a treatment field will suffer ovarian failure. Shielding can sometimes maintain function but despite this, 30–50% of women lose ovarian function after irradiation.[99] The effect of this is that reproductive function is lost and women lose their child-bearing ability. It may also induce early menopause, with premature ageing and feelings of diminished femininity.[100] Men treated with pelvic radiotherapy rarely report having discussed the possibility of infertility as a result of radiotherapy. Often they are considered too old for this to matter by medical and nursing staff, but Schover[94] found that this was a significant source of distress. The focus with men undergoing radiotherapy is on the subsequent ability to have an erection, but this is not the only significant aspect of sexuality. As Burke[101] suggests, many individuals 'may find it difficult to separate the pleasurable, from the reproductive aspects of sexual intercourse, consequently, once the reproductive function has gone, the reason for having intercourse has disappeared as well'.

Gonadal shielding is available and moving the ovaries outside the radiation field is sometimes possible. Sperm banking is often not considered prior to radiotherapy as it has demonstrated little value to viable fertility. Many patients have reduced sperm counts before receiving therapy, but research is limited and for some individuals the opportunity to discuss the options is important and should not be dismissed.

Diminished interest in sex

In many studies, one of the most frequent reasons cited for reduction in sexual activity is loss of desire or interest in sex. Loss of libido may have physical causes, such as a reduction in the production of sexual hormones following ablative doses of radiotherapy, or adjuvant hormone treatment. Siebel and Graves,[88] however, have found that loss of libido was not directly associated with the biological and physical changes resulting from radiotherapy. In women, body image changes and worries concerning early menopause may add to the anxiety and distress, resulting in decreased libido. Sexual interest has been found to be at its lowest at completion of treatment, which suggests that it is a side-effect of treatment.[92] Symptoms such as fatigue,

diarrhoea, dysuria, cystitis, nocturia, and rectal bleeding contribute to a decrease in desire for sexual intimacy. Concerns after treatment can vary greatly. Some people are fearful that they may spread the cancer or radiation through intercourse.

Fears and responses

It is often difficult to separate fears from the physical symptoms. Anderson[98] reported that 60% of patients studied reported sexual dysfunction prior to a cancer diagnosis. A combination of physical effects of disease and anxiety were found to lead to a decline in sexual activity. Fear of the disease still being present and being caused by sexual intercourse are common beliefs. Women with cervical cancer may see a link between sexual activity and the cancer, viewing the disease as a punishment for sin or sexual promiscuity.[102] Radiotherapy is sometimes perceived as not curative and used as a last resort. Anderson[98] found that 17% of patients gave fear of recurrence as a reason for decline in sexual activity, believing cancer to be still in the body and that it would spread or damage their partner. For example, a patient with bladder cancer undergoing pelvic radiotherapy believed that the epithelial debris he saw in his urine was the cancer seeding. He refrained from sex as he believed that these cancer cells would infect his partner and subsequently put her at risk of cancer.[63] Understanding of how radiation affects such private and personal matters is often left unexplored by clinicians and these fears may contribute to sexual dysfunction. Sexual issues may cause strain to marriage and personal relationships. Andelusi[97] found that 36% of couples separated after a female partner had gynaecological radiation. However, it is not clear how this compares with the rate of marriage breakdown in the general population.

Management

Sexual dysfunction following radiotherapy is clearly a multifaceted problem, with both physical changes and psychological components influencing desire and function. There are many misconceptions in radiotherapy centres about the problem, and doubt about whether management of physical sexual dysfunction is appropriate or part of active symptom management. Information is often lacking about potential sexual problems and this area is rarely monitored. Information about sexual issues in radiotherapy is neglected. In one study, only 30% of patients were given any information about potential sexual problems.[103] When asked whether they would have liked information, 40% of informants indicated that they would. Why is it then that clinicians are reluctant to address this issue? Possibly it is because it is presumed that older women will be offended, or assumptions are made that sex is no longer of interest to older women, particularly if they do not have a partner. Studies, however, have shown that a majority of older people may be sexually active.[104]

Lack of adequate information regarding sexual issues may also relate in part to the fact that information is often given prior to the start of treatment when worries and concerns surround side-effects and anxieties are about coping with the radiotherapy. Sexual issues may not be a concern until after therapy, when professional support is limited. In an interview study of men who were having or had had pelvic radiotherapy for prostate or bladder cancer, sexual concerns such as lack of libido or impotence were often ranked as a lower priority than urinary problems during and immediately after treatment. At 6 months post-treatment, however, loss of interest in sex was third in priority.[63] Sexual functioning and desire for sex may not be seen as important, when other side-effects are at their peak. Not uncommonly, the question of fertility or sexual function arises after side-effects of treatment have diminished. All too often, no pre-treatment counselling is offered and loss of fertility or potency comes as a bitter disappointment. The difficulty also arises when action has been delayed, fibrosis or strictures have developed, and intervention is often too late. The focus of health professionals is often on provision of information, but practical strategies as well as psychological insight need to be considered as integral to any intervention.

One of the most effective ways of preventing vaginal stenosis and adhesions is to use a vaginal dilator and douche as part of sexual rehabilitation after gynaecological radiotherapy.[105] Dilators need to be used over a long time period unless the patient has regular sexual intercourse,[90] although their use can be difficult and painful. The use of lubrication for a dry vagina reduces irritation and pain.

Decreased vaginal elasticity and scarring may make particular sexual positions uncomfortable, so suggesting different positions may help to increase comfort and satisfaction. For men, careful assessment of the cause of erectile dysfunction may help in providing solutions to the cause of diminished sexual potency; Doppler ultrasound studies can show whether the cause of erectile dysfunction is due to arterial changes. Penile implants, drug therapy, pumps, or prostheses may be used if dysfunction is permanent.[106]

Many individuals find discussing sexual issues embarrassing, although the opportunity to discuss sexual issues is reported to be helpful.[103] Women who are well informed during gynaecological treatment have been found to be more motivated towards recovery.[107] Although practical suggestions for women and men are available, it is clear that nurses and clinicians find difficulty with discussing sexual issues and that this impedes sexual rehabilitation. Counselling patients and partners has been shown to have beneficial effects. A crisis counselling service and intervention programme for women with genital malignancies has been demonstrated to be extremely effective in promoting sexual functioning when counselling was initiated shortly after diagnosis.[108]

Support following radiotherapy is important; however, sexual problems for many are all too frequently ignored. Providing information about potential sexual problems that may be experienced during and after radiotherapy legitimises this as an area of care that is possible to discuss. Assessment and appropriate referral for sexual counselling is an essential element of the role of the nurse in the radiotherapy department.

Mucositis and radiation therapy

Mucositis resulting from radiation to the head and neck area is considered an inevitable consequence of radiation cancer treatment.[109] Terms such as stomatitis and mucositis are often used interchangeably; both mean mucosal damage in the oral or pharangeal cavity. The degree of mucositis depends on many factors, such as the extent and dosage of radiotherapy treatment, and also the individual's pre-treatment health and general oral hygiene. Although it is a symptom that occurs during radiation treatment and heals rapidly after therapy is finished, it can be distressing and is often identified by radiotherapy nurses as being difficult to manage. Mucositis is exacerbated by changes in saliva and taste, and affects eating and nutrition. Mucositis causes pain and sometimes sensations of coughing and choking, which can be frightening.

Physiological changes

Changes in the mucosal membranes occur early in radiotherapy treatment, as fast-growing cells such as those in the mouth are vulnerable to damage. They tend to appear in the beginning of the second week of treatment and persist for 2–3 weeks after completion of radiotherapy.[110] The homeostatic balance between new and old cells is lost. As cells are lost they are not replaced, causing denudation of the mucosal layers, with epithelial and vascular changes.[111] The direct damage caused by radiotherapy may also exacerbate infection or previous mouth problems.[112]

Different areas of the oral cavity are more sensitive than others to radiation treatment and therefore the distribution of radiation side-effects may occur only in specific areas. The pharyngeal walls, tonsils and buccal membranes are most vulnerable. The extent of mucosal reaction depends on several factors: those related to the treatment and those that relate to the patient's pre-existing problems. Acute radiation mucositis, including soreness and epithelial changes, often quickly recovers once therapy is finished. Longer term effects such as saliva changes and dental problems or radionecrosis may never heal.[109] Although these longer term problems occur in less than 5% of patients, radiotherapy to the head or neck carries a small risk of side-effects persisting long after treatment has finished.[109,110]

The extent of mucosal reactions depends on:

- radiation regimen
- dose
- fractionation
- area and volume
- anatomic location.

How treatment is delivered has important implications for how quickly side-effects are manifested. The shorter the time between doses the greater the severity of the reactions. For example, in hyperfractionated schedules, individuals develop mucositis that is severe and often require a planned break in therapy to allow for some recovery before continuing treatment. Although treatment factors determine the extent of radiation mucositis, indirect factors such as the general health of the individual impact on the healing and treatment of mucositis.

Individual factors that increase vulnerability to mucositis include:

- oral hygiene
- smoking/alcohol
- poor dental hygiene
- traumatising agents, i.e. dentures
- large amalgam fillings
- chemotherapy
- fungal infections.

Constant use of the mouth through talking, breathing, eating, and drinking makes any changes more noticeable. Distinct changes in taste and saliva flow are noticed within a few weeks of starting therapy.[113]

Mucositis begins with changes in feeling in the mouth. These may be subtle changes in saliva flow or consistency. As radiobiological damage occurs, more visible changes are seen with a whitish discoloration in areas of the mucosal membrane. Mild erythema occurs with epithelial cells diminishing, as well as inflammatory changes due to cell damage.[114] This causes redness and pain when eating or cleaning the mouth.

Erythema is less obvious with a reddish appearance; red patches occur with small white patches, sometimes in conjunction with ulceration. Often a fibrous exudate covers areas of mucositis, and ulcers underneath cause pain and bleeding. The first signs occur frequently in the second week of radiotherapy, but this may be more rapid in hyperfractionated treatment regimes. Patients complain of pain, burning and discomfort in the mouth, which is exacerbated by swallowing, eating, and breathing. Thickening of saliva is also a consequence of treatment as a result of damage to the salivary glands. Saliva helps in moistening the mouth, digesting food, and in preventing infection. Loss of saliva (xerostomia) is one of the key problems and exacerbates other symptoms.[115]

The distress of mucositis is sometimes under-estimated. Changes in saliva, taste, and soreness and pain have an important effect on quality of life. The focus of studies is often on healing and agents used in dealing with mucosal ulceration; however, it can be the additional symptoms that are particulary hard for people to deal with. Gamble,[116] in a study of how patients felt while undergoing head and neck radiotherapy, describes the trauma that these additional symptoms can cause:

> One lady having head and neck radiotherapy found that her saliva had changed during treatment: she was coughing up copious nasty tasting and sticky saliva: 'If I had known that something like that was going to happen I would have been prepared for it . . . I mean I could fill a carrier bag with this stuff in the night . . . when I was going on the tube . . . I used to get quite err, agitated, because you know this coughing used to sound so dreadful.'

Wells[80] found that these enduring unpleasant symptoms were a vicious circle for patients. She describes the effects that radiation symptoms have on the people she interviewed:

> Mucositis changes affected one man's throat early in the radiotherapy. He wrote in his diary, 'Woke up at 4 am and had a fit of coughing, made my throat bleed' [day 3].
>
> Others describe described having a 'choked up feeling' that affected sleep. One man at interview described 'the biggest trouble was at night I couldn't sleep because of my throat'. Taste changes were also a distressing symptom. One man said 'everything bland like mashed potato . . . you cannot describe what it's like losing your taste, that was the worse thing . . . you don't feel like eating and that makes you worse because you are not getting enough nourishment so you get tired, it's a sort of vicious circle . . .'
>
> Taste changes not only affect appetite but reduce the pleasure of eating and can result in a poor diet. One man said: 'I thought I was going to fade away, that's the only thing that worried me, I would have hated it for people to say to me, you do look ill, you're losing weight.'

The combination of symptoms can result in feeling depressed and in social isolation. Thus patients undergoing head and neck irradiation need considerable support to cope with oral symptoms.

The management of radiation-induced mucositis
Oral care has been well addressed in the literature but knowledge about this radiation side-effect is still limited. It is difficult to manage and healing will not occur while an individual is having radiotherapy treatment. Often the issues are different from mucositis due to chemotherapy. The aims are primarily to provide support, to give symptomatic relief, and to prevent secondary infection.

Much of the focus of research has been on which agents or chemicals are best used to rinse the mouth and provide oral care. However, it is often routine assessment and simple preventive strategies that are most effective in mediating patient symptoms. There are no clear answers in the research literature but it would appear that the distress from symptoms can be reduced by providing information, early assessment and support to help patients with pain, and saliva, and nutrition, and taste changes (see Table 12.10).[117]

Radiation mucositis cannot be avoided but its impact can be reduced and prevented by assessment of the oral cavity prior to treatment and elimination of sources of infection and chronic irritation. It is important that mouth care is performed frequently and consistently and this is now considered more important than the specific oral care agents used.[118] Many of the mouth rinses that are anti-plaque or anti-bacterial (such as

Table 12.10 Helpful and unhelpful strategies for managing decreased saliva[121]

Unhelpful strategies
Smoking
Alcohol
Spicy foods
Very hot or cold foods
Citrus juices
Commercial mouthwashes
Coarse or hard foods

Helpful strategies
Keeping your mouth clean after eating
Taking frequent sips of water
Use synthetic saliva when mouth feels dry
Sucking on hard sugarless sweets or gum
Using a cool mist vaporiser

chlorehexidine) are ineffective, as the active ingredients require saliva to be effective. It is also important to brush teeth regularly, as reduction in saliva can cause plaque and dental problems. Encouraging fluids and regular sipping of water can help in reducing the unpleasantness of reductions in saliva. Studies have shown that artificial saliva is of minimal benefit for those with acute symptoms.[119] In a cross-over randomised trial, 12 out of 17 patients thought pilocarpine was more helpful.[120] Problems with managing associated drug symptoms such as nausea and sweating have diminished the likely value of pilocarpine. Assessing an individual's associated medications can also have substantial benefits on saliva flow.[120] Managing symptoms such as pain from the mucositis with either systemic analgesics or local analgesics such as sprays (e.g. Difflam) is important. Pain also affects swallowing and reduces nutritional intake. Preventing secondary infection is essential, and studies suggest that the use of nystatin pastilles is useful in reducing the development of fungal infections.[115]

Research to date has focused on cleansing agents, timing of mouth care and protective coatings. Sucraflate shows promise as a protective coating to prevent damage; it also improves comfort and reduces pain, and early studies have shown better healing.[122] Studies exploring pain relief have found anti-inflammatory and steroid preparations of benefit in reducing inflammatory changes and delaying the onset of symptoms.[123]

It is clear that there are no easy answers to the problems of radiation-induced mucositis; like many side-effects of therapy, their intense nature can cause great distress. What is important is to provide information and education for the patient in providing oral care. Unrealistic expectations of what mouth rinses and medications can provide do not help patients to cope with these distressing symptoms. It is vital to start preventive strategies at the onset of treatment, rather than waiting for problems to occur. Symptom management should encompass not only the mucosal reactions but also the decrease and changes in saliva. Research is currently underway in the USA to investigate the benefits of aloe vera and its anti-inflammatory properties.

The role of supportive care: can this make a difference to radiation side-effects?

Supportive care has been a key element in the discussion of the management of the radiation side-effects in cancer care. Supportive care is defined as the provision of information, counselling, social support, and side-effect management, with the aim of reducing radiotherapy morbidity. It is clear from the literature that few studies have been conducted to contribute to the knowledge that is required to provide evidence-based radiotherapy practice, and reflect the value or benefits of different approaches. The lack of consistency across the country and internationally in radiotherapy treatment strategies is also reflected in how adverse effects of therapy are managed. Many nurses and health care professionals are unaware of the problems patients experience as a result of treatment and much of what we know in terms of nursing or supportive care interventions has been focused on specific areas.

This is not to say that supportive care has little impact; it is just that many of the studies in the literature have had only minimal effect in influencing service provision. Questions as to the best and most appropriate symptom management, follow-up services and surveillance during radiotherapy treatment are not adequately studied. The interface between follow-up care, physical and psychological needs, and community services has been a neglected area. Supportive care is a Cinderella area in radiotherapy and the literature attests to this, with less than 1% reflecting quality of life assessments or the impact that treatment can have on the individual, but it is clear that radiotherapy treatment can have a substantial impact on the person with cancer. The evidence about whether supportive and nursing care can make a difference to the individual, not only in terms of physical symptoms but also in terms of psychological distress, is as yet not clear, but it is likely to be of considerable benefit to well-being, recovery, and the experience of symptoms associated with radiotherapy treatment.

References

1. Rotman M., Rogow L., DeLeon G. and Heskel N. (1977). Supportive therapy in radiation oncology. *Cancer* **39**, 744–750.

2. Hall E.J. (1988). Time, dose and fractionation in radiotherapy. In Hall E. (ed.) *Radiobiology for the Radiologist.* Philadelphia, PA: Lippincott, pp. 239–259.

3. Hill R.P. (1987). Cellular basis of radiotherapy. In Tannock I. and Hill R. (eds.) *The Basic Science of Oncology.* New York: Pergamon, pp. 237–277.

4. Leibel S.A. (1998). *Textbook of Radiation Oncology.* Philadelphia, PA: W.B. Saunders.

5. Powell S. and McMillan T.J. (1990). DNA damage and repair following treatment with ionizing radiation. *Radiotherapy and Oncology* **19**, 95–108.

6. McMillan T. (1989). The molecular basis of radiosensitivity. In Steel C., Adams G. and Horwich A. (eds.) *The Biological Basis of Radiotherapy.* Amsterdam: Elsevier, pp. 29–44.

7. Withers R.H. (1992). Biological basis of radiation therapy for cancer. *Lancet* **339**, 156–159.

8. Hopewell J.W., Calvo W. and Reinhold H.S. (1989). Radiation effects on blood vessels: role in late normal tissue damage. In Steel C., Adams G. and Horwich A. (eds.) *The Biological Basis of Radiotherapy.* Amsterdam: Elsevier, pp. 101–112.

9. Burnet N.G., Nyman J. and Turesson I. (1992). Prediction of normal tissue tolerance to radiotherapy from in-vitro cellular radiation sensitivity. *Lancet* **399**, 1570–1571.

10. Bentzen S.M., Overgaard M. and Overgaard J. (1993). Clinical correlations between late normal tissue endpoints after radiotherapy: implications for predictive assays of radiosensitivity. *European Journal of Cancer* **29A**, 1373–1376.

11. Trott K.R. and Kummermehr J. (1985). What is known about tumour proliferation rates to choose between accelerated fractionation and hyperfractionation? *Radiotherapy and Oncology* **3**, 1–9.

12. Saunders M.I. and Dische S. (1990). Continuous hyperfractionated accelerated radiotherapy (CHART) in non small cell carcinoma of the bronchus. *International Journal of Radiation Oncology, Biology, Physics* **19**, 1211–1215.

13. Price P., Hoskin P.J. and Easton D. (1986). Prospective randomized trial of single and multi-fraction schedules in the treatment of painful bone metastasis. *Radiotherapy and Oncology* **6**, 247–255.

14. Dodd J., Barrett A. and Ash D. (1992). *Practical Radiotherapy Planning,* 2nd edition. London: Edward Arnold.

15. Eardley A. (1986). Expectations of recovery. *Nursing Times* 23 April, 53–54.

16. Forester B.M., Kornfield D.S. and Fleis J. (1985). Psychiatric aspects of radiotherapy. *American Journal of Psychiatry* **142**, 22–27.

17. Peck A. and Boland J. (1977). Emotional reactions to radiation treatment. *Cancer* **40**, 180–184.

18. Ward S., Viergutz G., Tormey D., DeMuth J. and Paulen A. (1992). Patients' reactions to completion of adjuvant breast cancer therapy. *Nursing Research* **41**, 6, 362–366.

19. Norcross Weintraub F. (1992). Coping with cancer treatment: patient and family response to radiation therapy. In Hassey Dow K. and Hilderly L.J. (eds.) *Nursing Care in Radiation Oncology.* Philadelphia, PA: W.B. Saunders, pp. 45–56.

20. Eardley A. (1986). After the treatment's over. *Nursing Times*, 30 April, 40–41.

21. Gottschalk L.A., Kunkal R., Wohl T.H., Saenger E.L. and Winger C.N. (1969). Total and half body irradiation: effects on cognitive and emotional processes. *Archives of General Psychiatry* **21**, 574–580.

22. Holland J.C., Rowland A., Lebovitz A. and Rusalem R. (1979). Reactions to cancer treatment: assessment of emotional response to adjuvant radiotherapy as a guide to planned intervention. *Psychiatric Clinics of North America* **2**, 347–358.

23. Eardley A. (1990). Patients' needs after radiotherapy: the role of the general practitioner. *Family Practice* **7**, 39–42.

24. Mitchell G.W. and Glicksman A.S. (1977). Cancer patients' knowledge and attitudes. *Cancer* **40**, 61–66.

25. Holland J.C. and Tross S. (1989). Psychological sequelae in cancer survivors. In Holland J.C. and Rowland J. (eds.) *Handbook of Psychooncology.* Oxford: Oxford University Press.

26. Herbert D. (1977). The assessment of the clinical significance of non compliance with prescribed schedules of irradiation. *Journal of Radiation Oncology, Biology, Physics* **2**, 763–772.

27. Strohl R.A. (1988). The nursing role in radiation oncology symptom management of acute and chronic reactions. *Oncology Nursing Forum* **15**, 429–434.

28. Anderson B. and Tewfik H. (1985). Psychological reactions to radiation therapy: reconsideration of the adaptive aspects of anxiety. *Journal of Personality and Social Psychology* **48**, 1024–1032.

29. Wells M. (1994). Unpublished case study, University of London.

30. Ash D.V. (1999). Breast radiation injury litigation and RAGE. *Clinical Oncology* **11**, 138–139.

31. Haylock P. and Hart L. (1979). Fatigue in patients receiving localised radiation. *Cancer Nursing* **2**, 461–467.

32. Greenberg D., Sawicka J., Eisenthal S. and Ross D. (1992). Fatigue syndrome due to localised radiotherapy. *Journal of Pain and Symptom Management* **7**, 38–45.

33. King K., Nail L., Kreamer K., Strohl R. and Johnson J. (1985). Patients' descriptions of the experience of receiving radiation therapy. *Oncology Nursing Forum* **12**, 55–61.

34. Larson P., Lindsey A., Dodd M., Brecht M. and Packer A. (1993). Influence of age on problems experienced by patients with lung cancer undergoing radiation therapy. *Oncology Nursing Forum* **20**, 473–480.

35. Piper B. and Dodd M. (1991). Self initiated fatigue interventions and their perceived effectiveness. *Oncology Nursing Forum* **18** (Abstract 189), 39.

36. Nail L. (1993). Coping with intracavity radiation treatment for gynaecologic cancer. *Cancer Practice* **1**, 218–224.

37. Faithfull S. (1991). Patients' experiences following cranial radiotherapy: a study of the somnolence syndrome. *Journal of Advanced Nursing* **16**, 939–946.

38. Fobair P., Hoppe R., Bloom J., Cox R., Varghese and Spiegle D. (1986). Psychosocial problems among survivors of Hodgkin's disease. *Journal of Clinical Oncology* **4**, 908–914.

39. Kobashi-Schoot J. (1985). Assessment of malaise in cancer patients treated with radiotherapy. *Cancer Nursing* **8**, 306–313.

40. Faithfull S. and Brada M. (1998). Somnolence syndrome in adults following cranial irradiation for primary brain tumours. *Clinical Oncology* **10**, 250–254.

41. Munro A.J., Biruls R., Griffin A.V., Thomas H. and Vallis K.A. (1994). Distress associated with radiotherapy for malignant disease: a quantitative analysis based on patients' perceptions. *British Journal of Cancer* **60**, 370–374.

42. Richardson A. (1995). Fatigue in cancer patients: a review of the literature. *European Journal of Cancer Care* **4**, 20–32.

43. Winningham M. (1991). Walking program for people with cancer: getting started. *Cancer Nursing* **14**, 270–276.

44. Pearce S. and Richardson A. (1994). Fatigue and cancer: a phenomenological study. *Journal of Cancer Nursing* **3**, 381–382.

45. Graydon J., Bubela N., Irvine D. and Vincent L. (1995). Fatigue-reducing strategies used by patients receiving treatment for cancer. *Cancer Nursing* **18**, 23–28.

46. Chrumratanakul S., Wirzba B., Lam T., Walker K., Fedorak R. and Thompson A.B. (1990). Radiation and the small intestine: future perspectives for preventive therapy. *Digestive Disease* **8**, 45–60.

47. Flickinger J.C., Bloomer W.D. and Kinsella J. (1900). Intestinal intolerance of radiation injury. In Galland R. and Spencer J. (eds.) *Radiation Enteritis*. London: Edward Arnold, pp. 51–65.

48. Danielsson A., Nyhlin H., Stendahl R., Stenling U. and Suhr O. (1991). Chronic diarrhoea after radiotherapy for gynaecological cancer: occurrence and aetiology. *Gut* **32**, 1180–1187.

49. Kinsella T.J. and Bloomer W.D. (1980). Bowel tolerance to radiation therapy. *Surgical Gynaecology and Obstetrics* **151**, 273–284.

50. Yeoh E.K., Lui D. and Lee N.Y. (1984). The mechanism of diarrhoea resulting from pelvic and abdominal radiotherapy: a prospective study using selenium-75 labelled conjugated bile acid and cobalt-58 labelled cyancobalamin. *British Journal of Radiology* **57**, 1131–1136.

51. Sullivan M.F. (1962). Dependence of radiation diarrhoea on the presence of bile in the small intestine. *Nature* **195**, 1217–1218.

52. Newman A. (1974). Breath-analysis tests in gastroenterology. *Gut* **15**, 308–323.

53. Stryker J.A., Hepner G.W. and Mortel R. (1977). The effect of pelvic irradiation on ileal function. *Radiology* **124**, 213–216.

54. Gray G.M. (1975). Carbohydrate digestion and absorption: role of the small intestine. *New England Journal of Medicine* **292**, 1225–1230.

55. Mennie A.T., Dalley V.M., Dinneen L.C. and Collier H.O. (1975). Treatment of radiation induced gastrointestinal distress with acetysallcylate. *Lancet* **ii**, 942–943.

56. Martenson J.A., Hyland G., Moertl C.G., Maillard J., Fallon J., Collins R. *et al.* (1996). Olsalazine is contraindicated during pelvic radiation therapy: results of a double blind, randomized clinical trial. *International Journal of Radiation Oncology, Biology, Physics* **35**, 299–303.

57. Yeoh E. and Horwitz M. (1988). Radiation enteritis. *British Journal of Hospital Medicine* **June**, 498–504.

58. Potish R.A. (1990). Factors predisposing to injury. In Galland R.B. and Spencer J. (eds.) *Radiation Enteritis*. London: Edward Arnold, pp. 103–119.

59. Perez C.A., Camel M.H., Kuske R.R., Galakatos A., Hederman M.A. and Powers W.E. (1986). Radiation therapy alone in the treatment of carcinoma of the uterine cervix: a 20 year experience. *Gynaecolic Oncology* **23**, 127–140.

60. Levi S. and Hodgson H.J. (1990). In Galland R.B. and Spencer J. (eds.) *Prevention of Radiation Enteritis*. London: Edward Arnold, pp. 121–135.

61. Green N., Iba G. and Smith W.R. (1975). Measures to minimise small intestine injury in the irradiated pelvis. *Cancer* **35**, 1633–1640.

62. Padilla G.V. (1990). Gastrointestinal side-effects and quality of life in patients receiving radiation therapy. *Nutrition* **6**, 367–382.

63. Faithfull S. (1995). 'Just grin and bear it and hope that it will go away'. Coping with urinary symptoms from pelvic radiotherapy. *European Journal of Cancer Care* 4, 158–165.

64. Hassey Dow K. (1987). Radiation therapy for rectal cancer and the implications for nursing. *Cancer Nursing* 10, 311–318.

65. Bosaeus I., Andersson H. and Nystrom C. (1979). Effect of low-fat diet on bile salt excretion and diarrhoea in the gastrointestinal radiation syndrome. *Acta Radiologica Oncologica* 18, 460–464.

66. Chary S. and Thomson D.H. (1984). A clinical trial evaluating choletryramine to prevent diarrhoea in patients maintained on low fat diets during pelvic radiation therapy. *International Journal of Radiation Oncology, Biology, Physics* 10, 1885–1890.

67. Dini D., Macchia R., Gozza A., Bertelli G., Forno G., Guenzi M. *et al.* (1993). Management of acute radiodermatitis. *Cancer Nursing* 16, 336–370.

68. Barkham A. (1993). Radiotherapy skin reactions and treatments. *Professional Nurse* 8, 732–736.

69. McDonald A. (1992). Altered protective mechanisms. In Hassey Dow K. and Hilderley L.J. (eds.) *Nursing Care in Radiation Oncology.* Philadelphia, PA: W.B. Saunders, pp. 96–124.

70. Thomas S. (1992). Current practices in the management of fungating lesions and radiation damaged skin. Bridgend Hospital: Surgical Materials Testing Laboratory.

71. Lavery B.A. (1995). Skin care during radiotherapy: a survey of UK practice. *Clinical Oncology* 7, 184–187.

72. Hilderley L. (1983). Skin care in radiation therapy: a review of the literature. *Oncology Nursing Forum* 10, 144–162.

73. Sitton E. (1992). Early and late radiation induced skin alterations: Part 1. Mechanisms of skin changes. *Oncology Nursing Forum* 19, 801–807.

74. Sitton E. (1992). Early and late radiation induced skin alterations: Part 2. Nursing care of irradiated skin. *Oncology Nursing Forum* 19, 907–912.

75. Bomford C.K., Kinkler I.H. and Sherriff S.B. (1993). *Walter & Millers Textbook of Radiotherapy: Radiation Physics, Therapy and Oncology,* 5th edition.

76. Dunne-Daly C.F. (1995). Skin and wound care in radiation oncology. *Cancer Nursing* 18, 144–162.

77. Turesson I. and Thames H. (1989). Repair capacity and kinetics of human skin during fractionated radiotherapy: erythema, desquamation and telangiectasia after 3 and 5 years follow up. *Radiotherapy and Oncology* 15, 169–188.

78. Moody M. (1993). Radiation damaged skin: which treatment option and why? *Wound Management Supplement* 4, 86–87.

79. Lawton J. and Twoomey M. (1991). Skin reactions to radiotherapy. *Nursing Standard* 6, 53–54.

80. Wells M. (1995). *The Impact of Radiotherapy to the Head and Neck: A Qualitative Study of Patients After Completion of Treatment.* London: Institute of Cancer Research, Centre for Cancer and Palliative Care Studies, pp. 1–76.

81. Campbell I. and Ilingworth M.H. (1992). Can patients wash during radiotherapy to the breast or chest wall? A randomised controlled trial. *Clinical Oncology* 4, 78–82.

82. Morgan D. (1993). Is there a role for antiseptics? *Journal of Tissue Viability* 3, 80–84.

83. Crane J. (1993). Extending the role of the new hydrogel. *Journal of Tissue Viability* 3, 98–99.

84. Margolin S., Breneman J., Denemn J., LaChapelle P., Weckbach L. and Aron B. (1990). Management of radiation induced moist skin desquamation using hydrocolloid dressing. *Cancer Nursing* 13, 71–80.

85. Decker W.H. and Schwartzman C. (1962). Sexual functioning following treatment for carcinoma of the cervix. *American Journal of Obstetrics and Gynecology* 83, 283.

86. Perez C.A., Fair W.R. and Ihde D.C. (1989). Carcinoma of the prostate. In DeVita V.T., Hellman S. and Rosenberg S. (eds.) *Cancer Principles and Practice of Oncology.* Boston, MA: Jones and Bartlett, pp. 1023–1058.

87. Abbitol M. and Davenport J. (1974). The irradiated vagina. *Obstetrics and Gynaecology* 44, 249–256.

88. Siebel M. and Graves W. (1982). Sexual function after surgery and radiotherapy for cervical carcinoma. *Southern Medical Journal* 75, 11–15.

89. Hubbard J. and Singleton H. (1985). Sexual function of patients after carcinoma of the cervix treatment. *Clinical Obstetrics and Gynaecology* 12, 247–264.

90. Cartwright-Alcarese F. (1995). Addressing sexual dysfunction following radiation therapy for a gynaecologic malignancy. *Oncology Nursing Forum* 22, 1227–1231.

91. Lamb M. (1985). Sexual dysfunction in gynaecological oncology patients. *Seminars in Oncology Nursing* 1, 9–17.

92. Flay L.D. and Matthews J.H. (1995). The effects of radiotherapy and surgery on the sexual function of women treated for cervical cancer. *International Journal of Radiation Oncology, Biology, Physics* 31, 399–404.

93. Dembo A.J. and Thomas G.M. (1994). The ovary. In Cox J.D. (ed.) *Moss Radiation Oncology.* St Louis, MO: Mosby, pp. 712–733.

94. Schover L. (1987). Sexuality and fertility in urologic cancer patients. *Cancer* 60, 553–558.

95. Goldstein I., Feldman M.L., Deckers P., Babayan R. and Krane R. (1984). Radiation associated impotence: a clinical study of its mechanism. *Journal of the American Medical Association* **251**, 903–910.

96. Auchincloss S.S. (1989). Sexual dysfunction in cancer patients: issues in evaluation and treatment. In Holland J.J. and Rowland J.H. (eds.) *Handbook of Psychooncology: The Psychological Care of the Patient with Cancer.* New York: Oxford University Press.

97. Andelusi B. (1980). Coital function after radiotherapy for carcinoma of the cervix uteri. *British Journal of Obstetrics and Gynaecology* **87**, 821–823.

98. Anderson B.L. (1987). Sexual function in women with gynaecological cancer. *Cancer* **60**, 317–323.

99. Schuster E., Unsain A. and Goodwin M. (1982). Nursing practice in human sexuality. *Nursing Clinics of North America* **17**, 345–349.

100. Shell J. (1990). Sexuality for patients with gynaecologic cancer. *Clinical Issues in Perineal Women's Health Nursing* **1**, 479–514.

101. Burke L.M. (1996). Sexual dysfunction following radiotherapy for cervical cancer. *British Journal of Nursing* **5**, 239–244.

102. Glasgow M., Haltin V. and Althausen (1986). *Sexual Response to Cancer.* New York: American Cancer Society.

103. Jenkins B. (1988). Patients' reports of sexual changes after treatment for gynaecological cancer. *Oncology Nursing Forum* **15**, 349–354.

104. Starr B.D. and Weiner M.B. (1981). *The Starr–Weiner Report on Sex and Sexuality in the Mature Years.* New York: McGraw Hill.

105. Bransfield D., Herriot J. and Abbitol A. (1984). A medical chart for information about sexual functioning in cervical cancer. *Radiotherapy and Oncology* **1**, 317–323.

106. Hendry W.F. (1986). Cancer therapy and fertility. In Horwich A. (ed.) *Oncology: A Multidisciplinary Textbook.* London: Chapman and Hall, pp. 213–221.

107. McMullin M. (1992). Holistic care of the patient with cervical cancer. *Nursing Clinics of North America* **27**, 847–858.

108. Capone M.A., Good R.S., Westie K.S. and Jacobson S. (1980). Psychosocial rehabilitation of gynaecological oncology patients. *Psychosocial Medical Rehabilitation* **61**, 364–372.

109. Calman F.M. and Langdon J. (1991). Oral complications of cancer: preventative treatment is vital and many specialities are required. *British Medical Journal* **302**, 485–548.

110. Dreizen S. (1990). Description and incidence of oral complications. *NCI Monographs* **9**, 11–15.

111. Maciejewski B., Zajusz A., Pilecki., Switnicka J., Skladowski K., Orr W. *et al.* (1991). Acute mucositis in the stimulated oral mucosa of patients during radiotherapy for head and neck cancer. *Radiotherapy and Oncology* **22**, 7–11.

112. Squier C.A. (1990). Mucosal alterations. *NCI Monographs* **9**, 169–172.

113. Greenspan D. (1990). Management of salivary dysfunction. *NCI Monographs* **9**, 159–161.

114. Martin M.V. (1993). Irradiation mucositis: a reappraisal. Oral oncology *European Journal of Cancer* **29**(B), 1–2.

115. McIlroy P. (1996). Radiation mucositis: a new approach to prevention and treatment. *European Journal of Cancer Care* **5**, 153–158.

116. Gamble K. (1998). Communication and information: the experience of radiotherapy patients. *European Journal of Cancer Care* **7**, 153–161.

117. Unit T.M. (1995). *Managing Oral Care Problems Throughout the Cancer Illness Trajectory.* London: Cancer Relief Macmillan Fund, The Institute of Cancer Research, The Royal Marsden NHS Trust.

118. Crosby C. (1989). Method in mouth care. *Nursing Times* **85**, 38–41.

119. Davies A.N. and Singer J. (1994). A comparison of artificial saliva and pilocarpine in radiation induced xerostomia. *Journal of Laryngology and Oncology* **108**, 663–665.

120. Leslie M.D. and Glaser M.G. (1993). Impaired salivary gland function after radiotherapy compounded by commonly prescribed medications. *Clinical Oncology* **5**, 290–292.

121. Trinque J. and Meers K. (1992). Oral care of patients receiving radiation therapy to head and neck: practice corner. *Oncology Nursing Forum* **19**, 940–941.

122. Makkonen T., Bostrom P., Vilja P. and Joensuu H. (1994). Sucraflate mouth washing in the prevention of radiation-induced mucositis: a placebo-controlled double-blind randomized study. *International Journal of Radiation Oncology, Biology, Physics* **30**, 177–182.

123. Abdelaal A.A., Barker D.S. and Fergusson M.M. (1987). Treatment for irradiation-induced mucositis. *Lancet* **i**, 97.

CHAPTER THIRTEEN

Endocrine therapies

Deborah Fenlon

The experience of endocrine (or hormone) therapy will depend on the context in which it takes place. For some, hormone treatment has little or no impact on life; others will achieve remission from their disease and so find that their quality of life is greatly improved. Others will find that the benefit they gain from treatment of the disease is countered by significant side-effects, which are of such magnitude that treatment may be considered unacceptable.

The view that society holds of hormones is centred around the sex hormones and is associated with gender. An individual's identity is inextricably linked to being male or female and the sex hormones confer the degree of femininity or masculinity. Within a culture that values and rewards these attributes, there is a fear of altering them by treatment. A man may not be able to think of himself as a man unless he is fully virile, able to have intercourse and to engender children. Masculine attributes such as courage, power, fighting spirit, justice, and technical achievement may be jeopardised or threatened as a result of hormonal treatment. Worse still, hormone therapy may even confer female attributes, such as enlarged breasts and hot flushes.

Femininity is associated with the ability to conceive children. Identity as a woman is tied up in her roles of wife and mother. Femininity is demanded in the way one looks. When a woman's hormones are altered as a result of cancer treatment, she risks losing all of this. Youth, beauty, sexual attractiveness, and mothering may be threatened.

Hormone treatment may result in the loss of the capacity to conceive and the onset of premature symptoms of menopause.

While cancer inspires fear, the very treatments that are offered may strike at the root of an individual's being and cause questions about his or her identity and place in society.

How endocrine therapy works

As long ago as 1616, William Harvey noted that prostatic atrophy occurred after castration and in 1896[1] it was observed that surgical removal of the ovaries of premenopausal women caused regression of breast cancer.

Tumours arising in organs that are normally under endocrine control may be influenced by manipulating hormonal status. This has subsequently been used as the basis for treatment of cancers of the breast, prostate, thyroid, and uterus. Other tumours, such as renal cell carcinoma and malignant melanoma, have shown responses to hormone therapies but they are not widely used in this context. Hormonal treatments, particularly steroids, have also been shown to enhance the effect of chemotherapy.

Endocrine therapy is not normally regarded as a curative treatment. It causes disease regression, but does not eliminate disease altogether. This is probably due to tumours being comprised of mixed cell populations, where some of the cells are sensitive to hormone deprivation and therefore die, while others are not sensitive and grow and spread.

However, where a cancer becomes resistant to one hormone treatment, another treatment may still cause a response, by affecting a different cell population.

Normal physiology

Hormones are chemicals that are produced by endocrine glands and circulate in the body to affect other tissues; they are used to control many different functions in the body. The hormones of most importance in cancer treatment are those produced in the hypothalamus, anterior pituitary, adrenals, and gonads. The hypothalamus governs the activity of the anterior pituitary gland via small polypeptide hormones such as thyrotrophin-releasing hormone (TRH) and luteinising hormone-releasing hormone (LHRH). In response, the anterior pituitary gland produces more complex hormones such as thyroid stimulating hormone (TSH), adrenocorticotrophic hormone (ACTH), follicle stimulating hormones (FSH) and the luteinising hormone (LH). These hormones then stimulate the target gland to produce its own hormones. The thyroid gland releases thyroxin, the adrenal gland produces corticosteroids, and the gonads produce oestrogens or androgens. High levels of end hormones, such as oestrogen, will provide negative feedback and inhibit the activity of the hypothalamus; consequently, the stimulatory system will be switched off so that a constant balance of hormones in the blood stream can be maintained. The purpose of these hormones is to control the growth and maturation of organs such as the breast, uterus, and prostate gland, as well as having more general effects on development and metabolism in the whole body.

Hormone receptors

Hormones exert their effect by acting on individual cells in the target gland. Protein hormones do not enter the cell but bind to receptors on the surface of the cell and the receptor mediates the effect. Steroid hormones do enter the cell but need to combine with cytoplasmic receptors in order to enter the nucleus and exert their effect. Each hormone has its own receptor, which cannot be activated by another hormone and only the tissues that have specific hormone receptors will be affected by that particular hormone. Tumours that have hormone receptors are more likely to be responsive to hormone manipulation.

In breast cancer, the overall response rate to hormone therapies is 30%, and of those that are oestrogen receptor positive (ER +ve) the response rate is 60%.[2] ER +ve tumours are more common in postmenopausal women and are associated with better prognosis, a longer disease-free interval and longer survival. Oestrogen receptor negative tumours are much less likely to respond to hormone treatment but about 10% may have a useful response.

Prostate tissue contains androgen, oestrogen, and progesterone receptors and, as with breast cancer, those with high levels of hormone receptors are more likely to respond to hormonal therapy.

Steroid hormones

The steroid hormones are related to cholesterol and include the sex hormones, such as androgen and oestrogen, and hydrocortisone. Hydrocortisone (cortisol) is produced by the adrenal glands and has an effect on the metabolism of all tissues in the body. Artificial replacements include cortisone (which is converted to hydrocortisone by the liver), prednisolone, dexamethasone, and betamethasone. Androgens are largely made by the testes and oestrogens and progesterone are produced by the ovaries. However, the testes do produce small amounts of oestrogens and the ovaries produce small amounts of androgens, and some sex hormones are also produced in subcutaneous fat under the control of the adrenal gland. Male hormones are involved in the development of male genitalia and body hair (androgenic effect) and the development of muscle and skeletal tissues (anabolic effect). Oestrogens and progesterone are responsible for the development of the breasts and the endometrium and are involved in the control of the processes of menstruation, pregnancy, and lactation.

Clinical use of endocrine therapy

The use of endocrine therapy was largely developed in the treatment of metastatic disease and is still most widely used in this area. Cure is not possible, so the best quality of life is being sought. For many, endocrine therapy can bring about disease regression and relief of symptoms. However, for some the side-effects from treatment are perceived as great, therefore an accurate assessment of the unwanted effects is important when considering whether to continue or to change therapy.

The chance of achieving a response with endocrine therapy varies according to the type of cancer. In breast cancer it is about 30–40%, although with prostate cancer this may be as high as 80%.[3] Where a response is seen to one endocrine treatment, it is more likely that a second-line hormone will also achieve a response, although this decreases with each subsequent treatment. The disease is often slow to respond, so a rapidly progressing illness should be treated with chemotherapy.

Endocrine therapy can also be used in the adjuvant, neo-adjuvant, and preventive setting. A synthetic anti-oestrogen, tamoxifen, is now being given as an adjuvant treatment alongside primary surgery for breast cancer, as it has been demonstrated to delay relapse and prolong survival time.[4]

It has also been suggested that tamoxifen may be able to prevent breast cancer. Evidence from animal data shows that tamoxifen protects mice exposed to a carcinogenic agent from developing breast cancer.[5] The incidence of a second primary breast cancer is reduced in women who received tamoxifen as an adjuvant for a first case of breast cancer.[6] Studies are now underway to investigate the role of tamoxifen in women at high risk of developing breast cancer.[7] Early reports suggest that tamoxifen may reduce the risk of breast cancer in high-risk women by as much as 45%.[8]

Endocrine treatments for different cancer sites

Breast cancer
Clinical and laboratory evidence now supports the theory that oestrogens play a primary role in

Table 13.1 Endocrine treatment for pre-menopausal women with breast cancer

Treatment	Drug name and dose	Mechanism of action	Unwanted effects
Oophorectomy		Decreases oestrogen production by 90% by surgical removal of ovaries.	Menopause, including hot flushes, infertility, dry vagina.
LHRH analogues		Decrease oestrogen production by preventing release of LH.	As above.
Leuprorelin	Prostap (3.75 mg s.c. once per month)		
Goserelin	Zoladex (3.6 mg s.c. once per month)		
Chemotherapy		Suppresses ovarian function.	As above.
Oestrogen antagonists		Oestrogen receptor antagonist.	Hot flushes, weight gain, changes in menstrual flow, thrombosis, endometrial hyperplasia, endometrial cancer,[13] retinopathy, tumour flare.
Tamoxifen	Nolvadex, tamofen (20 mg daily)		
Raloxifene			

Table 13.2 Endocrine treatment for post-menopausal women with breast cancer

Treatment	Drug name and dose	Mechanism of action	Unwanted effects	Notes
Oestrogen antagonists				
– tamoxifen	Nolvadex Tamofen (20 mg daily)	Competitive inhibitor of oestrogen, with some oestrogenic activity.[12]	Hot flushes, weight gain, thrombosis, endometrial hyperplasia, endometrial cancer,[13] retinopathy, tumour flare.	
– toremifene	Fareston (60 mg daily)			
– raloxifene	Evista			
Aromatase inhibitors				
– aminoglutethimide	Orimeten (250 mg daily)	Enzyme inhibition, preventing post-menopausal production of oestrogen.	Lethargy, N&V, skin rash and fever, ataxia[16]	Cortisone production also affected; need to give hydrocortisone replacement.
– trilostane	Modrenal (960 mg daily)		Diarrhoea, abdominal discomfort.	
Aromatase inhibitors				
– formestane	Lentaron (250 mg i.m. every 2 weeks)	As above.	Pain at injection site, rarely dizziness, lethargy, hot flushes.[17]	
– letrozole	Femara (2.5 mg p.o. daily)		Very mild side-effects, possibly arthralgia, fatigue, headache, nausea.[18]	
– anastrozole	Arimidex (1 mg p.o. daily)			
Progestins				
– medroxyprogesterone acetate				
– megestrol acetate	Farlutal, Provera (500 mg daily) Megace (160 mg daily)	Activation of the progesterone receptor affects oestrogen activity.	Stimulate appetite, weight gain, fluid retention, thromboembolic disorders, vaginal bleeding, tremors, sweating, Cushing-like features, muscular cramps, N&V.[19]	
Oestrogens				
– stilboestrol	Stilboestrol (10–20 mg daily)	?Blocking oestrogen receptors or negative feedback on pituitary gland.	Nausea, fluid retention, thrombosis, withdrawal bleeding, tumour flare.	
Androgens				
– testosterone	Viromone (100 mg i.m. 2–3 times per week) Primotestan Depo (250 mg i.m. every 2–3 weeks)	Synthetic hormone with androgenic activity.	Oedema, nausea, dizziness, rash, facial hair, male pattern hair loss, headache, depression, deepening of the voice, increase sebum, increase in libido.	

the maintenance of growth of at least some breast carcinomas.[9] Many endocrine treatments in breast cancer are therefore aimed at either reducing the synthesis of oestrogen or opposing its action (see Tables 13.1 and 13.2). Surgical or radiation oophorectomy reduces oestrogen production by 90%. Ovaries can now be switched off by the use of highly potent synthetic LHRH analogues, which initially stimulate the pituitary to produce LH, causing a rise in oestrogen levels. This may cause a 'flare', or worsening of disease-related symptoms. However, after the initial stimulation of the pituitary, the high potency of these analogues causes overstimulation of the pituitary and no further LH is released so that the ovaries are effectively switched off. This process is reversible, so that if treatment is discontinued ovarian function will return.

Adjuvant chemotherapy often causes inhibition in menstruation and the nearer the woman is to her natural menopause, the less likely it is that her periods will return. Adjuvant chemotherapy has been shown to confer a greater survival benefit on pre-menopausal women than on post-menopausal women[10] and it has been suggested that this added benefit may be due to the suppression of ovarian function caused by chemotherapy.[11]

Anti-oestrogens act by binding to oestrogen receptors, making them unavailable to endogenous oestrogens, without stimulating cell division. Tamoxifen is the major anti-oestrogen. However, it appears that tamoxifen does have some oestrogenic activity,[12] continuing to cause proliferation of the lining of the womb, which may affect menstrual flow in pre-menopausal women. Most pre-menopausal women continue to ovulate and menstruate while on tamoxifen, although women who are near the natural menopause may be 'tipped into it' by tamoxifen. Tamoxifen has also been shown to be associated with a slightly higher incidence of endometrial cancer.[13] For this reason, women should be encouraged to report abnormal bleeding. It has also been suggested that tamoxifen protects against coronary heart disease and osteoporosis.[4,14] Newer, purer anti-oestrogens or selected oestrogen receptors modifiers (SERMs) such as raloxifene and idoxifene, have been identified and their role in the treatment of breast cancer is currently being investigated.[15]

Subsequent to the menopause, some oestrogen is still made in subcutaneous fat under the control of the adrenal gland, by the conversion of androgens by aromatase enzymes. A group of drugs called aromatase inhibitors can prevent these enzymes from working and inhibit the production of post-menopausal oestrogens. However, some of these drugs (e.g. aminoglutethimide) also interfere with enzyme action in the adrenal gland and so corticosteroid replacement is necessary. These drugs also tend to have severe side-effects and so more specific aromatase inhibitors, such as formestane and anastrozole, have been developed, which are associated with very few side-effects.

Other hormones that are effective in breast cancer, such as progestogens and androgens, appear to oppose the action of oestrogen. Androgens are now rarely used owing to the severity of their side-effects. Aromatase inhibitors are now generally preferred to progestogens, although in pre-menopausal women progestogens continue to be the second-line treatment.

Male breast cancer

Breast cancer is much more rare in men than in women, accounting for less than 1% of all breast cancer cases. There are about 170 cases per year in Britain, resulting in about 90 deaths. It also occurs later in life and does not start to appear until the age of 55.

Endocrine therapy is effective in men with metastatic breast cancer. A high percentage of male breast cancers is oestrogen receptor positive and approximately 79% of patients will respond to orchidectomy for an average duration of 30 months.[20] LHRH agonists are usually used in preference to surgery. Tamoxifen and the aromatase inhibitors may also be useful second-line therapies.

Prostate cancer

Prostate cancer is the second most common cancer in men, accounting for 90% of cancer cases in men over the age of 65. In the USA, 132 000 new cases are diagnosed each year,[21] while in the UK in 1988 there were 13 974 new cases.[22] Endocrine therapy in prostate cancer is generally reserved for use in metastatic disease; however, as 50–60% present with metastatic disease, a substantial number will therefore be treated with hormone therapy. Endocrine

Table 13.3 Endocrine treatment for prostate cancer

Treatment	Drug name and dose	Mechanism of action	Unwanted effects
Bilateral orchidectomy		Prevents androgen production.	Loss of sexual drive.
LHRH agonists			
Goserilin	Zoladex (3.6 mg s.c. once per month)	Decrease androgen production by preventing release of LH.	Tumour flare, hot flushes, decreased libido, impotence, depression.
Leuprorelin	Prostap (3.75 mg s.c. once per month)		
Buserilin	Suprefact (500 μg s.c. three times daily for 1 week, then intranasal six times daily)		
Triptorelin	De-capeptyl (3 mg i.m. every 4 weeks)		
Anti-androgens Steroidal:			
Cyproterone	Cyprostat (300 mg daily)	Block androgen receptors and inhibit release of LH.	Hepatotoxicity in long-term use.
Non-steroidal:			
Flutamide	Drogenil (250 mg daily)		Hot flushes, gynaecomastia, and breast tenderness, pruritus and N&V.
Bicalutamide	Casodex (50 mg daily)		
Oestrogens			
Stilboestrol	Stilboestrol (1–3 mg daily)	Reduction in testosterone by negative feedback on the pituitary.	Gynaecomastia, weight gain, fluid retention, N&V, impotence cardiovascular disease, tumour flare.
Fosfestrol	Honvan (100–200 mg daily)		

treatments can achieve a response in 40–80% of men treated.[23] This high response rate makes it the treatment of choice for metastatic prostate cancer. However, as with breast cancer, this does not represent a cure, and most men will subsequently relapse after treatment with endocrine therapy (see Table 13.3).

Over 60 years ago, Huggins and Hodges[24] observed that the prostate gland is dependent on androgens and demonstrated a response in patients with advanced prostatic cancer to orchidectomy. Androgen deprivation can produce symptomatic relief in 80–85% of patients, with a mean duration of response of about 18 months.[25] The use of LHRH analogues suppresses the function of the testes in the same way as ovarian function is suppressed in women, resulting in a medical orchidectomy and depriving the tumour of androgens. After either of these treatments, men will usually lose their sex drive and ability to develop erections. Many will also suffer hot flushes. A smaller num-

ber (one study reported an incidence of 4.8%) will experience breast swelling.[23] LHRH analogues used are buserilin, goserelin, leuprorelin, or triptorelin.

Because of the initial stimulation of the pituitary, up to 5% of patients may suffer an increase in symptoms or 'flare' in the first 1–2 weeks of treatment.[23] The effect of this 'flare' can be blocked by giving an anti-androgen, such as flutamide, for several days before and for 2 weeks after commencing treatment with LHRH analogues.[26]

Following treatment with either LHRH analogues or orchidectomy, testosterone may still be produced by the adrenal glands. This normally constitutes about 5% of circulating testosterone.[21] Anti-androgens may be used to oppose the action of this testosterone: these compete with androgens for binding sites at the androgen receptor in the nucleus of prostate cancer cells.

There are two classes of anti-androgens: the steroidal, such as cyproterone acetate (Cyprostat) and the non-steroidal, such as flutamide (Drogenil), nilutamide, or bicalutamide (Casodex). It is unclear whether the non-steroidal anti-androgens are as effective as castration when they are used as single agents, but they are becoming more widely used because of the chance of retaining sexual function. Side-effects include nausea, vomiting, and gynaecomastia, but sexual function may be maintained. Breast tenderness also occurs.[26] The steroidal anti-androgens not only block androgen receptors, but also inhibit the release of LH, causing a reduction in testosterone production. They may be used as a first-line treatment instead of orchidectomy or LHRH analogues. Sexual potency may also be retained. Side-effects include results of androgen deprivation, and liver dysfunction and fatigue have also been reported.[21]

The administration of oestrogens, such as stilboestrol and fosfestrol tetrasodium (Honvan), causes a reduction in testosterone levels due to negative feedback on the pituitary. There may also be a direct effect as there are oestrogen receptors in the prostate. Oestrogens may therefore be used in place of orchidectomy, but the side-effects are greater, including feminisation (such as gynaecomastia), as well as erectile dysfunction, penile and testicular atrophy, weight gain, fluid retention, nausea, vomiting, and impotence. Anti-coagulation therapy, such as aspirin or low-dose warfarin, may be given to reduce cardiovascular complications. Cardiovascular disease is a major problem with oestrogen therapy, so that oestrogens are now rarely used for prostate cancer. However, for those men who prefer to have an alternative to castration it is one of the options that may be considered.

Corticosteroids may have a use in those who have relapsed after first-line hormonal treatment as they reduce concentrations of ACTH and so interfere with the production of adrenal androgens. Second-line treatments have the much lower response rate of 30% at best.[21]

Endometrial cancer

The primary treatment for cancer of the womb is surgery and radiotherapy. Hormone therapy may be given as an adjuvant treatment, but the evidence to support this is poor and hormone therapy is usually reserved for treatment of metastatic disease. However, endometrial cancer is hormone dependent and responds to progestogens such as medr-oxyprogesterone acetate (100–500 mg daily) or megestrol acetate (40–320 mg daily). Responses to LHRH analogues are also recognised. There is a 20–30% response rate with hormone therapy and useful palliation of metastatic disease may be obtained. Tamoxifen and Danazol may also be useful.

Endocrine tumours and paraneoplastic syndromes

Tumours arising in endocrine glands may cause disturbances to normal hormonal levels, including tumours of the pituitary, thyroid, and adrenal gland (such as phaeochromocytoma) and carcinoid tumours. Treatment is usually by surgery and subsequent replacement and monitoring of hormone levels. Some tumours also produce inappropriate hormones and cause endocrine abnormalities not directly associated with the tumour. This is most common with lung cancer, where 12% produce endocrine abnormalities.[27] The hormones secreted include ACTH, ADH (anti-diuretic hormone) and PTH (parathyroid hormone). These can cause effects such as Cushing's syndrome, hyponatraemia, and hypercalcaemia. Gynaecomastia, hyperthyroidism, and acromegaly may also be seen.

Carcinoid tumours

Carcinoid tumours arise from enterochromaffin cells, which may be scattered throughout the body, but mostly occur in the intestine and the main bronchi. They are often multi-hormonal and secrete hormones such as ACTH, 5-HT (serotonin) and 5-HTP (hydroxytryptophan). Excess levels of these hormones may result in carcinoid syndrome, which is characterised by cutaneous flushing (especially in the face and neck), diarrhoea, wheezing, and valvular heart disease. Where possible the tumour is treated by surgery. Carcinoid syndrome can be treated by the somatostatin analogue octreotide (Sandostatin).

Thyroid cancer

The treatment of thyroid cancer is thyroid ablation, usually by surgery or radiotherapy, followed by physiological hormone replacement therapy. This prevents hypothyroidism and maintains TSH at low levels to minimise the chance of recurrence of a TSH-dependent tumour. Elderly patients who are unfit for surgery and have small, well-differentiated tumours that are dependent on TSH for growth may be treated by thyroxin alone, which inhibits the secretion of TSH by negative feedback control.

Renal cancer

Progestogens can be used in renal cancer with some effect, e.g. medroxyprogesterone acetate in a dose of 100–500 mg daily, but the chance of response is very low and may be less than 10%.

Pituitary adenomas

Tumours arising in the pituitary gland may cause disturbances in normal hormone levels. The pituitary may underfunction, resulting in a lack of growth hormone and gonadotrophins. Pressure on the hypothalamus may result in a lack of regulation of hormones, characterised by an increase in prolactin levels. The tumour cells may secrete excess amounts of hormones, such as growth hormone, prolactin, or ACTH. Treatment is primarily surgical, and will result in lifelong endocrine regulation and hormone replacement therapy.

Corticosteroid hormones

Corticosteroid hormones have an anti-tumour effect and may cause regression of breast cancer. They have a marked effect in acute lymphoblastic leukaemia, Hodgkin's disease, and non-Hodgkin's lymphomas and are sometimes used in conjunction with chemotherapy regimens in order to boost their effectiveness. A more common use in oncology is for acute symptomatic relief or palliative care due to their suppression of inflammatory and allergic disorders. The use of chemotherapy may result in patients requiring support in the form of multiple platelet and blood transfusions and, as a consequence, they are more vulnerable to reactions from transfusion and so hydrocortisone is routinely used to prevent allergic reactions in these patients.

Large doses or prolonged use may exaggerate some of the normal actions of corticosteroids. The mineralocorticoid effects are fluid retention, potassium loss, and hypertension. Glucocorticoid effects include diabetes, osteoporosis, myopathy, transient euphoria followed by depression, muscle wasting, and peptic ulceration. High doses may result in Cushing's syndrome, with moon face, redistribution of body fat, skin striae, and acne. Corticosteroids predispose to infection and they may mask signs and symptoms of infection.

Hydrocortisone is topically active and has a relatively low incidence of side-effects as it is the least active of this group, and is therefore used for inflammatory skin conditions, such as radiation inflammation. Prednisolone is most commonly used by mouth for long-term administration and has few mineralocorticoid effects. Dexamethasone is a very potent anti-inflammatory with virtually no mineralocorticoid effects, making it very useful where fluid retention would cause a problem, such as with cerebral oedema. Symptoms from brain tumours can be rapidly relieved by high doses of dexamethasone. Brain irradiation will initially cause an increase in inflammation and so dexamethasone cover will normally be continued throughout a course of treatment.

Pain control

Corticosteroids act as co-analgesics. That is, they are not true analgesics in the pharmacological sense, but contribute to pain relief by inhibiting production of prostaglandins and thereby reducing inflammation and oedema associated with tumour deposits. They are particularly useful in the treatment of neurological disturbances, such as raised intracranial pressure and brachial plexus damage, and are also effective in treating pain due to bone metastases or where capsular stretching occurs, as with liver disease. Commonly used drugs are prednisolone (30 mg), dexamethasone (4 mg), and hydrocortisone (120 mg).[28] They may also be used to combat difficult pain problems, such as bladder or rectal pain, particularly where there is thought to be a neuropathic component.[29] However, side-effects from long-term use are generally unacceptable, so corticosteroids will usually only be used for short-term pain relief.

Breathlessness

Because of their anti-inflammatory action, corticosteroids also have a useful role to play in relieving the distress caused by breathlessness. They can reduce problems such as airways obstruction, tracheal tumour that causes stridor, lymphangitis carcinomatosis, pneumonitis, and SVC obstruction.[30]

Nausea and vomiting

The anti-emetic activity of steroids is unexplained, but may have a direct effect on the vomiting centre in the brain stem. It is particularly useful for chemotherapy-related nausea or where nausea is associated with hepatic involvement. It is best used in conjunction with other anti-emetic agents as it enhances their effects.[31]

Other uses include the treatment of hypercalcaemia, stimulating the appetite, and a general improvement in mood and malaise.[32] The wide application of corticosteroids makes them very useful agents in the control of advanced disease; however, their toxicity can be severe in the long term, so they should be used with caution. Many of the beneficial effects are also short lived, so steroids should only be used for short periods. Patients taking high doses of steroids for acute episodes may also suffer a number of changes, which may be distressing. The typical round cheeks of the cushingoid syndrome are a marked feature, which can be very noticeable and, in the eyes of the patient, a significant indicator of severe disease.

Problems faced by women having endocrine treatment

Many women are very aware of hormonal changes in their body as they have been accustomed to marking the changes caused by the menstrual cycle. They are familiar with the 'bloating' effect of progesterone due to fluid retention prior to menstruation and the nausea and increased appetite during pregnancy. They are aware that significant body changes take place as a result of hormone changes, such as changes in the skin and hair, fluctuations in weight, and changes in the distribution of body fat. These changes are often unwelcome in the normal course of life and many women may, therefore, anticipate difficulties in adjusting to hormone therapies and will be looking for familiar signs.

Within current Western society, images of what is thought to be beautiful are conveyed powerfully and constantly by the media. Fashion magazines give an endless flow of advice to women about how to maintain their hair, skin, and 'youthful looks'. The 'body beautiful' is young, sexy, and thin. Hormone therapies affect every part of this image. Those that induce the menopause bring signs of ageing; many will reduce libido, induce vaginal discharge, bleeding or dryness, and a frequent side-effect is weight gain. Some therapies may even induce masculinising changes, such as facial hair and hair loss from the head. At the same time as affecting a woman's self-image and self-esteem, her role as wife, lover, or mother is also affected. The experience of cancer itself may make a woman less fit and physically able to undertake her normal activities in life and, in addition to this, hormone therapy may render her infertile, interfere with her sexuality, or affect her relationship with her partner.

For many women, the relief from symptoms caused by the disease may make hormone therapy well accepted. For others, especially those having hormone therapy as adjuvant treatment, the side-effects may be much more unacceptable and these problems may easily be underestimated by medical staff.

Menopause

Canney and Hatton[33] have shown that 70% of women under the age of 65 having adjuvant treatment for breast cancer will experience menopausal symptoms. From many studies it has been shown that chemotherapy given as an adjuvant treatment to surgery can decrease mortality. Therefore, it is now normal practice for most women in this group to be offered chemotherapy, especially in the presence of poor prognostic factors, such as the grade of tumour and the presence of affected lymph nodes. Chemotherapy will suppress ovarian function and, for most women, menstruation will cease altogether. Menopause induced in this way will have the same effects in terms of hot flushes, night sweats, vaginal dryness, and other problems associated with a normal menopause, and it is possible that a suddenly precipitated menopause may be associated with more symptoms than a normal one.[34]

As oestrogen is thought to have a part to play in stimulating the growth of breast cancer, many pre-menopausal women are offered oophorectomy, or drug-induced suppression of the ovaries, which will also induce the menopause. The drugs used would be LHRH agonists such as leuprorelin. Even for post-menopausal women there is the chance of suffering menopausal symptoms. Those that have been taking hormone replacement therapy (HRT) will be advised to stop, with the consequence that menopausal problems may return. Tamoxifen is widely used as an adjuvant treatment in this group owing to its efficacy in reducing mortality[6] and its principal side-effect is hot flushes.[7] For women who are having a combination of chemotherapy and tamoxifen, it is very difficult to separate out the causes of their symptoms and it is possible that the symptoms may even be exacerbated.

Experience of menopause

The experience of menopause is a very different transition for each woman. For some it is a time of major role change, when children are leaving home, and the menopause is a reminder of ageing, which may make them feel less attractive as a sexual partner. For others, it is dominated by physical effects such as hot flushes and night sweats, which interfere with their lives and make them feel unwell. The medical response has been to regard the change as abnormal, a cessation of normal function, and therefore a condition to be treated with medication. Many women find that there is a dearth of information to help them to adjust or even to know what they should expect as normal. However, it has been suggested that the menopause should, more constructively, be considered as a complex event, with physical, psychological, and social components, and that peri-menopausal distress has many causes.[35] The following is an account illustrating one woman's experience of menopause induced by cancer treatment:

> Whilst I was having the chemo and for a couple of months after it was absolutely dreadful . . . . I was tremendously cold all the time, in fact this is a feature of it, I got very, very cold before I started sweating . . . I had been sitting on the side of the bed from one o'clock that morning and it went on to five o'clock and I couldn't get dry. I was in a towel and I literally could not – it was just wave after wave of sweating and I was frozen. It was not hot sweats, now I'm getting hot sweats and um I think that helps because obviously your skin is warm and it cools your skin off . . . I went to bed in the end in towels ummm . . . couldn't wear night clothes because they would get absolutely soaking.

Hot flushes/night sweats

In a normal menopause up to 80% of women suffer from hot flushes.[36] One study showed the number of flushes to range from two to 247 per day,

with 87% being perceived as mild or moderate and only 13% perceived as severe.[37] There is no literature to describe whether drug-induced menopause or flushes are any different. However, Feldman[38] showed that 92% of women suffered hot flushes if they had undergone a surgical menopause. Some women find that the daytime flushes are quite bearable, but that being woken many times during the night soaked in sweat is much more distressing.

Images of ageing

As part of the 'beauty myth', old age is dreaded by many women in Western society. As Simone de Beauvoir[39] said, 'old age looms ahead of us like a calamity'. Menopause is regarded by many as the time when old age starts and that the resulting changes will rapidly appear as soon as oestrogen levels are depleted. With this kind of image in a woman's mind as she is being offered treatment that brings about menopause, it is not surprising if she thinks twice about the necessity of such a treatment.

A medical description of post-menopausal changes runs as follows:

> After menopause . . . the breasts begin to shrivel and sag . . . the breasts become pendulous, wrinkled and flabby. Often the skin of the breasts coarsens and is covered with scales. The breasts lose their erotic sensitivity and sometimes do not respond to pain stimuli. Only timely oestrogen can prevent this premature decline of a woman's symbol of femininity.[40]

Infertility

Endocrine therapies, which are designed to bring about menopause and consequently cause infertility, include oophorectomy and the use of LHRH analogues. Chemotherapy may also bring about an early menopause. Some of these changes are reversible and others are not. Initially it is not possible to know whether a woman has been rendered infertile and so it is important to advise the continued use of contraception. Barrier methods must be used as the contraceptive pill may interfere with the action of the endocrine treatments. It is important to consider whether the loss of fertility is an issue for the woman and to take this into consideration when commencing treatment.

Interventions for menopausal symptoms

Hormone replacement therapy

There is some confusion as to whether it is safe to give HRT to women who have had breast cancer. HRT of combined oestrogen and progestin has been associated with a slightly increased risk of causing breast cancer.[41] Other studies do not show this increased risk.[42] However, a meta-analysis suggests that HRT could promote breast cancer[43] and recent reviews support this view.[44] While there is some uncertainty of the place of HRT in causing breast cancer, its role in women who have already had breast cancer is even more uncertain. It is received wisdom that it is contraindicated, as it is known that low doses of oestrogen stimulate the growth of breast cancer.[45] However, there is no evidence about how combinations of oestrogen and progesterone affect breast cancer cells. Scientists are now beginning to postulate theories as to the safe use of HRT in breast cancer patients[46] and studies are emerging to investigate this area.[47]

Other drugs therapies for the relief of hot flushes

The most effective treatment to relieve menopausal symptoms is HRT, although this does not always bring complete relief. Other medications, such as clonidine, propanolol, phenobarbitones, bromocriptine, and naloxone, have been proposed, but are not generally very effective, and are associated with side-effects that may make them unacceptable.[48,49] Megestrol acetate has been shown to be effective to control hot flushes; however, the safety of its use in women with breast cancer has been questioned and is not widely used.[50] It has been suggested that cessation of smoking may help.[51]

Alternative therapies for the relief of hot flushes

Menopause is clearly an event that is experienced in many different ways and cannot be reduced to one single physical cause. It is likely that women will find relief in different ways, so that helping to explore what menopause means and discussing different strategies to cope with it will enable each woman to find her own way of coping. Stress can cause a woman to suffer from more hot flushes[52,53] and there is some evidence to suggest that practising relaxation methods can help to reduce the number and intensity of hot flushes suffered.[54] There may be a simple physiological cause and effect being demonstrated here or it may be a more complex mixture of psychological and physiological effects. Other alternative remedies, such as acupuncture and homeopathy, have been suggested. Gannon et al.[52] showed an increase in hot flush activity with alcohol consumption. Other dietary recommendations are reducing caffeine and increasing vitamin E and B intake.[55,56] Herbal remedies include evening primrose oil, ginseng, and dong quai.[57] Ginseng and dong quai contain plant hormones and may be contraindicated.

Practical measures for the relief of hot flushes

Helping a woman to talk through her experience of hot flushes may help her to put them into context with her life and make the experience more bearable. Many have no idea what to expect as 'normal' and what to attribute to their disease, their treatment, or the menopause. For example, formication (a crawling sensation under the skin of the upper chest) may be taken to be cancer recurrence or the result of chemotherapy working against cancer. It may also help to discuss how the woman copes with the flushes when they occur. For example, many find that they pass more easily if they sit down and relax instead of trying to fight it. Simple measures such as layered clothing, particularly cotton to help absorb excess moisture, fans, and scented sprays or wipes may all help to alleviate discomfort.

One woman's experience of menopausal symptoms was described in the following terms:

> In fact she decided that it was a little like New York City summer heat: the more you fought against it, the worse it became. The only thing to do was to surrender yourself to it totally, let it flow through you.[58]

A summary of strategies to help with problems induced by hormone therapies is shown in Table 13.4.

Other problems for women on hormonal therapies

Changes in mood state

Alterations in hormones can have a profound effect on mood state. An increase in progesterone or testosterone will cause an initial feeling of well-being. This can be useful in the terminal stages of disease, but is not generally useful otherwise, owing to the effect being short-lived. Other changes, particularly a reduction in testosterone, may cause depression. This has also been noted with the use of some of the aromatase inhibitors. There is a general belief that menopause can cause depression, although it is unclear whether this is due to biological changes or whether it is largely the result of concurrent changes in lifestyle. This time of life is often associated with children gaining independence and, for women who have adopted the role of wife and mother as their major role in life, this can be a blow to their self-esteem. Individuals who perceive that their bodies are changing and becoming less attractive due to hormonal therapies, may also suffer from lowered self-esteem and this too can result in depression. For both men and women these difficulties may be secondary to concerns about cancer and their mortality, but they may all contribute to a depressive state. It is important to assess an individual who suffers from depression carefully and to note whether this coincides with commencing hormone therapy, as for some it may be a major contributory factor.

Weight gain

Progestins and steroids can cause weight gain, which can be difficult to control as they are associated with an increased appetite as well as fluid retention. The increased gain in weight is often seen in a cushingoid distribution, with the typical 'moon face'. This may be distressing in the way it alters appearance. Tamoxifen has also been connected with weight gain, but the causes are unclear. It has been demonstrated that a high percentage of women treated for breast cancer with chemotherapy, with or without tamoxifen, gain weight, while those on tamoxifen gain more weight.[59,60] Premenopausal women put on more weight (3–4 kg) than post-menopausal women (1–2 kg). Part of the explanation for women with breast cancer may be a change in lifestyle, since after a cancer diagnosis, women may take less exercise and are less rigorous about dieting. Many women search for ways in which they can regain control over their lives after breast cancer and advice about diet can help in this area. When giving advice, it is important to help women look not only at what they eat, but also at

what else is happening in their lives and what physical activity they are able to undertake. However, it is also possible for women to feel guilty if they are unable to keep their weight at their accepted norm. If it is not acknowledged that tamoxifen contributes to this gain, then this may be perceived as another burden to bear.

Vaginal bleeding

Vaginal bleeding is reported as the most distressing side-effect of hormonal therapy, followed by weight gain and hot flushes.[61] It is not known whether this distress is found only when patients are not warned that bleeding is a possibility, as they will then be concerned about the cause. Tamoxifen can cause irregular periods in pre-menopausal women – either heavier or lighter – and can induce a discharge or bleeding in post-menopausal women. Progestins and oestrogens can also cause bleeding. Some hormones are associated with a withdrawal bleed, so that women should be warned about the possibility of bleeding as they discontinue the drug. Abnormal bleeding may be a sign of gynaecological cancers and tamoxifen can cause a slight increase in the incidence of endometrial cancer.[13,62] For this reason, women need to be warned about the possibility of unusual bleeding and to report this to their doctor.

Sexuality

Combined with a loss of confidence and self-esteem following cancer diagnosis and treatment, physical changes may also occur which affect sexuality. Ganz et al.[63] have demonstrated poorer sexual functioning in breast cancer survivors whose therapy has caused them to stop menstruating. Reduction in oestrogen may cause a decreased libido, although this is gradual. This may exacerbate the effects of treatments such as chemotherapy or surgery. Loss of oestrogen also results in more fragile, less well lubricated vaginal mucosa and may be accompanied by irritation or itching. For some women the change in the acid balance of the vagina can lead to an increase in infections, such as thrush (*Candida albicans*). Over a period of time the vagina becomes shorter and narrower.

One woman's comments on her experience of sex after hormonal treatments were as follows:

Table 13.4 Strategies to help with problems induced by hormone treatments

Problem	Strategy
Hot flushes	• Reduce trigger factors (e.g. alcohol, spicy food, hot drinks) • Wear thin layers of adjustable cotton clothing and bed linen • Carry a small electric fan, cooling wipes, or spray • Reduce smoking • Regular gentle exercise • Utilise coping strategies, such as distraction • Practise relaxation • Dietary supplements, such as vitamin B and E, evening primrose oil • Complementary medicine (e.g. homeopathy, acupuncture) • HRT as advised by physician • Clonidine
Weight gain	• Advice regarding changing lifestyle following cancer diagnosis • Encourage appropriate exercise • Reduce diet (refer to dietician if required)
Female sexual difficulties Dry and/or painful vagina	• Increase foreplay to increase lubrication • Recommend continued sexual activity to prevent narrowing of the vagina • Suggest that woman adopt superior position to increase comfort • External lubricants, such as K-Y jelly, Senselle, Replens[64] • Oestrogen creams (may not be advised due to absorption of oestrogen)
Itchy vagina	• Exclude and treat infection, such as *Candida albicans* • External lubricants, such as K-Y jelly, Senselle, Replens[64]
Male sexual difficulties Inability to achieve erection	• Consider use of phentolamine/papaverine injection into base of penis[65] • Alprostadil (MUSE, Caverject, Viridal) may also be given by intra-urethral application • Consider vacuum therapy – using vacuum cylinder to mimic natural process of creating and maintaining an erection[66] • Consult with physician re penile implants
Partial erection	• Viagra (Sildenafil) is now available • Try new coital positions, e.g. place a pillow under partner's hips to elevate pelvis and allow for easier penetration • Massage the penis – pressure on the major blood vessels will hold blood in the penis

I know all the way through he was absolutely wonderful, but when it came to any sexual activity I don't think he fancied me very much. I really don't and I've put on a lot of weight. He's not a man to push himself forward any way too much so er . . . it affected me, I mean it still does, I still have no libido. And I've had thrush and all sorts of things you know which I'm trying to get rid of at the moment and that doesn't help much either.

If one or other partner finds it a problem then it is a problem, but if you've both adjusted then it's not. The vagina is dryer. It takes longer to be comfortable. One is getting older.

Tumour flare

Some drugs may cause an initial worsening of symptoms, known as a 'tumour flare'. This is particularly important for those with bone disease. Initially bone pain may become more severe, but bone destruction can result in hypercalcaemia or spinal cord compression. Individuals at risk should be warned of relevant symptoms and watched carefully for these problems.

Much of the nursing care required for women facing these problems is rooted in helping to give realistic information about what they should expect, what is 'normal', and what practical measures they might be able to implement to help. However, listening and talking through their difficulties may provide a positive focus for improving very difficult problems.

Problems faced by men having endocrine treatment

Many of the problems for men are similar to those faced by women. For those with breast cancer there may also be the added stigmatisation of suffering from a 'female' disease, as well as the feminising effects that can occur with some of the treatments.

Alterations in sexuality

Lion[67] has defined sexuality as:

> . . . all those aspects of the human being that relate to being woman or man, and is an entity subject to lifelong dynamic change. Sexuality reflects our human character, not solely our genital nature.

Therefore, in caring for a man having treatment that will affect his sexuality, it is important to consider both his ability to perform the sexual act and his feelings about sexuality, which are closely aligned to masculinity. Hormonal treatments or surgical interventions such as orchidectomy and prostatectomy not only directly affect the ability to function sexually (for example, the ability to have an erection) but are also profoundly threatening to masculinity, self-image and esteem.

Hormonal treatments can have feminising effects. Loss of androgens, or treatment by oestrogen, can cause development of the breasts and the reduction in body and facial hair. Little research appears to have been done on how this may make a man feel; however, it is suggested that that this

may be construed as a further insult to his masculinity and self-esteem.

The research that has been conducted in this area has largely been carried out in men who have had orchidectomy for testicular cancer. In this case only the affected testis is removed and therefore sexual functioning is unlikely to be affected. For these men the priority was shown to be one of having their cancer treated, while issues of fertility and sexuality were secondary, although some did express concern about losing their manhood.[68] However, even among testicular cancer survivors it has been shown that a significant proportion suffers treatable sexual problems long after treatment has been discontinued.[69]

Where men have undergone radical prostatectomy for prostate cancer, it may be assumed that they have already lost sexual function. However, nerve-sparing techniques have reduced the incidence of impotence from nearly 100% to about 32%.[69]

By offering information about sexuality and fertility, without waiting for the subject to be raised, nurses can help men to talk over problems that may be worrying. They can also help to redefine sexuality in broader terms, such as sharing, communication, and intimacy. Nurses may also be able to help consider choices about treatment that may affect sexuality. For example, given the choice, most men would prefer castration through drug treatment rather than surgical removal of the testes, although many who are suffering symptoms choose the surgery, since relief of symptoms may be achieved more quickly.[70] Where symptoms are severe, such as spinal cord compression due to bone metastases, it may be considered necessary for surgical intervention to obtain a speedy response. In the absence of severe disease, one approach could be to use medical treatment to ascertain whether a hormonal response is likely, and follow up with surgical treatment if it proves to be effective. For those where there is no response, surgery would be spared and the effects of hormonal treatment could be reversed. Since the majority of patients with prostate cancer is elderly it is often assumed that sexuality is not an issue for them. This assumption is erroneous; the elderly can enjoy continued sexual interest, function, and satisfaction until the end of life[71] and hormonal therapies have a profound effect on sexual function, which should not be dismissed.

Hot flushes

Hot flushes have been reported to occur in over 75% of men who have undergone orchidectomy and these interfere with their quality of life.[72] This may be relieved by oestrogen therapy or cyproterone acetate, an anti-androgen with progestogen properties. It has also been shown that megestrol acetate can reduce the incidence of hot flushes by 50% or more in 74% of sufferers.[50]

Infertility

The assumption may often be made that as prostate cancer occurs in the older age group, most men with prostate cancer will not wish to father children. However, it is not uncommon for older men to marry women considerably younger than themselves and so the possibility of preservation of sperm should not be dismissed. The threat of loss of fertility is also an issue for men whenever this occurs, even when they have had children, just as it is for women. Since men do not usually completely lose their fertility even into old age, this loss may be difficult.

Conclusion

Endocrine therapy can bring about useful palliation of symptoms and, in breast cancer, has a role to play in early disease. In general, it is regarded as non-toxic and easily tolerated, bringing about symptom relief in many. The side-effects that do occur may be made tolerable by information, understanding, and appropriate intervention. However, it is important to remember that the perception of what is tolerable will be moderated by the knowledge that this treatment cannot cure and that the disease will inevitably return, with or without treatment.

References

1. Beatson G.T. (1989). On the treatment of inoperable cases of carcinoma of the mamma: suggestions for a new method of treatment with illustrative cases. *Cancer Journal* **2**, 303–306.
2. Powles T.J. (1983). The role of aromatase inhibitors in breast cancer. *Seminars in Oncology* **10**, Suppl. 4, 4.
3. Hardy J. (1995). Endocrine therapy in advanced malignancy. *European Journal of Palliative Care* **2**, 151–154.
4. Medical Research Council Scottish Trials Office (1987). Adjuvant tamoxifen in the management of operable breast cancer: the Scottish trial. *Lancet* **ii**, 171–175.
5. Jordan V.C. (1986). *Estrogen/Antiestrogen Action and Breast Cancer Therapy.* Madison, MA: Wisconsin Press.
6. Early Breast Cancer Trialists Collaborative Group (1988). Effects of adjuvant tamoxifen and cytotoxic therapy on mortality in early breast cancer. An overview of 61 randomized trials among 28,896 women. *New England Journal of Medicine* **319**, 1681–1692.
7. Powles T.J., Jones A., Ashley S. *et al.* (1994). The Royal Marsden Hospital pilot tamoxifen chemoprevention trial. *Breast Cancer Research and Treatment* **31**, 73–82.
8. Smigel K. (1998). Breast cancer prevention trial shows major benefit, some risk. *Journal of the National Cancer Institute* **90**, 647–648.
9. Dowsett M. (1991). Reproductive endocrinology and endocrine effects of therapy. In Powles T.J. and Smith I.E. (eds.) *Medical Management of Breast Cancer.* London: Martin Dunitz.
10. Padmanabhan N., Howell A. and Rubens R.D. (1986). Mechanisms of action of adjuvant chemotherapy in early breast cancer. *Lancet* **ii**, 411–414.
11. Baum M. and Afifi R. (1991). Adjuvant endocrine therapy. In Powles T.J. and Smith I.E. (eds.) *Medical Management of Breast Cancer.* London: Dunitz.
12. Jackson I.M., Litherland S. and Wakeling A.E. (1991). Tamoxifen and other antioestrogens. In Powles T.J. and Smith I.E. (eds.) *Medical Management of Breast Cancer.* London: Dunitz.
13. Fornander T., Rutqvist L.E. and Cedermark B. (1989). Adjuvant tamoxifen in early breast cancer: occurrence of new primary cancers. *Lancet* **i**, 117–120.
14. Costantino J.P., Kuller L., Ives D., Fisher B. and Dignam J. (1997). Coronary heart disease mortality and adjuvant tamoxifen therapy. *Journal of the National Cancer Institute* **89**, 776–782.
15. Pace P., Jarman M., Phillips D., Hewer A., Bliss J. and Coombes R. (1997). Idoxifene is equipotent to tamoxifen in inhibiting mammary carcinogenesis but forms lower levels of hepatic DNA adducts. *British Journal of Cancer* **76**, 700–704.
16. Coombes R.C., Powles T.J. and Easton D. (1987). Adjuvant aminoglutethimide therapy for postmenopausal patients with primary breast cancer. *Cancer Research* **47**, 2496–2499.
17. Coombes R.C. (1991). Clinical studies with 4-hydroxy-androstenedione in advanced breast cancer. In Coombes R.C. and Dowsett M. (eds.) *4-Hydroxyandrostenedione – A New Approach to Hormone Dependent Cancer.* London: Royal Society of Medicine Services.
18. Dombernowsky P., Smith I., Falkson G. *et al.* (1998). Letrozole, a new oral inhibitor for advanced breast cancer: double-blind randomized trial showing a dose effect and improved efficacy and tolerability compared with megestrol acetate. *Journal of Clinical Oncology* **16**, 453–461.

19. Pannuti F., Martoni A., Zamagni C. and Melotti B. (1991). Progestins I: medroxyprogesterone acetate. In Powles T.J. and Smith I.E. (eds.) *Medical Management of Breast Cancer.* London: Dunitz.

20. Judson I. and Powles T.J. (1988). Endocrine therapy. In Tiffany R. (ed.) *Oncology for Nurses and Health Care Professionals*, Vol. 1, *Pathology, Diagnosis and Treatment,* 2nd edition. Beaconsfield: Harper and Row.

21. Dearnaley D. (1994). Cancer of the prostate. *British Medical Journal* **308**, 780–784.

22. Cancer Research Campaign (1996). Factsheet 3.1.

23. Denis L. (1993). Prostate cancer: primary hormonal treatment. *Cancer* **71**, 1050–1058.

24. Huggins C. and Hodges C.V. (1941). Studies on prostatic cancer. I. The effects of castration, or of oestrogen and of androgen injection on serum phosphatases in metastatic carcinoma of the prostate gland. *Cancer Research* **1**, 293–297.

25. Shearer R. and Davies J.H. (1991). Studies in prostatic cancer with 4-hydroxyandrostenedione. In Coombes R.C. and Dowsett M. (eds.) *4-Hydroxyandrostenedione – A New Approach to Hormone Dependent Cancer.* London: Royal Society of Medicine Services.

26. McLeod D. (1993). Antiandrogen drugs. *Cancer* **71**, 1046–1049.

27. Bunn P. and Ridgeway E.C. (1989). Paraneoplastic syndromes. In De Vita V., Hellman S. and Rosenberg S. (eds.) *Principles and Practice of Oncology,* 3rd edition. Philadelphia, PA: Lippincott.

28. De Conno F. and Foley K. (1995). *Cancer Pain Relief: A Practical Manual.* Dordrecht: Kluwer.

29. Hanks G., Portenoy R., MacDonald N. and O'Neill R. (1993). Difficult pain problems. In Doyle D., Hanks G. and MacDonald N. (eds.) *The Oxford Textbook of Palliative Medicine.* Oxford: Oxford University Press.

30. Ahmedzai S. (1993). Palliation of respiratory symptoms. In Doyle D., Hanks G. and MacDonald N. (eds.) *The Oxford Textbook of Palliative Medicine.* Oxford: Oxford University Press.

31. Allen S. (1993). Nausea and vomiting. In Doyle D., Hanks G. and MacDonald N. (eds.) *The Oxford Textbook of Palliative Medicine.* Oxford: Oxford University Press.

32. Portenoy R. (1993). Adjuvant analgesics in pain management. In Doyle D., Hanks G. and MacDonald N. (eds.) *The Oxford Textbook of Palliative Medicine.* Oxford: Oxford University Press.

33. Canney P. and Hatton M.Q.F. (1994). The prevalence of menopausal symptoms in patients treated for breast cancer. *Clinical Oncology* **6**, 297–299.

34. Chakravarti S., Collins W.P., Newton J.R., Oram D.H. and Studd J.W. (1977). Endocrine changes and symptomatology after oophorectomy in pre-menopausal

women. *British Journal of Obstetric Gynaecology* **84**, 769–775.

35. Fugate Woods N. (1982). Menopausal distress: a model for epidemiological investigation. In Voda A.M. (ed.) *Changing Perspectives on Menopause.* Austin, TX: University of Texas Press.

36. Levine-Silverman S. (1989). The menopausal hot flush; a procrustean bed of research. *Journal of Advanced Nursing* **14**, 939–949.

37. Voda A.M. (1981). Climacteric hot flush. *Maturitas* **3**, 73–90.

38. Feldman M.F., Voda A. and Gronseth E. (1985). The prevalence of hot flush and associated variables among perimenopausal women. *Research in Nursing and Health* **8**, 261–268. Oxford: Oxford University Press.

39. De Beauvoir, S. (1970). *Old Age.* London: Penguin Books.

40. Wilson R.A. (1966). *Feminine Forever.* London: W.H. Allen.

41. Bergqvist L., Adami H.O., Persson I., Hoover R. and Schairer C. (1989). The risk of breast cancer after estrogen and estrogen–progestin replacement. *New England Journal of Medicine* **321**, 293–297.

42. Nachtigall M., Smilen S., Nachtigall R.D., Nachtigall R.H. and Nachtigall L. (1992). Incidence of breast cancer in a 22-year study of women receiving estrogen–progestin replacement therapy. *Obstetrics and Gynecology* **80**, 827–830.

43. Sillero-Arenas M., Delgado-Rodriguez M., Rodigues-Canteras R., Bueno-Cavanillas A. and Galvez-Vargas R. (1992). Menopausal hormone replacement therapy and breast cancer: a meta-analysis. *Obstetrics and Gynecology* **79**, 286–294.

44. Colditz G. (1998). Relationship between estrogen levels, use of hormone replacement therapy, and breast cancer. *Journal of the National Cancer Institute* **90**, 814–823.

45. Powles T.J. (1988). Treatment of menopausal symptoms in breast cancer patients. *Lancet* **ii**, 345.

46. Stoll B.A. (1990). Hormone replacement therapy for women with a past history of breast cancer. *Clinical Oncology* **2**, 309.

47. Marsden J. and Sacks N. (1997). Hormone replacement therapy and breast cancer. *Endocrine Related Cancer* **4**, 269–279.

48. Laufer L.R., Erlik Y. and Meldrum D.R. (1982). Effect of clonidine on hot flushes in postmenopausal women. *Obstetrics and Gynecology* **60**, 583–586.

49. Lichtman R. (1991). Perimenopausal hormone replacement therapy: a review of the literature. *Journal of Nurse-Midwifery* **36**, 30–46.

50. Loprinzi C., Michalak J., Quella S. *et al.* (1994). Megestrol acetate for the prevention of hot flushes. *New England Journal of Medicine* **331**, 347–352.

51. Greenwood S. (1987). *Menopause the Natural Way: Looking Forward to the Future.* London: MacDonald Optima.

52. Gannon L., Hansel S. and Goodwin J. (1987). Correlates of menopausal hot flushes. *Journal of Behavioural Medicine* **10**, 277–286.

53. Swartzman L., Edelberg R. and Kemmann E. (1990). Impact of stress on objectively recorded menopausal hot flushes and on flush report bias. *Health Psychology* **9**, 529–545.

54. Germaine L.M. and Freedman R.R. (1984). Behavioural treatment of menopausal hot flushes: evaluation by objective measurements. *Journal of Consulting and Clinical Psychology* **52**, 1072–1079.

55. Scharbo-DeHaan M. and Brucker M. (1991). The Perimenopausal period: implications for nurse-midwifery practice. *Journal of Nurse-Midwifery* **36**, 9–16.

56. Barton D., Loprinzi C., Quella S. *et al.* (1998). Prospective evaluation of vitamin E for hot flushes in breast cancer survivors. *Journal of Clinical Oncology* **16**, 495–500.

57. Davis P. (1993). *A Change for the Better: A Woman's Guide through the Menopause.* Saffron Walden: C.W. Daniel.

58. Sands G. (1993). *Is It Hot In Here or Is It Me?* London: Bloomsbury.

59. Demark-Wahnefried W., Winer E. and Rimer B. (1993). Why women gain weight with adjuvant chemotherapy for breast cancer. *Journal of Clinical Oncology* **11**, 1418–1429.

60. Hoskin P., Ashley S. and Yarnold J. (1992). Weight gain after primary surgery for breast cancer – effect of tamoxifen. *Breast Cancer Research and Treatment* **22**, 129–132.

61. Leonard R.C.F. and Lee L. (1995). *Choice of endocrine treatment for advanced breast cancer: clinicians and patients perspectives.* Fourth Nottingham International Breast Cancer Conference, Zeneca.

62. Stearns V. and Gelmann E. (1998). Does tamoxifen cause cancer in humans? *Journal of Clinical Oncology* **16**, 779–792.

63. Ganz P., Rowland J., Desmond K., Meyerowitz B. and Wyatt G. (1998). Life after breast cancer: understanding women's health-related quality of life and sexual functioning. *Journal of Clinical Oncology* **16**, 501–514.

64. Loprinzi C., Abu-Ghazaleh S. and Sloan J. (1997). Phase III randomized double-blind study to evaluate the efficacy of a polycarbophil-based vaginal moisturizer in women with breast cancer. *Journal of Clinical Oncology* **16**, 969–973.

65. Floth A. and Schramek P. (1991). Intracavernous injection of prostaglandin E, in combination with papaverine: enhanced effectiveness in comparison with papaverine plus phentolamine and prostaglandin E alone. *Journal of Urology* **145**, 56–59.

66. Nadig P.W. (1990). Vacuum erection devices: a review. *World Journal of Urology* **8**, 114–117.

67. Lion E.M. (1982). *Human Sexuality in Nursing Process.* New York: John Wiley.

68. Jones L. and Webb C. (1994). Young men's experiences of testicular cancer. In Webb C. (ed.) *Living Sexuality: Issues for Nursing and Health.* London: Scutari Press.

69. Ofman U. (1993). Psychosocial and sexual implications of genitourinary cancers. *Seminars in Oncology Nursing* **9**, 286–292.

70. Chadwick D., Gillatt D. and Gingell J. (1991). Medical of surgical orchidectomy: the patients' choice. *British Medical Journal* **302**, 572.

71. Butler R.N. and Lewis M.I. (1987). Myths and realities of sex in the later years. *Provider* **13**, 11–13.

72. Charig C.R. and Rundle J.S. (1989). Flushing. Long-term side effect of orchiectomy in treatment of prostatic carcinoma. *Urology* **33**, 175–178.

CHAPTER FOURTEEN

Complementary therapies

Nicola Beech

Complementary and alternative therapies are increasingly used in promoting health and well-being and in managing some minor illnesses, as well as major illnesses such as cancer. Indeed, a vast and growing parallel system of individually assessed and frequently self-managed alternative health practices exists, which is undocumented and largely unknown (or only partially known) to conventional care and treatment services.

As the British Medical Association[1] acknowledges, adult citizens are entitled and choose to make choices and decisions as to the form and manner of health care they receive. Increasing demand and utilisation of alternative and complementary therapies may be due in part to the changing health and social needs of society. Illnesses are often more chronic in nature, due to improvements in methods and efficiency of treatment. Similarly, illness may often be caused or exacerbated by societal or environmental factors, such as the effect of pollution on asthma, or the link between inadequate dietary fibre intake and colorectal cancer. The more holistic patterns of care associated with complementary therapies cater for wide-ranging health needs, rather than the more mechanistic, mainstream view of diagnoses and treatment required by people who are ill. Limited resources are resulting in changing health policies, which focus on preventative health care or support, which minimises reliance on hospitals as the main providers of care. Self-help and choice are increasingly emphasised. One result of this is that complementary or alternative therapies are increasingly utilised to supplement medical care or to maximise independence, and such care is located outside traditional hospital settings.

Definitions

Orthodox or conventional medical treatment relates to that treatment based on the philosophy and understanding of disease and treatment taught in established medical schools, practised by doctors and regulated by their governing authorities.[2] The definition and differences between alternative and complementary therapies are more complex. Many therapies can fall under both definitions, depending upon the circumstances and conditions of their use. Generally, the term 'complementary therapies' relates to those treatments that may be used concurrently and in conjunction with orthodox medical treatment. These can include a wide-ranging group of therapies, which primarily aim to enhance or promote health and well-being. 'Alternative therapies' have been termed unproven, unorthodox, unconventional, questionable; they are those therapies that are used in place of orthodox medical treatment.

All therapies aim, to differing degrees, to enhance or stimulate the self-healing capacities of the body.[3] Many therapies, such as acupuncture, herbalism, and homoeopathy, incorporate theories of diagnosis, investigation, and treatment, and can be used independently of orthodox treatment, but may also be sought as a complement to conventional treatment.

Other therapies aim to be therapeutic, in that they promote feelings of well-being and minimise symptoms; for example, aromatherapy and massage. The British Medical Association[1] distinguishes between types of therapy; differentiating between self-help therapies such as yoga, re-educational therapies such as the Alexander technique, non-invasive therapies such as massage, and intervention therapies such as acupuncture. In order to practise using one of these therapies, a foundation training course, varying in length from a short weekend course to several years of academic study, is generally required. Although little regulation exists regarding statutory requirements in order to practice these therapies, such regulation varies considerably across Europe.

The complexity in defining complementary and alternative therapies has been compounded by the diversity of the therapies. Current definitions and classifications rely on banding all the therapies together, not because they share any underlying common principles, but because they fall outside the teaching and practice of orthodox medical treatment. For example, acupuncture is founded on the belief of energy channels that run throughout the body. If the energy flow through one of the channels is interrupted or restricted, then illness results. Some therapies are linked to more 'conventional' beliefs of illness and health; for example, massage is believed to work on the mechanism of the pain pathways. As a result, the most commonly used definitions distinguish alternative or complementary medicine as 'anything given to or done to a patient by a practitioner whose interventions are based on a body of consistent practices and teachings outside the limits of conventional medicine'.[2]

Terminology used to define differing professionals offering the therapies is also complex. Some call themselves therapists, while others prefer to be termed practitioners. Pietroni[4] suggests that a key feature separating practitioners from therapists is their respective approaches to health care. Practitioners have distinctive systems of health care, including a theoretical base for diagnosis and treatment, whereas therapists do not claim diagnostic skills.

Therapies fall outside what is traditionally recognised as conventional Western orthodox medicine. At present, many argue that as these therapies serve to supplement traditional and mechanistic methods of treatment, they are fulfilling a valuable role within a health service aiming to provide holistic care. Strong emphasis is placed on the term 'complementary', rather than 'alternative' when discussing these therapies, since in cancer care they are used alongside more orthodox treatment.

Complementary therapies commonly used by people with cancer are shown in Table 14.1.

History and development

Use of complementary therapies has increased dramatically over the past 30 years. Knowledge of other forms of health care have become more widespread, particularly those offered in countries such as China, as a result of improved political relations and terrestrial communication.[5] The 1970s saw a rise in the number of centres offering training and education in complementary therapies, but it was not until the 1980s that real developments occurred. As Fulder and Munro comment,[6] if the trend towards the increasing use of complementary therapies continues, conventional medical care will have to be more pluralistic and holistic, necessitating changes in the planning and administration of health care.

Sceptics of the value of complementary therapies argued that there was little or no evidence of the method in which the therapies worked, nor of any benefit to patients.

Dietary therapies are widely used by people with cancer. Hunter[7] identifies several reasons for the popularity of these, such as media publicity, sales techniques utilised by the product manufacturers and claims of the curative properties of some therapies. It is felt that since poor diet can cause cancer, a good diet can cure the disease. The common principles of the therapies rely on a strict vegan or vegetarian diet, with large amounts of raw food, low sugar and fat content, and high doses of vitamins, minerals, and enzymes. While these principles mimic a healthy diet, Hunter suggests that in someone already undernourished because of the effects of cancer and treatment, adhering to a low calorie and fat diet can exacerbate weight loss, weakness, and depression, and lead to feelings of guilt and anger if the therapies fail to produce the expected cure.

Montbriand[8] studied the use of alternative therapies in an American cancer population and found that 76% of the 300 people studied were using

Table 14.1 Summary of key complementary therapies

	Contraindications for cancer patients	Indications for cancer patients
Acupuncture – life energy (Chi) flows through the body through 14 channels (meridians). Stimulating points on the meridians can influence the flow of energy through the channels to the organs of the body. Illness is an imbalance within the energy flow throughout the body.	Friable or broken skin, or radiotherapy sites along insertion points. Patients with severely depleted energy reserves may require more sessions.	Pain of many origins and nature. Digestive disorders including nausea, vomiting and constipation. Psychological symptoms including insomnia, stress and anxiety. Lethargy and fatigue.
Aromatherapy – use of natural aromatic essences or oils extracted from wild or cultivated plants. Dilute doses of specific oils are blended with a carrier oil.	Many oils should not be used in specific conditions/ailments. Oils must be purchased from a reputable supplier. Oils must always be diluted before application to the skin with the exception of lavender and tea tree oil.	Pain of many origins and nature. Oils must never be taken internally unless prescribed by medically trained practitioner. Digestive disorders including nausea, vomiting, and constipation. Psychological symptoms including insomnia, stress, anxiety, depression. Lethargy and fatigue. Therapists can advise of oils suitable for nearly all symptoms/ailments.
Art therapy – aims to enable the individual to express himself/herself in a visual way.	Patients may require psychological support during and following the sessions, particularly if distressing issues arise from their work.	The opportunity for self-exploration and expression, valuable for patients with difficulties in communicating verbally.
Herbalism – the use of the whole plant in remedies to promote healing and in the maintenance of health.	Many herbs still require scientific testing. Skin preparations must not be used on broken or friable skin. Patients must consult a registered practitioner, and advise their own doctor if they are following a course of treatment.	Many physiological disorders, particularly those of a chronic nature. Infections.
Homoeopathy – uses highly diluted, small doses of substances where larger doses of the same substance would actually cause the illness in a healthy individual.	Patients should consult a registered practitioner, and advise their own doctor if following a course of treatment.	Long-term, chronic conditions including digestive disorders such as constipation, nausea, and vomiting. Some aromatherapy oils may be incompatible with homoeopathic treatment. Pain including migraines and headaches. Skin conditions.

(Contd)

Table 14.1 Summary of key complementary therapies (*contd*)

	Contraindications for cancer patients	Indications for cancer patients
Massage – systematic methods of touch.	Massage should not be used on or around areas of broken or friable skin, underlying fractures, tumour sites, thrombosis, radiotherapy sites, infection sites. Massage should be used with caution when patients have temperatures of unknown origin.	Pain of many origins and nature, including chronic, muscular pain, arthritis. Psychological symptoms including insomnia, headaches, stress, anxiety and depression. Constipation.
Nutritional therapies – use of diet to correct ill health. The belief is that good health is directly related to the quality of food eaten by an individual.	Patients should consult a registered practitioner and advise their doctor if they are following a course of treatment. Patients must be cautious of using extreme doses.	Digestive disorders including constipation, irritable bowel syndrome. Psychological symptoms including headaches, migraines, lethargy, fatigue.
Relaxation – involves the slowing down of the physical and psychological systems of the body.	No contraindications.	Particularly useful for psychological symptoms including stress and anxiety, insomnia, lowered self-esteem. May be beneficial for chronic pain.
Music therapy – includes both listening to live or recorded music and the patient's participation in making music.	No contraindications.	Similar to relaxation.
Reflexology – use of pressure to particular acupuncture points on feet. The points on the feet relate to specific parts of the body and control the energy flow.	Should not be used when there are circulatory disorders, broken or friable skin, radiotherapy sites, or tumour sites around feet and lower legs.	Pain of many origins and nature, including headaches and migraines. Psychological symptoms including stress, anxiety, depression, insomnia. Constipation.
Shiatsu – the application of pressure to the acupuncture points on meridians to restore the flow of Qi (energy).	Temperatures, haematological disorders such as low platelet count, should not be used with over areas of disease site, bone secondaries.	Psychological symptoms including stress, anxiety, insomnia. Headaches and pain.

complementary therapies, including dietary therapies, herbs, megavitamins, and over-the-counter remedies from health food shops. Little evidence, however, exists regarding the effectiveness of these remedies in relation to controlling cancer. In addition, some of the therapies may be harmful taken in the doses recommended within the therapy. For example, megavitamin therapy refers to taking 10 times the recommended daily intake. Since many vitamins are water or fat soluble and are not secreted by the body, toxicity may result from their accumulation. Montbriand concludes that lay consumers are seldom in a position to select or accurately identify a high vitamin dose that is appropriate for a specific medical condition and are therefore suggestible to the inaccurate information they may obtain from some therapists or literature.

Dietary therapies may be beneficial to people with cancer when used as a complement to conventional treatment. Most hospitals employ dieticians who recommend dietary supplements, such as vitamins, minerals, and fibre. Increasing the intake of these with an increased calorie intake may assist in maximising the body's immune system, enhancing energy levels, maximising well-being, and reducing symptoms such as constipation or infection.

The use of certain therapies that can be self-prescribed and purchased easily gives cause for concern. Many herbal remedies are accepted as legal medicines under the Medicines Act, and can therefore be prescribed by doctors. However, as many as 80% have not been through rigorous testing procedures.[9] The influx of contaminated herbs from Asia, South America, and China has also caused concern. The British Herbal Medical Association insists on its members adhering to established good manufacturing practices, including aspects of safety, quality, and efficacy. Despite these recommendations, the public may often purchase over-the-counter remedies, or those from less reputable dealers that fail to adhere to these recommendations.

Despite the possible negative consequences of following certain therapies, when prescribed by a qualified practitioner and used to complement conventional treatment, many of these therapies offer positive benefits to people with cancer. These benefits can include increased feelings of well-being, enhanced personal control over health, and reduction of certain symptoms.

The separation between orthodox and complementary therapies was highlighted in the speech by The Prince of Wales when he became the President of the British Medical Association in 1983. The speech was widely reported, highlighting what he saw as the limitations of conventional medicine and its neglect of the personal needs of the person who is ill. In 1986 the British Medical Association[10] commissioned an inquiry into alternative medicine. The report concluded that there was little evidence to support the use of alternative and complementary therapies. The result was a storm of protest from therapists, who saw the report of the inquiry as flawed and unfair. The British Medical Association had failed to provide adequate time for the therapists to provide information and to review all the evidence. In response, a new body was formed – the Council for Complementary and Alternative Medicine. One of its primary objectives was to provide a forum for discussion and enquiries into complementary medicine.

In 1993, the British Medical Association published its second report into the practice and use of complementary therapies within the UK. In contrast to the previous one, this report was positive and supportive of the development and use of therapies, while recognising that registration and professional standards must be addressed and legislated for within the professional groups. The report advocated increased resources for evaluation of therapies, and that training and education in complementary therapies should be included in undergraduate medical curricula. More recently, proposals have been made regarding how complementary and alternative therapies might become integrated into mainstream health care.[11]

Demand for therapies

The exact numbers of complementary therapists and people seeking complementary therapies are unknown, although it is known that these are increasing rapidly. Surveys are unable to determine the number of practitioners owing to the lack of regulatory bodies and registration details. Likewise, it is impossible to assess how many people receive complementary therapies, because of differences in the methods of estimating and recording numbers and the lack of central registries. Results from studies are difficult to assess because of some of the methods and approaches adopted.[12] The majority of studies employs questionnaires, some supplementing this information with follow-up interviews. The majority of studies reported is American, although a few have been conducted in the UK and continental Europe.

Fulder and Munro[6] conducted the first large-scale survey in the UK. On the basis of demographic information collected from five geographical regions, they calculated that there are 12.1 practising complementary and alternative medical practitioners and therapists per 100 000 of the population. Healing, acupuncture, chiropractic, and osteopathy were the most commonly used therapies, with women aged 21–60 years from social groups I and II representing the largest group of users (i.e. those who are most affluent). The survey did not explore reasons for people seeking therapies; the average length of time spent consulting therapists was six times longer than that spent with general practitioners. The highest levels of complementary care were found in areas well served medically, indicating a substantial subsidiary system.

In 1985[13] a survey of 28 000 members of the UK Consumer Association found that 1 in 7 had used complementary therapies; in 1991,[14] this number had increased to 1 in 4, and a third survey in 1997[15] examined the perceptions of the general public towards the use of complementary therapies. Of those responding, 92% were very satisfied with the therapy they used, and 84% claimed that the therapy had improved their condition. The most popular therapy was osteopathy. The most common symptom for which people sought complementary therapies was back pain (41%).

A survey of 3500 Americans estimated that nearly 10% (almost 25 million people) of the general public used alternative therapies.[16] Poor health was associated with the use of therapies, and users of alternative therapies were found to have a higher level of unmet need for conventional health care (12.9% versus 4.9% for non-users of therapies). The most commonly used therapies were chiropractic (17.6 million users), massage (8 million users), relaxation (3.5 million users), and acupuncture (1 million users). The level of use of chiropractic may reflect medical insurance covering the costs of the therapy. Interestingly, over 70% of people using relaxation, massage, and acupuncture were also receiving conventional medical care.

Another study conducted in America used a random digit-dialling telephone survey of 36 000 American households.[17] Over 5000 people provided information and 9% of the population had used unorthodox alternative therapies. There was a linear correlation between higher income or higher education levels and the use of such therapies.

Attitudes of health professionals toward complementary therapies

Studies exploring the perceptions of health professionals have focused predominantly on general practitioners and physicians; little evidence exists regarding the attitudes of nurses.

Reilly[18] explored the attitudes of 86 trainee general practitioners and found that the majority had positive attitudes toward complementary therapies. Acupuncture and hypnosis were believed to be the most useful therapies, and 70 of the general practitioners personally wanted to train in at least one therapy. They indicated that they were more likely to refer a patient for a therapy if they had used the therapy themselves (50%) than if they were a non-user (32%), and only two thought that therapies were of no benefit.

Similar results were found in a study by Wharton and Lewith.[19] They administered a questionnaire to 200 general practitioners and received responses from 145. Three-quarters ($n = 110$; 76%) had referred patients to medically trained therapists and 104 (72%) had referred patients to non-medically trained therapists. Over one-third ($n = 55$; 38%) had had some training in therapies themselves, and 22 (15%) wanted training.

Personal experiences and recommendations from others fostered a positive attitude for these doctors and only a very small percentage had negative views concerning the effectiveness of the therapies. The doctors raised important concerns relating to the legislation and training requirements for therapists, and appeared to overcome these concerns by referral to therapists they knew personally or who had been recommended to them.

Gray *et al.*[20] conducted a smaller study using

open-ended interviews to elicit the attitudes of Canadian physicians; 19 out of 40 responded to the study, including general practitioners, oncologists and one surgeon. All the doctors agreed that they needed greater access to information concerning therapies so that they could accurately and comprehensively inform people in their care. They perceived that therapies were used to increase personal control over an individual's own health. The physicians cited limitations of conventional care due to time constraints and the effective and sometimes misleading marketing strategies used for complementary therapies as other factors. The physicians stated support for the use of therapies in conditional terms, in that they would support the use of complementary therapies as long as this was used in parallel with, rather than to replace, conventional care.

A study undertaken on behalf of the American Society of Clinical Oncology[17] interviewed 104 cancer physicians; over half (64%) of the physicians stated that when they were aware that patients were using therapies, they actively tried to dissuade them. They would recommend therapies in only 2% of cases, but ultimately went along with an individual's decision in 37% of cases. The term 'questionable treatments of cancer' was used in the interviews, which may have elicited more negative comments and responses from the physicians. Several studies have reported that it is common for people not to tell their doctor if they are receiving complementary therapies, because they are worried about the negative response. Given the attitudes expressed by cancer physicians, this seems unsurprising.

Despite the small size of the studies, the largely positive response from UK general practitioners observed by Reilly[18] and Wharton and Lewith[19] warrants further exploration. In particular, useful comparisons could be made between UK and American family doctors to determine whether these doctors act as co-ordinators of care, referring or directing patients towards complementary therapists. The negative views held by some specialist and hospital doctors may be partly in response to the observation that their patients refuse conventional treatment in preference to alternative therapies. General practitioners, in contrast, appear to see the use of complementary therapies

as a true complement to the treatment and care they offer.

Sharma[21] studied the nature of complementary medicine within England. Nearly one-third of complementary practitioners had previously worked in health care and moved into complementary medicine because they were interested in holistic care and preferred autonomous working. No specific details were available as to the positions held by these practitioners while working in the National Health Service. The study highlighted the need for communication between orthodox and non-orthodox health care professionals, particularly at a local level.

The National Association of Health Authorities and Trusts[22] conducted a survey in the UK of the attitudes towards the availability of complementary therapies by authorities providing and funding health care. In general, they had a positive attitude towards complementary therapies, with more than 70% of family health service authorities and general practitioner fund-holders, and 65% of district health authorities believing that some or all therapies should be available on the National Health Service. Thirty-nine authorities/fundholders, and seven general practitioner fund-holders did not believe that complementary therapies should be available on the National Health Service, because of concerns relating to lack of evidence of efficacy of the therapies, lack of proven cost-effectiveness, resource constraints, and a perceived lack of demand from the public or from general practitioners.

There are few data available to indicate how many nurses use complementary therapies within their practice, nor how many patients use these therapies as part of care. However, many hospitals now employ complementary therapists, and nurses may use complementary therapies within their clinical practice. The UK Royal College of Nursing Special Interest Group for Complementary Therapies has seen a rapid increase in membership, suggesting that many of these nurses are either practising therapies themselves, or caring for individuals receiving complementary therapies.

Rankin-Box[23] conducted an informal survey of the members of the Royal College of Nursing special interest group, administering a questionnaire to all the members (*n* = 1662). Despite a very low response rate (n = 178; 9.3%) some interesting results emerged. The most common therapies used were massage, aromatherapy, and reflexology. A small number of nurses also used acupuncture homoeopathy, shiatsu and hypnosis. Nearly half of the respondents worked within the National Health Service, although there were no details of place of employment provided by 18% of the sample. The staff working within the private sector reported having more time available to practise therapies, which may be related to higher staffing levels. Several nurses reported that they used complementary therapies in addition to their daily workload, rather than as an integral part of care. This could be viewed as a source of conflict when nurses aim to work with a philosophy of holistic care. It may also suggest that the use of complementary therapies is not seen as a valid component of nursing duties. Nearly half of the nurses reported that their employer did not have a policy relating to the use of complementary therapies; it appeared that nurses were practising therapies without locally agreed policies and standards. The nurses reported that few of their employers had a formal audit and evaluation programme for the use of therapies, indicating a lack of control and regulation of therapies within nursing practice.

Nurses are the largest group of health care providers and owing to the diversity of their roles, they are in an ideal position to incorporate complementary therapies into their practice.[24] They also have an important role in initiating changes in the attitudes of other professionals and patients towards holistic care, because of their responsibility for the co-ordination of care and for providing direct and indirect care.[25]

Complementary therapies and cancer

Complementary therapies may be used as a pleasant intervention to enhance quality of life and complement or counteract the effects of conventional cancer treatment. Particular therapies may also be sought for relief of specific symptoms, such as acupuncture for pain relief and massage for tension release. As most complementary therapies are non-invasive and have been designed to be utilised alongside conventional treatment regimes, they can be used at a time when other interests or lifestyle activities have to be reduced, for example the use of aromatherapy by a person with poor mobility who is housebound. Many nurses are now integrating complementary therapies into their practice, as they emphasise the art of nurturing and caring for the whole person, reflecting an increasing focus on a holistic model of care.[26] Complementary therapies may also contribute to well-being, by restoring feelings of control, assisting with adjustment to the changing circumstances imposed by cancer, and enhancing quality of life.[25]

Montbriand's studies[27,28] used interviews to explore the use of alternative therapies by American patients with cancer. The studies explored the attitudes towards the use of specific therapies by nearly 400 people with cancer. Over three-quarters used physical therapies such as diet or healing, choosing these therapies partly in response to influence from their social groups, and because of anger and disillusionment with conventional medical systems. Montbriand also found that those using therapies cited a desire for control as a strong reason for seeking them. The issue of control appears to be a recurring theme within the studies and warrants further exploration. An interesting criticism of conventional care was the difficulty they experienced in accessing comprehensive and understandable information concerning the use and applicability of therapies from their conventional care doctors. Many also commented that they were secretive about the use of their therapies and rarely disclosed that they were using these to their family doctor.

Kelvinson and Payne[29] compared patients seeking health care for pain control from a complementary therapy centre in the UK with those receiving conventional care from a National Health Service hospital. The results of the study are inconclusive, partly as a result of the small samples sizes used (n = 60). The study did not report the cause and nature of the pain experienced by the patients, which may have influenced the interpretation of the results. Those seeking complementary therapy had less favourable attitudes towards conventional medicine, perhaps as a result of conventional care failing to resolve their need for pain control. They also had a higher score for personal control over their own health, relying less on powerful others (health professionals) and chance.

Downer *et al.*[30] found that 16% (*n* = 65) of 415 people with cancer in the UK had used complementary therapies: healing, relaxation, visualisation, diets, homoeopathy, vitamins, and herbalism were most commonly used. The users tended to be younger, of higher social economic groups, and female. Of those using complementary therapies, 14% had been dissatisfied with conventional treatment, owing to the severe side-effects of treatment and the low hope of a cure. The group using therapies had higher internal locus of control scores over origin or cause of illness, similar to the results found by Kelvinson and Payne.[29] Twenty-six said that their doctor was unaware that they were using complementary therapies. The major dissatisfaction experienced by those using complementary therapies related to dietary therapies. Specific comments stated that the diets were unpalatable, took time to prepare, and precipitated severe weight loss. These findings support the comments made by Hunter.[7] No conclusions can be drawn as to the relatively low numbers who were using complementary therapies, but the sample was drawn from two London hospitals. It is not clear whether those using therapies received them from the National Health Service or had to fund them privately.

Moore *et al.*[31] found that pain was the most common reason for attending a complementary therapy centre. A high number stated that failure of conventional care in alleviating symptoms was the prime reason for attending. Fifty-nine per cent of respondents felt that their symptoms had improved after 4 weeks of treatment. Although the exact diagnosis and cause of the symptoms were not identified, the majority was suffering from chronic conditions that had failed to be resolved by conventional care.

Yates *et al.*[32] explored the extent of, and commitment to, the use of alternative therapies by people with advanced cancer. The interviews elicited four categories of user of therapy: those who made conventional modifications to their lifestyle, those who relied on religious faiths, uncommitted users of therapies, and committed users of therapies. The committed users consulted a wide variety of therapists and adhered to the recommended treatments, whereas the uncommitted users consulted the therapists but did not follow the treatment. Those who made conventional modifications adopted the therapies and treatments, which required only minor moderations to their existing lifestyle, for example, dietary changes.

Generally, those who used alternative therapies were found to be younger, with a higher income, a more positive belief in the alternative causes of cancer, a strong desire for control, and a strong will to live.

Risberg *et al.*[33] conducted a comprehensive longitudinal study of the use of complementary therapies by people with cancer in Norway. Most new users of complementary therapies commenced the therapies within the first year after diagnosis, although during the 5-year follow-up, 45% of the whole sample used a therapy at least once. Women were the most common users, and the majority were aged 30–59 years. Three-quarters of the sample used spiritual therapies, either alone or in conjunction with non-spiritual therapies such as homoeopathy, zone therapy, and dietary therapies. The study found that people may dramatically change their health behaviours over the course of their disease, and therefore cross-sectional studies may underestimate the use of complementary therapies by people with cancer.

While these studies provide interesting results in relation to the numbers of people seeking therapies and the types of therapies often chosen, they do not provide great detail about the reasons for seeking therapies or about their effectiveness. The issue of personal control over health arose in a few studies and warrants further attention. The use of complementary therapies to reduce or relieve the symptoms caused by disease and treatment also needs to be explored in greater depth, to identify key therapies and how they may assist people who have cancer.

Costings and resources

There is scant evidence in the literature as to the costs and resources required to provide complementary therapies although, as Smith documents,[34] the cumulative National Health Service budget for complementary therapies is believed to be approximately £1m per year. This figure is likely to be an underestimate, as many therapies are now included in other health costings, for example, acupuncture in pain clinics.

The National Association of Hospitals and Trusts report[22] stated that despite a lack of agreed policies in the majority of family health service authorities and district health authorities, many were purchasing or funding the provision of complementary therapies. Eleven family health service authorities had detailed policies, including funding strategies and information on how practices could obtain funding. A further eight had more limited policies, either funding therapies as pilot projects or actively encouraging practices to apply for funding.

General practitioners were able to offset the cost of commissioning complementary therapies on a sessional basis as a result of health promotion clinic payments from their family health service authorities. Fifty-five family health service authorities had been approached to fund health promotion clinics, of whom 44 had approved. Five out of the remaining 10 had not believed it was appropriate to fund complementary therapies through the National Health Service. The most common therapy funded was acupuncture (for smoking cessation and pain control for musculoskeletal disorders).

In total, 92 district health authorities were funding complementary therapies, of which 38 were able to provide details of the costings. Costings varied from £120 000 to £269 000, with a sum total of £975 438. This figure is likely to be an underestimate because the majority of district health authorities were unable to identify funding figures, as they were included in mainstream specialty contracts. Costs to general practitioner practices were lower, as the majority of therapy provision was provided by a member of the practice. Fourteen practices used the services of independent therapists, of whom half provided their services for free.

Despite the provision of therapies by some family health service authorities and district health authorities, the majority of people using complementary therapies have to pay themselves. This may result in inequality of care, in that many of those who may benefit the most may be unable to afford to pay; for example, those with chronic disabilities who are unable to work and rely on state disability benefits, or the elderly. The increasing emphasis on holistic care within the traditional health service and the upsurge in the provision of complementary therapies within hospital settings and community practices may serve to alleviate some of the direct costs to the public. The family health service authorities and district health authorities in the National Association of Hospitals and Trusts survey[22] were committed, and intended to continue to purchase complementary therapies, although they were unable to confirm specific future plans owing to the changing structure and policies within the health service. Many felt that moneys would be used from the research and development budget, although they emphasised that priority would be given to funding essential staff and other treatments. One-quarter of the family health service authorities, district health authorities, and general practitioner fund-holders expressed concern about funding issues, suggesting that this may become a prime issue in a health service already under financial constraint.

Complementary therapies are increasingly being offered within the National Health Service, through primary and secondary health care providers. Many medical schools in America, and increasingly in the UK, are including education relating to complementary and alternative therapies within their curricula.[11] Increasing numbers of general practitioners in the UK appear to be training in at least one therapy, or have contracts with therapists to whom they can refer their patients. Hospitals, particularly those with cancer centres or units, often employ complementary therapists or staff who are able to provide complementary therapies.

The demand for complementary therapies creates a potential for escalating costs and resource requirements. This is a factor that needs to be addressed within health care.

Education and training

The Foundation for Integration of Medicine[11] has identified several concerns with the present situation in the UK, namely, that many orthodox doctors may have a basic understanding of complementary therapies but they have no mechanism by which to ensure practitioners are competent, qualified, and experienced to offer therapies to their patients. Similarly, many therapists have little or no training in key principles of basic medicine and may therefore fail to refer a patient to an appropriately trained professional.

Other European countries have different legislation and training policies. For example, several countries require alternative therapy practitioners also to be medically qualified.[21] In other countries such as Germany and Switzerland, certain therapies such as chiropractic are considered to be part of conventional care. However, with the move towards consensus within Europe in relation to health care provision, many countries are reviewing their policies towards legislation and training for complementary and alternative therapists.[35]

Two key areas are apparent in relation to education and training issues, the first being that health professionals working within conventional health care practice are seeking and needing comprehensive information about the various therapies available. The second consideration is that of the standardisation and development of accredited and statutory courses for complementary or alternative therapies.

Training and qualification of therapists

The British Medical Association survey[1] identified that there is a considerable range of standards and levels of training for practitioners of complementary therapies. Training courses range from those offered at higher education establishments, including university access courses, to short or modular courses offered by complementary therapy colleges. Certain therapies have established professional bodies and developed rigorous educational programmes; for example, acupuncture, chiropractic, herbal medicine, homoeopathy, and osteopathy.[5] These five have also made major developments towards the accreditation of their educational courses. However, a high proportion of courses offered at university level is not accredited by an independent regulatory body for the profession concerned.[11]

The British Medical Association report[1] outlines several requirements for any educational or training course, including the establishment of a core curriculum, which states the basic competencies for the practice of that therapy, and includes a medical science foundation. It continues to state that a regulatory body must assume responsibility for the clinical and professional accreditation of the training establishments. Accreditation would include a rigorous assessment programme to ensure that the training establishment is externally monitored.

Strong similarities exist between the specific recommendations for course content advocated by the British Medical Association report[1] and the Foundation for Integration of Medicine.[11] Both groups recommend that the common elements to be included in any curriculum would include basic anatomy, physiology, and pathology, principles of conventional medicine and specific therapies, the variety of therapies and their potential uses, holistic models of health care, and the planning and recording of courses of treatment. Some aspects of the core curriculum could be jointly studied by students training within the health professions or as complementary therapists.

Many of these issues also need to be addressed by colleges offering specialist courses in complementary therapies. Short or modular courses, separate from those linked to health professional training, require the development of levels of competence, with courses being accredited by the professional therapy body.

Following the development of a core curriculum for all health care training, the continuing educational needs of both therapists and health care professionals will need to be addressed. Further education could enhance professional development through an increased awareness of therapies and their uses, within the framework of holistic care.[11] The development of more collaborative working, and communication between orthodox and nonorthodox professionals could also be included.

Needs of health professionals

Health professionals, including doctors and nurses in primary and secondary health care, need to be informed as to the uses, applicability, and effects of a variety of therapies. Education and information are required throughout health professional training, at both undergraduate and postgraduate level.[18,19,30] Purchasers of health care have identified that they have lacked knowledge about what the therapies involve, the principles and theoretical basis for the therapy, appropriate qualifications and training of therapists, and the medical and legal implications.[22] These same areas were also identified by health professionals within the literature.[20,21,36]

This information could ideally be offered throughout continuing education programmes, providing the depth and detail required by health professionals. Many trainee general practitioner courses now include information relating to complementary therapies, perhaps because of the apparently positive attitude towards therapies held by this group, but also because they represent the key health professional acting as a resource for and co-ordinator of care.

All health professionals have a responsibility to act as advocates for people with cancer and to provide full and accurate information to enable patients to make informed decisions and choices.[17] Despite some doctors' concerns and reservations about the efficacy of therapies, they have a duty to inform people with cancer fully and to assist them in choosing appropriate forms of health care.[30]

Legislation

The lack of legislation and formal registration of complementary therapists is an area requiring action.[1] There are few systematic methods by which patients or health professionals can identify appropriately trained and qualified therapists. Consequently, the real fear is that people may unwittingly be treated by 'charlatans'. The reality is that anyone in the UK can set up as a complementary therapist, with or without any formal training, and practise under common law.[37] These therapists are subject only to provisions of statutes such as Medical, Dental, Professions Supplementary to Medicine, and Medicines Acts.[11] Nonetheless, all therapists have a legal duty of care towards patients.[38] The potential harm incurred by patients while using some therapies includes the costs of obtaining treatment (which may be large), the potential of severe side-effects (for example, some dietary therapies), and the indirect harm of delay in seeking and obtaining orthodox, proven therapies. The legal standard of care is a duty to act in accordance with a practice accepted as proper by a body of professional opinion. However, this is complex because few therapists' organisations have stated comprehensive standards and qualifications.[38] The British Medical Association[1] recommends the development of different categories of therapies because of the diverse nature of the therapies and their potential to do harm or benefit. It advocates this view in order to distinguish between therapies requiring long, comprehensive training courses and those only requiring short periods of study. It suggests the categories devised by Pietroni:[39] complete systems including homoeopathy, osteopathy, herbal medicine, and acupuncture; diagnostic methods including iridology, kinesiology, and hair analysis; therapeutic modalities including massage, shiatsu, and reflexology; and finally self-care approaches including meditation, yoga, and relaxation.

A survey of complementary therapy organisations conducted in the UK found that many groups were in the process of developing high standards of training, regulation, and clinical practice.[11] However, further developments are required, including the establishment of statutory self-regulatory bodies for those professions who may put patients at risk of harm, such as acupuncture or herbal medicine. Voluntary self-regulation may be sufficient for the majority of therapies not utilising invasive techniques or less likely to cause the patient harm, such as massage. To conclude, patients seeking a complementary therapist should ask the following questions: Is the therapist registered with a professional organisation?; Does the organisation have a public register?; Does it have a code of practice, effective disciplinary procedure, or complaints mechanism? Conventional health professionals, including doctors and nurses, must also be aware of these issues and inform or direct patients to those therapists fulfilling these criteria.

Stone[38] identifies that many medical professionals are concerned as to whether they themselves will retain legal liability for recommending therapies that may have an adverse outcome. Stone continues to discuss the legal implications of the differences between referring or delegating a patient's care to another professional. When a doctor refers a patient to another professional, that professional then takes responsibility for assessing and treating that patient. Providing that the doctor has made a responsible referral, the professional who has received the referral then assumes professional and legal responsibility for treating the patient. In the delegation model, the doctor transfers the patient to another individual for care, but retains clinical accountability.[39] For many patients, referral to a complementary therapist occurs when their condition is not amenable to conventional treatment and the treatment provided by the therapist is likely to be outside the domain and expertise of the referring doctor. It therefore seems inappropriate for this to be termed a delegation as recommended by the health minister, Steven Dorrell, in 1991.[38] This is an issue warranting further attention within the debate concerning legislation of therapies.

The issue for nursing is slightly less complex, although issues relating to legal liability, accountability, and health and safety must be addressed.[35] At present, UK nurses may undertake training and practise complementary therapies so long as they adhere to the United Kingdom Central Council code of professional conduct.[40] Individual hospitals and health care settings may have specific policies relating to the use of therapies by their staff, but these are not standardised. Difficulties arise if a nurse has an approved qualification in a particular therapy, but perhaps does not have the level of professional expertise within a specific practice environment. For example, a nurse working in an oncology unit may have a massage certificate but have little clinical experience in that area. Specific issues arise when considering the application of massage with a patient who may be immunosuppressed, suffering from secondary fractures, or receiving certain chemotherapy regimes. It would seem that individual hospitals may need to develop their own policies, regulated and assessed within specific health services. Rankin-Box[41] suggests the development of specialist therapeutic nurses who undertake accredited complementary therapy training. These specialists could then develop their professional expertise in the appropriate health setting, gaining an understanding of the issues and factors applicable to the use of specific therapies within identified patient groups.

Research and evaluation

The lack of rigorous testing and validation of the benefits, hazards, and cost of complementary therapies has hindered their widespread introduction into conventional health care. One London health authority that had previously been referring more than 500 patients a year for homoeopathic treatment decided to stop the funding as there was a lack of scientific evidence to support its use.[42] It was reported that many patients and health professionals were disappointed by the decision, but the fact remains that even if studies have been conducted, they have often used unsound methods. Nurses have been incorporating therapies such as massage or reflexology into their practice, often with few guidelines for practice and little 'scientific' evidence of the effects of this therapy:

> Whilst there is tremendous potential for the use of complementary therapies within orthodox nursing, there are a number of considerations and challenges to be addressed before certain practices are promoted as part of mainstream nursing practice.[25]

Research evaluating specific therapies

At present, there has been limited rigorous evaluation of complementary therapies and in particular their use for people who have cancer. Massage and aromatherapy have received the most attention within the nursing literature, although many of the reports are anecdotal or based on limited research methods. A review of 14 research studies aiming to evaluate massage identified several concerns with the methods used and the conclusions to be drawn from the studies.[43] The review concluded that there were many differences between studies in terms of the designs utilised and therefore comparison between the results was problematic. When viewed individually, all the studies appeared to suggest that massage was beneficial but the limitations of the designs used and the lack of comparison between studies mean that the results of the studies have to be viewed as tentative. Cawley[43] concludes with key recommendations for future research, including: replication of previous studies; the use of experimental or quasi-experimental studies to demonstrate therapeutic effects; the use of a control groups; larger sample sizes; longitudinal studies; and the use of interventions. The study by Corner et al.[44] (Research study 14.1) is offered as an example of a nursing research study, which adheres to some of these recommendations.

Research study 14.1: An evaluation of the use of massage and massage with the addition of essential oils on the well-being of cancer patients[44]

Aim of study
To evaluate the effects of massage with or without the addition of essential oils on cancer patients' perceptions of their quality of life, symptom distress, and levels of anxiety and depression.

Design
Quasi-experimental research, using a three group, before-and-after design.

Sample
Fifty-two patients with cancer, stratified according to disease site, sex, and performance status.

Measurement tools
Quality of Life and Symptom Distress Scale (Holmes and Dickerson, 1987); Hospital Anxiety and Depression Scale (Zigmond and Snaith, 1983).

Interviews
Semi-structured interviews focused on patients' reasons for choosing massage, their expectations and beliefs about massage and their perception of effects of massage.

Interventions
Two treatment groups received eight weekly massages of 30 minutes' duration, with up to 30 minutes' rest following the massage.

The carrier oil group received massage using sweet almond oil; the essential oil group received massage using a blend of lavender, rosewood, lemon, rose, and valerian.

The control group received no intervention.

Method
Interviews and tools were administered at baseline, prior to first massage. The two treatment groups completed the measurement tools before and after every massage over the next 8 weeks; the control group completed the measurement tools once weekly.

Results
The group receiving massage with essential oils had a reduction in anxiety scores ($p = 0.05$), and improvements in pain, mobility, tiredness, function, and ability to earn. The group receiving massage with carrier oil had an improvement in feelings about the future, concentration, mood, and appearance. The control group had improvements in tiredness, appearance, and ability to eat.

Massage appeared to have a cumulative effect on anxiety, with the maximum effect after three or four sessions.

Qualitative analysis of the interview data provided an illustration of the patients' experiences during the massage therapy:

> It was wonderful, I completely forgot about everything that was being done to my body, and got lost in the gentle music and massage.

> I felt very good, the pain seemed to go out of the body. Massage did definitely help very much. I wanted to cry all the time, and I began to feel I was drifting and floating away, that was very nice.

Aromatherapy is one of the therapies most widely practised by nurses. Despite the lack of evidence of the effect of aromatherapy oils, there are increasing data available about the effects and toxicity of specific oils.[45,46] However, these oils require testing for appropriateness to patients with cancer. Nursing research is required to explore the effects of essential oils on people with cancer in relation to a variety of symptoms.

Relaxation is another therapy that may be easily incorporated into nursing practice. Although there have been several studies exploring the use of relaxation for a variety of symptoms, including anxiety,[47–49] side-effects of chemotherapy,[50,51] and general well-being,[52] there has been little systematic analysis of the results of these studies.

Acupuncture is one of the most widely researched complementary therapies, although most of the evidence is medically based. Studies have examined acupuncture's effect on pain,[53,54] nausea and vomiting,[55] and breathlessness,[56] amongst others. A comprehensive review of the literature examining the effects of acupuncture on anti-emesis has been conducted by Vickers,[57] who examined 33 controlled trials, of which 27 were statistically superior in their analysis. Eleven of these trials showed consistent effects of stimulation of the P6 point, using a total sample of nearly 2000 patients. Vickers concludes that acupuncture appears to have an effect on anti-emesis, and researchers are now faced with the choice between deciding that acupuncture has a specific effect, and changing from 'Does acupuncture work?' to more practical questions, or deciding that

Table 14.2 Possible areas for research development

Use and demand for therapies	Research methods
Provision of therapies (National Health Service, private sector, primary and secondary health care).	Surveys, audit, focus groups.
Needs among practitioners, purchasers, providers.	Surveys, interviews, co-operative inquiry, action research, reflective practice.
Evaluation of therapies: mechanisms of work, effectiveness and applicability.	Randomised controlled trials, quasi-experiments, observation, outcome studies, action research, case studies.

the evidence does not provide enough proof and specifying what would constitute acceptable evidence.

The Foundation for the Integration of Medicine[11] states that the first aim must be to set priorities for the development of research and evaluation. Several areas must be addressed, namely: the use and demand for therapies; the provision of therapies within the National Health Service and private sector, including primary and secondary health care settings; the needs of practitioners, purchasers, and providers of care; and the evaluation of therapies including the mechanisms by which they work, their effectiveness, and applicability. Issues also arise about the location in which to conduct this research, and about which methods best enable this research to be conducted. One of the criticisms of research in complementary therapies is the lack of the use of randomised, controlled trials. However, this method is not always suitable to assess the varied and individual response to therapies, and the use of a placebo control group and double-blinding are not always possible.[24] Surveys and observation research designs are valuable and can be more appropriately used when addressing specific areas of complementary therapy research. For example, large-scale surveys that ascertain the use of therapies by the general population, and also by specific patient groups, are required. Similarly, surveys may also be useful in exploring the use of and attitudes towards complementary therapies by professional groups, including generic and specialist doctors and nurses. Qualitative methods are also valid when evaluating the spiritual and emotional aspects of a therapy, as the value of complementary therapies for patients may often lie in their subjective and individual perceptions.[58] Table 14.2 offers possible research studies and methods that could be developed.

Integration of complementary therapies

Several authors have documented their experiences of incorporating complementary therapies into more conventional health care services. These services include a cancer centre, general practices, and a specialist hospital. While many other hospitals and health settings offer complementary therapies as an adjuvant to conventional care, these services are unique in that they have formally set out to incorporate complementary therapies and include them within the total package of care available to patients.

One of the key aims for all these integrated services is that of education and enabling and encouraging self-help when appropriate. Two of the services employ general practitioners alongside complementary therapists.[59,60] The benefits of this approach are cited as improved and speedier access to all forms of care for patients, and providing more holistic, patient-centred care. The multidisciplinary team is involved in the assessment and planning of care, and the person receiving care is an active participant in the process. However, this can cause conflicts for patients, as reported by the Marylebone Health Centre,[59] in that there is a potential for patients to be faced with too many choices. The Cavendish Centre[60] overcame this issue by having the general practitioner act as the co-ordinator of care.

The positive effects for health professionals involved in the integrated model of care relate to improved communication and understanding between team members. However, for this to be achievable, clear guidelines and policies are required for defining the roles of the team members, their accountability and responsibilities, and the development of a common, uniting purpose and philosophy.[61]

Conclusion

Complementary therapies are being increasingly used by patients with cancer, and practised by nurses. However, several important areas require attention for the future development and integration of complementary therapies into more conventional health care services. Key recommendations relating to research and evaluation, education and training, legislation, and practice are identified below. As Burke[61] comments, the many and varied therapies need to be integrated into conventional care in a organised way, and chosen by and for patients depending on their acceptability and therapeutic value. To achieve this, comprehensive evidence about the effects and applications of complementary therapies within cancer care is required. This will involve the development of research studies to evaluate specific therapies and assess their efficiency within a variety of clinical conditions. Although large-scale surveys to assess the prevalence and use of complementary therapies are of interest, there can be little doubt that many people with cancer will seek therapies as an adjuvant to their conventional care. Therefore, the exploration and development of integrated models of health care that provide complementary therapies alongside conventional care must be expanded.

Complementary therapists have begun the process of developing legislative and validated professional bodies; however, this is an ongoing process. Nurses must be aware of the issues when advising patients who wish to access complementary therapies and ensure that patients consult a qualified, registered practitioner. Although many nurses may not personally provide complementary therapies, it is their professional responsibility to provide accurate and comprehensive information about the choices and care available to them. Nurses also have a duty to advise patients to inform their conventional care doctors of any complementary therapy they may be receiving. The development and use of complementary therapies within cancer care is likely to continue and nurses may be increasingly involved in patients' decisions to access these therapies.

References

1. British Medical Association (1993). *Complementary Medicine: New Approaches to Good Practice.* London: British Medical Association.
2. Buckman R. and Sabbagh K. (1993), *Magic or Medicine?: An Investigation into Healing.* London: Macmillan.
3. Fulder S.J. (1988). *Handbook of Complementary Medicine.* Oxford: Oxford University Press.
4. Pietroni P.C. (1991). *The Greening of Medicine.* London: Victor Gollanz.
5. Mills S. (1993). The development of the complementary medical professions. *Complementary Therapies in Medicine* 1, 24–29.
6. Fulder S.J. and Munro R.E. (1985). Complementary medicine in the United Kingdom: patients, practitioners, and consultations. *Lancet* ii, 542–545.
7. Hunter M. (1988). Unproven dietary methods of treatment of oncology patients. *Recent Results in Cancer Research* 108, 235–238.
8. Montbriand M.J. (1994). An overview of alternate therapies chosen by patients with cancer. *Oncology Nursing Forum* 21, 1547–1554.
9. Doyle C. (1995). The hazards of herbal remedies. *Daily Telegraph* (Health), 14th June.
10. British Medical Association (1986). *Report of the Board of Science and Education on Alternative Therapy.* London: British Medical Association.
11. Foundation for Integration of Medicine (1997). *Integrated Healthcare: A Way Forward for the Next Five Years?* London: Foundation for Integrated Medicine.
12. Sharma U. (1992). Who uses complementary medicine? In Sharma U. (ed.) *Complementary Medicine Today; Practitioners and Patients.* London: Routledge.
13. Consumers' Association (1986). Magic or medicine? *Which* October, 443–447.
14. Consumers' Association (1992). Regulation of practitioners of non-conventional medicine. *Which* Magazine.
15. Consumers' Association (1997). Complementary medicine: what works? *Which,* June, 1–3.
16. Paramore L.C. (1997). Use of alternative therapies: estimates from the 1994 Robert Wood Johnson Foundation National Access to Care Survey. *Journal of Pain and Symptom Management* 13, 83–89.

17. American Society Clinical Oncology (1997). The physician and unorthodox cancer therapies. *Journal of Clinical Oncology* **15**, 401–406.

18. Reilly D.T. (1983). Young doctors' views on alternative medicine. *British Medical Journal* **287**, 337–339.

19. Wharton R. and Lewith G. (1986). Complementary medicine and the general practitioner. *British Medical Journal* **292**, 1498–1500.

20. Gray R.E., Fitch M., Greenberg M. *et al.* (1997). Physician perspectives on unconventional cancer therapies. *Journal of Palliative Care* **13**, 14–21.

21. Sharma U.M. (1991). Complementary practitioners in a Midlands locality. *Complementary Medical Research* **5**, 12–16.

22. National Association of Health Authorities and Trusts (1993). *Complementary Therapies in the NHS.* Research Paper No. 10. Birmingham: NAHAT.

23. Rankin-Box D. (1988). Therapies in practice: a survey assessing nurses' use of complementary therapies. *Complementary Therapies in Nursing and Midwifery* **3**, 92–99.

24. Ersser S.J. (1995). Complementary therapies and nursing research: issues and practicalities. *Complementary Therapies in Nursing and Midwifery* **1**, 44–50.

25. Burke C. (1993). Cancer nursing: complementary/conventional approaches combine. *Complementary Therapies in Medicine* **1**, 158–163.

26. Williams S.M. (1989). Holistic nursing. In Stallier D. and Glymour C. (eds.) *Examining Holistic Medicine.* New York: Prometheus.

27. Montbriand M.J. (1993). Freedom of choice: an issue concerning alternate therapies chosen by patients with cancer. *Oncology Nursing Forum* **20**, 1195–1201.

28. Montbriand M.J. (1995). Decision tree model describing alternate health care choices made by oncology patients. *Cancer Nursing* **18**, 104–117.

29. Kelvinson R. and Payne S. (1993). Decision to seek complementary medicine for pain: a controlled study. *Complementary Therapies in Medicine* **1**, 2–5.

30. Downer S.M., Cody M.M., McCluskey P. *et al.* (1994). Pursuit and practice of complementary therapies by cancer patients receiving conventional treatment. *British Medical Journal* **309**, 86–189.

31. Moore J., Phipps K., Marcer D. and Lewith G. (1985). Why do people seek treatment by alternative medicine? *British Medical Journal* **290**, 28–29.

32. Yates P., Beadle G., Clavarino A. *et al.* (1993). Patients with terminal cancer who use alternative therapies: their beliefs and practices. *Sociology of Health and Illness* **15**, 199–216.

33. Risberg T., Lund E., Wist E., Kaasa S. and Wilsgard T. (1988). Cancer patients use of nonproven therapy: a 5-year follow-up study. *Journal of Clinical Oncology* **16**, 6–12.

34. Smith I. (1996). More than pin money. *Health Service Journal,* 25 January, 24–25.

35. Rankin-Box D. (1992). European developments in complementary medicine. *British Journal of Nursing* **1**, 103–105.

36. Thomas K.J., Carr J., Westlake L. and Williams B.T. (1991). Use of non-orthodox and conventional health care in Great Britain. *British Medical Journal* **302**, 208–210.

37. Trevelyan T. and Booth B. (1993). Fringe benefits. *Nursing Times* **89**, 30–33.

38. Stone J. (1996). Complements slip. *Health Service Journal,* 25 January, 26–27.

39. Pietroni P. (1992). Beyond the boundaries: relationships between general practice and complementary medicine. *British Medical Journal* **305**, 564–566.

40. United Kingdom Central Council (1992). *The Scope of Professional Practice.* London: United Kingdom Central Council.

41. Rankin-Box D. (1993). Innovation in practice: complementary therapies in nursing. *Complementary Therapies in Medicine* **1**, 30–33.

42. Wise J. (1997). Health authority stops buying homeopathy. *British Medical Journal* **314**, 1574.

43. Cawley N. (1997). A critique of the methodology of research studies evaluating massage. *European Journal of Cancer Care* **6**, 23–31.

44. Corner J., Cawley N. and Hildebrand S. (1995). An evaluation of the use of massage and essential oils on the well-being of cancer patients. *International Journal of Palliative Nursing* **1**, 67–73.

45. Buckle J. (1992). Which lavender oil? *Nursing Times* **88**, 54–55.

46. Tisserand R. (1988). *The Essential Oil Safety Data Manual.* Brighton: Tisserand Institute.

47. Pender N.J. (1985). Effects of progressive muscle relaxation training on anxiety and health locus of control among hypertensive adults. *Research in Nursing and Health* **8**, 67–72.

48. Gift A.G., Moore T. and Soeken K. (1992). Relaxation to reduce dyspnoea and anxiety in COAD patients. *Nursing Research* **41**, 242–246.

49. Houldin A.D., McCorkle R. and Lowery B.J. (1993). Relaxation training and psychoimmunological status of bereaved spouses: a pilot study. *Cancer Nursing* **16**, 47–52.

50. Lerman C., Rimer B., Blumberg B., Cristinzio S., Engstrom P.F., MacElwee N. *et al.* (1990). Effects of coping style and relaxation on cancer chemotherapy side effects and emotional responses. *Cancer Nursing* **13**, 308–315.

51. Scott D.W., Donahue D.C., Mastrovito R.C. and Hakes T.B. (1986). Comparative trial of clinical relaxation and an antiemetic drug regimen in reducing chemotherapy related nausea and vomiting. *Cancer Nursing* 9, 178–187.

52. Larsson G. and Starrin B. (1992). Relaxation training as an integral part of caring activities for cancer patients: effects on wellbeing. *Scandinavian Journal of Caring Science* 6, 179–185.

53. Lewith G.T., Field J. and Machin D. (1983). Acupuncture compared with placebo in post-herpetic pain. *Pain* 17, 361–368.

54. Hidderley M. and Weinel E. (1997). Effects of TENS applied to acupuncture points distal to a pain site. *International Journal of Palliative Nursing* 4, 185–191.

55. Dundee J.W., Chestnutt W.N., Ghaly R.G. and Lynas A.G.A. (1986). Traditional Chinese acupuncture: a potentially useful antiemetic? *British Medical Journal* 293, 583–584.

56. Filshie J., Penn K., Ashley S. and Davis C.L. (1996). Acupuncture for the relief of cancer-related breathlessness. *Palliative Medicine* 10, 145–150.

57. Vickers A.J. (1996). Can acupuncture have specific effects on health? A systematic review of acupuncture antiemesis trials. *Journal of Royal Society of Medicine* 89, 303–311.

58. Byrne C. (1992). Research methods in complementary therapies. *Nursing Standard* 6, 54–56.

59. Reason P., Chase H.D., Desser A. *et al.* (1992). Towards a clinical framework for collaboration between general and complementary practitioners: discussion paper. *Journal of the Royal Society of Medicine* 85, 161–164.

60. Peace G. and Simons D. (1996). Complementing the whole. *Nursing Times* 92, 52–54.

61. Burke C. and Sikora K. (1992). Cancer – the dual approach. *Nursing Times* 88, 62–66.

CHAPTER FIFTEEN

Hereditary cancer

Audrey Ardern-Jones and Rosalind Eeles

Cancer genetics is a new and emerging speciality in cancer care. Although at the cellular level cancer is always a genetic condition, it is not always an inherited genetic disorder. Indeed, only 5–10% of cancers are inherited but for families with an inherited cancer susceptibility, the risk of developing cancer is very high compared with the normal population cancer risk. The importance of genetics in cancer care is to elucidate the reality of the cancer risk and to relate this to families seeking advice for prevention strategies. Families who carry an identified cancer gene need specialist care and understanding. The implications of living with a known cancer gene are far-reaching and although not all family members carrying cancer predisposition genes develop cancer, the concern for the whole family is paramount.

The genetic material

Humans, as well as all living organisms, are composed of cells. Each nucleated cell of an individual contains the entire human genome, which has been estimated to contain 35 000 genes. The human genome is composed of DNA (deoxyribose nucleic acid), a long, complex molecule in the form of a double helix. The basic element of DNA is a nucleotide, which is a carbon sugar (deoxyribose) with an attached phosphate group and a base, which may be a purine (adenine, A, or guanine, G) or pyrimidine (cytosine, C, or thymine, T). The nucleotides are joined together by phosphodiester bonds between the sugar molecules to form a linear strand. The double helix is formed by two DNA strands linked together with the sugar phosphate backbones on the outside of the molecule and the bases on the inside, orientated such that hydrogen bonds form between opposing purine and pyrimidine bases.

The base pairing is strict, with A always pairing with T and C always pairing with G. This strict base pairing results in two DNA strands, which are termed 'complementary' to each other.

The linear sequence of bases is important as it codes for specific amino acids. Each group of three adjacent bases (codon) is a code for a single amino acid or a stop signal; hence, the linear DNA sequence forms the genetic code for the formation of specific proteins, which are composed of these amino acids. Proteins direct the function of cells and therefore the entire organism; hence the DNA structure stores all the necessary information for the correct functioning of an individual.[1]

A gene is a sequence of DNA, which can code for a specific protein or have a specific function, such as regulating the expression of other genes. The gene sequence may contain both coding areas for amino acids (exons) and non-coding areas (introns). It is interesting to note that only 3–5% of the DNA in the human genome is used to code for proteins. The function of the remaining 95% of the genome is not well understood, but is likely to be involved with the structure and maintenance of the genome. The sequence of adjacent base pairs in a gene may vary between individuals.

This may be a normal variation, which results in the differences observed between two individuals and is termed 'genetic polymorphism', or an abnormal alteration in the sequence of adjacent base pairs in a gene, termed a 'mutation'.

Different types of mutations exist in genes; for example, a change that alters only one single base to another is known as a point mutation. Alternatively, other mutations include the deletion of an existing base and insertions or deletions of multiple bases, or even the rearrangement of the correct bases into an incorrect order. All types of mutations can result in the incorrect amino acid(s) being incorporated into a protein, therefore changing the structure and/or function of the protein. Alternatively, a mutation may result in the formation of a stop codon, which terminates the coding sequence and results in a shortened or truncated protein. These changes from the normal may result in an abnormal protein that does not function correctly. Fortunately, not all genes are functional (gene expression), so mutational changes in the genetic code may not always cause abnormal proteins.

Mutations in the DNA sequence of a gene are copied and transferred from parent to daughter cells through the process of mitosis. If a mutation occurs in a somatic cell [that is, all the cells of the body other than the reproductive cells of ova and sperm (germ cells)], then only the daughter cells from the original cell will contain this abnormality and all the other cells of the organism will have a normal genetic code. This is termed a 'somatic mutation' and is the likely mechanism of formation of sporadic (non-inherited) cancers. As the germ cells are normal, then the somatic mutation will not be passed to subsequent generations of the organism. If a mutation affects a germ cell, a germ-line mutation, then the abnormal gene may be passed to the next generation and this forms the mechanism of familial predisposition to specific cancer syndromes.[1]

Genetic inheritance

Humans are diploid organisms; that is, they contain two copies of the entire genetic code in each cell, one copy from each parent. The genetic code is in the form of chromosomes, which are long lengths of DNA condensed into a compact structure. Each copy of the genetic code consists of 22 autosomal chromosomes and one sex chromosome, hence the full genetic complement consists of 44 autosomal chromosomes and two sex chromosomes. The term 'homologous chromosomes' refers to a pair of matching chromosomes, one from each parent. These matching chromosomes are not exact copies of each other, but are similar in that the positions of specific genes (loci) are aligned in the same way on each homologous chromosome, but the actual genes are of different sequences due to genetic polymorphism. The term 'allele' refers to a version of a gene; hence, each nucleated cell contains two alleles for each gene. The genetic code inherited by an individual is termed the 'genotype', whereas the appearance of an individual (for example, hair colour) is termed the 'phenotype'.[1]

The major contributor to the understanding of the role of inheritance was Gregor Mendel in 1865. Indeed, it was through his novel experiments on plant breeding that he discovered statistical ratios that made sense in calculating averages. These ratios have achieved high status and indeed Mendel's laws on inheritance are known as dominant, recessive, or sex-linked. Dominant inheritance refers to the expression of a phenotype determined by the inheritance of a single allele; Huntington's chorea is an example of this type of inheritance. Recessive inheritance refers to the expression of a phenotype determined by the inheritance of two identical alleles; if only one is inherited then that phenotype is not expressed, as the recessive allele is dominated by the homologous allele. Cystic fibrosis is the most common recessive inherited genetic disease in UK Caucasians and both parents must be carriers of the recessive gene in order to produce a child with cystic fibrosis. Sex-linked inheritance is the inheritance of genes carried by the sex chromosomes and haemophilia is a well-described X-linked disease that is passed down through the female on the female X chromosome.

It must be remembered that except for sex-linked inheritance, the inheritance of a germ-line mutation in a gene is not dependent on the sex of an individual; male and females may equally be carriers. However, the phenotypic expression of the gene may depend on the sex of the individual. For example, men and women can inherit breast and ovarian cancer predisposition genes, but men rarely develop breast cancer and cannot develop ovarian cancer, but can still pass on the gene to the next generation.

The phenotypic expression of an inherited gene depends on the penetrance of the gene. A highly penetrant gene is one that is usually expressed if inherited. For example, a carrier of either of the recently identified breast cancer genes known as BRCA1 or BRCA2[41] has a 40–85% lifetime expectancy of development of breast cancer, depending on ethnicity. The penetrance of a gene will depend on many factors, but may include the sex of the individual (a male carrying the BRCA1 gene rarely develops breast cancer), the presence of carcinogens such as smoking, or the interplay of other genes. The penetrance of germ-line cancer predisposition genes has been estimated, but the estimations are continually refined as further knowledge of cancer genetics is gained.[3]

Cancer predisposition genes

Cancer predisposition genes are genes in which germ-line mutations can predispose to the development of cancer in individuals who have inherited the mutation. The understanding of these genes and the developments in the field of cancer molecular biology have been extraordinarily rapid in the last decade. Three types of cancer genes have been identified.

Oncogenes

Oncogenes are genes that may cause cancer if present in a mutated form. They are usually mutated forms of normal genes (proto-oncogenes), which commonly have important cell regulatory functions; mutations will therefore tend either to increase gene expression or to lead to uncontrolled activity of the proteins encoded by the oncogene. Germ-line oncogenes tend to show a dominant pattern of inheritance and the only examples currently identified in the human are the *ret* and *met* oncogenes in multiple endocrine neoplasia[4] (MEN) and familial papillary renal cell cancer syndromes. Current opinion is that somatic oncogene activation is an important step in sporadic tumour carcinogenesis.

Tumour suppressor genes

In contrast to oncogenes, tumour suppressor genes have an opposite effect in that if they are inactivated, cancer may develop. The normal function of tumour suppressor genes is to inhibit cell proliferation and growth; hence loss of function will result in uncontrolled proliferation and growth. Germ-line mutations in tumour suppressor genes tend to show recessive genetic inheritance at the cellular level, as both copies of the gene have to be inactivated before cancer can develop, otherwise the remaining normal copy of the gene will still be able to produce adequate quantities of the relevant protein for the normal functioning of a cell.

However, the phenotype of inheritance is dominant as during the lifetime of an individual, the remaining normal copy of the gene is altered. This second change is known as the 'second hit' or Knudson's hypothesis[5] and undergoes a somatic mutation in a single cell and thereby renders that cell null for the normal tumour suppressor gene. This cell has now lost all suppressor function of that particular gene. Recessive genetic inheritance by phenotypically dominant inheritance is a difficult concept to introduce in genetic counselling; the inherited mutation on its own is not sufficient to cause cancer and often it is unknown which factors result in the mutation of the remaining normal allele. These factors may include diet, chemicals, viruses, and occupational exposure to carcinogens. Many identified inherited germ-line cancer predisposition genes appear to show this type of inheritance, the most well characterised being the breast and colon cancer predisposition genes.

Repair genes

These are also called DNA repair genes and are involved in correcting DNA replication errors, which are common events during the natural process of DNA replication. Similar to tumour suppressor genes, repair gene mutations tend to show a recessive genotypic inheritance, but a phenotypically dominant expression as a somatic mutation of the remaining normal copy of the gene commonly occurs during the lifetime of the individual in at least one somatic cell. The main example in humans is the hereditary non-polyposis colon cancer syndrome, where germ-line alteration in the several genes that have so far been identified can cause this syndrome, characterised by colon carcinomas and other tumours.[6]

Cancer genetics clinics and genetic counselling

Background and historical perspective

Genetic counselling can be regarded as advice about patterns of inheritance and may be seen as cross-cultural. For example, in ancient as well as modern Japan, marriage brokers are most concerned about 'familial diseases' and therefore take great care to understand and analyse family pedigrees. Familial clustering of common cancers is said to have been recorded as an important fact in Roman times. Cancer clustering has also been reported by various authors, including Paul Broca,[7] Napoleon's physician, who referred to a particular family called Madame Z and described four generations that included many breast cancer cases who had died at a very early age. The suspected number of breast cancer deaths in this family amounted to at least 15 and Broca commented on the possibility of a genetic component to the disease and the difficulty of understanding the genetic explanations in smaller family clusters.

Interest in patterns of family inheritance was first described and formulated by Francis Galton.[8] His approach was mathematical and he devised ways of measuring human traits, including measuring hand grips and intelligence. He developed the theory 'that intelligence was inherited' and this was explained in the collected pedigree analysis of generations of successful families. This theory included the notion that undesirable characteristics such as criminality and mental illness were also inherited. Both he and his followers believed that the social and health problems related to nineteenth-century English society were caused by high fertility amongst the undesirable and lower fertility amongst intelligent families. He became a champion of a new movement to change this balance and he devised a new social campaign to rectify the problems.

The eugenics movement began in 1907 and soon became international, promoting selective breeding by moral influence, incentive, or legislation (i.e.

enforced sterilisation of the 'feeble-minded'). This movement in both Europe and America was considered to be part science and part social engineering and as a movement it was well supported in the early years of its inception by distinguished Cambridge scientists, churchmen, and dignitaries. The period of the unchallenged dominance of the eugenecists in human genetics came to an end in 1930. Galton developed the word 'eugenic', while Mazumadar,[9] for example, has recently argued that human geneticists are the successors of the eugenecists.

The significance of the new genetics of the 1930s is that it allowed for the repudiation of the principles underpinning the eugenics movement. The arguments regarding inheritance raged and the pedigree methodology was criticised. New methods used distinct clinical and biological traits, e.g. analysis of blood groups or haemophilia, to replace pauperism and the social problem group. It was not until the 1950s, with the coming of the post-war welfare state and the end of the Poor Law, that the eugenics movement was finally to dissolve.

Following the decline of this movement doctors interested in advising parents about their concerns related to genetic conditions used the terms 'consultation' and 'advice' on 'genetic hygiene' when talking to family members who were concerned about genetic risk. Interestingly, in 1947 a turning point came in America when the speciality changed the titles 'genetic consultation', 'genetic advice', and 'genetic hygiene' to the specialist title 'genetic counselling'.[10] The reason for this change was to remove the stigma and association with the past, as the former names were deemed inappropriate because they could be perceived as eugenic.

The term 'genetic counselling' has evolved over the years to include psychosocial issues that are paramount as part of the process of counselling.[11] The complex process of genetic counselling involves problems associated with diagnosis, risk assessment, and the explanation of all the possible options available to help with the burden associated with genetic risk.[12] The essence of genetic counselling is to make known to the counsellee(s) the information about an inherited disorder that is of concern, and to help to evaluate the alternative options stemming from the many concerns that may be raised by the counsellee during the session. This may include advising the person seeking genetic counselling about the different services (i.e. screening or support) that are available to both the patient and the family.

Cancer development

The origin and development of cancer are due to inherited susceptibility and environmental influences or a combination of both. The global incidence

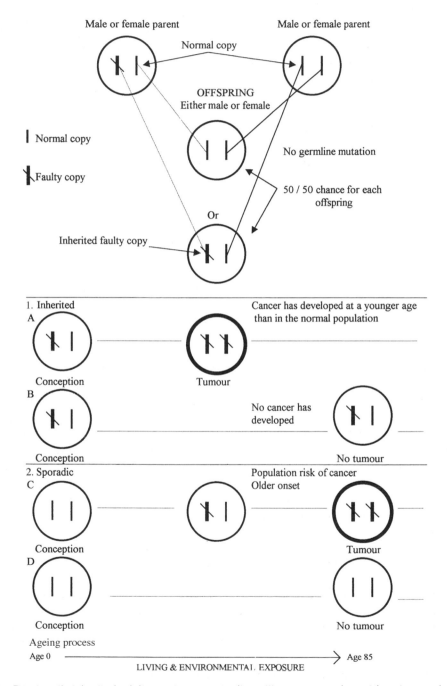

Figure 15.1 Dominantly inherited adult-onset cancer predisposition gene, e.g. breast/ovarian syndrome.

of cancer is increasing, mainly due to increased longevity. By the year 2020 there may be 20 million new cancer patients each year.[13] Once completed, the Human Genome Project will bring sophisticated genetic risk analysis, which will need very careful consideration with regard to screening programmes that already exist.

Hereditary cancer varies considerably and develops in different ways; for example, in terms of the ages at which people develop the disease, differences in tumour grading and clinical staging, and length of survival. Cancer inheritance can be predicted from an informative family history either on the maternal or paternal side of the family or, in rare instances, on both sides of the family where people have intermarried.

In the UK, the first clinical genetics service was established in 1946 and it is only in the last two decades that cancer genetics clinics have become part of this service. In the UK, genetic testing for rare cancer genes is a relatively new phenomenon. As a result of recent developments in this field it has been necessary to define these services and a government multi-disciplinary working party has been set up to report and advise on the provision, professional expertise, and educational training needed for these rapidly developing services.[14]

Understanding a cancer family history and detecting who is at risk

It is estimated that one in three persons will develop cancer in their lifetime. Included in these numbers are people with a hereditary predisposition to cancer. More than 200 types of hereditary cancer syndromes are known and these account for 5–10% of all cancers diagnosed.[15] Families who have a hereditary predisposition have a high risk of developing cancer and if they have already developed one cancer, have a high risk of developing a second cancer. However, included in these families may be family members who have developed cancer by chance alone (sporadic cases or phenocopies).

Analysing a family history is a complex process. There are certain features that a counsellor will recognise as typical of an inherited cancer syndrome. For example, if several family members on either the maternal or paternal side in any generation have developed the same or related cancers, in particular two or three first-degree relatives, then this pattern is highly suggestive of the presence of a cancer predisposition gene. Another important factor to consider when analysing a family pedigree is the principle that the younger the age of onset of a particular cancer the more likely it is that the cancer has developed due to an inherited susceptibility. Furthermore, the phenotypic appearance of the individual attending the clinic is also of great importance. It is therefore necessary to take note of any significant features of a family member that may implicate a known hereditary condition; for example, large circumference of the head and skin tricholemmomas, which can occur in Cowden's syndrome. This rare syndrome may predispose families to the development of both breast and thyroid cancers.[16]

Cancer risk counselling is provided where family members believe that the cancers in their families are due to hereditary factors. Therefore the most important task when collecting a family history is to collect enough information to estimate whether or not the family member seeking genetic counselling is at risk of inheriting the cancer that is in the family. Commonly, the histories that people give in the clinic are inaccurate and further research and collection of histological reports are necessary. The ages of family members and dates when the cancer was diagnosed in the family are essential. Sensitive handling of family members during this part of the consultation is of paramount importance. Family members have often experienced bereavement and simply talking about past experiences is profoundly disturbing.

Through the counselling process, it is necessary to make estimates of environmental exposures such as sun exposure and smoking, as well as to clarify the ethnic groups of the family members seeking counselling. For example, Ashkenazi Jewish women who have developed breast cancer at <40 years have a higher chance of carrying a specific alteration in two of the breast cancer susceptibility genes (BRCA1 and BRCA2) than a woman from another ethnic group.[17] Unaffected family members need to inform the counsellor of their age and information should be given about routine screening. If family members have died, it is wise to collect copies of death certificates to establish the cause of death. All the information is collated on a family tree and this is known as the family pedigree.

The meaning and presentation of risk and screening issues

Epidemiological studies of many human cancers have demonstrated a modest (two- or threefold) increase in risk of cancer amongst first-degree relatives of individuals with a similar cancer.[18] Family members may well be advised to seek screening for these cancers. Genetic cancer risk is multi-dimensional and hard to define. The risk may consist of the probability and consequence of a cancer developing; also important is the possible effect of knowing and how it may impact on a person's behaviour (for example, the decision to take preventive action or no action at all).[19] The way people perceive their risk is complex. Several psychological studies[20,21] have shown that many people at a high risk of developing cancer do not understand their risk of cancer and tend to overestimate it.

Many factors contribute to risk perception, not least the subtle differences in the framing of risk information given by health professionals, which in itself may have dramatic effects on perceptions of risk and health behaviour.[22] Many health risks are considered to be the result of deliberate decisions by individuals who understand what they perceive to be their risk and then according to their best beliefs either take action or not.[22] For example, a smoker may justify his smoking habit by believing that his father had smoked all his life and had died of a heart attack rather than cancer, thereby convincing himself that smoking was not cancer causing for his family. He continues to smoke with little concern for a potential cancer diagnosis.

The role of contextual factors in risk perception relates to lay constructions of genetic risk.

Several studies have shown that people have their own beliefs regarding cancer genetic risk. For example, using in-depth interviews as part of the methodology both Kelly[23] and Mahon and Casperson[24] found that some high cancer risk families had special needs for information and support. Women consulting about their own risks of breast cancer or the risk to their sisters and daughters required more than a risk percentage or ratio, no matter how carefully these were presented. Their feelings regarding the threat of developing cancer were not helped by quantitative numerical risk figures given as a result of assessment. Feelings

of the inevitability of cancer developing in the future were common and genetic risk was misconstrued.

The presentation of information regarding cancer risk needs to be tailored to an individual's background, sociodemographic status, and psychological profile. The interpretation of information regarding risk will depend on cultural background and subjective understanding of the situation. Understandably, perception of risk involves more than disclosure of information or presentation of the mathematically determined probabilities. Indeed, over 200 years ago the philosopher Kant[25] stated, 'We see things not as they are but as we are.'

Personal account 15.1

Susan has a 50% chance of inheriting a breast cancer susceptibility gene that exists in her family. Understandably anxious about her cancer risk, her feelings were as follows:

> I feel that I have a rush here, rush there attitude to life . . . I am making the most of it because I don't know how long . . . . now that I have hit thirty . . . I used to think that I am on a time bomb as soon as I hit 29. If I am going to get past 29 . . . I am going to be all right because that's when my sister was diagnosed . . . I feel that I am just ticking away, ticking away in the sense that I knew that we had this hereditary problem in the family . . .[26]

One of the most important reasons for identifying hereditary cancer is to enable family members who are not affected by cancer to seek preventive strategies for the future; that is, to seek screening, surveillance, or surgery. There is evidence to show that early detection may prevent the onset of metastatic cancer. In addition, by providing cancer risk information it may be possible to facilitate informed choices of anti-cancer treatments or surveillance programmes.

Common psychological reactions to genetic cancer risk information include denial, low self-esteem, anxiety, and guilt. This is not surprising given that cancer has been elegantly depicted as a disease that is despicable, dirty, and self-inflicted.[27] Interestingly, the methods used to assess the impact of risk information appear to affect the outcome of the particular study. For example, using quantitative methods, Lerman[21] found that there was a high level of anxiety in women who were first-degree relatives of breast/ovarian cancer patients. In contrast, a qualitative study revealed that women did not have high levels of anxiety about cancer risk, although 'peaks and troughs' were reported. Anxiety was at its peak as women approached the age of their relative's death.[28]

Cancer risk notification is fraught with ethical dilemmas. There is little more to offer the majority of 'at risk' family members other than surveillance or change in diet. Given the climate of present-day health care and rationing, the implications of cancer screening[29] are controversial. As well as the psychological and social costs, screening is expensive and benefits are not proven for all the screening programmes. Genetic counsellors are involved in planning screening programmes for family members at risk of hereditary cancer, and a referral to a clinic for this purpose can be seen by some members of the medical profession to have little benefit to the patient. This may cause disruption and anxiety for people who believe that a prevention programme is important.

Personal account 15.2

The following is the personal account of a family member seeking screening for hereditary colon cancer:

> I think that, as a lot of people feel, that if you have somebody close to you . . . [that has developed cancer] you immediately start to worry . . . but it didn't worry me unduly . . . until my mother's sister died and I thought no, all three sisters in the family, that is a bit too much . . . I thought I might be in line for it . . . . the thought of cancer frightens me . . . I had to press [my GP] very hard . . . and I had to go to another doctor . . . he had never written to the hospital . . . . I don't think that he particularly wanted me to go to the hospital . . . I don't have much confidence in that doctor.[26]

The following is an excerpt from a referral letter to the genetics department for the same woman:

> . . . she understands from various literature sources that a regular colonoscopy is sometimes suggested . . . however, there is an argument to suggest that this is not a cost effective means . . . however, if you feel it would be appropriate given her gross family history . . . .[26]

In fact, the patient referred to in this letter came from a high-risk hereditary non-polyposis colorectal cancer family and colonoscopy screening is clearly recommended as a beneficial procedure with proven benefits.[30]

The informational needs of individuals and families are different and vary according to the cancer risk. Some family members only want an explanation of their risk and screening options, whereas others choose to consider genetic testing. Explaining risk to a family requires considerable expertise as each person perceives risk in an individual way.

Therefore, it is important to understand an individual's level of understanding and to provide a comprehensible explanation of the risk. In a recent study of numerical risk explanation, family members were asked, prior to visiting the cancer genetics clinic, what they considered to be the best way of presenting risk for them to understand. Interestingly, the percentage risk (for example, telling someone that they have a 30% lifetime chance of developing hereditary cancer) seemed to provide a less threatening explanation than numerical risk.[31]

This is illustrated by the account of one Mrs S:

> 30 percent sounds easier because it sounds a lot less than 1 in 3.

However, she continued:

> I think if I wanted real factual information, and this is what we are talking about, I think that 1 in 3 would be better for me.

Recently, Hallowell et al.[32] argued in their study that risk information was best appreciated by use of quantitative formats. The researchers used a qualitative approach and interviewed 46 women in the study to assess the preferred format for risk information. The counsellors presenting the risk information used quantitative formats that included proportions, percentages, odds ratios, and comparisons with population risks. The women who had been counselled in the clinic answered a questionnaire following their consultation and were asked 'What do you think of using numbers as a way of describing your chance of developing cancer?' All the women except for one person found numerical risk estimates helpful and informative. However, only 40 women were interviewed following genetic counselling and 22 of these women spontaneously expressed that the use of quantitative formats was helpful. A recurring theme emerging from these interviews was that numerical risk seemed to clarify the risk both for the person being counselled and for others.

Screening

Most cancer genetic risk prevention programmes include screening as a tool to detect early signs of cancer so that it may then be cured. Screening is planned in accordance with age and may need to be followed for long periods of time.

There may be concerns that the advances in genetic technology and susceptibility will be translated into screening services and offered to those at risk without consideration of the consequences. The possible harm (for example, anxiety) that may arise from a screening test for any person may be very small in comparison with the potential harm from not offering screening, and screening may be life-saving by enabling treatment of a potentially fatal cancer. However, despite the wide publicity and optimism amongst the lay public about regarding the benefits of screening, some families may have problems with their family doctors arranging a referral for appropriate screening.

David (whose wife has a family history of colo-rectal cancer) comments:

I am surprised at the low level of interest the medical profession takes . . . once you have identified a problem, you need to find an answer to it . . . otherwise it saps away at everything . . . Penny is the target area at the moment, but it does affect all subsequent generations . . . if there is a gene related . . . she is the target, but behind that is the family . . . emotionally, you have got one person continuously involved but socially you have got the whole extended family, the cousins and their families . . . it is quite extended for people who should possibly be screened . . .[26]

Ethical issues associated with genetic counselling and testing

It is only in the last few years that laboratory tests have made it possible to detect those individuals who have an increased hereditary risk of cancer. This new knowledge in molecular biology is becoming more available with recent developments for genetic testing for common cancer susceptibility genes.

However, for most cancer families testing is not available. Genetic testing is a process whereby a blood sample is taken after full counselling from a person, usually in a family with multiple cases of cancer. Cancer genetic counselling involves providing the person seeking genetic testing with a full understanding of the implications of the testing process. For a person who has already developed cancer there are many issues that may face him or her should a mutation be found. These include serious associated prognostic factors such as the possibility of developing further cancers and the risks to their offspring (see below).

Box 15.1: Genetic testing

Cancer genetic testing usually starts with counselling a person who has already developed cancer in a family where there is a high chance of finding an alteration in a known cancer gene that relates to the patterns of cancers in the family.

Testing for a cancer-causing mutation may not find an alteration in the gene – the individual must be aware of this. This may be for several reasons, including the fact that modern technology is still in its infancy, not all areas of the gene may be screened, or the wrong gene may be tested, as familial cancer even at one site can be due to more than one gene.

It may take many months, even years, to complete the search for the gene. A negative result does not mean that there is no alteration, merely that it has not been found. This may mean that there is another gene yet to be discovered responsible for all the cancers in the family, or merely that the alteration is in a part of the gene that current technology cannot reach. If a mutation is found, this means that this is likely to be the reason for the development of the particular cancer in the individual concerned. This may have predictive implications factors for other cancers.

For example, the breast/ovarian cancer gene BRCA I confers a high risk for contralateral breast cancer, as well as the development of both breast and ovarian cancer, and a small increased risk of other cancers.

The individual who has had the test may wish to inform his or her brothers and sisters, children and other eligible family members of the result. All first-degree family members have a 50/50 chance of inheriting the same mutation in the family. This may or may not cause concerns and worries for other family members.

Counselling sessions for genetic testing may include several consultations with the individual, who may need to take time before undergoing such a test. Talking through all the implications with the multidisciplinary team members is important. The preparation time is described overleaf.

Box 15.2: Predictive genetic testing

In this case, a known mutation in the family has been identified and a person who has not developed cancer is seeking a test to know whether or not they carry this same mutation.

Informed consent
Full understanding of the implications of finding out whether or not the individual seeking testing carries the mutation in the family is required.

Session 1
Here, the risks and benefits of the test and the current risk factors associated with becoming a known carrier of the disease are explained. This is important, as statistical evidence associated with gene penetrance does change. Informing the person about insurance implications and explaining all the options that are available for them should they find that they are a carrier is important. Assessing that they have not been coerced into undergoing such a test and that they do not have any suicidal ideation is also necessary.

Session 2
This involves further discussion regarding all the emotional implications surrounding such a test. Is there anything bothering them about taking this test? This session should include time to establish a good relationship with the genetic counsellor, who will be there when they have their results. Part of the process is preparing for both a positive result and a negative result. Plans for either result may be mapped out on paper. This plan includes all the screening options, chemoprevention, and surgical options. When the person seeking the testing is confident and comfortable with all his or her information, a blood sample can be taken. If there is a known mutation in the family, the predictive test does not take very long (between 2 and 3 months).

Session 3
Test results are given, arrangements are made for follow-up support, and the planned programme is arranged for screening, surgery, or chemoprevention options.

Genetic technology is still in its infancy and many people who give blood for genetic testing may never have an informative result. Testing for genes and looking for the mutation in the family takes many months, even years. Family members need to be informed about this as part of the testing process. Information is given in the counselling process about the real chances of finding a mutation and the length of time that it may take. A negative test result following the search for a

mutation from a person with cancer in a high-risk cancer genetic family does not mean that there is no alteration in the suspect gene present, merely that current scientific discoveries have not managed to confirm all mutations in known cancer genetic families. This may change in the future as technology improves. However, at present a considerable proportion of cancer patients giving a blood sample for genetic analysis will not receive any answers. If, however, a mutation is found in an affected person, other blood family members in the family may choose to have a predictive genetic test.

When a person receiving genetic counselling considers having genetic testing, several counselling sessions are made available to the individual before a sample of blood is taken to ascertain whether or not the mutation that has been found in the family exists. This process aims to ensure that the person who is choosing to find out information that may profoundly affect them, does so on the basis of factual information about risk management and screening options.

Studies involving genetic testing of adult-onset dominantly inherited disorders are modelled on conditions such as Huntington's disease. This disorder, which is similar to cancer (in that it manifests itself in adult life), is known as Huntington's chorea. The difference between a cancer predisposition gene and the Huntington's chorea gene is that while the cancer predisposition gene may be inherited, there is still some chance that cancer will not have developed by the age of 80. Conversely, the Huntington's chorea gene, if inherited, means that the disease will always ultimately develop and furthermore there is no known cure for this disease. Indeed, testing for this disease has shown that those people at risk of developing it who did not receive test results, either because they declined or because results were uninformative, had significantly higher levels of distress at a 12-month follow-up evaluation than either those who carried the gene or those who had been tested and found to be non-carriers of the gene.[33] Among relatives of breast cancer patients, anxiety regarding cancer risk has been found to interfere with full understanding of factual risk and recommended screening programmes.[34]

Most of the ethical issues surrounding genetic testing concern confidentiality issues and the duties of the individuals sharing information with their family. For example, who should take the responsibility for informing other family members about a possible genetic risk or a 'positive' genetic test, and is there a duty to do so? If the patient does not wish to warn relatives about cancer risk, does the problem then become one for the professional? In general, this important consideration related to the professional ethics of genetics is difficult if one assumes that genetic testing is always a 'family affair'. Arguably, although it is assumed to be a family affair, the individual rights of the person seeking genetic counselling for him or herself need to be considered. After all, one brother or sister may wish to know and another may not wish to know, because of the fear of discrimination. The rights of an individual to decide to know or not are paramount.

The dilemma of communication within families in relation to genetics has been debated both by the Nuffield Council on Bioethics[35] and the House of Commons Science and Technology Committee.[36] Release of genetic information about cancer susceptibility inevitably has many considerations that include family members, health professionals, and researchers. Releasing information about an individual's mutation status provides a route for other family members to have the chance to consider genetic testing. However, in the interests of a person's right to confidentiality, results are not released to other family members about their risk status. Indeed, the House of Commons Science and Technology Committee rejected the notion that family members should be contacted in the interest of other family members. More recently, the Human Genetic Advisory Commission[37] has been asked to advise ministers on the complex issues surrounding the rapid advances in genetics and genetic testing. This commission has a facilitative and advisory role and aims to improve the level of informed debate about the implications of the development of human genetics. The aim is to minimise discrimination for those people with genetic disorders. Family communication may differ between ethnic groups or those with different cultural backgrounds. Indeed, the culture of a given group may be very different from another culture. For example, many African Americans are symbolised by family sharing and a sense of spirituality[38] and this contrasts with the ethic of many Europeans whose values are based on the notions of the individual and his right to choose for himself.[39]

Individuals should be involved in deciding whether or not the genetic test that they are considering is worth taking. The decision must be a joint one with the counsellor as part of the pre-test informed consent process. On the one hand, establishing the test itself is a scientific process, and on the other hand, the level of predictive power that justifies the test is a professional ethical question.[40] Assessing the test and its value includes requiring a professional judgement about the clinical significance of any of the results that may affect not only the individual, but also the family.

There is a probability component in estimating whether or not an individual who chooses to have a predictive cancer genetic test will develop cancer or not. Certainly, the knowledge that an individual may have inherited a cancer susceptibility gene provides important information. This information is of clinical significance, as preventive procedures may reduce morbidity and mortality in a known gene carrier. It is as well to note that there is an element of probability and uncertainty in clinical advice given concerning many cancer genes. The main considerations attributable to predictive cancer genetic testing are the knowledge that probability does not equate with certainty and that individuals who are otherwise healthy are faced with the knowledge of carrying a genetic mutation that they may or may not pass to their offspring with associated risk of developing cancer. This knowledge is linked in with modifying factors, which not only are genetic but have environmental influences. For example, if a woman carries either of the two known breast cancer genes (BRCA1 or BRCA2 genes), it is not certain that she will develop breast or ovarian cancer but merely that she has an estimated cancer risk from the latest gene penetrance studies.[41]

The example below illustrates the fear and concern associated with a genetic test.

Anna said:

> When I was asked if I would like to find out if I had the gene . . . I discussed it with my sisters . . . and I said my reaction is that I don't want to know, and they said 'I'd agree with you . . . I wouldn't want to know either, because like what are you going to do . . . if you find out you've got the gene . . .?[26]

Penny felt:

> I am not sure [about genetic testing] . . . it is one of those things that I am trying not to think much about because I am not sure what my answer would be . . . I would be quite happy to have the test, if there is a fair chance that it was going to be negative . . .[26]

Prophylactic surgery

Prophylactic surgery is debated as an option for the treatment of individuals at a high risk of developing cancer. In certain areas of cancer risk management, surgery has an established preventive role; for example, for the treatment of patients with multiple endocrine neoplasia type-2 syndrome. Prophylactic total thyroidectomy is advocated to prevent the development of medullary thyroid cancer. Prophylactic colectomy is normally advised for family members who have familial adenomatous polyposis and surgery prevents the inevitable progression of colonic adenomas to invasive cancers.[6] A small residual risk (3%) is left following prophylactic oophorectomy for ovarian cancer risk.[42] There is some evidence that the reduction in risk of breast cancer from prophylactic breast surgery may be as high as 90%, but such studies contain inherent bias and this may be an overestimate.[43]

Although surgery offers high preventive rates for some of these inherited cancer syndromes, it is never without trauma, fear, and an impact on an individual's life when they opt for what may be considered a 'life-saving option'. The long-term follow-up of family members who have opted for surgery should continue and the family history remains along with the continued concern for others in the family who may have already developed cancer. Surgery is extensive and should never be underestimated. The cost of prophylactic surgery in psychological terms has yet to be fully studied and understood.

Personal account 15.3

Susan (whose sister died at the age of 29, as did her mother and three sisters) said:

> Now that I am thirty-two . . . I am thinking . . . oh well there is hope because I am going to have this mastectomy . . . so I pin all my hopes on that mastectomy . . . and if it means that I do not have two lumps around my body

that didn't work for me . . . [she could not breast feed her child], as far as I am concerned [they are] two big bombs waiting to go off . . . I can't see another way . . . I wanted to have a baby before I died . . . I wanted to have that emotion . . . I could not face death without having a child . . . which is selfish because I was going to leave that child behind . . . I wasn't going to wait for the cancer to get me . . . I was going to get the cancer before it got me . . .[26]

Husband Mike commented:

> She has come to her own decision that she will go through the operation . . . she appreciates that it is not the be all and end all . . . and that she can obviously contract cancer . . . in a different form, but it takes away one area of the problem that could actually have an impact on her . . . if she suddenly woke up and found that she has breast cancer . . . So I think that in that sense it doesn't worry me in the slightest that she has made that decision . . . I am wholeheartedly behind her and will support her . . .[26]

The field of molecular genetics is rapidly developing, and understanding of whether or not radical surgical procedures such as prophylactic surgery reduce cancer risk is still emerging. The excerpt from Susan used in Personal account 15.2 was taken from a woman seeking such a procedure without knowing whether she carried a genetic risk for breast cancer, as no mutation could be found in the family to enable a test to be offered. Current genetic technology is not able to identify all the alterations that may be present in a cancer susceptibility gene.

Recently, while counselling three sisters with a very low breast cancer genetic risk (15% compared to the normal population risk of 10%) they wished to discuss the option of prophylactic breast surgery, since the premature death from breast cancer of their mother had led them to have a distorted perception of their own risk. Such profound fears are well recorded in the psychosocial literature and have been likened to the 'sword of Damocles'. The influence of the media and television had promoted an idea that it would be better for these young girls (aged 20, 21, and 22) to seek this option, despite a low calculated genetic risk. These findings have been echoed through the literature and Kelly[23] refers in her paper to the anguish of a low-risk person whom she has followed up for 20 years in her cancer risk clinic: 'Please God, I know I am going to die of breast cancer, but not this year'.

There is a dilemma for those people who consider cancer genetic testing, because there are no clear direct answers for them. If an individual tests positive, he or she does not know for sure that cancer will develop in the family, and if he or she tests negative there is always the sporadic cancer risk. Lerman[44] argues that not having the breast/ovarian cancer genetic test when it is available to you may produce depression as a consequence, and family members who choose not to have the test should be carefully followed up. Therefore, nurses looking after the whole family have a duty to care and consider those members in the family who have not come forward for testing but who may be silently very depressed.

Culture and the media's influence on families with cancer genetic risk

The media's influence on the culture of cancer is documented in the literature. Its depiction as 'the killer disease'[45] strikes vivid images of cancer that provide a negative response. The language of warfare is regularly described in newspaper journals and on television programmes, fuelling anxiety for many people, especially those with a cancer risk. Cancer becomes a disease that personifies death itself. In this context, time is particularly needed in the complex process of cancer genetic counselling. The language of warfare is very often reflected in the language used by families discussing their cancer risk. The metaphoric personification of cancer as the 'enemy' is profound and linked with images from the media and film world. For example:

> Cancer is such an awful illness and it still keeps evading every doctor, research scientist as to a cure, as to why it happens . . . it must be one hell of a disease . . . it reminds me of Dr Hannibal in The Silence of the Lambs, he was a psychopathic killer, who used his victims through their brains, he got to them through the way he spoke . . . I thought he was a very clever, very, very, clever guy . . . and that is how I feel about cancer, it is clever, it is a smart cookie . . .[26]

The cancer nurse is most suited to deconstructing and understanding stories and myths long believed by the devastated families with inherited cancers. Telling the story, listening to the story, and

empathising and understanding that cancer is a complicated illness is important. Lay people very often misinterpret the metastatic cancer process and believe that other organs that are invaded many years after a primary cancer diagnosis are new cancers. In this way individuals fear for themselves, believing that they are in line for many different types of cancers. Explanation of this process may decrease anxiety for some family members. Understanding the disease, the treatments, and the illness process is important. Some family members have never had the chance to do this and therefore feel a sense of confusion: they 'haven't liked to ask Dad' about the real truth about a family member's illness.

The following in an extract from Lisa's view of her genetic risk:

> I think [my grandmother's death] never really was explained to me . . . I just knew she was very ill and it was a cancer . . . but exactly what and why I didn't know . . . I didn't really register anything, that there might be a genetic link . . . so what can you do about it . . .?[26]

This example highlights the fact that some people are unaware of the cancer development in another family member and Lisa lives in a family with a dominantly inherited colon cancer gene. Her mother is terrified of developing the disease that killed her mother and her two sisters. Cancer remains confusing to her and the genetic link has been her mother's prime concern. Screening for colon cancer is recognised as a positive management strategy for hereditary colon cancer risk.[6]

Family dynamics are very important and one should establish with the family involved in the genetic counselling process the social relationships within the family. This is helpful to both the counsellor and the family member, as other members of the family may seek genetic counselling. Social relationships can be drawn in the format of a genogram (a family tree that shows the social relationship patterns in the family). It is essential to provide a confidential place of knowledge giving. All family members visiting the cancer genetics clinic are assured of their privacy with regard to the genetic counselling process. Any information about a cancer diagnosis or medical matter concerning a person who is alive should be given with written consent from the individual to whom the information pertains.

Psychological morbidity

It is important to be aware of any psychopathology that may occur as part of the experience of belonging to a cancer family. The many bereavements in the family and in particular the loss of a parent may make it difficult for people to accept their own personal cancer risks. Unresolved bereavement, cancerphobia, or excessive anxiety states all need expert assessment by a clinical psychologist.

Discrimination and insurance

Discrimination exists for people known to be at high risk of developing cancer. This most commonly occurs in the context of an individual's ability to obtain life insurance, and with his employers or potential employers. These issues raise practical questions about advising patients. The most important factor that is involved in the genetic counselling process is the information that should be provided outlining the possible dangers or harms that the individual could encounter as a direct consequence of a genetic test. Against the backdrop of risk discrimination, there is a need to warn patients that testing of apparently healthy persons for a hereditary gene may possibly have potential problems for many years and needs very careful consideration.

Insurance companies are debating the implications of genetic testing and in particular testing for cancer genes. Discrimination is a profound and understandable fear for families concerned for their children's future. Companies want to avoid unnecessary discrimination and adverse publicity. In the UK, there is currently a debate regarding the assessment of personal insurance, and the increase in predictive genetic testing is challenging the insurance market. It seems likely that risk-related premiums will be seen as discriminating against already vulnerable members of our society.[46] This topic has received considerable attention in the media and, understandably, this is one of the many concerns that families have when considering genetic testing.

In the UK the Human Genetics Advisory Commission has been set up to create a feeling of confidence that scientific genetic research is being monitored for the public good, but contrary to this practice the insurance industry aims to institutionalise insurers' rights to genetic information about potential clients.

Conclusions

Cancer genetics is a new and developing speciality. Nurses who choose to work in cancer genetic clinics need to understand the state of flux of knowledge, along with the many psychosocial implications that affect not only the person seeking the counselling but also other family members. This knowledge is both predictive and prognostic and has many implications for families.

The language of cancer genetics needs to be explained to family members seeking counselling. The changing and cutting-edge nature of this speciality is both exciting and symbolic of the complexities associated with a rapidly developing technological age. These developments are interlinked with cost-cutting budgets and constraints in practice. Scientific discoveries leading to improving cancer care need careful consideration and understanding from a holistic perspective. The scientific discoveries are moving at a great pace and by understanding the molecular basis of the mechanics of the genetic changes, there is hope for further discoveries leading to new treatments, useful screening, and perhaps a cure for inherited cancer. As this is a fast-moving field, the absolute risk figures can change with time as more knowledge becomes available.

If, however, predictions for improved diagnosis are true, then it is essential to process the knowledge in human terms. Understanding cancer risk is complex and each individual has their way of believing the facts and relating to them in meaningful ways according to experience. One of the main nursing concerns is understanding the individual for whom one is caring within the context of their predicament.

References

1. Suzuki D.T., Griffiths A.J.F., Miller J.H. and Lewontin R.C. (1986). *An Introduction to Genetic Analysis,* 3rd edition. New York: W.H. Freeman.
2. Jones S. and van Loon B. (1993). *Genetics for Beginners.* Cambridge: Icon Books.

3. Easton D. (1996). From families to chromosomes: genetic linkage, and other methods for finding cancer predisposition genes. In Eeles R.A., Ponder B.A.J., Easton D.F. and Horwich A. (eds.) *Genetic Predisposition to Cancer*. London: Chapman and Hall.

4. Ponder B. (1996). Multiple endocrine neoplasia. In Eeles R.A., Ponder B.A.J., Easton D.F. and Horwich A. (eds.) *Genetic Predisposition to Cancer*. London: Chapman and Hall.

5. Knudson A.G. (1985). Hereditary cancer, oncogenes and antioncogenes. *Cancer Res* **45**, 1437–1443.

6. Murday V.A., Bishop D.T. and Hall N. (1996). Familial colon cancer syndromes and their clinical management. In Eeles R.A., Ponder B.A.J., Easton D.F. and Horwich A. (eds.) *Genetic Predisposition to Cancer*. London: Chapman and Hall.

7. Broca P.P. (1866). *Traite des Tumeurs*. Paris: P. Asselin.

8. Galton F. (1983). Hereditary talent and character. *Macmillans Magazine* **12**, 157–327.

9. Mazumudar P.M.H. (1992). Eugenics, human genetics and human failings. *Millbank Quarterly* **68**, 497–525.

10. Haller M.H. (1963). *Eugenics: Hereditarian Attitudes in American Thought*. New Brunswick, NJ: Rutgers University Press.

11. Griffin M.L., Kavanagh C.M. and Sorenson J.R. (1976). Genetic knowledge, client perspectives and genetic counselling. *Social Work in Health Care* **2**, 177–180.

12. Muller H., Scott R. and Weber W. (1995). *Hereditary Cancer* London: Karger.

13. Imperial Cancer Research Fund (1995). *A Vision for Cancer*. London: Imperial Cancer Research Fund.

14. Harper P. (1996). *Report of a Working Group for the Chief Medical Officer*. London: Department of Health.

15. McKusick V. (1998). *Mendelian Inheritance in Man*. Baltimore, MA: Johns Hopkins University Press.

16. Eng C. (1998). Genetics of Cowden syndrome: through the looking glass of oncology. *International Journal of Oncology* **12**, 701–710.

17. Abeliovich D., Kadouri L., Lerer I. *et al.* (1997). The founder mutations in 185delAG and 5382insC in *BRCA*1 and 617delT in *BRCA*2 appear in 60% of ovarian cancer and 30% of early-onset breast cancer patients among Ashkenazi women. *American Journal of Human Genetics* **60**, 505–514.

18. Easton D.E. and Peto J. (1990). The contribution of inherited predisposition to cancer incidence. *Cancer Surveys* **9**, 395–416.

19. Evers-Kiebooms G., Cassiman J.-J., van den Berghe H. and d'Ydewalle G. (eds.) (1987). *Genetic Risk, Risk Perception and Decision Making*. New York: Liss.

20. Evans D.G.R., Burnell L.D., Hopwood P. and Howell A. (1993). Perception of risk in women with a family history of breast cancer. *British Journal of Cancer* **67**, 612–614.

21. Lerman C. and Schwarz M. (1993). Adherence and psychological adjustment among women at high risk for breast cancer. *Breast Cancer Research and Treatment* **67**, 612–614.

22. Lerman C., Rimer B. and Engstrom P.F. (1991). Cancer risk notification psychosocial and ethical implications. *Journal of Clinical Oncology* **9**, 1275–1282.

23. Kelly P.T. (1992). Breast cancer risk analysis: a genetic epidemiology service for families. *Journal of Genetic Counselling* **1**, 155–167.

24. Mahon S.M. and Casperson D.S. (1995). Hereditary cancer syndrome: part 2. Psychosocial issues, concerns and screening – results of a qualitative study. *Oncology Nursing Forum* **22**, 775–782.

25. Kant E. (1789). *The Critique of Pure Reason*. (trans. Kemp-Smith N., 1929). London: Macmillan.

26. Ardern-Jones A.T. *Living with a cancer legacy – the experience of hereditary cancer in the family*. Unpublished M.Sc. thesis, University of London, Institute of Cancer Research.

27. Sontag S. (1991). *Illness as Metaphor and AIDS and its Metaphors*. London: Penguin Books.

28. Green J., Murton F. and Statham H. (1993). Psychological issues raised by a familial ovarian cancer register. *Journal of Medical Genetics* **30**, 101–105.

29. Stewart-Brown S. and Farmer A. (1997). Screening could seriously damage your health. *British Medical Journal* **314**, 533–534.

30. Vasen H.F.A., Mecklin J.-P., Meera-Khan P. *et al.* (1991). The International Collaborative Group on Hereditary Non-Polyposis colorectal cancer (ICG-HNPCC). *Diseases of the Colon and Rectum* **34**, 424–425.

31. Ardern-Jones A.T., Louw G. and Eeles R.A. (1999). Presenting cancer risk – is there a best way? Unpublished study, The Royal Marsden NHS Trust, London.

32. Hallowell N., Statham H., Murton F., Green J. and Richards M. (1997). Talking about chance – the presentation of risk information during genetic counselling for breast and ovarian cancer. *Journal of Genetic Counselling* **5**, 269–286.

33. Tibben A., Frets P.G., van de Kamp J.J.P. *et al.* (1993). On attitudes and appreciation six months after predictive DNA testing for Huntington disease in the Dutch program. *American Journal of Human Genetics* **48**, 103–111.

34. Lerman C., Narod S., Schulman K. *et al.* (1996). *BRCA*1 testing in hereditary breast–ovarian cancer families: a prospective study of patient decision-making and outcomes. *Journal of the American Medical Association* **275**, 1885–1892.

35. Nuffield Council on Bioethics (1993). *Genetic Screening Ethical Issues*. London: Nuffield Council on Bioethics.

36. House of Commons Science and Technology Committee (1995). *Human Genetics: The Science and its Consequences,* 3rd report. London: HMSO.

37. Human Genetic Advisory Commission (1998). First Annual Report of the Human Genetic Advisory Commission. *Journal of Medical Ethics* **20,** 12–18.

38. Martin J.N., Hecht M.L. and Larkey L.K. (1994). Conversational improvement strategies for interethnic communication: African American and European American perspectives. *61 Comm, Monographs* **236, 237** 353–372.

39. Lerman C., Peshkin M.S., Hughes C. and Isaacs M.D. (1998). Family disclosure in genetic testing for cancer susceptibility: determinants and consequences, *Journal of Health Care, Law and Policy* 353–372.

40. Geller L.N., Alper J.S., Billings P.R., Barash C.L., Becwith J. and Natowicz M. (1996). Individual family and societal dimensions of genetic discrimination: a case study analysis. *Science and Engineering Ethics* **2,** 71–88.

41. Ford D., Easton D.F., Stratton M.R. *et al.* (1998). Genetic heterogeneity and penetrance analysis of the *BRCA*1 and *BRCA*2 genes in breast cancer families. *American Journal of Human Genetics* **62,** 676–689.

42. Struewing J.P., Watson P.L. and Easton D.F. (1994). Effectiveness of prophylactic oophorectomy in inherited breast/ovarian cancer families. *American Journal of Human Genetics* **55,** A70, 384.

43. Hartmann L.C., Schaid D.J., Woods J.E. *et al.* (1999). Efficacy of bilateral prophylactic mastectomy in women with a family history of breast cancer. *New England Journal of Medicine* **340,** 77–84.

44. Lerman C., Hughes C., Lemon S.J. *et al.* (1998). What you don't know can't hurt you: adverse psychological effects in members of *BRCA*1-linked and *BRCA*2-linked families who decline genetic testing. *Journal of Clinical Oncology* **16,** 1650–1654.

45. Birmingham News (1995). Prostate cancer a killer. *Birmingham News,* 16 August 1995, p. 1.

46. Wilkie T. (1998). Genetics and insurance in Britain: why more than just the Atlantic divides the English-speaking nations. *Natural Genetics* **20,** 119–121.

CHAPTER SIXTEEN

Developments in cancer treatment

John Bridgewater and Martin Gore

Cancer treatment is one of the most rapidly moving fields in health care because of ever-increasing scientific knowledge about its biology, genetics, and epidemiology, as well as changes in political, ethical, and social attitudes to cancer. The incidence of cancer is increasing, but this is not just confined to the increasing elderly population. As the numbers of cancer survivors increase, the incidence of secondary malignancies also increases, as do problems of long-term toxicity and psychological sequelae.

New developments in approaches to treatment mean that established drugs are experiencing a renaissance and there is an increasingly large number of new and helpful drugs available for use in treatment. The potentially large financial gains for the pharmaceutical industry and benefits to patients from successful cancer treatments, and the development of new cytotoxic drugs, chemoprotective agents, cytokines, or anti-emetic agents make oncology a highly competitive area for both academia and industry. Recent technical advances in molecular biology and immunology have enabled scientists to decipher some of the genetic causes of malignancy and to propose strategies for overcoming the primary genetic abnormalities responsible for the development of cancer.

New developments in chemotherapy

Infusional chemotherapy

The availability of portable pumps or non-mechanical infusors and long-term intravenous catheters (for example, Hickman or PICC lines) has made domiciliary infusional chemotherapy possible,

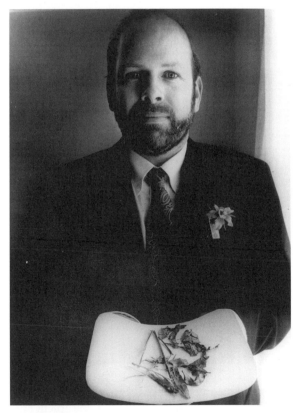

Figure 16.1 Novel drugs from natural sources. Dr Dai Chaplin of the Gray Laboratory, Mount Vernon Hospital, holds some African willow bark from which the novel anti-vascular agent combretastatin-A4 prodrug is derived. Development of drugs from natural sources has led to the discovery of novel effective agents such as taxanes and campothecans, which generate considerable public interest (with kind permission of the Independent Newspaper Publishing plc).

and is revolutionising chemotherapy treatment by enabling people to have their treatment at home, while maintaining their normal life. Most portable pumps/infusors are no larger than a personal stereo and, with support, bags or infusors can be changed by the person being treated; this means that chemotherapy treatment can continue without the need to attend hospital. The intravenous catheters used to deliver anti-cancer drugs into the bloodstream are normally kept patent using warfarin to prevent thrombosis. However, complications such as thrombosis or infection can occur and monitoring for these needs to be part of the care given.[1]

The infusion of chemotherapy over long periods may offer improved efficacy when compared to the same agent given as a bolus. The best example is 5-fluorouracil (5-FU), which inhibits thymidylate synthetase, an enzyme essential in cell metabolism. By virtue of its high cell turnover and metabolic rate compared to normal tissue, the tumour is more susceptible to thymidylate synthetase enzyme inhibition by 5-FU than normal tissue, and this can lead to relatively more tumour death. Infusional 5-FU therapy further exploits this differential between cancer and normal tissue because the constant level of the drug allows an overall greater dose intensity (dose per unit time) than when given as a single dose.[2] This increased dose intensity and anti-tumour efficacy is achieved without the toxicities associated with higher bolus doses because the relatively low levels of circulating drug allows normal tissue recovery. Using this approach, there is less myelosuppression as a result of treatment, although there is a higher incidence of stomatitis, diarrhoea and plantar–palmar erythrema (see Figure 16.2).[3]

The improved activity of infused 5-FU has been demonstrated for many tumour types, in particular metastatic colorectal cancer.[4,5] Infusional 5-FU has also been used in combination with epirubicin and cisplatin given at intervals as bolus treatments; for example, in the ECF regime. This regime exploits the recognised synergies of this combination. Bolus doses of epirubicin and cisplatin are given every 3 weeks and 5-FU is administered continuously for a period of 18 weeks. This regime has demonstrated remarkable efficacy in breast,[6] gastrointestinal,[7] hepatobiliary,[8] and ovarian cancers.[1]

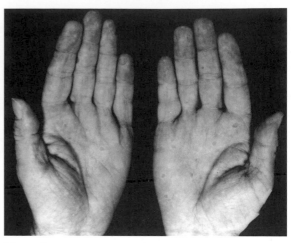

Figure 16.2 Novel uses of conventional drugs have led to novel adverse reactions. Infusional 5-fluorouracil (5-FU) can lead to a hand–foot–mouth syndrome comprising punctate lesions on the hands and feet with oral mucositis. Neutropenia, seen with bolus 5-FU, is not a feature of infusional 5-FU.

Infusional paclitaxel has been employed both to exploit the cell cycle specific toxicity of taxanes and to avoid hypersensitivity reactions, which are common with shorter infusions.[9] Anthracycline cardiotoxicity is a limiting factor in its use. Infused doxorubicin may have less cardiotoxicity than bolus doxorubicin, but the requirement of central venous access for infused doxorubicin is less convenient.

Chronotherapy, or the circadian timing of chemotherapy, has been developed from the experimental observation that when chemotherapy is given at certain times of the day it is more effective and less toxic.[10] This phenomenon has been explained by a number of scientific observations; for instance, some human cell types divide in the evening and may be more sensitive to chemotherapy at that time. In addition, there is increased evening activity of enzymes to which chemotherapy can be targeted.

A number of drugs in infusional therapy uses 5-FU, leucovorin and oxaliplatin, a novel platinum complex compound.[11,12] The effectiveness of these drugs was evaluated when given through a multi-channel programmable ambulatory pump equipped with four channels, each with a syringe programmed to give pulsed doses of 5-FU, maximal at 04.00 hours, decreasing to a minimum at 10.00 hours and recommencing at 22.00 hours. In contrast, oxaliplatin would begin at 10.00 hours, be maximal at 16.00 hours and cease by 22.00 hours, in a cycle that would repeat for 5 days. Data showed significant decreases in toxicity and a small but significant increase in survival when compared to continuous infusion of the same doses of drugs. To date, the relative complexity and modest benefit of giving chronotherapy has limited its use to a few oncology units in Europe.

High-dose chemotherapy

High-dose chemotherapy employs a single administration of chemotherapy at five to six times the dose of a conventional single dose, with the aim of overcoming drug resistance in situations where conventional chemotherapy has failed, or is likely to fail. A consequence of such high doses of chemotherapy is profound bone marrow suppression leading to prolonged neutropenia. Bone marrow or peripheral blood stem cells are harvested prior to treatment, and administered following high-dose chemotherapy so that haematological recovery can occur.[13] In the past 20 years, high-dose chemotherapy has been assessed primarily in chemosensitive cancers among the young and fit in order to improve the cure rate.

Advances in the support of profoundly neutropenic patients have transformed the use of high-dose chemotherapy from a treatment with considerable morbidity and mortality (5–10%) to a safe, commonplace procedure. The use of peripheral stem cell support, rather than harvested bone marrow, growth factors to enhance neutrophil recovery, broad-spectrum antibiotics to support people through episodes of sepsis, and improved methods of caring for mucosal surfaces have reduced the total morbidity and the period of absolute neutropenia to between 10 and 12 days and a total in-patient stay of less than 2 weeks. This is remarkable given the intensity and toxic nature of treatment. Such is the reduction of morbidity that two or more high-dose treatments can be given to individuals, although with repeated or higher doses, organ toxicities become a problem. The ben-

efit of higher intensity and multiple treatments is uncertain and few randomised controlled trials of high-dose chemotherapy compared with conventional chemotherapy have been undertaken to allow proper evaluation of these treatments. With the exception of acute leukaemias, myeloma, and non-Hodgkin's lymphoma, the value of high-dose chemotherapy in improving survival remains largely unproven.

Myeloma and non-Hodgkin's lymphoma
For 30 years, alkylating agents and steroids have been the mainstay of treatment for multiple myeloma and have achieved a response rate of between 40 and 60%. Despite numerous trials of new drug and biological treatments there has been no alteration in the prognosis for these diseases, with a median survival period of less than 3 years. Intensive protocols employing vincristine, doxorubicin, melphalan and prednisolone,[14] and maintenance IFN[15] have shown only marginal effects on survival. Recently, a French Intergroup trial has demonstrated a significant survival advantage with high-dose chemotherapy following conventional chemotherapy, particularly for people under the age of 50 years.[16] Newer strategies to improve the still very poor prognosis include the use of interleukins, retinoids, and anti-idiotype vaccination.

The value of high-dose chemotherapy in non-Hodgkin's lymphoma has been extensively investigated. In a randomised French trial of induction chemotherapy and high-dose chemotherapy in those at high risk of relapse, at 5 years, the rate of event-free survival was 46% in the transplantation group and 12% in the group receiving chemotherapy without transplantation, and the rates of overall survival were 53% and 32%, respectively;[17] however, this difference was only marginally significant. In an Italian study, in a poor prognosis group undergoing similar treatments, those given high-dose sequential therapy, as compared with those treated with conventional chemotherapy, had significantly higher rates of response and disease-free survival.[18]

Breast cancer and germ cell tumours
A recent review by the Autologous Blood and Marrow Transplant Registry of North America revealed that between 1989 and 1995, the number of

autografts for breast cancer increased by six times and constituted one-third of all autografts performed in North America.[19] This is surprising since there is little evidence to demonstrate advantages of high-dose chemotherapy over conventional chemotherapy. Bezwoda *et al.*[20] reported a study of high-dose chemotherapy as primary treatment in metastatic breast cancer. Women receiving high-dose chemotherapy compared with conventional chemotherapy had a greater response rate, disease-free survival, and long-term survival. The improvement in survival was due almost entirely to those who achieved a complete response with high-dose chemotherapy; however, these women also received tamoxifen, whereas the women receiving standard treatment did not. At present, there is a large

number of randomised trials ongoing in both Europe and the USA, which are attempting to determine the value of high-dose chemotherapy in adjuvant treatment and for metastatic breast cancer.

Future directions for research include the evaluation of sequential high-dose treatments and the use of novel growth factors; for example, the use of growth factors to protect and encourage re-establishment of gastrointestinal epithelium damaged by the chemotherapy.[21] In order to engineer resistance to chemotherapy in white cell precursors, gene therapy strategies are being evaluated, which aim to deliver genes for drug resistance.[22] The rationale is that white cells would recover more rapidly from high-dose chemotherapy and allow greater or sequential doses to be given. However, data from multiple dose protocols suggest that with increasing dose, the toxicities are no longer related to marrow toxicity but to organ failure,[23] suggesting that these strategies are unlikely to allow dramatic increases in dosage. Other studies are examining the use of high-dose chemotherapy in other cancers, such as epithelial ovarian cancer.

Neoadjuvant therapy

Neoadjuvant chemotherapy or primary medical therapy for cancer aims to reduce the size of the primary tumour using chemotherapy or radiotherapy following histological confirmation of cancer, before traditional treatments such as surgery or radiotherapy. This has the effect of 'downstaging' the tumour and may allow more conservative surgery where tumours were initially inoperable. There are some data to suggest that the tumour is more likely to respond to chemotherapy prior to surgery.[24] Although results have demonstrated improved disease-free survival, in many cases survival benefit is unclear. This treatment may lead to benefits in quality of life for women with breast cancer and allow less mutilating surgery.

Bladder cancer

Combination treatment with neoadjuvant chemotherapy, maximal resection of bladder tumour, radical radiotherapy and radical cystectomy have been combined in the treatment of high-risk, locally advanced, and inoperable transitional cell carcinoma of the bladder to improve survival and blad-

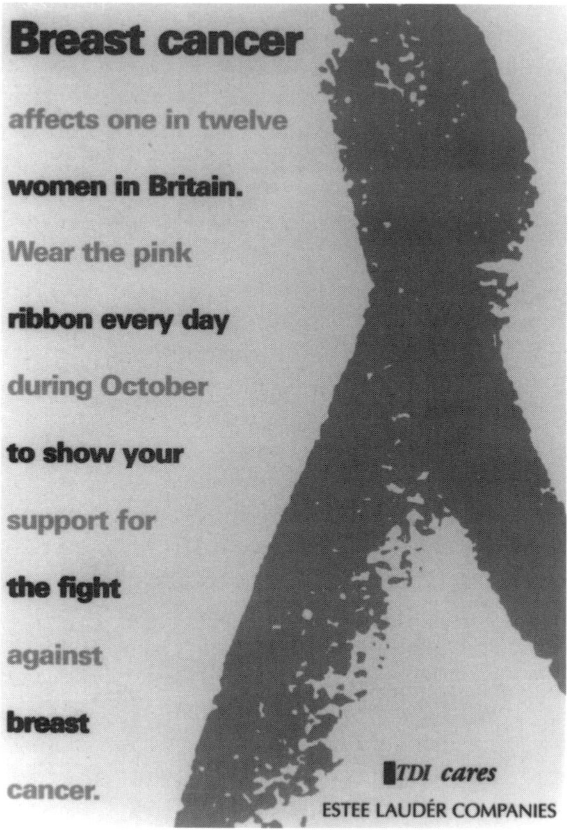

Figure 16.3 Public interest in cancer has escalated. Pink ribbons were fashion accessories de rigeur during this public awareness programme in 1997. Criticisms of public awareness campaigns include concern about the unnecessary anxiety (with kind permission of Estee Laudér Companies).

der preservation. Radical cystectomy is considered when there is penetration of muscle by tumour. The local control rate and 5-year survival for bladder cancer are poor at 30–50% and 20–40%, respectively, primarily because of undetected local and systemic disease.

As transitional cell carcinoma is intrinsically chemosensitive, several randomised trials have been undertaken to determine the value of neoadjuvant chemotherapy using cisplatin in combination with other agents, evaluating the effects of this on disease-free survival, survival, and bladder preservation. The trials reported have found increased bladder preservation in selected cases[25] and improved disease-free survival,[26] but opinions differ on survival. As a result, combined modality therapy with neoadjuvant chemotherapy is favoured for selected high-risk patients.

Neoadjuvant therapy for breast cancer
Neoadjuvant chemotherapy or primary medical therapy for breast cancer aims to reduce the size of the primary tumour following histological confirmation before surgery or radiotherapy. This 'downstaging' of the tumour size may allow conservative breast surgery for women whose tumours are larger than 3 cm, or allow conservative breast surgery, which was previously not cosmetically possible. Data suggest that breast tumours are more likely to respond to chemotherapy prior to surgery.[24] A drawback of downstaging the primary tumour is the additional downstaging of axillary lymph nodes that may confound prognostic information following resection. Protagonists of neoadjuvant chemotherapy argue that local control with axillary radiotherapy rather than lymph node resection is more appropriate.

Neoadjuvant chemotherapy for breast cancer has been demonstrated with numerous regimes similar to those used in metastatic disease and as adjuvant chemotherapy. Smith and colleagues[24] investigated the efficacy of continuous infusion 5-FU with 3-weekly epirubicin and cisplatin (ECF) as primary chemotherapy instead of immediate mastectomy for women with large, potentially operable, breast cancer. Of 50 women, 49 achieved an overall response (98%), including 33 complete response (66%). Only three women (6%) still required mastectomy. Tumour cellularity was

markedly reduced on repeat needle biopsy following 3 weeks of chemotherapy in 81% of women receiving ECF, compared with only 36% in women after conventional chemotherapy.

A randomised trial comparing neoadjuvant and adjuvant chemotherapy with four cycles of doxorubicin and cyclophosphamide concluded that in women receiving neoadjuvant treatment there was a high clinical response rate of 79%, 'downstaging' of both tumour and nodes occurred, and that neoadjuvant chemotherapy was safe. Although survival was improved in the neoadjuvant chemotherapy group, this improvement was not statistically significant.

Neoadjuvant chemotherapy for carcinoma of the cervix
Despite the decreasing incidence of locally advanced carcinoma of the cervix secondary to effective screening programmes in the Western world, carcinoma of the cervix remains a major worldwide health problem and 5-year survival of patients with stage IIB–IVA carcinoma of the cervix (primary tumour larger than 4 cm and up to the pelvic side wall) remains poor at 35–70%.[27] The value of neoadjuvant chemotherapy for carcinoma of the cervix prior to radiotherapy or surgery remains controversial. Although some studies claim little advantage for chemotherapy and radiotherapy over radiotherapy alone,[28–30] some trials suggest an advantage for chemotherapy prior to surgery.[31–33] Current practice tends towards neoadjuvant chemotherapy and surgery for stages IB to IIB (IIIA in some centres) and concomitant chemoradiotherapy for more advanced tumours where radiotherapy would be the standard treatment.

Neoadjuvant chemotherapy for non-small-cell lung cancer
Non-small-cell lung cancer has been demonstrated to be chemosensitive. A possible role for neoadjuvant chemotherapy in the treatment of non-small-cell lung cancer has been suggested where the tumour is potentially surgically resectable disease. Two studies compared chemotherapy followed by surgery with immediate surgery, and demonstrated a dramatic survival advantage for those receiving neoadjuvant chemotherapy.[34,35] However, both trials can be criticised for the small numbers in each trial (60 patients) and the unusually poor survival

in the immediate surgery arm. In addition, other trials have not been able to demonstrate a survival advantage and show increased toxicity in the combined therapy arms.

Further randomised trials are being performed to evaluate fully this controversial treatment. An MRC/EORTC trial is comparing MVP chemotherapy (mitomycin-C, vinblastine and cisplatin) or MIC chemotherapy (mitomycin-C, ifosfamide and cisplatin) followed, as feasible, by surgery or radiotherapy, with radiotherapy alone in stage IIIA non-small-cell lung cancer.

New developments in radiotherapy

Developments in radiotherapy have concentrated on the improved targeting of radiation (conformal radiation), the delivery of greater doses without increased toxicity (hyperfractionation), the use of drugs and carbon dioxide to increase sensitivity of tumour to radiation, and the re-organisation of radiotherapy services to ensure uniformity in quality of care (quality assurance).

Conformal radiotherapy
The goal of conformal radiotherapy is to conform the high-dose region of the radiation dose to the target, maximising the dose to tumour and minimising irradiation to normal tissue. It has been estimated that doses could increase by 20–25% and result in significantly improved response rates and local control.[36–38] This is often achieved by rotating the radiotherapy beam or shaping the beam. Efficacy has yet to be shown, although early indications are that local control is improved.

Hyperfractionation
The rationale for hyperfractionation is to increase dose intensity by using smaller fractions of radiotherapy more frequently, allowing normal tissue recovery without tumour re-growth. This technique, known as continuous hyperfractionated accelerated radiotherapy (CHART), was demonstrated extensively in animal models[39] and then trialled in inoperable head and neck cancer[40,41] and non-small-cell lung cancer. CHART required treatments to be given three times per day and also at weekends. Although the increased resource requirements meant greater cost and the frequency of dosage was

inconvenient for people, the total time for treatment was reduced from 6 weeks to 12 days. Toxicity was tolerable and equivalent to standard radiotherapy. For head and neck cancer, local control was improved, particularly for larger tumours, but survival was unchanged. In non-small-cell lung cancer[41] survival for those receiving CHART radiotherapy after 2 years was 29%, compared to 20% for conventional radiotherapy. A current trial compares CHARTWEL (CHART weekend less or hyperfractionated radiotherapy during weekdays only) to CHART. Data from this study will help to decide whether hyperfractionation will become standard practice for some tumour types.

Radiosensitisation
Radiosensitising agents increase the toxicity of radiation to tumour without affecting normal tissue. The mechanism of action of radiosensitisation is uncertain, but examples include compounds that are not normally tumour toxic, such as metronidazole, misonidazole, and nimorazole, as well as commonly used cytotoxic agents, such as cisplatin and 5-FU. With the exception of hydroxyurea in cervical cancer,[42] radiosensitising agents have not been shown to improve response or survival, but newer drugs with improved hypoxic tissue penetration are being evolved.

Radiotherapy is known to be less effective against hypoxic tumour, a problem in solid tumour kill as most tumours over 5 mm in size become hypoxic. In an attempt to improve oxygenation through carbon dioxide-related blood vessel dilatation and hence radiation kill of hypoxic tumour, the use of carbogen (5–10% carbon dioxide in air) exploits a non-pharmacological mode of tissue sensitisation and is currently being investigated. Breathing carbogen for 2 hours prior to radiation therapy and a combination of carbogen and pharmacological enhancers of tissue oxygenation are currently being investigated.

Concomitant chemoradiation
The concomitant administration of chemotherapy and radiotherapy aims to combine or enhance the efficacy of each modality without enhancing toxicity. Used in combination with radiosensitising chemotherapy, standard or hyperfractionated radiotherapy schedules may be followed by surgery that

has been rendered more conservative by neoadjuvant chemotherapy and radiotherapy. Such complex protocols require careful evaluation in randomised trials. Nevertheless, dramatic benefits for chemoradiation have been claimed for many tumour types. Following publication of data from a recent randomised trial, chemoradiation has become standard treatment for anal carcinoma. Although early morbidity was increased for the chemoradiation group, late effects were equal and chemoradiation has enabled conservative surgery in many.[43–45]

It is uncertain whether locally advanced inoperable cervical carcinoma should be treated with chemoradiation. Data from randomised phase III trials are few, but the results of large trials should be available soon. Phase II trial data do describe increased morbidity, particularly diarrhoea and neutropenia in the short-term, especially with the use of concomitant 5-FU.

Head and neck cancer is an inherently chemoradiosensitive cancer, but the natural history is of eventual failure of local tumour control. Radiotherapy is the standard treatment where the lesion is not operable; phase III trials have compared the addition of chemotherapy to standard or hyperfractionated regimens.[46,47] Most studies report improved survival and disease-free survival but increased short-term toxicity, particularly when chemoradiation is given sequentially.[48,49] Further studies with concomitant chemoradiation will confirm its potential role as standard treatment, also using novel drug combinations such as taxanes. Recently, improved local control and survival has been demonstrated by an Intergroup trial in chemoradiation for nasopharyngeal cancer.[50]

Surgery is the standard treatment for early oesophageal cancer but despite improvements in surgical mortality, 5-year survival is between 5 and 50% for stages I–IIB, with failure of treatment both locally and at distant sites. Phase III trials using cisplatin and 5-FU in combination with radiation prior to surgery gave complete response rates of up to 40% prior to surgery.[51] There have been conflicting data about overall survival when chemoradiation is followed by surgery, but several large studies have reported no improvement in survival with three modalities compared to immediate surgery. Following the observation that those who

do not respond to chemoradiation have a very poor outcome and allowing for the known surgical mortality of 8–10%, investigators have concentrated on chemoradiation without surgery. Phase III studies have demonstrated improved overall survival,[52,53] although treatment is toxic. Further trials are underway to determine the benefit of chemoradiation alone in oesophageal cancer.

The value of concomitant chemoradiation for non-small-cell lung cancer is still debated, although several randomised trials demonstrate improved survival for combined modality treatment. Where there was unresectable disease, survival improvement was achieved through improved local control at an acceptable toxicity.

Quality assurance

Quality assurance in radiotherapy is a process of ensuring uniformity of care. The Radiation Therapy Oncology Group (RTOG)[54] is a multi-institutional co-operative organisation based in North America, which provides a quality control for all aspects of care for people with cancer, and in particular provides mechanisms to assure compliance with complex protocols. Requirements include staffing, imaging, treatment planning, simulation, dosimetry, computing, megavoltage, brachytherapy equipment, calibration, recording, quality assurance, and clinical profile of patients. A profile of radiotherapy units through Europe compiled through site visits and questionnaires by the EORTC detailed a number of similar requirements mandatory for centres wishing to conduct EORTC trials.[55,56] These requirements, in which the details of planning, treatment, and documentation feature strongly, are hoped to form the basis for quality control and assurance not only for research centres but also for standards in everyday practice.

Surgery

Less aggressive surgery?

Recently there has been a trend towards reducing the morbidity of extensive surgery; for example, in breast cancer. For breast cancer, the overriding concern used to be local control, but with the realisation that breast cancer is a systemic disease where early metastasis and the failure of local control are often a manifestation of systemic progression, the paramount role of surgery was questioned. Thus radical mastectomy has given way to simple mastectomy and in turn to lumpectomy followed by radiation. The rationale and development of breast-sparing surgery following neoadjuvant chemotherapy have been already addressed. Thus the role of surgery in breast cancer has gradually converted from the mainstay of management to a diagnostic role.

Stents

Obstruction of blood vessels, airways, and bowel causes many of the symptoms in advanced cancer. The development and increasing use of surgical stents to relieve obstruction can provide good symptomatic relief for prolonged periods. Stents may also be used as a temporary measure to relieve symptoms and enable treatment. Stents are normally inserted without the need for a major surgical procedure. Biliary stents to relieve obstruction from cholangiocarcinoma have been combined with intra-luminal radiotherapy with success. Such internal stents avoid drainage to skin and associated drainage bags. Bronchial stenting for large airway obstruction can relieve symptoms of obstruction, which include breathlessness and pulmonary infection distal to the obstruction. Stents for relieving colonic obstruction are under investigation. Prostatic stents allow for spontaneous voiding during hormonal therapy for prostate cancer and are inserted using guided fluoroscopy under local anaesthetic. Ureteric stenting for progressive renal failure from ovarian or prostatic tumour relieves symptoms of uraemia and allows formal tumour therapy in a fitter patient. Stenting in oesophageal cancer is often combined with laser treatment following stenting to control tumour ingrowth, as may the use of metal stents in place of plastic stents. Iliac vein stents have been used to relieve lower limb oedema in pelvic malignancy causing iliac vessel obstruction and thrombosis.

The surgical oncologist

Recent attention has focused on how all aspects of clinical outcome from quality of life to overall survival depend on the degree of specialisation of the lead physician. Essential to this range of specialisation is the appointment of surgical oncologists in breast, bowel, and gynaecological cancer for each region, so that not only is optimum care provided but the infrastructure for national and international clinical research is established.

Palliative care

New drugs and novel routes of administration are widening treatment options for palliative care physicians. The use of fentanyl patches,[57] ketamine infusions,[58] biphosphonates for bone pain and in the prevention of pathological fracture and spinal cord compression,[59,60] and a single daily dose of morphine (MXL) are new effective options in pain control for palliative care physicians. An advance in the palliation of intestinal obstruction is the use of octreotide. This is a somatostatin analogue that inhibits the secretion of gut peptides responsible for gut motility and secretion. Subcutaneous infusions of octreotide can reduce vomiting and distress and will provide a valuable adjuvant to the care of patients in intestinal obstruction.[61]

Screening programmes

Screening programmes are mainly aimed at common cancers. For a screening programme to be effective there must be a sensitive test that is able to pick up as many true positives (sensitivity) as possible without registering false positives (specificity). The test must be cheap and without risk, and result in a survival benefit, as well as being economically feasible and acceptable to the screened population. The consequences of screening must also be feasible: patients at risk or with early asymptomatic cancer must be cured with the least morbidity. Widespread inappropriate screening may set off a cascade of diagnostic and treatment procedures that may be expensive and ineffective, and involve considerable morbidity, both physical and psychological. The economic implications of screening programmes are increasingly important at a time when health rationing is inevitable: cost can only be justified if mortality and morbidity are reduced. Several examples of appropriate and inappropriate screening exist. Following the success of cervical screening in reducing the incidence of advanced cervical cancer in the Western world,[62] several other tumour types have been targeted.

Breast cancer

Some of the criteria for appropriate screening programmes are met by the recent breast cancer screening programme in the UK, a preliminary report of which has been published.[63] In 1988 a programme was initiated following the recommendations of the Forrest report,[64] commissioned by the Department of Health to address the high incidence of breast cancer and the relatively poor survival of women in the UK when compared to other European countries.[65] This programme involves mammography for 50–64-year-old women every 2–3 years to detect early cancers that would otherwise have been missed. Mammography is relatively sensitive, specific, cheap, and acceptable. Preliminary data indicate that the numbers of women undergoing screening has increased by 25% in the targeted age group but has remained the same for all other age groups. Mortality for breast cancer has fallen by 12% but this is thought to be consequent on the increased use of tamoxifen in the early 1980s rather than screening. Because of the long natural history of breast cancer, the efficacy of this programme will not be evident for 10 years or more.

Prostate cancer

Prostate cancer is the second most common cancer in men, causing 10 000 deaths a year in the UK. Over 95% of deaths are over 65 years of age and mortality is rising with the increasing life expectancy of men.[66] Detection is often late in the disease, with 40% being diagnosed with advanced disease. Disease detected early and localised to the prostate may be treated by radical prostatectomy, hormonal treatments, or radiotherapy; therefore prostate cancer may be a good candidate for a screening programme.[67] Screening using a combination of the tumour marker prostatic specific antigen (PSA),[68] digital rectal examination (DRE), and trans-rectal ultrasound (TRUS) has been investigated in a number of pilot studies. Difficulties with the screening methods include the relative insensitivity of rectal examination and ultrasound and the fact that PSA concentrations are elevated for 10 years before the clinical presentation of cancer.[69] In a large American study,[70] overall compliance with follow-up screening was good; 51% of men who were positive on all three criteria had a positive trans-rectal biopsy. Screening of nearly 3000 men annually over 5 years detected 203 cancers. Similar data emerged from a randomised European study.[71] There are problems in the interpretation of data from screening studies due to the long natural history of prostate cancer; data may not be meaningful without 20 years or more of follow-up. In addition, many men may have biochemically and radiologically detectable yet clinically silent disease for many years, which may never require treatment.[69] Complications of prostatectomy and radiotherapy to the prostate are common, and may outweigh the potential morbidity from prostatic cancer for that individual. Despite the uncertainties over cost-benefit and efficacy, patient-driven medicine, particularly in the USA, has made random screening for prostate cancer commonplace. A prostate screening programme has been proposed in the UK.[72]

Ovarian cancer

Over the past 15 years a series of trials has defined a role for the tumour marker CA125 and transvaginal ultrasound with Doppler studies as a means of detecting early, curable epithelial ovarian cancer.[73] Whether this detection leads to lives being saved is being investigated in several large multicentre trials in Europe and the UK. A central problem for this mode of screening is whether curable rather than advanced (and therefore incurable) cancers are detected. Another core issue is the cost analysis: is more screening ultimately cheaper because it saves lives?

Genetic screening for cancer

Recently familial breast and ovarian cancer genes BRCA1 and BRCA2 have been cloned.[74,75] Mutations in these genes are responsible for up to 5% of inherited cancers, conferring a 70% likelihood of developing breast and/or ovarian cancer by the age of 70 in an individual who is found to possess an abnormal gene.[76] A commercially available kit (Myriad, USA) can be used to determine germ-line abnormalities in BRCA1 and increasingly, asymptomatic, clinically disease-free women with a strong family history of breast or ovarian cancer will be having their DNA screened to find an abnormality in BRCA1. Thus scientific advances and improved technology have made the diagnosis of a genetic predisposition to cancer easy to detect.

Difficulties arise over who to offer screening and subsequent treatment to. For BRCA1 and 2, individuals who have two or more close family members with either malignancy or a single family member with cancer below the age of 40 years and who possess the gene are considered to be at high risk of developing breast or ovarian cancer. Treatment options include prophylactic mastectomy and oophorectomy, although at what stage such intervention should be taken and its effectiveness are uncertain. The pitfalls and difficulties in giving advice as to whether or not to have genetic testing are difficult, especially when the predictive value of a positive test is uncertain, combined with the uncertainty over whether treatment that is radical is effective, and cannot be over-emphasised.[77] Mastectomy only removes 90% of all breast tissue, does not eliminate the incidence of breast cancer from residual breast tissue on the chest wall, and does not affect undetected microscopic metastases. Oophorectomy would induce early menopause, possibly requiring hormone replacement therapy, and does not affect the occurrence of primary peritoneal carcinoma. Furthermore, obstetricians can obtain placental tissue for prenatal diagnosis of a familial cancer gene, giving the option of termination of that pregnancy.[78] Some could argue that termination of a pregnancy, when the yet unborn child has a 70% chance of developing cancer at some stage over a 70-year lifespan, is simply eugenics.

Quality of life and cancer therapy

The quality of life of patients undergoing cancer therapy has been addressed in a series of studies over the past 5–10 years.[79] Quality of life has become an important issue in cancer care because of increased knowledge and choice in treatment. In addition, quality of life is evaluated in clinical trials of new treatment programmes as an important consideration when assessing these. Effective treatment of the cancer is often the best means of improving quality of life both physically and psychologically, although this equation is never straightforward. Increasingly, an individual's assessment of their quality of life during treatment is taken into account, since often their perception of toxicity and efficacy differs from the physician's evaluation of efficacy.[80]

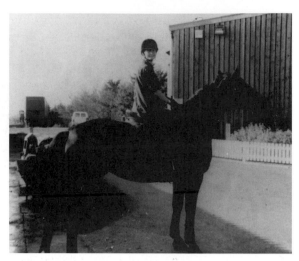

Figure 16.4 Novel drugs aim for efficacy with less toxicity than accepted treatment, thus maintaining quality of life during treatment and remission. Judith, pictured at her favourite hobby, was receiving paclitaxel chemotherapy (with kind permission of Judith and her husband).

An Australian/New Zealand breast cancer trial for people with advanced disease compared chemotherapy for three cycles of treatment with a further three cycles only when disease progressed, to six cycles of treatment from the outset.[81–83] Survival, response to treatment, and quality of life were all better for those who had continuous treatment. Although these data are likely to have reflected the poor quality of life experienced from a greater disease load, there may have been anxiety associated with stopping treatment. On the whole, despite significantly more side-effects and the lack of clinical benefit in those who are more intensively treated, quality of life was dramatically improved amongst those treated intensively, suggesting that there may be a sub-clinical response in addition to the positive contribution of hope and attention associated with treatment. Similar reasons may explain the unexpected popularity and well-being associated with alternative medicines.

Novel therapies and techniques

Novel chemotherapeutic agents

Recently there has been a number of novel chemotherapeutic agents entering clinical trial.

Most were isolated from natural sources as part of a screen of natural products initiated by the National Institutes of Health in the 1960s. All the drugs described have shown tumour activity in phase I, and for some, phase II trials, and are being assessed in phase III trials. Some of these novel agents have a different mode of action to that of conventional chemotherapeutic agents, making combination therapy with those agents an attractive option. Increasingly, strategies to exploit maximally the potential of new drugs, such as in infusional protocols, or the use of haemopoetic growth factors or chemoprotective agents to increase dosage, are being used.

Box 16.1: Novel chemotherapy agents

Taxanes
The taxanes are novel chemotherapeutic agents derived from the bark and leaves of yew trees. Paclitaxel is derived from the bark of the Pacific yew *Taxus brevifolia*, and docetaxol is a semi-synthetic product, derived originally from the needles of the common yew, *Taxus baccata*. These drugs show potent activity against breast, gastric, head and neck, non-small-cell lung, oesophageal, ovarian cancer and others. The primary toxicities of taxanes are hypersensitivity reactions, neutropenia and neurotoxicity, but in general, taxanes are tolerated well. Hypersensitivity does not occur if pre-medication with dexamethasone is used and neutropenia, although often profound, is rarely prolonged and uncommonly complicated by sepsis. Neurotoxicity is common, manifesting as peripheral neuropathy, particularly in patients pre-medicated with cisplatin. In most cases there is complete recovery following cessation of treatment. Although duration of remission following taxanes is often brief, overall survival is prolonged in many studies, a phenomenon poorly understood but thought to be related to a secondary anti-angiogenic action of taxanes on malignancy. Recent developments include using taxanes in intensive and high-dose protocols with stem cell support.

Campothecans
Irinotecan (CPT-11) and topotecan comprise members of a new group of anti-cancer agents known as campothecans, derived originally from alkyloids of the Chinese tree, *Campotheca acuminata*. Their mechanism of action is through inhibition of the enzyme topoisomerase I, which is essential in co-ordinating cell division and without which the cell is unable to repair its DNA. The main indication for irinotecan is colorectal cancer, where it has useful activity, including some activity in 5-FU-resistant disease. The main toxicities are

diarrhoea, which is controllable if treated vigorously and neutropenia, which can lead to life-threatening sepsis. Irinotecan is being compared to 5-FU in phase III trials. The main indication for topotecan is in ovarian cancer, where there is a 15–25% response rate in platinum-resistant disease. In contrast to irinotecan, topotecan is tolerated well, the primary toxicities being neutropenia, which rarely leads to sepsis, and mild alopecia. The main problem in use is scheduling, requiring a daily intravenous administration for 5 days, although an oral formulation is being tested. Activity is being investigated in small-cell lung cancer.

5-FU analogues
Tomudex (ZD1694) acts through inhibition of the enzyme thymidylate synthetase, an enzyme essential for the production of vitamin-based co-factors in metabolism. It was found to have similar activity to 5-FU in colorectal cancer and to have a more favourable safety profile, making it an attractive alternative to 5-FU if similar efficacy can be demonstrated. As 5-FU and tomudex have similar mechanisms of action, cross-resistance may limit their combined activity. Large-scale phase III trials comparing tomudex to 5-FU are being conducted at present. Capecitabine is a new oral fluoropyrimidine, which is a prodrug of 5-FU, being converted from the parent drug to active compound in gut then liver, and consequently avoids the gut toxicity of 5-FU. Phase II trials have demonstrated little toxicity and comparable efficacy to 5-FU and capecitabine is being tested in phase III trials.

Metalloproteinase inhibitors
Metalloproteinase inhibitors (batimastat and marimastat) have a novel mechanism of action that is cytostatic rather than cytotoxic. Metalloproteinases (MMP) are a group of cellular enzymes that act on and dissolve a number of cellular structural proteins that make up the fabric of the intercellular substance, such as collagens, proteoglycans, and fibronectin. Recent evidence suggested that the invasive potential of cancers was secondary to an imbalance between MMP and their natural inhibitors, allowing the dissolution of basement membranes and the invasion of tumour vasculature. Although the details of the complex balance between inhibitor and proteinase have not been fully elucidated, the pre-clinical activity of a number of synthetic MMP inhibitors, such as batimastat and marimastat, has been promising, particularly in the prevention of metastases. Metalloproteinase inhibitors are entering phase III trials following promising phase I data.

Other drugs
Gemcitabine is a novel drug that acts by mimicking nucleosides, the normal components of DNA. The drug becomes active once inside the cell by conversion to an active form, which is incorporated into DNA and terminates DNA replication, leading in turn to programmed cell death. Gemcitabine has shown activity in advanced breast cancer, non-small-cell

lung cancer, ovarian cancer, and small-cell lung cancer. The relative lack of toxicity and effective symptom relief (although without objective clinical response) in non-small-cell lung cancer has made gemcitabine a useful alternative in palliation. Gemcitabine is being tested in combination with conventional agents; for example, 5-FU and cisplatin for gastrointestinal and ovarian malignancies, respectively.

E09 is a novel bioreductive agent designed to be activated to a cytotoxic agent in hypoxic poorly perfused tissue. The activating enzyme for E09, DT diaphorase, is itself increased in tumour and hypoxia, as well as being more active in a hypoxic micro-environment. As tumour masses above 5 mm in size begin to show hypoxia, it was hoped that E09 would show selective activity against this hypoxic tumour rather than normally oxygenated tissue. Phase I trials showed some activity in adenocarcinoma of the lung with the main toxicity being proteinuria and salt and water retention, secondary to a minimal change glomerulonephritis. Phase II trials, conducted as an EORTC protocol, have initially proven disappointing but further data are awaited.

Anti-angiogenic agents
More biologically specific anti-angiogenic agents include the recent functional elucidation of two endogenous biological molecules such as angiostatin, which are very potent substances for suppressing tumour growth in many experimental systems. The anti-angiogenic effects of some other older drugs have resulted in their renaissance. Thalidomide, discarded because of its potent teratogenic effects, is being tested in phase II trials following demonstration of dramatic cases of tumour stabilisation.

Anti-vascular agents
Drugs aimed specifically at tumour vasculature are a novel group of compounds aimed at eliminating tumour bulk through vascular disruption and include flavone acetic acid (FAA), 5,6-dimethylxanthenone-4-acetic acid (DMXAA), and combretastatin A-4. Although the selectivity of these agents for tumour vasculature is poorly understood, the mechanism of action of FAA and DMXAA is through local cytokine production, particularly tumour necrosis factor (TNF-α). Although effective against murine tumour, FAA did not have activity in human disease and anti-vascular effects were seen only at half the maximal tolerated dose. This lack of activity was attributed to species differences in FAA activity and consequent cytokine production. DMXAA is currently in phase I trial and is a superior compound for several reasons. It has improved pharmacokinetics and solubility and is more potent than FAA, inducing cures and tumour delay in mice at doses of less than one-twelfth that of FAA. Combretastatin A-4 and its prodrug, derived originally from African willow bark, have been shown to induce dramatic changes in solid xenografts. These drugs have an anti-vascular effect through tubulin binding rather than cytokine production. An out-standing problem in the development and use of anti-vascular drugs is a residual rim of surviving tumour following vascular shutdown and tumour necrosis, whose oxygenation derives from surrounding normal tissue. Strategies to circumvent this problem will use agents specifically directed at both core and rim components of tumour.

Chemo-enhancing and chemoprotective agents
Leucovorin
Leucovorin (LV, folinic acid) is a co-factor in the activity of competitors of thymidylate synthetase (TS) and was shown experimentally to enhance the effect of 5-FU, a TS inhibitor. Early phase I data demonstrated that giving LV decreased 5-FU toxicity and increased the inhibition of TS, and concurrent administration was thought to enable a greater dose intensity. Clinical trials have shown an improved response rate and a small survival advantage; however, those patients receiving LV were more frequently hospitalised and the cost of LV was considerable. Trials are in progress to determine the optimum scheduling of 5-FU and LV, particularly with continuous infusion 5-FU and chronomodulation.

Desrazoxane
Desrazoxane (ICRF-187) is a novel cardioprotective agent that has shown much promise in clinical trial. Anthracyclines (doxorubicin and epirubicin) are active chemotherapeutic agents against many tumour types but their limiting toxicity is a cumulative cardiotoxicity that is irreversible. This toxicity is particularly critical in paediatric patients, who are more sensitive to doxorubicin cardiotoxicity and for whom long-term toxicity is an important factor in treatment strategy. Clinical studies showing the efficacy of ICRF-187 in both adults and children do so without a decrease in the anti-tumour effect and may lead to chemotherapy protocols that incorporate higher doses of anthracycline.

Amifostine
Amifostine (WR2721) is an organothiophosphate that selectively protects against the toxicities of radiation therapy, alkylating agents, and cisplatin. The mode of action for prevention of cisplatin toxicity is thought to be by prevention of cisplatin–DNA and cisplatin–protein complexes. This protective effect is greater in normal tissues than in tumour because of the increased rate of conversion of WR2721 to its active form, WR1065, and increased uptake of WR2721, two processes that are inherently poor in tumour. Amifostine has been shown to reduce toxicity without reducing efficacy in phase III trials and is being further assessed.

Biological response modifiers
Biological response modifiers are naturally occurring molecules, often cytokines, secreted by our own immune system and capable of enhancing the immune response to tumour and the

response of tumour to chemotherapy. Use of these seems logical in those inherently immunogenic tumours: those tumours that can rarely stimulate immunity and induce a spontaneous response, such as melanoma and renal cell carcinoma. One advantage of biological response modifiers is their different toxicity profile when compared to conventional chemotherapy, in some cases allowing the combined use of a biological response modifier and conventional chemotherapy without dose reduction in either. For example, the dose-limiting toxicities of interferon-α (IFN-α) are fatigue and malaise, and those of interleukin-2 (IL2) renal and cardiac insufficiency, compared to marrow toxicity for most chemotherapy agents. Despite much experimental evidence that suggests a role for biological response modifiers, clear indications for using these are few. IFN-α as adjuvant in high-risk melanoma has been described.

In most patients with chronic myeloid leukaemia (CML), symptoms and white cell counts can be controlled with busulphan and hydroxyurea, but these drugs do not affect survival. Allogeneic stem cell transplantation is currently the treatment of choice for young people with chronic phase CML. About 50% of those who undergo a transplant obtain a 5-year disease-free period, although it is uncertain whether this translates to cure.

In myeloma, adding continuous low-dose interferon to standard melphalan and prednisolone therapy may improve response rate or survival but response duration and plateau phase duration are prolonged. Toxicity is substantial and must be weighed by patients against the modest potential benefits in response duration and survival.

IFN-α was initially found to have a response rate of 54% in advanced lymphoma. Subsequently, randomised trials have demonstrated improved disease-free survival when IFN-α was used in addition to standard chemotherapy, although it was more effective in low-grade lymphoma. IFN-α as a maintenance therapy following remission also prolongs remission; however, the toxicity is considerable and many patients stop treatment.

Interleukin-2: melanoma and renal cell cancer

In the 1980s, Rosenberg and colleagues[84] dramatically changed the treatment options for metastatic malignant melanoma with the use of high-dose intravenous IL2. Although the toxicity was severe, with several cardiac deaths in the first cohort of patients, there were between 5 and 10% complete responders and 10–15% partial responses to IL2 [initially combined with lymphokine activated killer cells (LAK) or tumour infiltrating lymphocytes (TIL)] in a previously almost uniformly fatal clinical setting. As this work was repeated and further tested, it became clear that LAK cells did not add to benefit, and that benefit was often short lived at considerable toxicity. In selected good prognosis groups (low volume of disease and non-visceral disease), there appeared to be no benefit of more intensive regimens and

further regimens using IL2 for melanoma should only be in the context of a clinical trial.

For metastatic renal cell cancer response rates and durability of response are more favourable not only with high-dose treatment but also with domiciliary subcutaneous IL2 combined with IFN-α, particularly in those with a low volume of disease, good performance status, and a long interval between.

Biological response modifiers with chemotherapy

Many pre-clinical data suggested a synergy between IFN-α and conventional chemotherapy. Chemo-immunotherapy was feasible because of the different side-effect profile of IFN-α or IL2 and chemotherapy; this led to a series of trials of combined modality therapy in colorectal cancer using 5-FU and IFN-α and in metastatic melanoma with up to four drugs. These have been disappointing in efficacy in cervix cancer, colorectal cancer, metastatic melanoma and renal cell cancer, and often lead to increased toxicity. Many consider that chemo-immunotherapy should only be used in the context of a clinical trial.[85]

Monoclonal antibodies

Monoclonal antibodies are biological molecules, often generated in mice or rabbits against a human protein. In oncology this protein is expressed on tumour surface and tumour is targeted with toxins, radioactive conjugates, or enzymes as part of an enzyme prodrug complex to kill tumour. The anti-idiotype reaction, where an endogenous antibody is generated against tumour protein through a series of immune interactions, has been demonstrated clinically and is thought to constitute an important part of any anti-tumour effect. Monoclonal antibodies have been used as adjuvants in ovarian cancer, as well as primary treatment for metastatic disease. To date, successes have been limited, partly due to the problems with administering monoclonal antibodies. Since these are murine (derived from mice), an anti-murine antibody reaction develops following the first administration, limiting the number of times treatment can be given. 'Humanisation' or the modification of antibodies to display only human elements should overcome this. Currently, phase I trials evaluating ADEPT (antibody directed enzyme prodrug therapy),[86,87] where an enzyme is targeted to tumour by a moncolonal antibody, are being conducted. The enzyme makes tumour more sensitive to a prodrug delivered systemically, which is converted to a cytotoxic metabolite by the enzyme.

Tumour vaccines

Tumour vaccines attempt to stimulate immunity against tumour by returning tumour antigen as cells, lysates, or proteins in a modified attenuated form to avoid malignant potential, but yet to be able to stimulate immunity. The first vaccine incorporated non-specific adjuvants, such as that described originally by Coley.[88] Since that time, many biological vaccines have been tried without success, partly because of an inadequate understanding of the immune mechanisms involved and the absence of controlled trials. With increased understanding of vaccine biology and well-conducted randomised trials, vaccines are being tested in a controlled fashion and we may soon be able to evaluate their true potential.

Melanoma is a good target for vaccines as it has an intrinsic immunogenicity: an ability to generate an immune response in the patient. This is demonstrated by a spontaneous response rate of 1–2% and the common phenomenon of spontaneously resolving metastases, as well as a host of laboratory data demonstrating *in vitro* and *in vivo* immunogenicity.[89] The first series of tumour vaccines used irradiated autologous and allogeneic tumour combined with various biological stimulants, such as bacille Calmette Guérin (BCG), *Corynebacterium parvum* and chemical stimulants, with little success. Morton *et al.*[90] used a vaccine comprising three melanoma cell lines expressing a number of tumour antigens mixed with BCG in metastatic melanoma. Humoral antibody responses have been documented and immunised patients with metastatic disease show a survival advantage over historical controls. Livingstone and colleagues have used ganglioside vaccines comprising proteins normally present on the surface of melanoma, combined with BCG and a chemical adjuvant. The latter two vaccines are about to enter randomised clinical trial in the UK. A more experimental series of cancer vaccines comprises those engineered using gene transfer techniques.

Gene therapy

Gene therapy for cancer exploits the improved specificity that genetically engineered substances have over conventional treatments. It is now possible to deliver single or multiple genes to a target tissue to give expression and activate the protein coded for by that gene. However, genetic abnormalities leading to cancer are multiple and cellular 'normalisation' would require not only multiple genes to be introduced, a process at present technically difficult, but also the complete correction of every cancerous cell, as yet technically impossible. Most cancer gene therapy strategies have concentrated on delivery of cytokine genes capable of reversing the anti-tumour immunity inherent to metastatic tumour and suicide genes, which express an enzyme that converts a non-toxic prodrug into a cytotoxic metabolite, resulting in the suicide of that cell. The use of new technology to alter cells genetically has generated public interest with respect to the ethics and safety of gene ther-

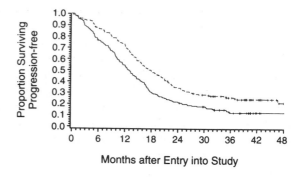

Treatment	No. Progression-free	No. with Treatment Failure	Total	Median Progression-free Survival (mo)
— Cisplatin + cyclophosphamide	28	174	202	13
- - - Cisplatin + paclitaxel	45	139	184	18

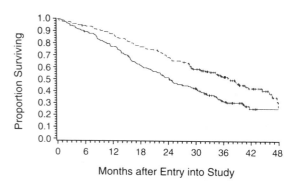

Treatment	No. Alive	No. Dead	Total	Median Survival (mo)
— Cisplatin + cyclophosphamide	65	137	202	24
- - - Cisplatin + paclitaxel	86	98	184	38

Figure 16.5 Cost–benefit is everything. These graphs demonstrating both improved disease-free interval and overall survival for patients treated with paclitaxel in addition to platinum have been the source of much controversy. The median survival benefit of 1 year requires 4 months of treatment, makes patients bald and cost approximately £15 000 per patient. Is it worth it? (with kind permission of Bill McGuire).

apy and the formation of an advisory body in the UK that monitors all the phase I trials (Gene Therapy Advisory Committee).

Vaccine tumour gene therapy is based on generating a cytokine-mediated immune response to genetically altered tumour.[91] By enabling tumour to secrete cytokine and generate a local immune response, it is hoped that this response will become systemic and lead to immunological kill not only of genetically altered tumour (the vaccine), but also of tumour that has not been modified. Commonly used cytokines include IL2 or IFN-γ but also IL4, IL12, tumour necrosis factor (TNF), granulocyte-macrophage colony stimulating factor (GMCSF) and any combination of these. IL2 is a cytokine produced by lymphocytes and mediates an inflammatory response through the stimulation of other cytokines but also non-specifically stimulates cytotoxic T-lymphocytes, thought to be essential in developing an anti-tumour immune response. Gene therapy protocols have concentrated on delivering the IL2 gene to tumour and through expression of IL2 both on tumour surface and in the immediate tumour microenvironment. In such experimental models, generated T-lymphocytes specifically target and eliminate tumour. In human trials, the IL2 is delivered to the tumour using viruses or chemical DNA complexes. At the Royal Marsden Hospital, a human gene therapy trial using autologous IL2 secreting melanoma has completed recruitment and is in the process of being analysed. Tumour was harvested from patients and modified in the laboratory, using a retrovirus carrying the gene coding for human IL2. The altered tumour is shown to express IL2, then returned to the patient following lethal irradiation. It is hoped that the IL2-secreting tumour will induce host immunity towards previously anergic tumour. IFN-γ is a cytokine that mediates inflammation and causes many of the symptoms experienced during a viral illness. When expressed in tumour, IFN-γ specifically enhances the expression of major histocompatibility complex (MHC) molecules, which in turn present immunogenic tumour antigens to the host immune response, presentation that is normally poor in tumour. By stimulating host immunity towards the tumour, it is hoped not only that the tumour will be modified to express cytokine but also that unmodified metastatic tumour will become sensitive to host immunity. Phase I trials using IFN-γ altered autologous and allogeneic tumour cell types are in progress.

Suicide gene strategies function through the delivery of an enzyme gene to tumour. The expressed enzyme converts a previously non-toxic prodrug into a toxic metabolite that kills the cell. This con-

cept, known as GDEPT (gene-directed enzyme prodrug therapy), is similar to ADEPT, but here the mode of delivery is viral and not with an antibody, and the delivered package is a gene rather than a protein. Essential to this strategy is the ability to kill not only modified cells but also neighbouring unmodified cells as current gene delivery systems can only deliver between 1 and 10% of the gene to a target cell population. This so-called bystander effect is generated partly through the passage of metabolites to neighbouring cells[92] and also through the generation of anti-tumour immunity following the prodrug-mediated killing of tumour. Oldfield *et al.* injected retroviral packaging cells into uncontrolled malignant glioma.[93] The packaging cells 'package' a retrovirus that delivers and expresses the herpes simplex thymidine kinase gene in tumour. The patient is then given the anti-viral drug ganciclovir, which is converted to a toxic metabolite. Early data have shown some partial responses but further improvements await the technical advances afforded by improved gene delivery.

After an initial wave of enthusiasm and a host of phase I trials, gene therapy for cancer is being evaluated and is awaiting improvements in the technical aspects of gene delivery and immune modulation. Few responses were obtained in phase I trials; thus, the main value of such trials lay in the demonstration of safety and clinically based scientific data on which to base further trials. Particular problems remain in the efficacy of gene delivery *in vivo,* particularly in GDEPT, and future GDEPT reagents will concentrate on more potent delivery mechanisms. Future directions in anti-tumour immunity will involve the use of more effective antigen presenting cells to stimulate immunity based on dendritic cells and the directed MHC-related expression of tumour antigens, such as the MAGE series in melanoma.

The Human Genome Project

The Human Genome Project (HGP) will undoubtedly accelerate the pace of research. This is a project under the auspices of the Human Genome Organisation (HUGO)[94] to encourage, co-ordinate and facilitate research into the genome without duplication of effort or unnecessary competition. This multinational project is supported by the European

Community, National Institutes of Health (USA), and various commercial and charitable bodies such as the Wellcome Foundation and the Howard Hughes Medical Trust, whose aim was to have sequenced the entire human genome by the year 2000. This will make available a large amount of information to facilitate molecular science and the rapid determination of molecular abnormalities responsible for cancer. An example of how highly efficient and rapid sequencing technology helps primary scientific research is the recent cloning of the BRCA2 gene.

The availability of the human genome has sharpened debates about the ethical and commercial implications of genomic research, in particular the patenting of gene sequences. Currently, most patents on the human genome have been filed by two companies, a SmithKline Beecham consortium called Human Genome Sciences and the pharmaceutical company Merck.[95] The debate concerns the desire of companies to restrict the use of gene sequences for their own development thus, in the eyes of academics, withholding a valuable resource from the public scientific community. Commerce holds the alternative view that patents are the only way to develop securely and fully a product based on the gene sequence. Religious and moral arguments concerning the ownership of human beings by others for commercial gain are unlikely to restrict the genome patent offices, one in Europe and one in the USA. Genes fulfil the criteria for being patentable: new, useful but without obvious developmental consequences, and their patentability is not under question but rather the conditions of that patent. The debate moves more on the consequences of gene patenting: if government funds have been used to map and sequence the human genome, why should the fruits of that effort be turned over to a single owner? Regulation of patent control seems a reasonable compromise but how that can be achieved is unclear.

Oncology is adapting to the novel technologies of molecular biology, to the rewards of new and possibly better drugs and their masters the pharmaceutical industry, to the increasing expectations of public and government, and to the painful constraints of fiscal policy at the start of the new millennium. Rarely has there been such an interesting, challenging, yet frustrating time for those who care for patients with cancer.

Box 16.2: A short history of the adjuvant therapy of breast cancer

Bonadonna, 1976	CMF improves survival in patients with breast cancer following radical mastectomy.
Fisher, 1975	L-PAM effective in the treatment of women with primary breast cancer, particularly those who are pre-menopausal.
Fisher, 1986	Chemotherapy treatment plus tamoxifen found to be effective for node-positive women only if oestrogen positive and >50 years, compared to chemotherapy alone.
Fisher, 1986	L-PAM and mastectomy more effective than mastectomy alone, particularly in women who are node positive and <50 years.
Mansour, 1989	CMF improves DFS in node-negative breast cancer (tumour >3 cm nd OR +ve, all OR −ve).
Fisher, 1990	Better outcome for node-positive breast cancer patients >50 years with chemotherapy compared to tamoxifen alone.
Fisher, 1990	Two months AC is equivalent to 6 months of CMF in node-positive breast cancer patients with tamoxifen non-responsive tumours.
EBCTG, 1992	Combined chemo–endocrine therapy improves DFS and OS in all women by 30–40%. In women >50, T seems more important, but in younger women, CT and ovarian ablation seem more important, although all treatments can contribute to either group. Node-positive and node-negative patients both benefit, but the absolute benefit for node-positive patients is greater.
EBCTG, 1995	Radiotherapy improves DFS but not OS following surgery. There is no difference between radical and breast-conserving surgery.
Bonadonna, 1995	CMF does not improve DFS or OS in OR +ve, node-negative tumours.
Fisher, 1996	Chemotherapy is better than lumpectomy alone and CMF is better than MF in node-negative, OR-negative women.
Rutqvist, 1996	Five years of adjuvant tamoxifen is more beneficial than 2 years in the treatment of post-menopausal women with oestrogen receptor-positive, early-stage, invasive breast cancer.
Fisher, 1997	NSABP-18 shows no difference in OS between pre- and post-operative ACx 4, with nodal and primary tumour downstaging and more breast-preserving surgery.

Box 16.3: Recent advances in the adjuvant therapy of colon cancer

Moertel, 1990	Levamisole and 5-FU for adjuvant therapy of resected colon carcinoma: DFS and OS benefit.
Wolmark, 1993	LV-modulated 5-FU (NSABP C-03) increases OS by 32% and DFS by 30%.
Riethmuller, 1994	OS advantage for adjuvant treatment with monoclonal antibody to UC-1 antigen.
Francini, 1994	OS and DFS improvement with LV and 5-FU over observation in Dukes C but not B.
Moertel, 1995	5-FU plus levamisole as effective adjuvant therapy after resection of stage III colon carcinoma, reducing OS by 33% and DFS by 40%. Intergroup study of 5-FU plus levamisole as adjuvant therapy for stage II/Dukes, B2 colon cancer shows DFS improvement only.
IMPACT, 1995	Efficacy of 6 months of adjuvant 5-FU and folinic acid in Dukes B/C colon cancer in improving DFS and OS.

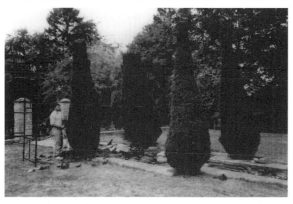

Figure 16.6 *Taxus baccata* or the common yew tree being pruned in north Oxfordshire. As of 1998, the author was able to sell fresh yew cuttings to entrepreneurs for 40p per kilogram. The needles provide the chemical basis for the semi-synthetic taxane docetaxel.

Acknowledgements

We would like to thank clinical and scientific colleagues who have given us a remarkable insight into the trials and tribulations of being an oncologist, particularly Mary Collins and Gordon Rustin.

References

1. Ahmed F.Y., King D.M., Nicol B. *et al.* (1995). Preliminary results of infusional chemotherapy (cisplatin, epirubicin and 5-fluorouracil, ECF) for refractory and relapsed epithelial ovarian cancer (meeting abstract). *Proceedings of the Annual Meeting of the American Society of Clinical Oncology* **14**.
2. Anderson N. and Lokich J. (1992). Controversial issues in 5-fluorouracil infusion use. Dose intensity, treatment duration, and cost comparisons. *Cancer* **70**, 998–1002.
3. Smith I.E., Jones A.L., O'Brien M., McKinna J.A., Sacks N. and Baum M. (1993). Primary medical (neo-adjuvant) chemotherapy for operable breast cancer. *European Journal of Cancer* **29a**, 1796–1799.
4. Pazdur R., Ajani J.A., Patt Y.Z. *et al.* (1990). Phase II study of fluorouracil and recombinant interferon alfa-2a in previously untreated advanced colorectal carcinoma. *Journal of Clinical Oncology* **8**, 2027–2031.
5. Tralongo P., Di Mari A., Scibilia G., Bosco V., Giudice A., Respini D. *et al.* (1995). Prolonged 5-fluorouracil infusion in patients with metastatic colon cancer pretreated with bolus schedule of the same agent. *Anticancer Research* **15**, 635–638.
6. Smith I. (1995). TOPIC: *A Randomised Trial of Infusional ECF (Epirubicin, Cisplatin and 5-FU) vs Conventional AC (Doxorubicin and Cyclophosphamide) as Primary (Neo-adjuvant) Chemotherapy for Patients with >3 cm Diameter Early Breast Cancer.* London: Royal Marsden NHS Trust.
7. Findlay M., Hill A., Cunningham D., Norman A., Nicolson M. and Ford H. (1994). Protracted venous infusion 5-fluorouracil and interferon-alpha in advanced and refractory colorectal cancer. *Annals of Oncology* **5**, 239–243.
8. Ellis P.A., Norman A., Hill A. *et al.* (1995). Epirubicin, cisplatin and infusional 5-fluorouracil (ECF) in hepatobiliary tumours. *European Journal of Cancer* **31A**, 1594–1598.
9. Catimel G., Spielmann M., Dieras V. *et al.* (1996). Phase I study of paclitaxel and epirubicin in patients with metastatic breast cancer: a preliminary report on safety. *Seminars in Oncology* **23**, 24–27.
10. Hrushesky W.J., von Roemeling R., Lanning R.M. and Rabatin J.T. (1990). Circadian-shaped infusions of floxuridine for progressive metastatic renal cell carcinoma. *Journal of Clinical Oncology* **8**, 1504–1513.
11. Depres Brummer P., Berthault Cvitkovic F., Levi F., Brienza S., Vannetzel J.M., Jasmin C. *et al.* (1995). Circadian rhythm-modulated (CRM) chemotherapy of metastatic breast cancer with mitoxantrone, 5-fluorouracil, and folinic acid: preliminary results of a phase I trial. *Journal of Infusion Chemotherapy* **5**, 144–147.

12. Levi F., Soussan A., Adam R. *et al.* (1995). A phase I-II trial of five-day continuous intravenous infusion of 5-fluorouracil delivered at circadian rhythm modulated rate in patients with metastatic colorectal cancer. *Journal of Infusion Chemotherapy* **5**, 153–158.

13. McElwain T.J., Hedley D.W., Burton G. *et al.* (1979). Marrow autotransplantation accelerates haematological recovery in patients with malignant melanoma treated with high-dose melphalan. *British Journal of Cancer* **40**, 72–80.

14. McElwain T.J., Gore M.E., Meldrum M., Viner C., Judson I.R. and Malpas J.S. (1989). VAMP followed by high dose melphalan and autologous bone marrow transplantation for multiple myeloma. *Bone Marrow Transplantation* **4** (Suppl. 4), 109–112.

15. Mandelli F., Avvisati G. and Amadori S. (1990). Maintenance treatment with recombinant interferon alpha-2b in patients with multiple myeloma responding to conventional induction chemotherapy. *New England Journal of Medicine* **322**, 1430–1434.

16. Attal M., Harousseau J.L., Stoppa A.M. *et al.* (1996). A prospective, randomized trial of autologous bone marrow transplantation and chemotherapy in multiple myeloma. Intergroupe Francais du Myelome. *New England Journal of Medicine* **335**, 91–97.

17. Philip T., Guglielmi C., Hagenbeek A. *et al.* (1995). Autologous bone marrow transplantation as compared with salvage chemotherapy in relapses of chemotherapy-sensitive non-Hodgkin's lymphoma. *New England Journal of Medicine* **333**, 1540–1545.

18. Gianni A.M., Bregni M., Siena S. *et al.* (1997). High-dose chemotherapy and autologous bone marrow transplantation compared with MACOP-B in aggressive B-cell lymphoma. *New England Journal of Medicine* **336**, 1290–1297.

19. Antman K., Rowlings R.A. and Vaughn W.P. (1997). High-dose chemotherapy with autologous haemopoetic stem-cell support for breast cancer in North America. *Journal of Clinical Oncology* **15**, 1870–1879.

20. Bezwoda W., Seymour L. and Dansey R.D.(1995). High-dose chemotherapy with haematopoetic rescue as primary treatment for metastatic breast cancer: a randomised trial. *Journal of Clinical Oncology* **13**, 2483–2489.

21. Leigh B.R., Khan W., Hancock S.L. and Knox S.J. (1995). Stem cell factor enhances the survival of murine intestinal stem cells after photon irradiation. *Radiation Research* **142**, 12–15.

22. Deisseroth A.B., Kavanagh J. and Champlin R. (1994). Use of safety-modified retroviruses to introduce chemotherapy resistance sequences into normal hematopoietic cells for chemoprotection during the therapy of ovarian cancer: a pilot trial. *Human Gene Therapy* **5**, 1507–1522.

23. Rodenhuis S., Westermann A., Holtkamp M.J. *et al.* (1996). Feasibility of multiple courses of high-dose cyclophosphamide thiotepa and carboplatin for breast cancer or germ cell cancer. *Journal of Clinical Oncology* **14**, 1473–1483.

24. Smith I.E., Walsh G., Jones A. *et al.* (1995). High complete remission rates with primary neoadjuvant infusional chemotherapy for large early breast cancer. *Journal of Clinical Oncology* **13**, 424–429.

25. Tester W., Caplan R., Heaney J. *et al.* (1996). Neoadjuvant combined modality program with selective organ preservation for invasive bladder cancer: results of Radiation Therapy Oncology Group phase II trial 8802. *Journal of Clinical Oncology* **14**, 119–126.

26. Einstein A.B., Wolf M., Halliday K.R. *et al.* (1996). Combination transurethral resection, systemic chemotherapy, and pelvic radiotherapy for invasive (T2–T4) bladder cancer unsuitable for cystectomy: a phase I/II Southwestern Oncology Group study. *Urology* **47**, 652–657.

27. Hoskins W., Perez C.A. and Young R.C. (1993). Gynaecologic tumours. In De Vita V. Jr, Hellman S. and Rosenberg S.A. (eds.) *Principles and Practice of Oncology.* Philadelphia, PA: Lippincott, pp. 1152–1226.

28. Kumar L., Kaushal R., Nandy M. *et al.* (1994). Chemotherapy followed by radiotherapy versus radiotherapy alone in locally advanced cervical cancer: a randomized study. *Gynecologic Oncology* **54**, 307–315.

29. Souhami L., Gil R.A., Allan S.E. *et al.* (1991). A randomized trial of chemotherapy followed by pelvic radiation therapy in stage IIIB carcinoma of the cervix. *Journal of Clinical Oncology* **9**, 970–977.

30. Tattersall M.H.N., Lorvidhaya V., Vootiprux V. *et al.* (1995). Randomized trial of epirubicin and cisplatin chemotherapy followed by pelvic radiation in locally advanced cervical cancer. *Journal of Clinical Oncology* **13**, 444–451.

31. Sardi J., Giaroli A., Sananes C. *et al.* (1996). Randomized trial with neoadjuvant chemotherapy in stage IIIB squamous carcinoma cervix uteri: an unexpected therapeutic management. *International Journal of Gynecological Cancer* **6**, 85–93.

32. Sardi J., Sananes C., Giaroli A. *et al.* (1993). Results of a prospective randomized trial with neoadjuvant chemotherapy in stage IB, bulky, squamous carcinoma of the cervix. *Gynecologic Oncology* **49**, 156–165.

33. Sardi J., Sananes C., Giaroli A., Maya G. and di Paola G. (1990). Neoadjuvant chemotherapy in locally advanced carcinoma of the cervix uteri. *Gynecologic Oncology* **38**, 486–493.

34. Rosell R., Gomez Codina J. and Camps Cea. (1994). A randomised trial comparing preoperative chemotherapy and surgery with surgery alone patients with non-small cell lung cancer. *New England Journal of Medicine* **330**, 153–158.

35. Roth J., Fosella F. and Komaki R. (1994). A randomised trial comparing preoperative chemotherapy and surgery with surgery alone patients in resectable stage III non-small cell lung cancer. *Journal of the National Cancer Institute* **86**, 673–680.

36. Bortfeld T., Boyer A.L., Schlegel W., Kahler D.L. and Waldron T.J. (1994). Realization and verification of three-dimensional conformal radiotherapy with modulated fields. *International Journal of Radiation Oncology, Biology, Physics* **30**, 899–908.

37. Fuks Z. (1993). Three-dimensional conformal radiotherapy. In De Vita V. Jr, Hellman S. and Rosenberg S.A. (eds.) *Principles and Practice of Oncology.* Philadelphia, PA: Lippincott, pp. 2614–2623.

38. Horwich A., Wynne C., Nahum A., Swindell W. and Dearnaley D.P. (1994). Conformal radiotherapy at the Royal Marsden Hospital (UK). *International Journal of Radiation Biology* **65**, 117–122.

39. Dische S. and Saunders M.I. (1990). The rationale for continuous, hyperfractionated, accelerated radiotherapy (CHART). *International Journal of Radiation Oncology, Biology, Physics* **19**, 1317–1320.

40. Saunders M., Dische S., Barrett A., Parmar M.K.B., Harvey A. and Gibson D. (1996). Randomised multicentre trials of CHART vs conventional radiotherapy in head and neck and non-small cell lung cancer: an interim report. *British Journal of Cancer* **73**, 1455–1462.

41. Saunders M., Dische S. and Barrett A. (1997). Continuous hyperfractionated accelerated radiotherapy (CHART) versus conventional radiotherapy in non-small cell lung cancer: a randomised multicentre trial. *Lancet* **350**, 161–165.

42. Rose P. *et al.* (1999). Concurrent cisplatin-based radiotherapy and chemotherapy for locally advanced cervical cancer. *New England Journal of Medicine* **340**, 1144–1153.

43. Cummings B, Keane T., Thomas G., Harwood A., Rider W., Cummings B. *et al.* (1984). Results and toxicity of the treatment of anal canal carcinoma by radiation therapy or radiation therapy and chemotherapy. *Cancer* **54**, 2062–2068.

44. Cummings B.J., Keane T.J., Wong C.S., Catton C.N., Tanum G., Tveit K. *et al.* (1991). Epidermoid anal cancer: treatment by radiation alone or by radiation and 5-fluorouracil with and without mitomycin C. *International Journal of Radiation Oncology, Biology, Physics* **21**, 1115–1125.

45. Cummings B.J., Rider W.D., Harwood A.R., Keane T.J., Thomas G.M., Erlichman C. *et al.* (1982). Combined radical radiation therapy and chemotherapy for primary squamous cell carcinoma of the anal canal. *Cancer Treatment and Research* **66**, 489–492.

46. Merlano M., Benasso M., Corvo R. *et al.* (1996). Five-year update of a randomized trial of alternating radiotherapy and chemotherapy compared with radiotherapy alone in treatment of unresectable squamous cell carcinoma of the head and neck. *Journal of the National Cancer Institute* **88**, 583–589.

47. Merlano M., Corvo R., Margarino G. *et al.* (1991). Combined chemotherapy and radiation therapy in advanced inoperable squamous cell carcinoma of the head and neck. The final report of a randomized trial. *Cancer* **67**, 915–921.

48. Pinnaro P., Cercato M.C., Giannarelli D. *et al.* (1994). A randomized phase II study comparing sequential versus simultaneous chemo-radiotherapy in patients with unresectable locally advanced squamous cell cancer of the head and neck. *Annals of Oncology* **5**, 513–519.

49. Urba S.G., Forastiere A.A., Wolf G.T., Esclamado R.M., McLaughlin P.W. and Thornton A.F. (1994). Intensive induction chemotherapy and radiation for organ preservation in patients with advanced resectable head and neck carcinoma. *Journal of Clinical Oncology* **12**, 946–953.

50. Al Sarraf M, LeBlanc M. and Giri P.G. (1996). Superiority of chemoradiation vs radiation in patients with locally advanced nasopharyngeal cancer. Preliminary results of Intergroup 0099 (SWOG 8892, RTOG 8817, ECOG 2388) randomised trial. *American Society of Clinical Oncology* **15**, 313.

51. Herskovic A., Leichman L., Lattin P. *et al.* (1988). Chemo/radiation with and without surgery in the thoracic oesophagus: the Wayne State experience. *International Journal of Radiation Oncology, Biology, Physics* **15**, 655–662.

52. Herskovic A., Martz K., Al Sarraf M. *et al.* (1992). Combined chemotherapy and radiotherapy compared with radiotherapy alone in patients with cancer of the oesophagus. *New England Journal of Medicine* **326**, 1593–1598.

53. Reddy S.P., Lad T., Mullane M., Rosen F., Carroll R. and Marks J.E. (1995). Radiotherapy alone compared with radiotherapy and chemotherapy in patients with squamous cell carcinoma of the oesophagus. *American Journal of Clinical Oncology: Cancer Clinical Trials* **18**, 376–381.

54. Rosenberg S., Lotze M.T., Muul L.M. *et al.* (1987). A progress report on the treatment of 157 patients with advanced cancer using lymphokine activated killer cells and interleukin-2 or high dose interleukin-2 alone. *New England Journal of Medicine* **316**, 889–897.

55. Bernier J., Horiot J.C., Bartelink H. *et al.* (1996). Profile of radiotherapy departments contributing to the Cooperative Group of Radiotherapy of the European Organization for Research and Treatment of Cancer. *International Journal of Radiation Oncology, Biology, Physics* **34**, 953–960.

56. van der Schueren E., Horiot J.C., Leunens G., Rubens R., Steward W., van Dongen J.A. *et al.* (1993). Quality assurance in cancer treatment. Report of a Working Party from the European School of Oncology. *European Journal of Cancer* **29a**, 172–181.

57. Miguel R., Kreitzer J.M., Reinhart D. *et al.* (1995). Post-operative pain control with a new transdermal fentanyl delivery system. A multicenter trial. *Anesthesiology* **83**, 470–477.

58. Mercadante S., Lodi F., Sapio M., Calligar M. and Serretta R. (1995). Long-term ketamine subcutaneous continuous infusion in neuropathic cancer pain. *Journal of Pain Symptom Management* **10**, 564–568.

59. Hortobagyi G.N., Theriault R.L., Porter L. *et al.* (1996). Efficacy of pamidronate in reducing skeletal complications in patients with breast cancer and lytic bone metastases. Protocol 19 Aredia Breast Cancer Study Group. *New England Journal of Medicine* **335**, 1785–1791.

60. O'Rourke N., McCloskey E., Houghton F., Huss H. and Kanis J.A. (1995). Double-blind, placebo-controlled, dose-response trial of oral clodronate in patients with bone metastases. *Journal of Clinical Oncology* **13**, 929–934.

61. Mangili G., Franchi M., Mariani A. *et al.* (1996). Octreotide in the management of bowel obstruction in terminal ovarian cancer. *Gynecologic Oncology* **61**, 345–348.

62. Clarke E.A. and Anderson T.W. (1979). Does screening by 'Pap' smears help prevent cervical cancer? A case–control study. *Lancet* **ii**, 1–4.

63. Quinn M. and Allen E. (1995). Changes in the incidence and mortality from breast cancer in England and Wales since introduction of screening. *British Medical Journal* **311**, 1391–1395.

64. Forrest Report (1986). London: Department of Health and Social Security.

65. Berrino F., Sant M., Verdecchia A., Capocaccia R., Halukinen T. and Esteve J. (1995). *Survival of Cancer Patients in Europe: The EUROCARE Study.* Lyons: International Agency for Research on Cancer.

66. Cancer Research Campaign (1994). *Incidence of Cancers in the United Kingdom.* In Factsheets. London: Cancer Research Campaign.

67. Hall R.R. (1996). Screening and early detection of prostate cancer will decrease morbidity and mortality from prostate cancer: the argument against. *European Urology* **29** (Suppl. 2), 24–26.

68. Armbruster D.A. (1993). Prostate-specific antigen: biochemistry, analytical methods, and clinical application. *Clinical Chemistry* **39**, 181–195.

69. Woolf S.H. (1995). Screening for prostate cancer with prostate-specific antigen. An examination of the evidence. *New England Journal of Medicine* **333**, 1401–1405.

70. Mettlin C., Murphy G.P., Babaian R.J. *et al.* (1996). The results of a five-year early prostate cancer detection intervention. Investigators of the American Cancer Society National Prostate Cancer Detection Project. *Cancer* **77**, 150–159.

71. Schroder F.H., Denis L.J., Kirkels W., de Koning H.J. and Sandaert B. (1995). European randomized study of screening for prostate cancer. Progress report of Antwerp and Rotterdam pilot studies. *Cancer* **76**, 129–134.

72. Parkes C., Wald N.J., Murphy P. *et al.* (1995). Prospective observational study to assess value of prostate specific antigen as screening test for prostate cancer. *British Medical Journal* **311**, 1340–1343.

73. Jacobs I. (1994). Genetic, biochemical, and multimodal approaches to screening for ovarian cancer. *Gynecological Oncology* **55**, S22–S27.

74. Miki Y., Swenson J., Shattuck Eidens D. *et al.* (1994). A strong candidate for the breast and ovarian cancer susceptibility gene BRCA1. *Science* **266**, 66–71.

75. Wooster R., Bignell G., Lancaster J. *et al.* (1995). Identification of the breast cancer susceptibility gene BRCA2. *Nature* **378**, 789–792.

76. Struewing J.P., Watson P., Easton D.F., Ponder B.A., Lynch H.T. and Tucker M.A. (1995). Prophylactic oophorectomy in inherited breast/ovarian cancer families. *Journal of the National Institute Monograph* **17**, 33–35.

77. Healy B. (1997). BRCA genes – bookmaking, fortune-telling, and medical care. *New England Journal of Medicine* **336**, 1448–1449.

78. Lancaster J.M., Wiseman R.W. and Berchuck A. (1996). An inevitable dilemma: prenatal testing for mutations in the BRCA1 breast – ovarian cancer susceptibility gene. *Obstetrics and Gynecology* **87**, 306–309.

79. Slevin M.L., Nichols S.E., Downer S.M. *et al.* (1996). Emotional support for cancer patients: what do patients really want? *British Journal of Cancer* **74**, 1275–1279.

80. Slevin M.L., Plant H., Lynch D., Drinkwater J. and Gregory W.M. (1988). Who should measure quality of life, the doctor or the patient? *British Journal of Cancer* **57**, 109–112.

81. Coates A., Forbes J. and Simes R.J. (1993). Prognostic value of performance status and quality-of-life scores during chemotherapy for advanced breast cancer. The Australian New Zealand Breast Cancer Trials Group. *Journal of Clinical Oncology* **11**, 2050.

82. Coates A., Gebski V., Bishop J.F. *et al.* (1987). Improving the quality of life during chemotherapy for advanced breast cancer. A comparison of intermittent and continuous treatment strategies. *New England Journal of Medicine* **317**, 1490–1495.

83. Coates A., Gebski V., Signorini D. *et al.* (1992). Prognostic value of quality-of-life scores during chemotherapy for advanced breast cancer. Australian New Zealand Breast Cancer Trials Group. *Journal of Clinical Oncology* **10**, 1833–1838.

84. Gallagher M.J. (1996). International quality control/quality assurance. *International Journal of Radiation Oncology, Biology, Physics* **34**, 965–967.

85. Legha S.S. and Buzaid A.C. (1993). Role of recombinant interleukin-2 in combination with interferon-alfa and chemotherapy in the treatment of advanced melanoma. *Seminars in Oncology* **20**, 27–32.

86. Bagshawe K.D. (1987). Antibody directed enzymes revive anticancer prodrugs concept. *British Journal of Cancer* **56**, 531–532.

87. Begent R.H., Verhaar M.J., Chester K.A.. *et al.* (1996). Clinical evidence of efficient tumor targeting based on single-chain Fv antibody selected from a combinatorial library. *Natural Medicine* **2**, 979–984.

88. Gore M. and Riches P.M. (1996). The history of immunotherapy. In Gore M. and Riches P.M. (eds.) *Immunotherapy of Cancer.* Oxford: Churchill Livingstone, pp. 1–23.

89. Bridgewater J.A. and Gore M. (1995). Biological response modifiers in melanoma. *British Medical Bulletin* **51**, 656–677.

90. Morton D.L., Foshag L.J., Hoon D.S. *et al.* (1992). Prolongation of survival in metastatic melanoma after active specific immunotherapy with a new polyvalent melanoma vaccine [published erratum appears in *Annals of Surgery* (1993) **217**, 309]. *Annals of Surgery* **216**, 463–482.

91. Bridgewater J. and Collins M.K.L. (1995). Vaccine immunotherapy for cancer. In Dickson G. (ed.) *Molecular and Cell Biology of Human Gene Therapeutics.* London: Chapman and Hall.

92. Bridgewater J., Knox R.J., Pitts J.D., Collins M.K. and Springer C.J. (1997). The bystander effect of the nitroreductase/CB1954 enzyme/prodrug system is due to a cell-permeable metabolite. *Human Gene Therapy* **8**, 709–717.

93. Oldfield E.H., Ram Z., Chiang Y. and Blaese R.M. (1995). Intrathecal gene therapy for the treatment of leptomeningeal carcinomatosis. GTI 0108. A phase I/II study. *Human Gene Therapy* **6**, 55–85.

94. Bodmer W.F. (1991). HUGO: the Human Genome Organization. *FASEB Journal* **5**, 73–74.

95. Caplan A. and Merz J. (1996). Patenting gene sequences. *British Medical Journal* **312**, 926.

Part 4

The Management of Cancer-related Problems

Introduction

Cancer causes a large range of difficult and distressing problems, as a result of either the disease process itself, or its treatment. In the preceding section on 'The Experience of Cancer Treatment', problems associated with treatment have been identified and nursing strategies for managing these examined. This section focuses more directly on those problems, which are primarily (although not exclusively) the result of the disease process. The problems and difficulties that often accompany cancer cannot be neatly divided into those resulting from treatment and those arising from the disease itself. These are not mutually exclusive, therefore a rather arbitrary distinction is made here. Several common cancer-related problems have been identified, however, and are explored with particular reference to the contribution that nursing could make to their control or management. A departure from the traditional notion of symptom management is made, and a more radical and person-centred approach is proposed.

Symptom management has been dominated by the successes achieved in cancer pain control using powerful drugs. This perhaps unintentionally set a path for the construction of care, which has placed heavy emphasis on a biomedical model of management, and the search for new and better drugs first for pain, and then for other symptoms common in cancer. This has led to the orientation of care around the 'relief' of the symptom experienced, and the neglect of other equally important aspects, such as suffering, distress, and ability to function independently.

The limitations of this model of 'symptom control' are well rehearsed in the literature, and surround the biomedical relationship to 'the body' since this:

- regards the body as an external object to the enquiries that yield knowledge of it
- assumes that the practitioner is in control of the body of the 'patient', and diagnosis and treatment therefore requires them to be subordinate to the practitioner
- deals with malfunctioning organs and related symptoms and not the 'body', which constitutes the actual person.[1,2]

A further limitation of the biomedical model of symptom management lies in its foundations in the epistemology of Cartesianism. Descartes' influence on Western thought has left us with the conception of the separate nature of mind and body, leaving only the body in the domain of medicine. The mind was originally the domain of the church (and more recently that of psychologists and psychiatrists); this has meant that biomedicine has worked within very narrow boundaries and neglects a real understanding of people and their problems.[3] The assumption that symptoms are reflections of disordered somatic processes, where the physician's task is to decode patients' descriptions of these in order to diagnose disease, is inadequate. Instead, a meaning-centred approach has been proposed,[4] which seeks to access an individual's interpretation of their illness and to assist them to construct new understanding of their illness. In this context, therefore, the term 'symptom' is highly problematic because of the assumption that this is universally defined and can be managed beyond the person by the health carer, with little reference to social or cultural influences. It also inherently excludes the person's own narrative and personal meanings from the therapeutic process. The terms 'problem' and 'need' are preferable, since these suggest something that is difficult to deal with or understand. The power for action and ownership of these, however, remains with the person experiencing the problem. Looked at in this way, it is possible to see that as health carers we have no right to 'manage' these problems, only to assist in their containment, and both the sufferer and health carer have a mutual need to understand them:[5]

> There is more to what people experience and know than they are able to express and we are able to hear.[6]

Problems associated with cancer and its treatment may be viewed both positively and negatively. Where a problem provides legitimisation to rest or temporarily to cease demanding activities, it may be interpreted as beneficial. More commonly it is interpreted as a sign of disease progression, failure of treatment, or imminent death. The meanings attributed to cancer-related symptoms and how people respond to and cope with problems are unique. These are influenced by an individual's life history and the wider culture in which understanding of illness develops.[7,8] Gender, personality traits, health beliefs, socio-economic status, environmental factors, and health carers themselves are all potent in either exacerbating or containing the problems that result from cancer.[9] This implies that health carers must disentangle what is 'really going on' from a person's account of their problem and any distress or difficulty associated with it. Their experience is of only secondary importance within the biomedical process of naming a symptom. Practitioners who use such a reductionist approach may respond to complex situations by applying a diagnosis based upon professional knowledge, discarding the subjective expressions of the person experiencing it since they do not 'fit' the diagnostic picture.[10]

Nurses have a tremendous contribution to make in helping people to articulate and interpret their problems and through this become better at managing them for themselves. Nurses' expertise lies not in telling people what ails them, but in working alongside them to clarify the totality of their experience. Even when cure is not possible, understanding the meaning problems hold for an individual can be a powerful source of support and comfort.

In this section, expert nurses have set out to articulate a way of working with people who have cancer in order to assist them in managing their problems. Many common problems are discussed. Some, such as pain, compromised nutrition, wounds, and the risk of infection, have been widely documented and researched. Others, such as breathlessness, ascites, confusion, and lymphoedema, have received less attention.

The section begins its consideration of the clinical management of cancer-related problems by focusing on nursing's contribution to the management of cancer pain. As one of the most commonly associated symptoms of cancer, it is not surprising that pain is often one of the most feared, and perhaps the most catastrophised, of all cancer symptoms. Despite the considerable attention paid by health care professionals to this phenomenon, pain continues to be inadequately controlled.

References

1. Lynon M.L. and Barbalet J.M. (1994). Society's body: emotion and the 'somatization' of social theory. In Csordas T.J. (ed.) *Embodiment and Experience.* Cambridge: Cambridge University Press.
2. Corner J. and Dunlop R. (1997). New approaches to care. In Clark D., Ahmedzai S. and Hockley J. (eds.) *New Themes in Palliative Care.* Milton Keynes: Open University Press.
3. Cassel E.J. (1982). The nature of suffering and the goals of medicine. *New England Journal of Medicine* **306**, 639–645.
4. Good B.J. and Delvecchio Good M.J. (1980). The meaning of symptoms – a cultural hermeneutic model for clinical practice. In Eisenberg I. and Kleinman A. (eds.) *The Relevance of Social Science for Medicine.* Dordrecht: Reidel.
5. Corner J. (1995). Innovative approaches to symptom management. *European Journal of Cancer Care* **4**, 145–146.
6. Halldorsdottir S. and Hamrin E. (1995). Experiencing existential changes: the lived experience of having cancer. *Cancer Nursing* **19**, 29–36.
7. Kleinman A. (1988). *The Illness Narratives: Suffering, Healing and the Human Condition.* New York: Basic Books.
8. Benner P. and Wrubel J. (1989). *The Primacy of Caring. Stress and Coping in Health and Illness.* Workingham: Addison-Wesley.
9. Vessey J. and Richardson B. (1993). A holistic approach to symptom assessment and intervention. *Holistic Nursing Practice* **7**, 13–21.
10. Schön D. (1983). *The Reflective Practitioner.* London: Maurice Temple Smith.

CHAPTER SEVENTEEN

Pain

Meinir Krishnasamy

It is estimated that only 10–15% of pain is satisfactorily managed, even though research evidence suggests that it is possible to relieve 80–90% of cancer pain.[1] Why is this and how can nurses contribute to an improvement in these statistics?

Pain is often the primary reason for seeking medical attention. For the individual subsequently diagnosed with cancer, it becomes a potent symptom, signifying the presence of disease or intimating its progression. Cancer, pain, and death may consequently become fused in the mind of the individual. Because of this, pain management will only be effective if a patient-centred approach to care is embraced by health professionals.[2] Unfortunately, there is little evidence to suggest that cancer pain management is either patient centred or holistic.[3]

The World Health Organisation[4] promotes the concept of 'total pain', which acknowledges that it has physical, emotional, social, and spiritual components.[5] Without attention to each of these facets of the pain experience, patient-centred care will continue to be an anomaly, and the statistics for unrelieved pain are unlikely to improve. As long ago as 1979, McCaffrey stated that 'everything written or said about pain is worthless in the hands of a practitioner who doubts that a patient has pain'.[5] The patient, she asserts, is 'the only authority about the pain he experiences'. An acceptance of pain, when reported by individuals, irrespective of whether or not there is verifiable tissue damage, is therefore fundamental to effective pain management.[6]

Pain is deeply personal – neither solely shaped nor confined by a biological reality.[3] It is a complex biocultural event and as such, one of nursing's greatest potential contributions to pain management is to facilitate the expression of each individual's experience of pain.[7]

Managing cancer pain

The aims and principles of cancer pain management are to:

- recognise and promptly assess pain in patients with cancer
- identify psychological and spiritual influences on pain perception and management
- alleviate pain at night, at rest, and on movement
- maximise independence and possible quality of life
- address and thus relieve current and future fears about pain
- provide support and encouragement for family members and friends and professional caregivers
- invite participation of the patient, family, and/or friends
- adopt a collaborative, multi-disciplinary approach
- design unique analgesic regimes tailored to each patient's needs and tolerance
- regularly follow up the outcome
- refer early to specialist services if pain control is not achieved.[8]

Without comprehensive assessment taking account of the many interdependent facets of pain it is unlikely that the principles outlined above will be met. An awareness of misconceptions that may hamper the process of assessment will facilitate effective nursing management.

Some common misperceptions about pain management are that:

- real pain has an identifiable, physical cause
- psychogenic pain (i.e. one better understood through the language of psychology rather than physiology) does not really hurt and may even be comparable to malingering
- members of the health care team are capable of making accurate inferences about the nature, severity, and existence of an individual's pain, based on professional knowledge and the patient's behavioural and physiological expressions of the pain
- the severity and duration of pain can be predicted by the nature of the cancer and the cause and location of the pain
- patients should be encouraged to have a high tolerance for pain
- patients in severe pain always look distressed
- pain can be understood in isolation solely as a facet of the cancer diagnosis.[6,9–11]

Box 17.1: Some factors affecting an individual's perception of pain[3,5,9,11]

- Fatigue
- Insomnia
- Discomfort
- Anxiety
- Depression
- Anger
- Fear
- Sadness
- Boredom
- Isolation
- Withdrawal
- Loneliness

- Perceptions of the significance of the pain and its meaning
- Cultural identity
- Cultural norms and expectations of pain expression and behaviour
- Religious or spiritual beliefs
- Familial support
- Social support network
- Perceptions of self
- Altered self-image and self-esteem
- Loss of income
- Professional expectations of causes of pain behaviour
- Professional expectations of pain behaviour
- Fear of being on 'a collision course with death'

Traditionally, medical management had involved identification of a relationship between pain and a noxious stimulus or abnormal neurophysiological activity.[5] When a cause for the pain is found, the doctor explains to the patient why he experiences pain and prescribes 'appropriate' analgesia. However, in the light of the factors affecting perception of pain, administering analgesia in isolation is clearly insufficient if pain relief is to be effective.

What happens when no cause for an individual's pain can be found? For many in this situation, their experience is left unverified and may ultimately result in stigmatisation or rejection by professionals, family, and friends. Exploring what pain means to the person experiencing it, and attempting to understand it within the context of social and cultural characteristics, is a means of overcoming the difficulty of identifying a cause. Unfortunately, there is currently little evidence of nurses' ability to enter into such profoundly therapeutic relationships with people in pain.

An appreciation of pain pathways and analgesic regimes (described later in this chapter) is central to effective nursing care. This may be especially important when complex pain syndromes such as bone and neuropathic pain impact on an individual's quality of life. However, nursing's critical contribution to cancer pain management will only be realised as we begin to nurture the therapeutic skills necessary to help others to articulate the experience of illness, as we begin to understand and work with what we are told about pain. Nevertheless, this is notoriously difficult as pain, like so many other symptoms discussed in this chapter, is deeply resistant to simple expression in everyday language or speech.[3] How many times have you been told, 'I just can't explain what it feels like' or 'I know it sounds stupid but I just can't point to where it is'?

As health care professionals, we may compound the unspeakable nature of pain, demanding acquiescence in an objective rhetoric so that symptoms may be validated, and the 'right' to help for them is justified.[12] Nurses are ideally placed to redress this bias. By directing assessment at the person and not the pain, we are likely to be effective in a way that has previously been unattainable (Care strategy 17.1).

Valuable questions to ask to try and evaluate a patient's pain include:

- When did you first notice you were ill?
- How have things been since you were told about the cancer?
- How have things been with and for your family or friends?
- What was happening in your life when the cancer was diagnosed?
- What plans or life events has it disrupted or destroyed?
- Did you experience any pain when you were first ill?
- When did you first experience any pain?
- Is the pain the same now or has it changed?
- What makes it worse and what makes it better?
- What are your expectations, fears and hopes for the future?
- What does the pain mean to you?

An overview of analgesic drugs

The World Health Organisation[4] has developed a guide for the selection of analgesic drugs to manage cancer pain. These steps, commonly referred to as the 'three-step analgesic ladder', have become the mainstay of pharmacological management of mild, moderate, and severe cancer pain.[14]

Box 17.2: The three-step analgesic ladder

Mild pain
Drugs of choice – non-narcotics:
- Paracetamol, aspirin, or non-steroidal anti-inflammatory drugs (NSAIDs)
- Combining paracetamol and NSAIDs is more effective than using either alone

Moderate pain
Drugs of choice – weak opioids:
- Dextropropoxyphene (Distalgesic), codeine, or dihydrocodeine

Severe pain
Drugs of choice – strong opioids:
- Morphine/diamorphine, papaveretum, methadone

Combining two strong opioids or mixing a weak and strong opioid is not advisable. Remember that most patients with cancer require strong opioids.

Adjuvant drugs/co-analgesics
- Corticosteroids for nerve and bone pain and for painful hepatomegaly and headache from raised intracranial pressure
- Antidepressants, anti-arrhythmic, and anti-convulsant drugs can all be used to alleviate nerve pain
- Anti-spasmodics for reduction of muscle spasm
- Biphosphanates for relief of bone pain
- Antibiotics or anti-rheumatic drugs for alleviation of co-existing pathologies.[4,13-16]

Unfortunately, there are many unwanted side-effects of these medications. The most prevalent are nausea, vomiting, and constipation. For those who are eating well or who have previously been taking opioids, an anti-emetic is less likely to be necessary. For some, nausea is only a problem for the first few days following initial prescription or while doses are being increased incrementally until pain control is achieved, while others may require indefinite anti-emetic cover. Nursing approaches to managing nausea and vomiting are discussed later in this chapter. Aperients should always be prescribed with opioids unless specific complications such as bowel obstruction contraindicate this. Combining a softening laxative (e.g. lactulose) with a stimulant (e.g. senna) may often be more effective.[17]

Drowsiness, urinary retention, confusion, hallucinations, itching, and bronchospasm have also been documented as side-effects of opioid medication.[8] Respiratory depression is not a problem when using strong opioids regularly by mouth to relieve pain. Indeed, circumstantial evidence suggests that the competent use of morphine to relieve pain facilitates better rest, dietary intake, and mobility, thus prolonging lives.[11] Addiction is not a problem when morphine is used to treat opioid-responsive pain[11] and this should not be used as a reason to withhold opioids from patients with cancer.[18]

Physical dependence, manifested as irritability, chills, sweating, abdominal pain, diarrhoea, and anxiety, if opioids are stopped suddenly, should not be confused with psychological addiction.[13]

Surgery, radiotherapy, nerve blocks, transcutaneous nerve stimulation (TENS), heat, cold, and cordotomy (although only occasionally used) are also effective methods of pain relief.[11] Increasing attention is being given to interventions, that rely more on psychological and cultural influences

Box 17.3: Guidelines for use of morphine for cancer pain in adults[19]

Administration

- The optimal route of administration of opioids is by mouth, but if patients are unable to swallow drugs, rectal and subcutaneous routes can be used, as the bio-availability and duration of action are the same. Morphine suppositories are widely available in several doses, but if you do have trouble accessing them, they can be prepared easily in hospital pharmacies.

  Morphine can be given *subcutaneously* every 4 hours or by continuous infusion. When converting from oral to subcutaneous morphine for chronic pain the dose should be divided by two (the precise ratio probably lies between 1:2 and 1:3). Other opioids such as *diamorphine* and *hydromorphone* may be preferred to morphine for parenteral use. However, neither drug is more effective than morphine, but both are more potent. The relative potency ratio of oral morphine to subcutaneous diamorphine is 1:3.

  Morphine should not be given intramuscularly for chronic cancer pain as subcutaneous administration is easier and less painful for the patient.

  If patients have generalised oedema, tend to develop erythema, soreness, or sterile abscesses with subcutaneous administration, have coagulation disorders or poor venous circulation, subcutaneous administration is contraindicated and intravenous (IV) administration should be considered instead. IV administration should also be considered if patients have indwelling central catheters or peripheral IV access. *The relative potency of oral to intravenous morphine is about 1:3.* Bolus IV doses of morphine will be higher in potency because of greater peak effects.

  Controlled release morphine tablets should not be crushed as this alters their dissolution and absorption characteristics. *Vaginal or rectal administration is also contraindicated* as reduced bio-availability and haphazard absorption are likely. Sublingual and nebulised routes of morphine administration for pain management are not recommended as there is little evidence of predictability of absorption rates.

- Dose titration should involve the prescription of immediate release morphine (oral morphine in solution or immediate release tablets) every 4 hours. The same dose should be used for breakthrough pain and can be given as frequently as required, e.g. every hour. There is no evidence to suggest that patients experience any significant adverse effects when the full dose is administered for breakthrough pain.

  If immediate release morphine is not available, the total daily dose requirement should be based on an individual's previous analgesic intake. Breakthrough pain should be managed with non-steroidal anti-inflammatory drugs or with another short-acting opioid. If available, morphine sulphate injection solution can be administered orally or rectally for breakthrough pain.

- *Controlled release morphine*, which provides cover over a 12-hour period, should not be used when attempting to titrate the analgesic dose, as its delayed peak plasma concentration makes it more difficult to assess the adequacy of the dose given, and to respond quickly to patients' needs. Several formulations are available but there is no evidence that they differ in their duration of effect or relative analgesic properties. However, care needs to taken if changing between preparations, as there may be possible variations in release profiles and bio-availability.

- *Once stabilised*, patients using a 4-hourly regimen based on immediate release morphine can continue to use the same dose for breakthrough pain. However, if a patient's pain is controlled using a 12-hourly regimen, the immediate release morphine dose used to counteract breakthrough pain should be *one-third of the regular 12-hourly dose*.

- If a patient's pain returns consistently before the next dose of regular analgesia is due, the 4- to 12-hourly prescription should be increased. Relying solely on breakthrough analgesia to 'top up' the analgesic requirement will not only result in greater inconvenience for the patient, but may also lead to increased adverse side-effects. For some patients, however, a 12-hourly regime is inadequate to control their pain, and controlled release morphine may be required an 8-hourly regime if their pain is to be effectively managed.

- Fentanyl, methadone and buprenorphine are well absorbed sublingually and may be used as alternatives to subcutaneous morphine. Buprenorphine is commonly used sublingually and may be a useful alternative for low-dose oral morphine where patients have difficulty swallowing. Evidence of efficacy in long-term use is limited. Early indications suggest that fentanyl provides continuous, controlled systemic delivery of analgesia for 72 hours via transdermal patches. It appears to be well tolerated and effective but further evidence of its place in the routine management of cancer pain is required.

- Advising a patient to take a double dose of their immediate release morphine at bedtime, to prevent night-time waking and disturbed sleep, is a widely accepted practice, which appears to have no adverse effects. However, no formal research evidence is available to support this practice.

(Reproduced with permission from the BMJ Publishing Group. Summarised from the Expert Working Group of the European Association for Palliative Care (1996). Morphine in Cancer Pain: Modes of Administration, *British Medical Journal* 312, 30 March, pp. 823–6.[14])

on pain.[20] It is beyond the scope of this chapter to discuss any of these in any depth, but the main non-pharmacological interventions featured in the literature are listed in Case strategy 17.2. Some recommendations for utilising relaxation in daily practice are outlined at the end of the chapter.

Care strategy 17.2

Examples of non-pharmacological interventions
- Relaxation
- Hypnosis
- Acupuncture
- Visualisation
- Art therapy
- Biofeedback
- Imagery
- Distraction
- Massage

Providing nursing care for a person experiencing cancer pain is a considerable nursing challenge. Its complexity demands that nurses open their minds to different ideas of ways in which to interact with people in pain.[3] This also involves relying on a process of individualising established components of pain relief.

- Don't wait until pain becomes severe before intervening.
- Use a variety of pain relief measures, but above all, include what the patient says works.
- How active does the patient want to be in managing his or her care and what means of patient education and information provision best suits his or her needs?
- How active can the patient be in managing his or her care and who else in the patient's support network should be involved?
- What are the individual's subjective perceptions of the severity of pain and the distress caused by it?
- What is the best way of assessing efficacy of pharmacological and non-pharmacological interventions? Are pain charts and/or patient diaries practicable?

Pain mechanisms

Of the many kinds of nerve, only a few are concerned with nociception and the transmission of impulses associated with pain. Some nerves carry nociceptive impulses, while others carry impulses that directly affect the perception of pain. Three types of neuron seem to be involved with pain transmission:

- large, heavily myelinated A-beta fibres: these respond to light pressure, and their stimulation leads to the sensation of tenderness
- smaller, thinly myelinated A-delta fibres, fine, unmyelinated C fibres: A-delta and C fibres are the principal transmitters of pain impulses, although other fibres may also be involved. Damage to these fibres results in intense pain. The A-delta fibres give rise to sharp pain, while the C fibres give rise to dull, persistent pain.

One of the earliest theories of pain was the specificity theory. It was postulated that there were special receptors for each type or modality of pain, e.g. Meissner's corpuscles responded exclusively to touch, Pacinian corpuscles to pressure, Ruffini and Krayse end-organs to heat and cold, and free nerve endings to pain. Melzack and Wall went on to show that these assumptions were over-simplified, assuming a 'rigid, fixed relationship between a neural structure and a psychological experience'.[20]

The pattern theory of pain followed the specificity theory. Criticised for discounting psychological aspects of the pain experience, the pattern theory was based on the belief that excessive stimulation of the skin receptors created particular patterns of nerve impulses that were summated in the dorsal horn of the spinal cord and consequently caused pain.

However, the most widely recognised pain theory is the gate control theory (GCT), first espoused by Melzack and Wall in 1965.[21] The theory proposes that:

- the transmission of nerve impulses is modulated by a spinal gating mechanism in the dorsal horn (substantia gelatinosa)
- larger fibres tend to close the gate (inhibit transmission), while smaller fibres tend to open the gate (facilitate transmission)
- descending impulses from the cerebral cortex influence the gate mechanism
- a system of specialised conducting fibres activates selective cognitive processes that influence the gating mechanism via descending fibres.

Pain occurs when spinal cord transmission exceeds a critical level. Despite its advantages over earlier pain theories, the GCT has been criticised for lacking detail about the interactions it proposes. Nevertheless, it is still the most important working model for pain researchers.[20–23]

Bone pain[24-29]

Bone metastases are the most common cause of cancer pain. Any part of the skeleton may be involved, but the axial skeleton and the proximal limb bones are particularly susceptible to metastatic disease. Approximately 50% of all bone metastases, usually resulting from bloodborne spread, arise from breast, lung, and prostate tumours.

Once inside the bone, pressure on the periosteum, nerves, and muscles surrounding the bone may lead to pain. Pain-sensitive nerve endings located in the periosteum or joints may be activated by mechanical stimuli, i.e. expansion of the tumour within the bone and/or chemical stimuli, e.g. prostaglandins. Prostaglandin production by bone metastases causes osteolysis and lowers the peripheral pain threshold.

Characteristics of bone pain

Base of skull metastases: metastatic spread to the head and neck (including orbital, parasagittal, middle fossa, jugular foramen, and clivus metastases, sphenoid sinus metastases and odontoid fracture) may result in aching facial pain, as well as severe headache, sometimes exacerbated by neck flexion (depending on sites involved). Diplopia, papilloedema, nasal stuffiness, a sense of fullness in the head, hoarseness, dysphagia, dysarthia, trapezius muscle weakness and ptosis, paralysis of the tongue, weakness of the sternomastoid, and stiff neck may also accompany bony metastatic spread to the head and neck region.

Bone metastases to C7–T1 may result in constant aching along the paraspinal areas radiating to both shoulders. One or other arm may also be affected where the patient experiences radiating pain to the ulnar region. The patient may also describe tenderness or pain when the spine is touched, parasthesia and numbness in the ulnar aspect of an arm, and progressive weakness of the triceps or hand.

L1 metastases may be accompanied by aching in the mid-back and sacroiliac joints and a radiating pain in the groins. Pain may be exacerbated when the patient lies down.

Aching pain in the sacral or coccygeal region characteristic of sacral metastases may be relieved by sitting or walking. Perianal sensory loss, bowel and bladder dysfunction, and impotence may also accompany sacral metastases.

Management

Although some bone metastases cause no pain, small localised metastases can cause severe pain where there is associated nerve involvement or damage. Alternatively, for other patients, disseminated bone diseases may result in only minimal discomfort or no pain.

Bone pain is generally only partly opioid responsive. A combination of non-steroidal anti-inflammatory drugs (NSAIDs) and morphine should therefore be used as first-line treatment. NSAIDs inhibit prostaglandin production stimulated by bone metastases. NSAIDs are classified under several different chemical classes, with marked variations reported in patients' analgesic response to the various drugs. Therefore, if bone pain is not controlled with one particular NSAID, there is merit in trying a different drug from a different class. However, there is never an indication to use two NSAIDs concurrently.

Corticosteroids (e.g. dexamethasone, with a starting dose of 8 mg) can be useful in the management of pain caused by bone metastases. However, their side-effect profiles make corticosteroids unacceptable as first-line or long-term therapy in the management of painful bone lesions.

Radiotherapy is the most effective single therapy for the treatment of local metastatic bone pain, with response rates as high as 80% consistently reported.[25] For some patients, radiotherapy can achieve complete pain relief, although the mechanisms by which pain control is achieved are poorly understood. Reduction of tumour bulk as cells are killed may result in a reduction in the pain experienced but it may also be that pain-mediating agents released as a result of treatment, in conjunction with osteoclast/osteoblast interaction, contribute to pain relief. When used to manage pain caused by localised metastasis, pain relief may occur within 2–3 days, with a maximum benefit seen at around 2–3 weeks following treatment. Immediate pain relief after local irradiation is rare. Therefore, it is important to continue with, and where necessary increase, the patient's analgesic regime throughout radiotherapy and for the immediate period following treatment.

Studies comparing the benefits of a single fraction of 8 Gy with a course of 5–10 fractions of 20–30 Gy have demonstrated few advantages of multiple fractionation over a single dose,[25] although multiple fraction regimes continue to be the treatment of choice where there is concern over possible fracture or nerve involvement. Radiotherapy has been demonstrated to help prevent pathological fractures and promote healing following a pathological fracture.

For patients with more widespread disease, hemi-body irradiation may be required, with a single dose of 8 Gy to the lower body or 6 Gy to the upper body, as appropriate. However, side-effects from hemi-body irradiation may be particularly distressing and up to two-thirds of patients may experience nausea, vomiting, or diarrhoea. The majority of patients will experience bone marrow suppression and in some instances, patients may experience radiation pneumonitis. Despite this, for patients whose pain is resistant to other forms of management, hemi-body irradiation has been shown to achieve effective pain relief, which, for the majority of terminally ill patients, may be maintained until death. In addition, pain relief may be achieved within 24–48 hours. As with any treatment, the side-effects of therapy must be balanced against patients' subjective wishes and the potential benefits of treatment.

For patients whose pain does not respond to radiotherapy or who relapse after an initial response, there is little evidence that re-treatment with radiotherapy is effective. Alternative approaches such as treatment with strontium-89 (SR-89)[28] or intravenous bisphosphonates[27] may be more appropriate.

Surgery may be useful in managing pain caused by a pathological fracture resulting from bone metastases or where there is a high risk of pathological fracture. Internal fixation is the preferred management when long bones are affected, but is not feasible for rib fractures or vertebral collapse, when local radiation should be used. As with any therapy, the benefits of treatment must be weighed against any possible costs to the individual. For patients in the advanced stages of illness, attempts at internal fixation with the associated demands of analgesia and risks posed by post-operative complications of bed rest may be inappropriate and

local irradiation should again be the treatment of choice.

Radioactive isotopes used in the management of multiple painful bone metastases have demonstrated some promising results. The most widely reported in the management of pain caused by bone metastases is strontium-89 SR-89. SR-89 is a calcium analogue with a half-life of 50.5 days. It is taken up by bone tissue and has the capacity to deliver therapeutic levels of radiation to a bone site for several months. It has been demonstrated to bring about equally effective pain relief when compared with five daily fractions or a single fraction of local radiotherapy given to patients with metastatic prostate cancer, and has also been shown to be an effective adjunct to local radiotherapy with the same cancer group.[28] Its potential to benefit terminally ill patients is limited as a period of 7–20 days is required before pain relief is achieved. Despite its radioactive properties, SR-89 poses a minimal threat to patients or health care professionals. Careful handling of any excreta is required, and gloves should be worn when disposing of any urine or faeces, or when blood is taken. Ideally patients should be discouraged from using bedpans and where a patient is incontinent of urine, sensitive explanation should be given prior to administration of the isotope, of the need to catheterise the patient for a period of 1 week after treatment.

Bisphosphonates, chemical analogues of pyrophosphate, are powerful inhibitors of osteoclastic function. They have become the treatment of choice when managing malignant hypercalcaemia and have also demonstrated some potential as analgesic agents in patients with multiple myeloma, prostate and breast cancer. The most widely used and evaluated to date is clodronate. Despite evidence to suggest that intravenous bisphosphonantes do relieve malignant bone pain, potential differences among them, the existence of dose-dependent effects, and lack of information relating to the long-term risks of their use have led to the conclusion that they should only be used at present with patients who have severe bone pain resistant to management with opioids, NSAIDs, and corticosteroids.[27]

Varying degrees of pain relief from bone metastases caused by breast and prostatic cancer have been reported as a result of chemotherapy. However, it is not clear whether symptom relief is brought by tumour regression or whether pain relief obtained as a result of chemotherapy administration occurs independently of tumour response.

Contradictory evidence of the efficacy of repeated doses of calcitonin in the management of bone pain characterises the current state of knowledge regarding its use as an adjuvant analgesic. As its benefits and long-term risks are unknown at this time, it should only be considered as an experimental treatment. Similarly, contradictory findings have been reported with L-dopa, and its use is currently not recommended for routine trials.

Neuropathic pain[30-32]

Neuropathic pain is non-nociceptive (i.e. visceral, somatic, or muscle spasm pain caused by stimulation of nerve endings), and may arise from disturbances of function or pathological change in peripheral and/or central nervous systems.

Neuropathic pain is therefore not a discrete entity. It may comprise:

- peripheral nerve injury (deafferentation pain), e.g. neuroma or nerve infiltration
- central nervous system injury, e.g. spinal cord compression
- mixed peripheral and central injury, e.g. post-herpetic neuralgia.

Distinguishing characteristics include the following.

- Abnormalities in pain quality – generally referred to as allodynia, hyperalgesia, and hyperpathia. Allodynia, hyperalgesia, and hyperpathia are commonly referred to as dysesthesia and associated sensations include tingling, prickling, electricity-like effects, burning, and lancinating pain.
Allodynia is pain caused by a stimulus that does not normally lead to pain, e.g. temperature or pressure; hyperalgesia refers to an increased response to a stimulus that does not normally cause pain; hyperpathia refers to pain caused in a relatively anaesthetic area of the body by an exaggerated reaction to a stimulus.

- Pain distribution consistent with neural damage.
- Evidence of neural injury or disease.

Major causes of neuropathic pain in patients with cancer

Neuropathic pain can be caused by compression or infiltration of nerves by tumour, nerve trauma due to diagnostic or surgical procedures, nervous system injury including spinal cord compression, and following chemotherapy or radiotherapy.

Specific causes include the following.

- Cranial nerve involvement due to base of skull metastases mainly from breast, lung or prostate cancers; leptomeningeal metastases; or infiltration from head and neck tumours.
- Post-herpetic neuralgia, frequently seen in association with malignancy, is a common cause of neuropathic pain.
- Intercostal nerve injury due to rib metastases.
- Tumour invasion of the sciatic notch.
- Epidermal tumour masses or leptomeningeal metastases, which may lead to dermatomal pain.
- Radiculopathy, which is exacerbated by coughing, and sneezing. Painful radiculopathy may be an indication of spinal cord compression and therefore requires urgent magnetic resonance imaging (MRI) scanning. Complaints of central back pain occurring in a rapid crescendo pattern may be an especially significant sign of probable cord compression.
- Brachial plexus infiltration, most commonly as a result of lymph node metastases from breast cancer or lymphoma, or direct infiltration from a pancoast tumour.
- Direct extension of colorectal or cervical carcinomas, sarcoma, lymphoma, or breast metastases, which may cause lumbosacral plexopathy.
- Neuronopathy or ganglionopathy, which may present with dysesthesias, parasthesias, and sensory loss in extremities, resulting in paraneoplastic peripheral neuropathy.
- High-dose intrathecal and epidural injections of opioids, which may result in neuropathic pains; approximately 20% of patients who receive anaesthetic epidural injections experience neuropathic pain.

- Chronic neuropathic pain, characterised by a burning or constricting sensation in the chest wall, axilla, or medial arm, has been reported to affect as many as 20% of women post-mastectomy. Patients undergoing surgery for head and neck tumours or thoracotomy for lung tumours may also experience considerable neuropathic pain, which varies in onset and duration. Thoracotomy and post-mastectomy pain usually develops shortly after surgery, while pain associated with neck block dissection may not occur for weeks or months after treatment.
- Radiotherapy may lead to myelopathy, plexopathy, and neuropathy. Radiation myelopathy most commonly occurs after radiotherapy for extraspinal tumours, while brachial plexopathy may follow chest wall and axillary radiotherapy. Sacral plexus irradiation has been reported to result in paresthesias, distal weakness, and pain in lower extremities.
- Vinca alkaloids (especially vincristine), and cis-platinum are known to cause painful neuropathy in some patients receiving chemotherapy. Paclitaxel and more rarely cytarabine have also been associated with the development of peripheral neuropathy. Withdrawal of the causative agent may result in resolution of the pain over some months; however, cisplatinum may cause persistent neuropathies even after withdrawal.
- Large doses of parenteral dexamethasone may be followed by a burning sensation in the perineum. This may be prevented by slow infusion.

Care strategy 17.3: Important factors to consider if neuropathic pain is suspected

1. Does the patient describe tingling or burning pain?
2. Do bed covers or underclothes cause severe pain?
3. Is the pain felt locally, does it radiate, cause an aftersensation, or is it a delayed sensation occurring some time after the stimulus?
4. Does the patient describe any associated weakness, vasomotor or dystrophic changes?
5. Does the patient have a primary tumour known to cause neuropathic pain as a consequence of metastatic spread or direct/primary infiltration/nerve damage?
6. Has the patient received cancer treatments with the potential to cause neuropathic pain?
7. Is the patient immunocompromised? Infection can cause peripheral neuropathy with intractable, escalating pain.
8. Does the patient have non-malignant degenerative disease of the spine, osteoporosis, aortic aneurysm, vasculitis, metabolic abnormalities, or nutritional deficiencies, all of which are known to cause central or peripheral neuropathies?

Analgesia

The use of opioids in the management of neuropathic pain remains controversial. Further evidence is required, which takes into account the plethora of aetiological and pathological mechanisms prevalent amongst heterogeneous groups of patients with cancer who present with neuropathic pain. Evidence available to date suggests a continuum of opioid responsiveness for patients and best practice guidelines advocate that a combination of opioid, non-opioid, and adjuvant analgesics be used judiciously, after a thorough examination of the patient, including computed tomographic and MRI scans where appropriate.

NSAIDs and adjuvant analgesics have been widely used in the management of neuropathic pain. Combinations of non-steroidals and an opioid are regularly used in clinical settings and their efficacy is widely acknowledged.

First-line adjuvant analgesia in the management of neuropathic pain

Adjuvant analgesics, i.e. drugs with primary indications other than analgesia, particularly tricyclic antidepressants such as amitryptyline, are accepted agents in the management of neuropathic pain. Evidence suggests that neuropathic pain responds more quickly to antidepressant medication than does depression and thus requires lower doses. However, full dosage may be necessary and should not be withheld. Other heterocyclic antidepressants, e.g. trazodone, may be less effective as they have different side-effect profiles to the tricyclics and should be used with caution (see Case strategy 17.4).

Care strategy 17.4: Recommended dose ranges of antidepressants/anticonvulsants

Tricyclic antidepressants
- Amitryptyline – start with 10–25 mg orally, increasing gradually to 150 mg.
- Desipramine – start with 10–25 mg orally, increasing gradually to 150 mg.

- Imipramine – start with 15.5 mg orally, increasing gradually to 150 mg.
- Clomipramine – start with 10 mg orally, increasing gradually to 150 mg.

Adjuvant anti-convulsants
- Carbamazepine – 200–400 mg three times a day (starting with 100 mg).
- Phenytoin – 300–400 mg (starting with 100 mg).

Anticonvulsant drugs such as carbamazepine have been found to be particularly effective in the management of lancinating pains. Phenytoin, valporic acid, and clonazepam may also be effective.

Second-line adjuvant analgesia

- Baclofen appears to be useful in trigeminal neuralgia. The usual dose is 20–120 mg.
- Oral local anaesthetics such as such as tocainide may be useful in either continuous or lancinating dysethesias. They may be helpful alternatives when patients experiencing continuous dysesthsias have not responded to tricyclic antidepressants.
- Neuroleptic drugs such as fluphenazine and haloperidol can be used in low does (2–8 mg per day) for neuropathic pain. However, the benefits of their prolonged use as adjuvant analgesics must be weighed against the risk of developing tardive dyskinesia.
- Anxiolytics such as alprazolam or clonazepam may also be useful in the management of neuropathic pain. Oral alprazolam (0.25–2 mg three times a day) has been shown to be helpful in some patients with phantom limb pain, while oral clonazepam (0.5–4 mg twice a day) may be useful in the management of lancinating pains.

Additional approaches to the management of neuropathic pain include: sympathetic blockade (e.g. nerve blocks); epidural injections (particularly bupivocaine, which has been shown to be effective with patients unresponsive to opioid treatment); neurosurgical interventions (although success rates are limited); and neurostimulation (e.g. TENS).

Care strategy 17.5: Relaxation – some recommendations for practice

Teaching a patient, family member or friend a relaxation technique is relatively quick and easy and the rewards can be significant. There are many forms of relaxation but progres-sive muscle relaxation (PMR) appears to be the most commonly used by nurses in their daily practice.[5] PMR involves tensing and then relaxing separate muscle groups throughout the body one after the other. Below are some basic phrases you may find helpful to use with patients and family members.

- Find yourself a quiet place. This may be your bedroom or a favourite spot in the garden.
- Make sure that you are sitting or lying comfortably and loosen any tight clothing.
- You may choose to have music playing or to sit in silence. Tell your family or friends that you are setting this time aside so that they do not disturb you. They may even choose to join you.
- You may choose to focus on a picture or a flower or just look at a distant point. You may prefer to close your eyes.

Most relaxation texts will emphasise the importance of deep breathing and of beginning the relaxation process by taking several deep breaths. For some patients with advanced disease, deep breathing may cause discomfort or even cause additional distress, e.g. patients with lung cancer who are breathless. Therefore, before beginning the relaxation process ask your patient about his or her breathing and find the most appropriate breathing pattern for him or her. If the patient is breathless try suggesting: 'Be aware of your breathing just for a moment and then just try to maintain a comfortable breathing pace throughout the relaxation period'.

If the patient can breath normally you may choose to say: 'As you breathe in count 1–2–3 slowly, hold your breath for 1–2–3 and breathe out 1–2–3–4–5–6'.

The next few steps are part of the process of progressive muscle relaxation. They are directed at relaxing the shoulders but can be applied to any part of the body.

- Once you have found a comfortable, well-supported position, slowly and gently draw your shoulders up towards your ears. Hold them in that position for as long as is comfortable for you (about half a minute to a minute).
- After you have felt the tension in your shoulders slowly let them relax, lowering your shoulders gently back to their usual position. Be aware of a release in tension as you do this.
- Some people talk about thinking of feelings of warmth and peace as they relax their shoulders, letting go of pain, fear, and anxiety.
- If you feel able, repeat this action a second time.

Some people prefer to set aside 20–30 minutes during the day to carry out relaxation of all muscle groups within the body. Others find that repeating some form of relaxation for as little as 5–10 minutes, two or three times a day, helps prevent tension from building up.

References

1. Hanks G.W. (1995). Problem areas in pain and symptom management in advanced cancer patients. *European Journal of Cancer Care* **31a**, 869–870.
2. Hiscock M. (1993). Psychological aspects of acute pain. *Professional Nurse,* December, 158–160.
3. Lanceley A. (1995). Wider issues in pain management. *European Journal of Cancer Care* **4**, 153–157.
4. World Health Organisation (1990). *Cancer Pain Relief and Palliative Care.* Geneva: World Health Organisation Report.
5. McCaffrey M. (1979). *Nursing the Patient in Pain.* London: Harper and Row, pp. 13–14.
6. Merskey H. (1976). Psychiatric aspects of the control of pain. In Bonica J.J. and Albe-Fessard D. (eds.) *Advances in Pain Research and Therapy,* Vol. 1. New York: Raven Press, pp. 711–716.
7. Bates M.S. (1987). Ethnicity and pain: a biocultural model. *Social Science and Medicine* **24**, 47–50.
8. Foley K.M. (1985). The treatment of cancer pain. *New England Journal of Medicine* **313**, 84–95.
9. Kleinman A. (1988). *The Illness Narratives: Suffering, Healing and the Human Condition.* New York: Basic Books.
10. Sternbach R.A. (1974). *Pain Patients: Traits and Treatment.* London: Academic Press, pp. 20–51.
11. Twycross R. (1988). The management of pain in cancer: a guide to drugs and dosages. *Oncology* **2**, 35–44.
12. Heath C. (1989). Pain talk: the expression of suffering in the medical consultation. *Social Psychology Quarterly* **52**, 113–125.
13. National Council for Hospices and Specialist Palliative Care Services (1994). *Guidelines for Managing Cancer Pain in Adults.* London: National Council for Hospices and Specialist Palliative Care Services.
14. Redmond K. (1996). Advances in supportive care. *European Journal of Cancer Care* **5** (Suppl. 2), 1–7.
15. Twycross R. (1984). Control of pain. *Journal of the Royal College of Physicians of London* **18**, 32–37.
16. Bruera E., Macmillan K., Hanson J. and MacDonald R. (1989). The cognitive effects of administration of narcotic analgesics in patients with cancer pain. *Pain* **39**, 13–16.
17. Sykes N.P. (1991). A clinical comparison of laxatives in a hospice. *Palliative Medicine* **5**, 307–314.
18. Schug S.A., Grond S., Zech D., Jung H., Meuser T. and Stobbe B. (1992). A long-term survey of morphine in cancer pain patients. *Journal of Pain and Symptom Management* **7**, 259–266.
19. Expert Working Group of the European Association for Palliative Care (1996). Morphine in cancer pain: modes of administration. *British Medical Journal* **312**, 823–826.
20. Wentworth Dolphin N. (1983). Neuroanatomy and neurophysiology of pain: nursing implications. *International Journal of Nursing Studies* **20**, 255–263.
21. Melzack R. and Wall P. (1988). *The Challenge of Pain.* London: Penguin Books.
22. Astley A. (1990). A history of pain. *Nursing* **4**, 33–53.
23. Melzack R. and Wall P. (1965). Pain mechanisms: a new theory. *Science* **150**, 971–979.
24. McDonald N. (1995). Principles governing the use of cancer chemotherapy in palliative medicine. In Doyle D., Hanks G. and MacDonald N. (eds.) *The Oxford Textbook of Palliative Medicine.* Oxford: Oxford University Press, pp. 105–117.
25. Hoskin P. (1995). Radiotherapy in symptom management. In Doyle D., Hanks G. and McDonald N. (eds.) *The Oxford Textbook of Palliative Medicine.* Oxford: Oxford University Press, pp. 117–129.
26. Portenoy R. (1995). Adjuvant analgesics in pain management. In Doyle D., Hanks G. and McDonald N. (eds.) *The Oxford Textbook of Palliative Medicine.* Oxford: Oxford University Press, pp. 187–203.
27. Ernst S., Brasher P., Hagen N., Paterson A., MacDonald C. and Bruera E. (1997). A randomized, controlled trial of intravenous clodrinate in patients with metastatic bone disease and pain. *Journal of Pain and Symptom Management* **13**, 319–326.
28. Kan M. (1995). Palliation of bone pain in patients with metastatic cancer using strontium-89 (Metastron). *Cancer Nursing* **18**, 286–291.
29. O'Brien T. (1993). Pain. In Saunders C. and Sykes N. (eds.) *The Management of Terminal Malignant Disease.* London: Edward Arnold, pp. 33–62.
30. Breitbart W. (1998). Psychotropic adjuvant analgesics for pain in cancer and AIDS. *Psycho-Oncology* **7**, 333–345.
31. Billings A. (1994). Neuropathic pain. *Journal of Palliative Care* **10**, 40–43.
32. Martin L.A. and Hagen N.A. (1997). Neuropathic pain in cancer patients: mechanisms, syndromes and clinical controversies. *Journal of Pain and Symptom Management* **14**, 99–117.

CHAPTER EIGHTEEN

Nausea and vomiting

Meinir Krishasamy

Cancer continues to be widely conceived of as an uncontrollable, capricious disease.[1] It may be suffused with feelings of fear, shame, and repulsion, feelings culturally and socially affiliated with physical manifestations such as vomit or malodorous wounds. Cancer and its treatment transpose many individuals to a world where previously private phenomena such as vomiting are moved into a public arena. It is unsurprising therefore that nausea, vomiting, and retching have repeatedly been identified by patients as being among the most disruptive, distressing, and feared side-effects of radiotherapy and chemotherapy.[2,3]

> While physicians are concerned with disease, clients are concerned with illness . . . This distinction defines a crucial domain for nursing. Nursing uses the model of illness and the model of disease and mediates the two.[4]

Disease refers to the way in which doctors and nurses frame illness within physiological and pathological theoretical models.[5] Illness refers to patients' perceptions, experiences, interpretations, and patterns of coping with symptoms or problems.[1] Inherent to any discussion of effective interventions for nausea and vomiting is the premise that the individual's experience of illness forms the cornerstone of nursing care. Regardless of the goal of treatment, whether it be prophylaxis or symptom control, the individual's beliefs and anxieties will strongly influence their ability to continue with any course of treatment, and to live with a life-threatening disease.[2] The importance of understanding the enormity of the impact of a symptom upon an individual's being is powerfully described by one young person:

> The severity of nausea and vomiting at times made the thought of death seem an almost welcome relief.[6]

For many, treatment becomes intolerable as a consequence of poorly controlled nausea and/or vomiting while for some, life itself may seem to be too high a price to pay for such anguish and suffering.[7] Persistent nausea and vomiting is known to be a factor in half of all missed appointments and delays in treatment and for some, leads to withdrawal from potentially curative treatment altogether.[6] Nausea and vomiting are among the most distressing side-effects of cancer therapy.[8–10]

Nausea, vomiting, and retching are discrete entities, and yet evidence suggests that patients are commonly invited to respond to questions, or to complete self-report measures, without prior clarification of the problem being explored.[2] Two-thirds of medical, surgical, gynaecological, and oncology patients are unfamiliar with the term nausea, using the term 'sick at stomach' instead, while the phrase 'throw up' is most frequently used to refer to vomiting.[10]

Assessment

Misunderstandings over terms such as nausea and vomiting may lead to confusion and subsequently to poor management. Careful exploration of the nature, duration, subjective feelings, and physical manifestations of the symptom being experienced

- *Nausea* – a subjective phenomenon; an unpleasant sensation experienced in the back of the throat and the epigastrium, which may or may not result in vomiting. It has been described as an autonomic response, a conscious recognition of a desire to vomit.
- *Vomiting* – the forceful expulsion of stomach, duodenum, or jejunum contents through the oral cavity. As the stomach contents become trapped between the forceful contractions of the muscles of the abdomen and diaphragm, intragastric pressure builds up, the oesophageal sphincters open, and vomiting follows.
- *Retching* – an attempt to vomit without bringing anything up. Retching is controlled by the respiratory centre in the brainstem. The respiratory centre lies near the vomiting centre. It shares the common neural pathway of the fifth, seventh, tenth, and twelfth cranial nerves, which are responsible for the changes in rate and depth of respiration that accompany nausea and vomiting.[2,11]

is fundamental. Measures of nausea and vomiting exist; however, these may not be either reliable or valid when used in everyday practice.

Objective observation tools used in studies measure the number of times emesis or retching occurs. They have several limitations. They fail to assess the perception of the distress caused by these symptoms and assume that nausea is an observable problem. The need for an observer to be present prevents measurement over time; observation is impractical in a busy ward or clinic setting. The advantages of using self-report questionnaires or diaries are clearly apparent. Visual analogue scales (VASs) offer a ready means of accessing subjective perceptions of symptoms, providing that the anchor statements at each end of the scale are meaningful to the person completing the tool. Although well recognised as being reliable, valid, and sensitive, visual analogue scales can be confusing and translating feelings into a quantifiable mark on a scale is difficult.[12] Guidance may need to be given on how to complete these. Where self-report measures such as visual analogue scales are to be used, it is important to ensure that they address both the occurrence of the symptom and the degree of distress caused by it.[10] For example, consider Figure 18.1.

I throw up:

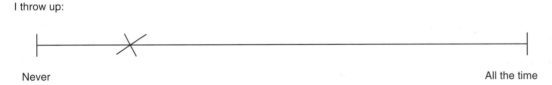

Never   All the time

This gives an idea of how often this person vomits but it doesn't tell us whether:

Throwing up:

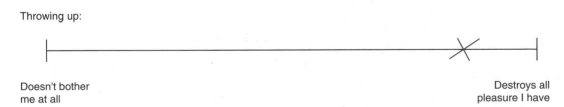

Doesn't bother   Destroys all
me at all   pleasure I have

Figure 18.1   Visual analogue scale.

From the first VAS shown in Figure 18.1, it could be assumed that this person vomits very little, and as such experiences minimal distress. However, each time he vomits, he might interpret it as a manifestation of worsening disease. Fearing that with greater disease activity vomiting might become persistent, the distress experienced may become so intense that it almost leads to a life perceived to be devoid of any pleasure. To date, we know little of the consequences of cumulative distress resulting from anticipatory and prolonged nausea and vomiting.[3] Without the added insight gained from the second VAS, or during skilled communication, management of the symptom and attempts at facilitating self-care may be ineffective.

Aspinall wrote in 1976:

> The many books and articles about nurse care planning and implementation generally start with the problem, which supposedly has already been identified in some way . . . they [the books] usually encourage the nurse to use another approach if her action is unsuccessful, rather than consider the possibility that the patient's disturbed or changed functioning may stem from a problem totally different from the one originally identified.[13]

If a nurse is to attach the correct diagnosis, facilitate subjective expression of the nature and meaning of the symptom, and plan effective care, then adequate theoretical knowledge and an ability to combine analytical and intuitive methods of thinking is needed. It is also important to draw upon what Benner and Wrubel[14] describe as 'perceptual awareness', where *knowing how* (theoretical knowledge) and *knowing that* (practical knowledge[15]) work to complement each other. In Figure 18.2, the physiological mechanisms (the knowing how) of nausea and vomiting are outlined. Pharmacological interventions for cancer-induced nausea and vomiting are outlined in Table 18.1.

Patterns of nausea and vomiting

Nausea and vomiting can be compounded by the memories of previous treatment cycles; anticipatory, acute post-treatment or delayed onset nausea and vomiting can complicate effective control. Personal account 18.1 illustrates this.

Personal account 18.1[20]

John, a 27-year-old mature student newly diagnosed with testicular cancer, arrived at the unit for his third course of combination chemotherapy. He looked pale and anxious as he sat in the day-room waiting for his chemotherapy to arrive from pharmacy. As I approached him with his anti-emetics, John told me that he had been vomiting at home throughout the morning, anticipating the smell of hospital and the sight of the infusion pump to which he would be 'locked' for the remainder of the day. He was distressed and frightened at the prospect of persistent nausea and vomiting following discharge home, and the 'dread' of going through the same experiences on each admission.

The emetogenic potential of cancer chemotherapy varies greatly (see Table 18.3). Most drugs do not cross the blood–brain barrier and therefore appear to initiate vomiting through mechanisms other than direct stimulation of the CTZ, such as irritation of the CTZ via a peripheral pathway.[2,16] Chemotherapy regimes that use several drugs associated with moderate to severe emetogenic potential are associated with higher risk of nausea and vomiting. John's combination chemotherapy regime placed him at greater risk of experiencing nausea and vomiting.

Anticipatory nausea and vomiting may occur moments before administration of the drug(s) or, as in John's case, at any time when the individual thinks of aspects of the chemotherapy experience. For John, it was the smell of the hospital and the sight of the infusion pump. Other patients have described tastes and sounds, even the sight of nurses or doctors involved with their care, as potentiating factors.[9] Factors associated with an increased risk of anticipatory nausea and vomiting are listed below. Many of these features were present for John and undoubtedly contributed to the onset of his anticipatory nausea and vomiting.

Box 18.2: Factors associated with increased risk of anticipatory nausea and vomiting[17]

- Being under 50 years of age
- Previously poorly controlled nausea and vomiting
- Subjective perceptions of the severity of the symptoms
- A sense of increased warmth and weakness following therapy
- A history of motion sickness.

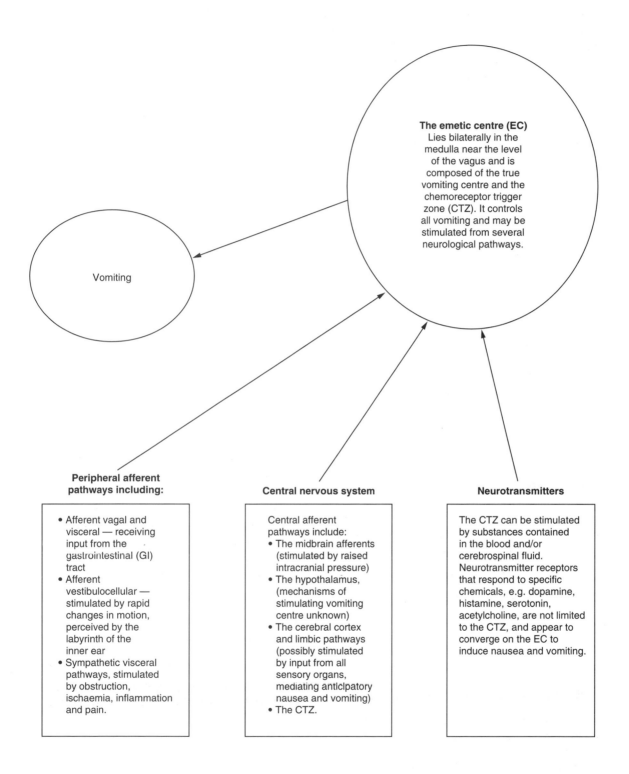

Figure 18.2 Physiological mechanisms of nausea and vomiting.[2,4,17]

Table 18.1 Pharmacological interventions for cancer-induced nausea and vomiting

Phenothiazines, e.g. prochlorperazine, chlorpromazine	They exert their primary effect as dopamine antagonists, inhibiting transmission in the CTZ. Associated with extrapyramidal reactions, acute dystonic reactions, autonomic and hypersensitivity reactions, they must be used with caution. Akathesia, described as feeling jittery and sleepy at the same time, is a common side-effect of phenothiazines and its occurrence warrants discontinuation of the drug.[2,10]
Serotonin antagonists, e.g. ondansetron, granisetron, tropisetron	They act by blocking serotonin-type receptors and have two possible sites of action; the vagal afferent peripheral nerve terminals and the central terminals of the same afferent nerves.[10] Although serotonin receptor antagonists have become first-line treatment in preventing acute post-chemotherapy nausea and vomiting, and have minimal side-effects, their ability to prevent delayed nausea and vomiting is less apparent.
Substituted benzamide, e.g. metoclopramide	Metoclopramide has been proven to be an effective anti-emetic against strongly emetogenic chemotherapy, including cisplatinum-based regimes.[2] It appears to have two modes of action, including dopamine antagonist activity and promotion of gastric emptying, limiting reflux and retching.[10] It has several potential distressing side-effects, including extrapyramidal reactions, diarrhoea, fatigue, and sleepiness.
Corticosteroids	Dexamethasone is commonly used in conjunction with other anti-emetics, especially ondansetron and metoclopramide, when aggressive treatment regimes are administered. The exact mechanism of action of corticosteroids is unknown but it is postulated that they manifest antiprostaglandin activity.[18]
Benzodiazepines, e.g. lorazepam, diazepam	Benzodiazepines appear to act at thalamic, limbic, and hypothalamic levels of the central nervous system, although their exact mechanism is not known. They produce anxiolytic, sedative, hypnotic, skeletal muscle relaxant and anti-convulsant effects.[10] As they are capable of producing all levels of central nervous system depression, they should be used with caution with elderly patients and with patients with poor respiratory function.
Antihistamines, e.g. diphenhydramine (Piriton)	Their primary site of action is in the CTZ, although they are ineffective as single-agent anti-emetics. They are most commonly used alongside phenothiazines or metoclopramide, incorporated into aggressive anti-emetic regimens to help prevent extrapyramidal reactions.[18]
Butyrophenones, e.g. droperidol, haloperidol	They act as dopamine antagonists in the CTZ and also have a sedating and anxiolytic effect. Hypotension and extrapyramidal reactions are significant side-effects.[18]
Cannabinoids, e.g. marijuana	Their mode of action is unknown but the anti-emetic effect may be related to the 'high' achieved by adequate blood concentration. Memory loss, mood changes, incoordination, euphoria, and hallucinations have all been documented as side-effects.[10]

Anxiety and hostility may also contribute to the development of anticipatory nausea and vomiting, although the relationship between anxiety, nausea, and vomiting remains unclear.[19]

As a 27-year-old man, as yet unmarried and without children, John was faced with potential future impotence and infertility and that, he told me, was only if he survived the cancer:

> Having cancer changes everything. What that little six-letter word, that incomprehensible diagnosis, that terrible thing you thought only happens to other people really means is that your life will be inexorably altered. Nothing, your daily routines, your relationships, your beliefs, or your future, will ever be the same again.[20]

Nurses play a crucial role in the prevention and early detection of anticipatory nausea and vomiting.[2] As illustrated in Personal account 18.2, thorough sensitive questioning, and an accepting and knowledgeable response, can avoid considerable suffering and enhance meaningful support given.

Personal account 18.2

Mark's father phoned me at home. 'He's just being sick all the time', he said, 'I don't think he can stand much more of it'. Mark is 20. He has Hodgkin's lymphoma, and is receiving radiotherapy to a mediastinal mass, on an out-patient basis. His radiotherapy field includes his oesophagus. He had been sent home with three metoclopramide tablets, which he tried to take following the onset of acute post-treatment vomiting. His vomiting becomes retching and they call me – and so it's long-distance intervention by telephone!

Radiation-induced nausea and vomiting is related to the dose and type of treatment. Radiotherapy to the upper gastrointestinal tract, as in Mark's case, results in vasculitis and direct irritation of the oesophageal mucosa, leading to nausea and vomiting.[2] Symptoms may occur early in the course of treatment and as quickly as within 2 hours of completing each radiotherapy fraction. Consequently, an individual's predisposition to anticipatory nausea

Table 18.2 Non-pharmacological interventions for nausea and vomiting

Non-pharmacological interventions	Rationale
Self-care facilitation	Orem[21] defines self-care as 'the personal care that individuals require each day to regulate their own functioning and development.' It has been suggested as a means of promoting enhanced symptom control and as a means of encouraging individuals with cancer to avoid the regression sometimes associated with the disease.[3,21] Nausea and vomiting may demand of an individual a new set of self-care actions. Where possible, the person will respond to these challenges, but when, as with a major life-event such as a diagnosis of cancer, self-care agency is overwhelmed, help is needed. Nurses have a key role to play in planning, designing, and evaluating new modes of self-care management.
Progressive muscle relaxation, humour, music, exercise, hypnosis, and systematic desensitisation	These activities re-direct an individual's attention away from nausea and vomiting.[10] Whether their success is due to cessation of the symptoms or to perceptual exchange is unclear, but currently available evidence supports their effectiveness and continued use.
Patient education and written information	Patient education is an integral part of symptom management and written instructions are often indispensable for a group of people bombarded by disease-related information and psychological trauma.[2]

Table 18.3 Emetic potential of commonly used cancer chemotherapy agents[22]

Highly emetogenic	Moderately emetogenic	Low emetogenic potential
Cisplatin	Doxorubicin	Etoposide (dose and route dependent)
Dacarbazine	Procarbazine	Hydroxyurea
Cychlophosphamide	Carboplatin	5-Fluorouracil (5FU)
BCNU	Mitomycin-C	Bleomycin
	Ifosfamide and mesna	Vinblastin
	Mitoxantrone	Vincristine
	Cytosine arabinoside	Methotrexate (dose related)
	Daunorubicin	Busulfan
	Carmustine	Taxol
	CCNU	Taxotere

and vomiting is great. For Mark, plans to deliver aggressive, combination chemotherapy on completion of radiotherapy were already underway. His anxiety concerning further treatment as a result of poorly controlled nausea and vomiting was therefore established very early on. Stomatitis, xerostomia, dysguesia, and abdominal cramping may all contribute to radiotherapy-induced nausea and vomiting[23] and for Mark, anorexia and persistent retching rapidly resulted in a sore, dry mouth and abdominal cramping Meticulous mouth care was therefore necessary, alongside prompt initiation of an effective anti-emetic regime.

Three days following the first telephone conversation Mark called me. His father had gone to the hospital 2 days earlier armed with a list of anti-emetics and Mark was now planning a weekend with some friends. He told me that he was coping with the diagnosis of cancer. He could cope with the hair loss, having to leave his job for an indefinite period of time, and the potential of prolonged isolation (resulting from future treatment plans). What made it intolerable, however, 'not worth the effort of trying to cope', was the vomiting. Mark's physical symptoms were quickly and easily resolved once appropriate intervention was initiated. The anxiety, anger, and resentment as a result of his past experiences are still with him.

Symptoms that persist or develop after 24 hours following chemotherapy are defined as delayed nausea and vomiting. Its aetiology is unclear but may be due to the ongoing effect that the anti-metabolites of cancer-related treatments continue to have on either the central nervous system or the gastro-intestinal tract.[18] As the blood levels of chemotherapeutic agents fall the neurotransmitters that mediate nausea and vomiting are no longer 'blocked'.[2] As illustrated by Mark's experiences, nurses need to develop tools to evaluate symptom management strategies for use at home. As increasing numbers of patients attend hospital on a day care basis, and political influences encourage the shift towards more home-based therapies, skilled care planning and meaningful nursing outcome measures are paramount.

Non-pharmacological interventions

Non-pharmacological interventions that may help with nausea and vomiting are shown in Table 18.2. The benefits of many of these measures rely on anecdotal evidence. These present nurses with many challenging and important areas for future research. Richardson[3] suggests several key areas for future research and these are outlined below.

Considerable research efforts over the past decade have significantly improved the management of cancer-induced nausea and vomiting. However, the application of these findings within a holistic model of care continues to present cancer and palliative practitioners with a substantial therapeutic challenge.

Areas for future nursing research

Potential areas for research include:[3]

- studies to explore the interface between pharmacological, behavioural, and self-care interventions in seeking to control chemotherapy-induced nausea and vomiting
- investigation of the potential relationships between intervening variables such as age, gender, diagnosis, cancer treatment, self-concept, self-care agency, locus of control, and the cancer patient's performance of self-care behaviour
- development and testing of valid and reliable measures of self-care behaviours performed and their effectiveness
- descriptive studies to assess how individuals monitor and react to symptoms over the course of chemotherapy, and relate such symptoms to self-care behaviour.

References

1. Donnelly E. (1995). Culture and meanings of cancer. *Seminars in Nursing Oncology* **11**, 3–8.
2. Hogan C.M. (1990). Advances in the management of nausea and vomiting. *Nursing Clinics of North America* **25**, 475–497.
3. Richardson A. (1991). Theories of self-care: their relevance to chemotherapy-induced nausea and vomiting. *Journal of Advanced Nursing* **16**, 671–676.
4. Dougherty M. and Tripp-Reimer T. (1990). Nursing and anthropology. In Johnson T.M. and Sargent C.F. (eds.) *Medical Anthropology: A Handbook of Theory and Method.* New York: Greenwood, pp. 174–186.
5. Kleinman A. (1988). *The Illness Narratives: Suffering, Healing and the Human Condition.* New York: Basic Books.
6. Stroudermire A., Contanch P. and Laszlo J. (1984). Recent advances in the pharmacologic and behavioural management of chemotherapy induced emesis. *Archives of Internal Medicine* **144**, 1029–1033.
7. Khan D.L. and Steeves R. (1995). The significance of suffering in cancer care. *Seminars in Oncology Nursing* **11**, 9–16.
8. Coates A., Abraham S., Kay S., Sowerbutts T., Frewin C. and Fox R. (1983). On the receiving end: patient perceptions of the side-effects of cancer chemotherapy. *European Journal of Cancer and Clinical Oncology* **14**, 203–208.
9. Nerenz D., Leventhal H. and Love R. (1982). Factors contributing to emotional distress during cancer chemotherapy. *Cancer* **50**, 1020–1027.
10. Rhodes V., Johnson M. and McDaniel R. (1995). Nausea, vomiting and retching: the management of the symptom experience. *Seminars in Oncology Nursing* **11**, 256–265.
11. Norris (1982). *Concept Clarification in Nursing.* London: Aspen.
12. Gift A.G., Plaut S.M. and Jacox A.K. (1986). Psychological and physiologic factors related to dyspnoea in subjects with chronic obstructive pulmonary disease. *Heart and Lung* **15**, 595–601.
13. Aspinall M.J. (1976). Nursing diagnosis – the weak link. *Nursing Outlook* **24**, 433–437.
14. Benner P. and Wrubel J. (1982). Skilled clinical knowledge: the value of perceptual awareness. *Nurse Educator,* May–June, 11–17.
15. Polyani M. (1962). *Personal Knowledge.* London: Routledge and Kegan Paul.
16. Fiore J.J. and Gralla R.J. (1984). Pharmacologic treatment of chemotherapy-induced nausea vomiting. *Cancer Investigations* **2**, 351–361.
17. Morrow G.R. (1984). Clinical characteristics associated with the development of anticipatory nausea and vomiting in cancer patients undergoing chemotherapy treatment. *Journal of Clinical Oncology* **2**, 1170–1179.
18. Gralla R.J. (1993). Antiemetic therapy. In DeVita V., Hellman S. and Rosenberg S. (eds.) *Principles and Practice of Oncology,* 4th edition. Philadelphia, PA: Lippincott, pp. 2238–2347.
19. Ingle R.J., Burish T.G. and Wallston K.A. (1984). Conditionability of cancer chemotherapy patients. *Oncology Nursing Forum* **11**, 97–102.
20. Eick-Swigart J. (1995). What cancer means to me. *Seminars in Oncology Nursing* **11**, 41–42.
21. Orem D. (1991). *Nursing: Concepts of Practice,* 4th edition. St Louis, MO: Mosby Yearbook.
22. Chabner B.A. (1993). Anticancer drugs. In DeVita V., Hellman S. and Rosenberg S. (eds.) *Principles and Practice of Oncology,* 4th edition. Philadelphia, PA: Lippincott, pp. 328–339.
23. Holmes S. (1991). The oral complications of specific anticancer therapy. *International Journal of Nursing Studies* **28**, 343–360.

CHAPTER NINETEEN

Fatigue

Meinir Krishnasamy

Fatigue is a nebulous concept, difficult to define and intensely personal. The North American Nursing Diagnosis Association defines fatigue as 'an unremitting and overwhelming lack of energy and an inability to maintain usual routines'.[1] Carpenito[2] describes fatigue as 'an overwhelming, sustained sense of exhaustion and decreased capacity for physical and mental work'. However, as a word, 'fatigue' seems to be insufficient to convey the experience of this distressing cancer problem. Individuals appear instead to talk of tiredness, lack of energy, general lethargy, weakness, exhaustion, inability to sustain exertion, impaired mobility, motivation and concentration span, sleepiness, drowsiness, heaviness, apathy, an inability to carry on, as well as many other subjective sensations.[3–8] The manifestations of fatigue identified in studies of cancer-related fatigue are outlined in Figure 19.1.

Models of fatigue have focused on its six distinct dimensions:[1]

- temporal
- sensory
- cognitive/mental
- affective/emotional
- behavioural
- physiological.

The temporal dimension refers to the timing of fatigue, its onset and duration, and its pattern.[1] Acute and chronic fatigue within the temporal dimension are differentiated. Acute fatigue is felt to have a protective function, is experienced in relation to exertion and has an identifiable cause. Its duration is usually short lived, lasting for no more than a few days or weeks. Chronic fatigue confers little benefit and commonly has no identifiable cause. It may be difficult to identify its onset but its presence may have been noted for a period of at least 1 month. Subjective experiences of fatigue, factors that exacerbate and alleviate it, and the presence of any concurrent problems, for example pain, nausea, or breathlessness, contribute to the *sensory dimension* of fatigue.[9]

The *cognitive/mental dimension* focuses on the ability to concentrate, changes in attention span, memory recall, and degree of alertness. Changes in mood, distress, and anxiety caused by the fatigue are considered within the *affective/emotional dimensions*, while functional status, ability to undertake work, social and recreational activities, changes in sleep pattern and nutritional intake are incorporated within the *behavioural dimension*. Findings from the medical history, including stage of disease and its symptoms, side-effects of malignancy and treatment, concurrent diseases, past coping mechanisms, and family history, form the core of the *physiological dimension*.[1,9,10]

Nursing studies have assumed that phenomena such as fatigue can be measured through objective assessment. This misconception has significantly hampered the development of nurse-led practice development initiatives. For the individual with cancer, fatigue may be the first sign of ill-health, leading him or her to seek medical advice. It may

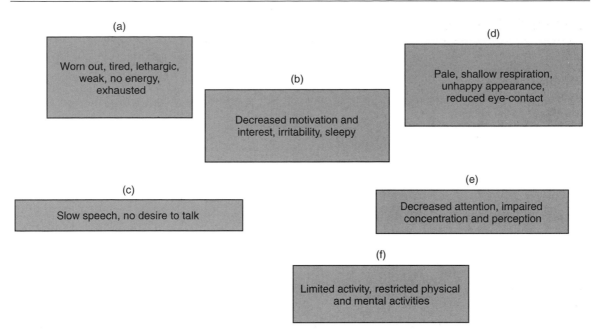

(a)

Worn out, tired, lethargic, weak, no energy, exhausted

(b)

Decreased motivation and interest, irritability, sleepy

(d)

Pale, shallow respiration, unhappy appearance, reduced eye-contact

(c)

Slow speech, no desire to talk

(e)

Decreased attention, impaired concentration and perception

(f)

Limited activity, restricted physical and mental activities

Figure 19.1 Manifestations of fatigue.[1,8,11,12]

therefore become a potent symbol of the presence of disease, possessing great significance for the patient and family. Despite a recognition of the prevalence of fatigue as a consequence of cancer and its treatment, little is known of the meanings inherent for the individuals experiencing it, and the families and professionals witnessing it. With a few exceptions, little has been documented of the experience of living with cancer-related fatigue.[8,13–17]

In a phenomenological study undertaken to describe the experiences of six individuals with chemotherapy induced fatigue, Pearce and Richardson[8] found that psychological and emotional distress were more commonly reported consequences of fatigue than were physical manifestations. They report one patient's experience of feeling extremely depressed and of having almost suicidal thoughts during her chemotherapy. She made sense of these extremely distressing emotions by stating: 'I think it may have been the realisation of my illness for the first time'. Other studies have found that physical limitations imposed by the fatigue are more commonly referred to.[16] Similarly, relatives and friends tend to describe the impact of fatigue in physical terms. Krishnasamy[17] undertook a detailed case study of 15 patients with advanced cancer who were expe-

riencing fatigue. The study also involved interviews with nominated friends or relatives and health professionals, and a case note analysis. Table 19.1 shows examples of these patients' and family members' descriptions of the fatigue accompanying advanced cancer.

The meanings inherent in these descriptions suggest that fatigue is much more than simply a physical problem; there are clear emotional, psychological, and social consequences of fatigue. This presents nurses with a considerable challenge, where the language used to describe the fatigue experience, especially within the last months of life, may convey little of its psychological distress. This remains hidden, and therefore nurses' ability to support patients experiencing distress will be limited.

Fatigue continues to be for the greater part a 'socially invisible'[18] consequence of cancer, the experience of which is far more complex than simply a lack of visibility.[19] It contributes to a complex world in which illness is a product of personal idealisation and social construction. It has a profound effect on an individual's ability to live a 'normal life', and their perception of self. All aspects of life may be affected, forcing withdrawal from

Table 19.1 Some descriptions of the fatigue of advanced cancer by patients, family members, and friends

Patient	Patient subjective descriptors	Relative or friend descriptors
David	*I just feel exhausted, no energy to do anything, you can sleep anytime.*	Just more and more tired, and losing weight, and not doing anything (Jennie, David's wife).
Michael	*It's like you're so heavy, drained of energy.*	It's just cut him off from everybody because it's too much of an effort, he's got no energy to spare (Judith, Michael's wife).
Ruth	*Some days I don't think I can physically get myself up out of bed, and I've got no energy.*	I feel for her so much because she wants to be busy, to see friends, but she's exhausted, just exhausted (Francis, Ruth's friend).
Beth	*I feel so tired but I want to be able to get up but I feel I physically can't.*	Some days you can almost feel the tiredness, it's so draining (Howard, Beth's husband).
Allan	*It's so heavy, like a weight coming down on you.*	He's just not the same person, always busy, but he tells me it's like a weight on him, and I think I can understand, like after I had an operation once, but I think it's very different too (Sandra, Allan's wife).
Enid	*It's a terrible tiredness, it makes you feel exhausted.*	She's got half, well not a quarter, of the energy she used to have, no get up and go (Frank, Enid's friend).

family, work, social, and recreational activities, all of which may previously have been powerful in reinforcing feelings of self-worth and self-esteem. As a consequence of this forced withdrawal from daily life, intense feelings of isolation and lack of motivation to continue to try to undertake normal functions have been described as a result of fatigue following chemotherapy.[8] Similarly, fatigue resulting from breathlessness has been found to cause withdrawal and isolation.[20] This may be especially true with tumours associated with extreme fatigue such as mesothelioma.

Krishnasamy[17] commented as follows in her research field notes after an interview with a gentleman with small-cell lung cancer:

> It seems to me that he felt the illness didn't show tiredness to begin with, he talked about things getting worse, of wanting to do things but not being able, I could feel his sense of dismay, knowing that there was more to come.

The consequences of social definition, interpretation, and judgement of obscure or 'invisible' phenomena such as fatigue[29] are powerfully demonstrated in this description of the impact of chronic disability:[30]

> It was not just that people acted differently towards me, but rather I felt differently towards myself . . . it [illness] left me feeling alone and isolated despite strong support from family and friends . . . a diminution of everything I used to be [pp. 71–76].

Evidence from the cancer literature suggests that fatigue has been hidden from the consciousness of well-meaning professionals and researchers, with little appreciation of the consequences of its obscurity for patients and relatives, or for the development of true patient-centred care:

> One cannot separate life experience from a person's unique interpretation of his or her illness and the ability and desire to get well. Expressions of hope, love, anger, fear, and loss provide the nurse with a lived dialogue, and offer the opportunity for interpretation of events in a way that has particular meaning for the patient.[31]

Further exacerbating nurses' inability to help patients and their families to manage cancer-induced fatigue is a lack of understanding of helpful behaviours identified by patients themselves. Although some work is now emerging within the field of chemotherapy- and radiotherapy-induced

Table 19.2 Strategies in alleviating fatigue

Helpful strategies identified by patients receiving chemotherapy and radiotherapy[1,27,28]
- Rest or sleep during the day
- Prioritise activities
- Read/listen to the radio/watch television
- Walk/gentle exercise
- Relaxation/massage
- Learning coping skills, e.g. goal planning, activity pacing
- Maintaining a diary or journal to map patterns of fatigue
- Information seeking
- Boosting nutritional intake
- Quiet or stimulating environment
- Social support, being with family or friends
- Effective management of physical symptoms, e.g. pain, nausea

Helpful strategies identified by patients experiencing the fatigue of advanced cancer, and their relatives, friends, and professional carers
- Talk to someone about it – tell them how awful it is
- Help to give it a language you can work with
- Help family and friends understand it
- Help patients describe the fears and meanings associated with the fatigue of dying.

fatigue much remains to be explored.[32–34] Table 19.2 lists activities reported as being helpful in alleviating fatigue. Few of these interventions have been evaluated through empirical research studies. Nevertheless, these accounts provide invaluable insight and information for planning future nursing intervention studies.

A comprehensive understanding of the possible causes and contributing factors of fatigue will lead to a precise nursing diagnosis.[9] At present, this is unlikely, as much research has yet to be undertaken before the nature of the relationship between factors contributing to fatigue and the resultant subjective experiences can be understood.

Figure 19.2 shows the complexity of the variety of factors thought to influence fatigue in cancer.

Patients treated with radiotherapy and chemotherapy often describe feelings of general malaise, incorporating feelings of lack of energy and tiredness.[39] Between 65 and 100% of patients receiving radiotherapy as a treatment for cancer experience fatigue with the most severe side-effects occurring during the last week of treatment.[3,10,39] For many, it may continue to be a problem for sev-

eral months after treatment has ended.[10] Studies involving patients receiving chemotherapy for a variety of different types of cancer report incidences of fatigue ranging from 59 to 82%.[40] There is considerable evidence documenting the occurrence of fatigue after surgery;[41] this may be especially problematic where adjuvant chemotherapy or radiotherapy may have to be administered prior to, or immediately following, surgery. Surgical procedures performed as palliative interventions for patients who may have already undergone months, even years, of anti-cancer treatment may confer considerable relief of acute symptoms, but at the expense of exacerbating profoundly debilitating fatigue.

Successive reports of the symptoms of advanced cancer suggest that fatigue is experienced by between 50 and 75% of patients.[42] Despite its prevalence, the impact of the fatigue of advanced cancer continues to be poorly understood as papers referring to it focus on a physiological consideration of asthenia. Asthenia is a medical term used to describe pathological fatigue associated with various diseases, and in particular with acute and chronic infections, as well as the fatigue of

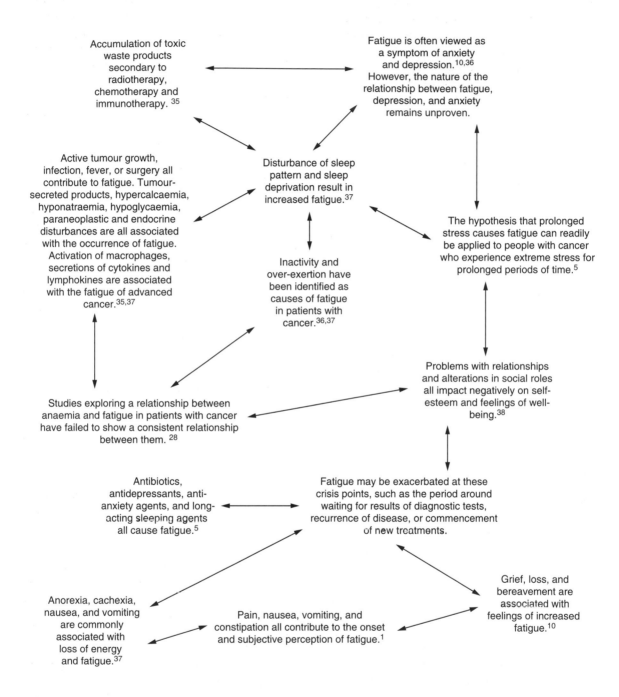

Figure 19.2 The complexity of fatigue in cancer.

advanced cancer. It is described as having two predominant symptoms – fatigue and generalised weakness – but no recognised body of knowledge about its aetiology or treatment currently exists.[35,42] Research to date has failed to differentiate between fatigue or tiredness as a component of cancer treatment, and fatigue or tiredness as a facet of advanced, terminal illness.

The ways in which fatigue is expressed and experienced are only just beginning to be explored. Fatigue as a feature of depression is one such area.[43] The perceptions of distress caused by fatigue and the intensely personal meanings attached to the phenomenon may play a significant part in altered mood state. Cimprich[44] concluded that subjects who report a depressed mood state tend to have lower self-ratings of attentional functioning than those with a more positive mood state. A relationship between perceptions of distress caused by unrelieved symptoms, and alterations in mood state is thought to exist.[45] The importance of working with patients to explore the meanings conferred by them onto their fatigue is therefore further supported. An in-depth interview study of 20 patients receiving a variety of ongoing treatments for cancer suggested that affective expressions of fatigue appeared to be strongly interwoven with its physical dimensions, leading us to question whether a factor such as sadness leads to tiredness (or vice versa), which then leads to decreased motivation and inactivity (or vice versa), with the inactivity then leading to sadness (or vice versa).[16] As nurses, we are ideally placed to begin to explore some of these fundamental problems with our patients.

There is currently little research to support specific interventions for managing fatigue induced by cancer treatments, and some of the most common interventions, such as the suggestion of rest, are based on little or no scientific evidence and may in fact prove to be detrimental.[46] Winningham warns that 'unnecessary bed rest and prolonged sedentarism can contribute significantly to the development of fatigue and may result in rapid and potentially irreversible losses in energy and functioning'.[46] Improved psychological status, decrease in fatigue and increased feelings of vigour have been reported in groups of women with breast cancer following initiation of exercise.[47,48] Nevertheless, there continues to be some conflicting evidence over whether people suffering from cancer can benefit from exercise[10] and although some guidelines and precautions relating to safe exercise have been developed,[46] there is little information to date to inform the practice of nurses, particularly when working with patients experiencing the fatigue of advanced cancer.

Energy conservation, enhancing energy sources, and preventing energy waste are three potential strategies for managing fatigue identified in the literature. Vincent[37] suggests that a multi-method fatigue therapy programme, including energy conservation activities, a planned exercise programme, stress reduction instruction, and nutritional counselling, may prove to be especially helpful for people with chronic fatigue. Stress management and energy conservation appear to be the two most widely reported facets of care currently employed. Stress management has been defined as incorporating 'counselling' (facilitating a trusting relationship with the person with cancer), patient education, meditation, exercise, muscle relaxation, biofeedback, time management, and diversional activities, e.g. games, music, or reading.[5] Energy conservation focuses attention on the value of rest, setting priorities in valued activities and roles, and delegating tasks. Their applicability to patients with advanced cancer is untested but insights gained from Krishnasamy's study[17] suggest that they may in fact be of little relevance to this group of patients:

> She told me it's no good all the things that used to help don't now. She listed lots of things like activity pacing and goal planning, although she didn't call them that, but they just didn't work for her anymore.

Activity pacing, goal setting, and identification of priority activities have repeatedly been identified as potentially helpful interventions to manage fatigue.[1] However, there is emerging evidence that goal setting and identification of priority activities may be less helpful for the fatigue of advanced cancer, as the very unpredictability and severity of the fatigue may preclude such planning.[7,17] For those experiencing chemotherapy- and radiotherapy-related fatigue, anticipating when fatigue is most likely to occur may allow forward planning. Activities can then be planned to avoid high fatigue times; routine rest periods can be set and requests for help with daily activities targeted effectively for patients and their families. Fatigue following radiotherapy has been found to occur most often in the afternoon and planning for a nap or rest periods at that time can be helpful.[10] Work by Corner *et al.*,[49] evaluating a nursing approach to managing breathlessness for patients with advanced lung cancer, presents as one of its therapeutic interventions the need to be able to help patients to plan and organise their days around prioritised activities. The notion of balancing daily activities in relation to a 'breathing cost' may have an important contribution to make to the development of a nursing strategy for helping patients to live with the fatigue of advanced cancer, where each activity incurs an 'energy cost'. One of the key therapeutic aspects of their intervention is a commitment to explore the existential meaning of the cancer and its many ramifications.

If we accept that caring is attending to a person's wholeness,[50] we must develop the skills to work with individuals in such a way that phenomena such as fatigue cannot be reduced to specific component parts. For individuals who experience cancer-related fatigue, it mediates between the 'I' of pre-cancer person and the 'me' as cancer patient. It becomes a representation of self:[30]

> . . . there is another aspect of my fatigue that cannot be eased by rest. This is a sense of tiredness and *ennui* with practically everything and everybody, a desire to withdraw from the world, to crawl into a hole and pull the lid over my head [p. 77].

Notes on selected cancer sites 19.1: Malignant pleural mesothelioma

The exact annual incidence of mesothelioma is unknown, as diagnosis, even when undertaken by expert pathologists, is difficult.[21] However, its incidence has been reported as rising by as much as 50% in the last decade and projection statistics suggest that it will continue to rise moderately into the 21st century.[22] As a result of legislation to reduce individuals' exposure to asbestos (the main cause of mesothelioma), the incidence of the disease is projected eventually to decline. Men are significantly more likely to be diagnosed with mesothelioma than are women and its incidence steadily rises with age. It is ten times more prevalent among men aged 60–64 than among those aged 30–34.[22]

Malignant pleural mesothelioma has a poor prognosis (median 4–18 months), and one of the key aspects of

diagnosis is to exclude other more treatable conditions.[23] Breathlessness, non-pleuritic chest pain, or both, are what usually leads patients to visit their doctor. Pleural fluid eventually becomes loculated as the tumour obliterates the pleural space and as disease progresses, fatigue and breathlessness increase out of proportion with any objective, measurable values.[24]

Despite increasing trends in incidence of mesothelioma, relatively few large-scale clinical trials have been undertaken.[25] Surgery has proved ineffective and removal of pleura and the lung fail to prevent recurrence. Use of radiotherapy is controversial and there is little evidence of overall benefit from chemotherapy.[22] For the majority of patients, survival figures and quality of life data appear to advocate supportive care alone.[26] Nurses have a significant contribution to make to expert symptom management for a group of patients for whom cure is not possible.

References

1. Piper B., Lindsay D. and Dodd M. (1987). Fatigue mechanisms in cancer patients: developing a nursing theory. *Oncology Nursing Forum* 14, 17–23.
2. Carpenito L. (1995). Fatigue. In Carpenito L. (ed.) *Handbook of Nursing Diagnosis,* 5th edition. Philadelphia, PA: Lippincott.
3. Haylock P. and Hart L. (1979). Fatigue in patients receiving localised radiation. *Cancer Nursing* 2, 461–467.
4. Varricchio C. (1985). Selecting a tool for measuring fatigue. *Oncology Nursing Forum* 12, 122–127.
5. Aistars J. (1987). Fatigue in the cancer patient: conceptual approach to a clinical problem. *Oncology Nursing Forum* 14, 25–30.
6. Pickard-Holley S. (1991). Fatigue in cancer patients. A descriptive study. *Cancer Nursing* 14, 13–19.
7. Armes J. (1995). *Cancer patients' experiences of fatigue in cancer.* Unpublished B.Sc. dissertation, University of Hull.
8. Pearce S. and Richardson A. (1996). Fatigue in cancer: a phenomenological perspective. *European Journal of Cancer Care* 5, 111–115.
9. Gall H. (1996). The basis of cancer fatigue: where does it come from? *European Journal of Cancer Care* 5 (Suppl. 2), 31–34.
10. Nail L. and King K. (1987). Fatigue. *Seminars in Nursing Oncology* 3, 257–262.
11. Grandjean E. (1968). Fatigue. Its physiological and psychological significance. *The Ergonomics Research Society* 11, 427–436.
12. Cimprich B. (1992). Attentional fatigue following breast cancer surgery. *Research in Nursing and Health* 15, 199–207.

13. Rhodes V., Watson P. and Hanson B. (1988). Patients' descriptions of the influence of tiredness and weakness on self-care abilities. *Cancer Nursing* **11**, 186–194.

14. Ream E. and Richardson A. (1997). Fatigue in patients with cancer and chronic obstructive airways disease: a phenomenological enquiry. *International Journal of Nursing Studies* **34**, 44–53.

15. Jamar S. (1989). Fatigue in women receiving chemotherapy for ovarian cancer. In Funk S., Tornquist E., Champagne M. *et al.* (eds.) *Key Aspects of Comfort: Management of Pain, Fatigue and Nausea*. New York: Springer, pp. 224–228.

16. Glaus A., Crow R. and Hammond S. (1996). A qualitative study to explore the concept of fatigue/tiredness in cancer patients and in healthy individuals. *European Journal of Cancer Care* **5** (Suppl. 2), 8–23.

17. Krishnasamy M. (1996). *An exploration of the nature and impact of fatigue in advanced cancer. A case study*. London: Macmillan Practice Development Unit, Centre for Cancer and Palliative Care Studies.

18. Alonzo A. (1985). An analytical typology of disclaimers, excuses and justifications surrounding illness. A situational approach to health and illness. *Social Science and Medicine* **21**, 153–162.

19. Thorne S. (1993). *Negotiating Health Care. The Social Context of Chronic Illness*. London: Sage.

20. Brown M., Carrierri V., Janson-Bjerklie S. and Dodd M. (1986). Lung cancer and dyspnoea: the patient's perception. *Oncology Nursing Forum* **13**, 19–24.

21. McDonald A.D. and McDonald J.C. (1987). Epidemiology of malignant mesothelioma. In Antman K. and Aisner J. (eds.) *Asbestos-related Malignancy*. Orlando: Grune & Stratton, pp. 31–55.

22. Antman K., Pass H., DeLaney T., Li F. and Corson J. (1993). Benign and malignant mesothelioma. In DeVita V., Hellman S. and Rosenberg S. (eds.) *Cancer. Principles and Practice of Oncology*, 4th edition. Philadelphia, PA: Lippincott, pp. 1489–1508.

23. Thatcher N. and Spiro S. (1994). *New Perspective in Lung Cancer*. London: British Medical Journal.

24. Elmes P.C. and Simpson M. (1976). The clinical aspects of mesothelioma. *Quarterly Journal of Medicine* **45**, 427.

25. Williams C. (1992). *Lung Cancer. The Facts*. Oxford: Oxford University Press.

26. Hulks G., Thomas J.S. and Waclawski E. (1980). Malignant pleural mesothelioma in Western Glasgow. *Thorax* **44**, 496–500.

27. Richardson A. (1995). Fatigue in cancer patients: a review of the literature. *European Journal of Cancer Care* **4**, 20–32.

28. Yarbro C. (1995). Interventions for fatigue. *European Journal of Cancer Care* **5** (Suppl. 2), 35–38.

29. Czechmeister C. (1994). Metaphor in illness and nursing: a two-edged sword. A discussion of the social use of metaphor in everyday language, and implications of nursing and nursing education. *Journal of Advanced Nursing* **19**, 1226–1233.

30. Murphy R.F. (1987). *The Body Silent*. London: W.W. Norton.

31. Ryder R. and Ridley M. (1990). The place from which the patient comes. *Journal of Professional Nursing* **6**, 255.

32. Richardson A. and Ream E. (1997). Self-care activities initiated by chemotherapy patients in response to fatigue. *International Journal of Nursing Studies* **34**, 35–43.

33. Nail L., Jones S., Greene D., Schipper D. and Jensen R. (1991). Use and perceived efficacy of self-care activities in patients receiving chemotherapy. *Oncology Nursing Forum* **18**, 883–887.

34. Graydon J., Bubela N., Irvine D. and Vincent L. (1995). Fatigue reducing strategies used by patients receiving treatment for cancer. *Cancer Nursing* **18**, 23–28.

35. Morant R. (1991). Asthenia in cancer patients: a double-edged inflammatory response against the tumour? *Journal of Palliative Care* **7**, 22–24.

36. Chen M. (1986). The epidemiology of self-perceived fatigue among adults. *Preventive Medicine* **15**, 74–81.

37. Vincent L. (1992). Management of fatigue in cancer patients. In Bailey C. (ed.) *Cancer Nursing – Changing Frontiers – 7th International Conference on Cancer Nursing*, 16–21 August, Vienna, Austria. Oxford: Rapid Communications, pp. 91–94.

38. Dunkel-Schetter C. and Wortman C. (1979). Interpersonal relations and cancer: a theoretical analysis. *Journal of Social Issues* **35**, 120–155.

39. Kobashi-Schoot J., Hanewald G., VanDam F. and Bruning P. (1985). Assessment of malaise in cancer patients treated with radiotherapy. *Cancer Nursing* **8**, 306–313.

40. Nerenz D., Leventhal H. and Love R. (1982). Factors contributing to emotional distress during cancer chemotherapy. *Cancer* **50**, 1020–1027.

41. Rhoten D. (1982). Fatigue and the postsurgical patient. In Norris C. (ed.) *Concept Clarification in Nursing*. Rockville: Aspen, pp. 277–300.

42. Bruera E. and MacDonald N. (1988). Overwhelming fatigue in advanced cancer. *American Journal of Nursing*, January, 99–100.

43. Visser M. and Smets E.M.A. (1998). Fatigue, depression and quality of life in cancer patients: how are they related? *Journal of Supportive Care in Cancer* **6**, 101–108.

44. Cimprich B. (1993). Development of an intervention to restore attention in cancer patients. *Cancer Nursing* **16**, 83–92.

45. Love R., Leventhal H., Easterling D. and Nerenz D. (1989). Side effects and emotional distress during cancer chemotherapy. *Cancer* **63**, 604–612.

46. Winningham M. (1991). Walking programme for people with cancer. Getting started. *Cancer Nursing* 14, 270–274.

47. Winningham M., MacVicar M. and Burke C. (1986). Exercise for cancer patients: guidelines and precautions. *The Physician and Sports Medicine* 14, 125–134.

48. Mock V., Dow K.H., Mears C.J. *et al.* (1997). Effects of exercise on fatigue, physical functioning, and emotional distress during radiation therapy for breast cancer. *Oncology Nursing Forum* 24, 991–1000.

49. Corner J., Plant H. and Warner L. (1995). Developing a nursing approach to managing dyspnoea in lung cancer. *International Journal of Palliative Nursing* 1, 5–11.

50. Picard C. (1991). Caring and the story: the compelling nature of what must be told and understood in the human dimension of suffering. In Gaut D. and Leininger M. (eds.) *Caring: The Compassionate Healer.* New York: National League for Nursing Press, 89–98.

CHAPTER TWENTY

Breathlessness

Christopher Bailey

Breathlessness is 'the sensation of difficult breathing' and a 'frequent and distressing symptom experienced by patients with chronic obstructive pulmonary disease'.[1] It has also been described as 'the sensation of difficult, uncomfortable breathing . . . the most reported and most incapacitating symptom of the patient with COPD [chronic obstructive pulmonary disease]'.[2] Ahmedzai, writing in the *Oxford Textbook of Palliative Medicine*, comments that,

> . . . it is helpful to think of dyspnoea as the major part of 'total respiratory distress' which would encompass the physical, psychological, and social manifestations.[3]

Breathlessness accounts for a high proportion of the disability, impaired life quality, and human suffering experienced by people with respiratory disease. Breathlessness is more than a sensation, more than unpleasant. It is difficult to think of it only in terms of ordered classifications, which are so useful when it comes to managing unruly thoughts and disordered emotions, the stuff of human experience.

Breathlessness does cause a lot of suffering, and though much of the literature on managing breathlessness derives from studies of patients with non-malignant disease, breathlessness is a major issue for people with cancer; 30% of people terminally ill with cancer and 65% of people with lung cancer experience breathlessness.[4] In the USA, a study by Reuben and Mor[5] indicated that 70% of terminally ill cancer patients were breathless at some time in the last 6 weeks of life.

Much of the effort to manage breathlessness has thus far focused on the treatment of underlying causes, or on pharmacological strategies. Surgery, radiotherapy, and chemotherapy, and administration of steroids, are important treatments for obstruction of the upper airways by primary or secondary tumours.[6] Mediastinal obstruction, or obstruction of the bronchus, can be treated with radiotherapy, chemotherapy, and again, steroids. Pleural effusions, most common in tumours of the lung or breast, can be drained (although fluid frequently reaccumulates), or pleuradesis performed. Lymphangitis, in which the lymphatic system of the lungs is affected by tumour, is unlikely to respond to treatment; palliation of lymphangitis may be achieved by a combination of dexamethasone and oral morphine.[6]

If it is not possible to reverse the cause of breathlessness, drug treatment is often seen as the principal means of alleviating the symptom. Bronchodilators may be useful for patients whose breathlessness is exacerbated by reversible airways disease. Reversibility can be assessed by measuring the patient's peak expiratory flow rate (PEFR) before and half an hour after a standard dose of a drug such as salbutamol. An improvement of more than 15% suggests that the patient will benefit from the appropriate bronchodilator.[6]

Respiratory sedatives are often recommended for alleviating breathlessness:

> In the palliation of dyspnoeic patients with advanced cancer, neurological disease, or cardiorespiratory disease,

the main benefit comes from the suppression of respiratory awareness [p. 361].[3]

Morphine has been the drug most commonly referred to in this respect. While the mode of action of morphine in breathlessness is not well understood, oral morphine has been shown to improve exercise tolerance in patients with COPD.[7]

A study[8] evaluating the work of terminal care support teams in Bloomsbury Health Authority, London, examined 14 items, agreed by support teams to be independent objectives of care and measures of the condition and further needs of dying patients and their families, graded on a seven-point scale.[8] Definitions for the score level were agreed and documented. In all, the symptoms of 86 patients were rated throughout the period that patients were under the care of the support teams. While pain was found to be the most common symptom at referral (41% of patients), assessment scores improved after the first week of care, and in the last week of life. By contrast, the 13 patients with breathlessness at referral all had breathlessness at death. In addition, five patients developed breathlessness after referral. Symptom control scores suggested that 'pain was controlled very early in care, while dyspnoea was not controlled at all'. The authors[8] point out that a full range of treatments, including opioids, bronchodilators, anxiolitics, and corticosteroids, was used by the support teams, and acknowledge that:

> . . . our results suggest that treatment may not be sufficiently effective. The existing measures may have poor efficacy, or they may be applied too late.

Chest physiotherapy is usually seen as alleviating breathlessness by removing excess secretions, but techniques of breathing control have also been developed to avoid breathlessness at rest or on exertion. Breathing control involves relaxing the upper chest and shoulders, and breathing at the normal rate using the lower chest (sometimes referred to as 'diaphragmatic breathing'). People who are breathless often attempt to climb stairs by breathing in, holding their breath, and making a dash for it, ultimately arriving panting at the top.[9] Breathing control can be used to climb stairs, breathing in as one step is climbed, and out as the next is climbed, and walking at a slightly slower pace, reducing the degree of breathlessness. The

technique can also be applied on hills or slopes, on level ground if necessary, or to recover the breath when stationary. Together with pursed lip breathing (PLB), lower chest breathing constitutes what is known as 'breathing re-training' or breathing control.[10] While PLB is thought to be a more effective pattern of respiration, it probably does not decrease the work of breathing. The source of symptom benefit from PLB may be due to decreased airway collapse, enlarged tidal volume, and slowed respiration.[11] The aims of breathing retraining are to:

- promote a relaxed and gentle breathing pattern
- minimise the work of breathing
- establish a sense of control
- improve ventilation at the base of the lungs
- increase the strength, co-ordination, and efficiency of the respiratory muscles
- maintain mobility of the thoracic cage
- promote a sense of well-being.

Often, breathlessness can lead a person to breathe with the upper chest and shoulders in a rapid, shallow manner.[1,12] Gasping for air increases the resistance to flow, which increases energy expenditure. Using accessory respiratory muscles, which are not as efficient as primary respiratory muscles, leads more quickly to fatigue, and to greater oxygen consumption. As the rate of breathing increases, the depth often decreases, creating a larger dead space in the lungs and reducing the amount of oxygen available to the body. In effect, this response to inadequate ventilation actually places even greater demands on the respiratory system.

Breathing retraining is intended to encourage as efficient a breathing pattern as possible, and to reverse as far as possible the ineffective response that has developed.

Breathlessness can be a frightening experience: anyone who has experienced, say, asthmatic attacks, or altitude sickness, or, indeed, anyone whose children have experienced breathlessness can testify to that. The experience of people whose breathlessness occurs in the context of cancer, more particularly in the context of lung cancer, must be powerful indeed. Roberts[13] has pointed out that,

> . . . patients' interpretations of what the signal of shortness of breath meant in relation to their disease seemed

. . . the predominant influencing factor in shaping their experience with dyspnoea.[13]

She describes one woman who avoided any activity that made her aware of her breathing, despite being able to bath, walk, and dress independently, because she believed that being breathless would make her cancer spread. Breathlessness, it seems, can represent a threat to life itself:

It starts to feel like you're choking. Someone's taking the breath away from me

and,

I panic a bit sometimes, because deep down I know that [this breath] could be my last one . . . It's an awful feeling.[13]

Both patients and nurses, Roberts claims, respond to breathlessness by decreasing and restricting activity. Steele and Shaver[14] also identify that breathlessness constitutes a serious threat:

. . . the experience of dyspnoea incorporates cognitive interpretation of the event as threatening

and suggest that this is why activity is circumscribed:

. . . motivation to alleviate threat through behaviours such as slowing or cessation of activities that evoke dyspnoea would be expected [p. 67].

While it is understandable that both patients and carers respond to breathlessness in this way, the objective of therapy remains to roll back inactivity, or loss of function, and to work with the heavy psychological burden that is so influential in restricting freedom.

Researchers at the Centre for Cancer and Palliative Care Studies in the Institute of Cancer Research, London, have been involved in developing and evaluating an intervention that addresses both the functional and the psychosocial aspects of breathlessness.[15] They refer to the importance of the suggestion that,

. . . dyspnoea might be more comprehensively viewed as a nociceptive phenomenon like pain, with motivational and affective dimensions expressed as distress . . . in addition to the sensory dimension.[14]

and acknowledge the relevance of the 'ecologic' model of dyspnoea, 'a framework for guiding nursing science', which:

. . . unlike the linear, reductionist biomedical model with notions of cause, disease, and cure, . . . acknowledge[s] the interactive effects of multivariate individual and environmental influences upon individual adaptations and health outcomes.[14]

Corner *et al.*[15] point out that Steele and Shaver[14] do, in fact, maintain some elements of the reductionist approach. In the nociceptive model of breathlessness, dimensions of effort and discomfort can be regarded as separate, and consequently capable of 'selective modification'. A process of long-term adaptation is envisaged, whereby:

. . . perception of the discomfort dimension of dyspnoea is selectively reduced so as to preserve function.[14]

Corner and colleagues[15] propose an 'integrative model', in which the emotional experience of breathlessness is considered as inseparable from the sensory experience and the biological mechanisms. They use this model as the basis for a non-pharmacological intervention for breathlessness, developed for the out-patient setting, which draws on breathing retraining, relaxation, and biofeedback techniques. The intervention, which was the subject of a randomised controlled trial in a specialised cancer centre,[16] consists of the strategies shown below.

- Detailed assessment of breathlessness and factors that ameliorate or exacerbate it.
- Advice and support for patients and their families on ways of managing breathlessness.
- Exploration with individuals of the meaning of breathlessness, their disease, and their feelings about the future.
- Rebreathing techniques for patients and families.
- Progressive muscle relaxation and distraction for patients (with tapes if desired).
- Goal setting to complement breathing and relaxation techniques, to assist in the management of functional and social activities, and to support the development and adoption of coping strategies.
- Early recognition of problems warranting pharmacological or medical intervention.

Findings of the study indicate that this approach is of value in enhancing the quality of life of patients with lung cancer who are experiencing breathlessness.[16] From the beginning, it was anticipated that the meaning of breathlessness in the context of severe, life-threatening illness would be an important factor in patients', experiences, and that managing breathlessness would involve working with its meaning.

A small study, conducted in parallel with the main evaluation study, was developed to record and assess nurse-researchers' perceptions of the intervention.[17] Using an exploratory single case design,[18] interviews were conducted with the three nurse-researchers working in the out-patients' clinic at that time. One nurse-researcher was interviewed three times, the other two twice each.

Evidence from interviews with nurse-researchers suggests that the deep emotional consequences of breathlessness in lung cancer have a profound influence on how the intervention is realised in practice. The value of breathing retraining is at least as great as the value of attention paid to psychosocial issues. As one nurse-researcher says:

> . . . the [practical] framework that we give people, actually helps them cope, and that has to . . . go alongside talking about emotional issues, and the difficulties . . .

Referring to a man she is seeing in the clinic, she gives an example of how this works in practice:

> . . . last week he was talking about . . . walking up the car park . . . it goes up a bank . . . it sort of steps up. Well, for all the people who attend it's a problem, because they have to park their cars on the third level, and having talked about the difficulties of any kind of incline they then have to climb up to get back to their car. So I walked back to his car with him, slowly, to see how it was for him . . . we had this little conversation while I went up to the car with him . . . the fact that I walked to the car with him obviously means something enormous . . . he actually lives with his son, who he feels a tremendous burden on . . . I always got a feeling . . . that they feel no-one really cares about them . . . I think this was like he did matter to me . . . almost a confirmation of it, 'cos I bothered to walk up to his car with him . . .

The opportunity to accompany this man to the car park is a means of rehearsing an aspect of breathing retraining in a practical situation. It is also a means of working socially with a client whose sense is that he is a burden because of his illness, and that he cannot make claims upon people's care. Being a burden, and being beyond the reach of care, are part of illness and breathlessness, and are

approached, with the physical experience of breathlessness, as a single, integrated phenomenon.

The same nurse-researcher refers to her clients' feelings of loss of worth again in another interview:

> . . . there is . . . this need to give something back . . . it's almost self-respect . . . to say that they are still wanted and needed . . . I had a really long conversation with him telling me the most economical way to use my washing machine . . . and another time he told me about cooking nectarines, well I thought it was just so important to listen to that.

Breathlessness has literally restricted this man's ability to carry out his customary daily personal and work-related activities, and it has also evoked a sense of being unable to fulfil a socially useful role. The nurse is addressing part of the overall effect of breathlessness when she acknowledges her client's domestic skills. The literal effects of breathlessness, evident in the man's difficulty in walking to his car, and the emotional ones, played out at home and in his relationship with his son, are lost elements of mastery within the domestic arena towards which she directs her attention and support.

Night-time panic attacks exemplify the way in which breathlessness is not a sensation, not an emotion, and not a physical process, but all three of these, at least, and also a dynamic, fluctuating state. Responding therapeutically to panic attacks makes great demands on both the client, and the nurse. The client experiences an escalating predicament in which normal breathing patterns collapse, awareness is acute, and fear takes hold. Sleep becomes impossible and panic rises. The essence of panic is that catastrophe is imminent and inescapable, and with breathlessness, panic frequently revolves around the idea of suffocation and death:

> . . . his breathing was bad, he used to come in at night with these panic attacks, he couldn't sleep . . . because he was so frightened, and a lot of the work I did with him was with strategies for coping with the night, and getting to sleep, and ways of calming himself down at night . . . he used to get breathless at night . . . it was just because he would go to bed and think about his breathing and think he wouldn't be able to breathe and then get in a panic about it . . .

It is, then, appropriate to apply the practical discipline of breathing retraining to a highly charged emotional situation such as this (and it is true to say that part of what the nurse is doing is responding to a pathological process). The nurse, however, is aware and involved in the predicament as a whole, and is called upon to work with a high level of distress.

Fabricius[19] suggests that being 'with' and 'for' the patient is a therapeutic response to distress:

> . . . by 'being for the patient' . . . I mean allowing the patient, to some extent, to use the nurse, psychically, as the sort of object he needs. Often this will be, to use Bion's term, as a container for whatever of his anxieties are at the moment intolerable to him, and of course this . . . is a maternal function.

Fabricius points out that nurses are often unable to meet the demands made on them by patients:

> . . . the sheer quantity, as well as force, of the projections that are thrust on them are too much for any human unless she herself is held in a supportive, containing structure.

She suggests that facilitated small group meetings for nurses to discuss anything to do with their relationships with patients and the feelings aroused by them represent progress towards such a structure.

The conceptualisation put forward by Corner *et al.*,[15] which treats the emotional experience of breathlessness as inseparable from the sensory experience and the biological mechanisms, demands a response that is less dependent on ordered and bounded categories and classifications. The nociceptive model described by Steele and Shaver[14] suggests that one dimension of a phenomenon, for example distress, can be reduced independently of another, for example, sensation. Corner *et al.*,[15] however, state that breathlessness can be,

> . . . understood holistically in the context of an individual's life, illness experience and its meaning.

The implication is that dimensions of a phenomenon cannot be generalised from individual to individual: that the experience is particular, not universal. What is demanded is not a separation of a symptom into discrete entities, defined by reference to established categories, or an appeal to strict cause and effect relationships. As one nurse-researcher said,

People don't even know that they're anxious . . . it's so much part of your physiological activity that you don't know what's doing what . . . it's impossible to start saying there are components of it, to even talk about components seems to be wrong . . . you have to treat it as a whole experience, and it must have intense meaning to people.

The essence of the response demanded by this conceptualisation is the 'containing, supportive structure' referred to by Fabricius,[19] which is extended by nurse to client and, as importantly, by co-workers and institution to nurse.

Breathlessness is not a symptom, a commodity: it is lived experience. For some patients with lung cancer, it is fear of dying, and therapy is an accepting response to that:

> . . . one lady . . . I turned to put the pulse oximeter, turned it on, and to put it on her, and as I turned my back to her, she said, 'Am I going to die of this?' And, I mean the fact that I'd done something, moved away to do something technical and turned my back, allowed her to say the thing that she really wanted to say, and it was about allowing that person to be in a totally private place with someone who appeared to be very comfortable and safe to ask that question of.

For some, often it is the same people, breathlessness is panic, and the things that cannot be accomplished, and therapy is tackling panic, and accomplishing some of those things:

> . . . teaching a few simple strategies to manage those attacks, and techniques and new ways of breathing . . . by the next session . . . he'd only had minor attacks of breathlessness at night, so he was beginning to master these awful panics . . . then . . . teaching a bit more, like how do you use these breathing techniques to manage stairs . . . he could recover quicker at the top by using diaphragmatic breathing . . . timing your breathing while you're walking . . . talking about sleeping and those sorts of things, and getting a bit further with them about what they both felt about it and the future . . .

Fabricius[19] asks how nurses can be psychotherapeutic, and what hinders them from being so. She likens the psychotherapeutic role to the actions of a mother 'holding' an infant, protecting it physically from harm and psychically from overwhelming distress.

Evidence suggests that there is scope for developing nursing roles within a framework that makes it possible to be more accepting of patients' 'conscious and unconscious demands', to employ nursing as therapy. The order of nursing situations, the routine; the way in which 'symptoms' are dealt with at a high level of abstraction; the prevalence of models or algorithms which 'stand for' human entities without expressing them; the splitting of human experience into neatly bounded categories, setting aside the undisciplined, disorderly whole; all of this stands in the way, provides a means to become detached, to leave painful things untouched.

Lung cancer

About 158 000 new patients are registered with lung cancer in the European Community each year,[20] with an excess of 100 000 deaths from lung cancer in the USA annually.[21] It is the most common of all cancers.[22] Over the past 20 years there has been a worldwide increase in deaths from lung malignancies, with death rates having doubled in women.[23] It has overtaken breast cancer as the number one killer of women and continues to be the most common cause of cancer death in men.[24]

It is well known that most deaths from lung cancer are caused by tobacco smoke and that it is not only those who smoke who are at risk. Hirayama[25] demonstrated that non-smoking wives of husbands who smoked heavily had an increased risk of lung cancer. Similar results were found in studies of children and adults exposed to environmental tobacco smoke in their homes.[26] There is little evidence of a dietary cause for lung cancer, but exposure to asbestos, radon, chromium, nickel, and inorganic arsenic compounds have been proven to increase an individual's risk of developing lung malignancy.[27]

Despite advances in understanding of lung cancer biology, mortality rates for patients with lung malignancies remain high, with a 5-year survival rate of less than 10% at all ages.[28] Notwithstanding improvements in the cure rate from 5% to 30% over the past 30 years, most patients still die from metastatic disease resistant to chemotherapy.[29] It is widely acknowledged that chemotherapy still has a long way to go in non-small-cell lung cancer (NSCLC), providing little advantage to patients with inoperable NSCLC in terms of survival and quality of life, over current best supportive treatment.[30] Although standard combination chemotherapy and thoracic radiotherapy regimes prolong survival in patients with small-cell lung cancer (SCLC) with limited disease, long-term survival rates are low, and toxicities often unacceptably high.[31] For patients with mesothelioma prognosis is especially poor, with very few individuals benefiting from either surgery, radiotherapy, or chemotherapy.[32]

Unfortunately, there appears to be little optimism surrounding future treatment developments. Randomised trials seem to offer the most effective way

Table 20.1 Common problems in lung cancer[33]

Some common signs problems and symptoms of lung cancer	Frequency of patients perceived
Cough	Identified by 71% of patients with lung cancer
Breathlessness	Identified by 59% of patients
General malaise	
Pain in the arm, chest, or back	Identified by 48% of patients
Weakness	
Fatigue/overwhelming tiredness	Identified by 84% of patients
Anorexia and weight loss	Identified by 57% and 54% of patients, respectively
Feeling wheezy/tight chest/stridor	
Haemoptysis	Identified by 84% of patients
Superior vena cava obstruction	
Chest infection/pneumonitis	
Lymphatic obstruction	
Reduced activity	Identified by 81% of patients

of identifying future lung cancer patients best placed to receive curative treatments, while also defining the minimum treatment required for palliation.[29,31] However, as much of the care provided for lung cancer patients is carried out by non-experts on an out-patient basis,[34,35] the number of patients being entered for randomised trials is limited. When asked, 37% (of a total group of 154) hospital-based surgeons, physicians, radiotherapists, and oncologists stated that they would choose to treat NSCLC patients themselves, with only 7% indicating referral to palliative care services as a management option. International attempts to evaluate the efficacy of screening for lung cancer have concluded that there is little, if any benefit from mass screening as a means of reducing the magnitude of the problem, or of improving therapeutic outcomes.[19] However, there appears to be consensus amongst lung cancer specialists that a person with a high risk for developing lung cancer might benefit from annual chest X-rays.

To date, however, given the limitations of current therapeutic options and the poor prognosis of lung cancer, the necessity for good palliative and terminal care, which focuses on physical symptom control and psychological care, is great. Patients with advanced lung cancer experience a multiplicity of symptoms incorporating pain, dyspnoea, anorexia, fatigue, and anxiety, symptoms recognised as being especially difficult to manage, and which impact considerably on the patient's quality of life.[22,36]

Notes on selected cancer sites 20.1: Lung cancer – classification and staging

- Non-small-cell lung cancer (NSCLC) accounts for approximately 74% of all lung cancers, while small-cell lung cancer (SCLC) accounts for approximately 25% and mesothelioma around 1%.[32]
- NSCLC may consist of squamous cell carcinoma, adeno-carcinoma, or large-cell carcinoma.
- Small-cell carcinoma may consist of oat cell carcinoma, intermediate cell carcinoma, or combined oat cell carcinoma.

Staging lung cancer
A very simple system of staging is used for SCLC:

- Limited disease refers to disease confined to one side of the chest (although disease may be very extensive on that one side) and to the draining lymph nodes on that side.

- Extensive disease refers to any other condition where the cancer has spread beyond that outlined above.

As chemotherapy is the mainstay of treatment for SCLC, the distinction between limited and extensive disease is more important in understanding the patient's outlook than on the possible choice of treatment.[32]

For patients with NSCLC, surgery is the most important treatment. Consequently, the staging system is far more precise and complicated.

NSCLC is staged according to the TNM system – tumour, nodes and metastases.

1. T refers to the primary tumour, which may be classified as being T1, T2, or T3.
   - T1 – a tumour must be less than 3 cm in diameter and surrounded by normal lung.
   - T2 – the tumour is more than 3 cm in diameter, or any size if invading the pleura, or associated with some lung collapse or infection.
   - T3 – the tumour may be of any size invading the chest wall, the diaphragm, the pericardium or aorta, be within 2 cm of the carina, or there may be collapse of an entire lung or a pleural effusion.
2. N refers to lymph nodes.
   - N0 – there is no spread to the lymph nodes
   - N1 – there is spread to the first group of draining lymph nodes
   - N2 – the tumour has spread into the nodes in the centre of the chest.
3. M refers to distant metastases.
   - M0 – there are no known metastases
   - M1 – distant metastases have been found.[32]

Staging tests for patients suspected of having lung cancer

NSCLC	SCLC
All patients: chest X-ray, blood tests, bronchoscopy, biopsy of gland or the tumour if present	All patients: chest X-ray, blood tests, bronchoscopy, occasionally a bone marrow aspiration, ultrasound or CT of liver and an isotope bone scan.
Patients eligible for surgery will also undergo CT scanning, mediastinoscopy or mediastinotomy, fine needle biopsy of the tumour, lung function tests, ultrasound or CT of liver and an isotope bone scan.	

Table 20.2 Comparison of the incidence of the top 13 problems related to physical, psychological, and interactional aspects, with reported associated suffering (patients with lung cancer)

Incidence	Reported suffering
Changed activities (63%)	Disability (50%)
Disability (54%)	Pain (40%)
Weakness/fatigue (50%)	Anxiety (34%)
Job problems (50%)	Changed activities (34%)
Pain (43%)	Weakness/fatigue (33%)
Coughing (43%)	Fear of disability (30%)
Nausea/vomiting (36%)	Nausea/vomiting (30%)
Anxiety (34%)	Depression (23%)
Fear of disability (34%)	Coughing (23%)
Changed appearance (33%)	Fear of recurrence (20%)
Depression (26%)	Job problems (20%)
Fear of recurrence (23%)	Powerlessness (17%)
Powerlessness (20%)	Changed appearance (10%)

Benedict[36] invited 30 patients with primary lung cancer from a haematology-oncology clinic to respond to a series of Likert scales aimed at quantifying individuals' perceptions of suffering associated with lung cancer. Prevalence of identified problems compared favourably with those outlined above and interestingly, there was considerable correlation between those problems occurring most frequently, and the degree of suffering associated with them.

Astoundingly, there was no mention of breathlessness or the suffering associated with it from the individuals in Benedict's study. It is unlikely that none of these individuals had experienced dyspnoea and it would be interesting to know whether dyspnoea was included within the Likert scales presented to them.

Acknowledgement

The material presented in was first published in the *European Journal of Cancer Care*, 1995, **4**, 184–190 and is reproduced with permission of Blackwell Science Ltd.

References

1. Gift A.G. and Cahill C.A. (1990). Psychophysiologic aspects of dyspnoea in chronic obstructive pulmonary disease: a pilot study. *Heart and Lung* **19**, 252–257.

2. Renfroe K.L. (1988). Effect of progressive muscle relaxation on dyspnoea and state anxiety in patients with chronic obstructive pulmonary disease. *Heart and Lung* **17**, 408–413.

3. Ahmedzai S. (1995). In Doyle D., Hanks G. and McDonald N. (eds.) *The Oxford Textbook of Palliative Medicine.* Oxford: Oxford University Press.

4. Twycross R.G. and Lack S.A. (1986). *Therapeutics in Terminal Cancer.* London: Churchill Livingstone.

5. Reuben D.B. and Mor V. (1986). Dyspnoea in terminally ill cancer patients. *Chest,* **89**, 234–236.

6. Cowcher K. and Hanks G.W. (1990). Long-term management of respiratory symptoms in advanced cancer. *Journal of Pain and Symptom Management* **5**, 320–330.

7. Light R.W., Muro J.R., Sato R.I., Stansbury D.W., Fischer C.E. and Brown S.E. (1989). Effects of oral morphine on breathlessness and exercise tolerance in patients with chronic obstructive pulmonary disease. *American Review of Respiratory Diseases* **139**, 126–133.

8. Higginson I. and McCarthy M. (1989). Measuring symptoms in terminal cancer: are pain and dyspnoea controlled? *Journal of the Royal Society of Medicine* **82**, 264–267.

9. Webber B. (1991). The role of the physiotherapist in medical chest problems. *Respiratory Disease in Practice,* **February/March**, 12–15.

10. Kersten L. (1989). *Comprehensive Respiratory Nursing.* Philadelphia, PA: W.B. Saunders.

11. Mueller R.E., Petty T.L. and Filley G.F. (1970). Ventilation and arterial blood gas changes induced by pursed lips breathing. *Journal of Applied Physiology* **28**, 784–789.

12. Gift A.G., Moore T. and Soeken K. (1992). Relaxation to reduce dyspnoea and anxiety in COPD patients. *Nursing Research* **41**, 242–246.

13. Roberts D., Thorne S.E. and Pearson C. (1993). The experience of dyspnoea in late-stage cancer: patients' and nurses' perspectives. *Cancer Nursing* **16**, 310–320.

14. Steele B. and Shaver J. (1992). The dyspnoea experience: nociceptive properties and a model for research and practice. *Advances in Nursing Science* **15**, 64–76.

15. Corner J., Plant H. and Warner L. (1995). Developing a nursing approach to managing dyspnoea in lung cancer. *International Journal of Palliative Nursing* **1**, 5–11.

16. Corner J., Plant H., A'Hern R. and Bailey C. (1996). Non-pharmacological interventions for breathlessness in lung cancer. *Palliative Medicine* **10**, 299–305.

17. Bailey C. (1995). Nursing as therapy in the management of breathlessness in lung cancer. *European Journal of Cancer Care* **4**, 184–190.

18. Yin R. (1994). *Case Study Research. Design and Methods,* 2nd edition. London: Sage.

19. Fabricius J. (1991). Running on the spot or can nursing really change. *Psychoanalytic Psychotherapy* **5**, 97–108.

20. Cancer Research Campaign (1991). *Factsheet. 17.1.* London: Cancer Research Campaign.

21. Bleehen N.M., Girling D.J., Gregor A., Leonard R., Machin D., McKenzie C. *et al.* (1994). Can long-term survival be improved in patients with small-cell lung cancer (SCLC) and good performance status? *British Journal of Cancer* **70**, 142–144.

22. Krech R., Davis J., Walsh D. and Curtis E. (1992). Symptom of lung cancer. *Palliative Medicine* **6**, 309–315.

23. Parkin D.M. (1989). Trends in lung cancer world-wide. *Chest* **96** (Suppl.), 5–8.

24. Charlton A. (1994). Tobacco and lung cancer. In Thatcher N. and Spiro S. (eds.) *New Perspectives in Lung Cancer.* London: British Medical Journal, pp. 1–18.

25. Hirayama T. (1981). Non-smoking wives of heavy smokers have a higher risk of lung cancer. *British Medical Journal* **282**, 183–185.

26. Sandler D.P., Wilcox A.J. and Everson R.B. (1985). Cumulative effects of lifetime passive smoking on cancer risk. *Lancet* **i**, 312–315.

27. Ginsberg R., Kris M. and Armstrong J. (1993). Non-small cell lung cancer. In DeVita V., Hellman S. and Rosenberg S. (eds.) *Cancer. Principles and Practice of Oncology,* 4th edition. Philadelphia, PA: Lippincott, pp. 673–721.

28. Office for National Statistic (1999). *Cancer Survival Trends in England and Wales 1971–1995: Deprivation and NHS Region.* Series SMPS No. 61. London: The Stationery Office.

29. Smith D.B. (1989). Sexual rehabilitation of the cancer patient. *Cancer Nursing* **12**, 10–15.

30. Maasilta P., Rautonen J., Mattson T. and Mattson K. (1990). Quality of life assessment during chemotherapy for non-small cell lung cancer. *European Journal of Cancer* **26**, 706–708.

31. Bleehen N.M. (1990). Lung cancer – still a long road ahead. *British Journal of Cancer* **61**, 493–494.

32. Williams C. (1992). *Lung Cancer. The Facts.* Oxford: Oxford University Press.

33. Hollen P.J., Gralla R.J., Kris M.G. and Potanovich L.M. (1992). Quality of life assessment in individuals with lung cancer. Testing the lung cancer symptom scale (LCSS). *European Journal of Cancer* **29** (Suppl. 1), 51–58.

34. Bristol-Myers Squibb Pharmaceuticals Ltd/Cancer Research Campaign (1991). *Lung Cancer Report.* Unpublished Report.

35. Standing Medical Advisory Committee (1994). *Management of Lung Cancer: Current Clinical Practices,* PL/CMO (94)9. London: Department of Health.

36. Benedict S. (1989). The suffering associated with lung cancer. *Cancer Nursing* **12**, 34–40.

CHAPTER TWENTY-ONE

Wound management

Meinir Krishnasamy

In his book *The Body Silent*, Murphy reminds us that illness is 'not simply a physical affair . . . it is our ontology, a condition of our being in the world' (p. 77).[1] Illness, especially when it is associated with disfigurement or alterations in body image, confers on people a loss of self-esteem, a stigma, resulting in a 'spoiled identity'.[2] When the disfigurement is associated with the disease of cancer, the potential for negative self-perception through acceptance of a subjectively created or objectively projected spoiled identity is enormous.[3] Where self-perception is altered by the presence of a physical wound, whether visible or otherwise, profoundly negative associations may occur. In extreme cases, a person may identify him or herself with the malignant wound, believing himself to be foul, odorous, or repulsive. The consequences for an individual's quality of life, self-esteem and well-being are enormous.

Skilled technical and physiological knowledge is necessary if avoidable wounds are to be prevented, wounds caused by any number of invasive procedures and treatments are to be managed effectively, uncomplicated wound healing is to be facilitated, or when complete healing is not feasible, if discomfort and distress are to be minimised. Alongside technical proficiency, nurses must also convey compassion, as illustrated in Personal account 21.1[4].

Personal account 21.1

I was so shocked when I saw the wound, it was leaking and black, and the smell was very strong. As soon as I began to unpack the items on the dressing trolley he fixed his eyes on me, waiting for me to show signs of repulsion, I think. I stopped and asked him if he minded me seeing the wound and him like this.

The wound had broken through, out onto his lower abdomen, but the area to be cleaned and dressed spread down to his genital area. He was very thin. He started to tell me how disgusting he found the wound and how he was ashamed of having it on his stomach. His wife sat quietly trying very hard to be absorbed in a book. He talked about it as though it were something alien that had taken over his body.

By the time he had finished talking, the technical dressing was over, but the effects of the interaction, of asking him what this wound meant to him were far-reaching. This time became an opportunity for intense personal interaction and over the course of the next ten days, the three of us began to talk about their sadness and fears about the future.

Wound healing

Irrespective of the nature or type of wound, the same basic processes are required to bring about wound healing, and yet wound care has altered so dramatically over the past 20 years that nurses often feel overwhelmed by the array of dressings and treatments available.[5]

Currently available wound dressings

- *Absorbent dressings*, e.g. gauze, gamgee, and lint, are highly absorbent, but have a tendency to adhere to wound surfaces, causing trauma and pain on removal.

- *Low-adherence dressings* are those that have one non-adherent surface intended for direct contact with the wound. They are for use on minor wounds with minimal exudate.
- *Tulle dressings* are sheets of gauze impregnated with various amounts of paraffin, antiseptics, or other agents. They too are best used with low-exudate wounds.
- *Semi-permeable dressings* consist of clear polyurethane film coated with adhesive. When used with low exudating wounds, they conform well and allow unimpeded observation of the wound site.
- *Polysaccharide dressings* work by exerting osmotic action at the wound surface. They are available as pastes, beads, and ointments and are intended to be used during the inflammatory phase of sloughy or infected wounds.
- On contact with the wound surface *hydrocolloids* form a gel, which creates an ideal, moist, wound-healing environment.
- *Hydrogels* are especially suited for use in cavities and are effective débriding/desloughing agents.
- *Alginates* are intended for use on moderately or heavily exudating wounds. On absorbing secretions they form a gel, creating optimum humidity and temperature for wound healing.
- *Foam dressings* are highly absorbent materials suitable for a wide range of granulating wounds.[6-8]

There are many types of wounds and several methods exist to classify them. However, there is to date no universally accepted classification system and wounds may be described as:

- mechanical injuries, incorporating abrasions, lacerations, penetrating wounds, bites, and surgical wounds
- burns and chemical injuries, incorporating superficial, deep dermal, and full-thickness thermal, chemical, electrical, and radiation burns
- chronic ulcerative wounds, which can be divided into decubitus ulcers (pressures sores), leg ulcers (venous, ischaemic, or traumatic), and ulcers arising from systemic infections, radiotherapy, or malignant disease[6]
- acute wounds, which include surgical and traumatic wounds

- chronic wounds, which include the ulcers, malignant and fungating wounds.[5]

Patients with cancer are at risk of developing any one of these many types of wounds.

Principles of wound healing

Damaged tissue passes through a number of phases of repair following injury. Inflammatory, destructive, proliferative, and maturation phases are characterised by numerous overlapping processes involving cell regeneration and proliferation, and collagen production.[9] In the surgical management of wound healing, four types of repair are recognised and a brief overview of the types of wound healing and phases involved is outlined below.[6]

Primary closure
Clean surgical wounds or newly inflicted traumatic injuries are managed by primary closure. When wounds heal by primary closure, granulation tissue and scar formation are visible. An acute inflammatory phase begins within a few minutes of injury, resulting in constriction of smooth muscle, reduced blood flow, and aggregation of collagen and platelets at the wound site.[10] Activation of the clotting mechanism occurs and results in the production of a clot or plug, which brings about haemostasis, while supporting and strengthening the injured tissue.[6] As the capillary walls at the damaged site become permeable, serum, leucocytes, erythrocytes, and antibodies pass into the wound. During the destructive phase of wound healing, and within hours of clot formation, polymorphonuclear leucocytes and macrophages begin the process of removing debris and bacteria from the wound site.[11] After a period of about 24 hours, epidermal cells begin to grow across the surface of the wound underneath the now dried scab, and depending on the nature and size of the wound, this process will continue for 2–3 days.

Open granulation
When drawing the edges of a wound together immediately is inadvisable, for example following major surgery or when there is a considerable risk

of infection, open granulation becomes the healing method of choice.[6] Open granulation is by necessity a slower process than primary closure, involving the progressive filling of the wound with granulation tissue. Granulation tissue is composed of collagen, a complex mixture of proteins and polysaccharides, salts, and other colloid materials.[6] When the wound cavity is almost filled with granulation tissue, the epithelium around the wound margin becomes active and strands of collagen are drawn across the surface of the wound.[11] This early collagen is very delicate and the wound needs to be stabilised to prevent damaging its delicate structure. Collagen growth is dependent upon a good supply of oxygen and an adequate supply of vitamin C.[9]

Delayed or secondary closure

Delayed primary closure occurs following infection, break down of the healing process, or when there is a poor blood supply.[6] Delayed primary closure involves leaving the wound open for 3–4 days before closure is undertaken, or involves resuturing of a previously closed wound.

During the maturation phase of healing, fibroblasts begin to leave the wound and as a result of dehydration and reorganisation of collagen fibres, the edges of the wound are drawn together through a process of contraction.[5] However, open granulation and contraction may be unacceptable where the scar left by the injury is to be visible, as contraction, especially of a facial wound, may result in distortion of surrounding features.

Grafting or flap formation

Grafting involves the removal of a portion of skin from one anatomical site, usually the thigh or buttock, to be placed onto a wound elsewhere. Despite offering rapid potential for healing, grafting results in the patient having two wounds instead of one. There is also considerable anecdotal evidence that donor sites cause greater pain than the original wound.

Skin flaps involve raising a portion of skin and subcutaneous tissue and rotating it to cover an area of skin loss.[6] Adequate blood supply, and prevention of infection and stress at the graft or flap site are essential factors in the success of these procedures.

Assessment

Nursing management of wounds will only be effective if based on informed decisions following a thorough assessment of objective and subjective information.[5] This requires a systematic approach to wound management and involves consideration of many inter-related variables. A key component of the assessment process is the nurse's ability and willingness to enter into a relationship with the patient, which engenders trust and a mutual respect (see Figure 21.1). The rationale for wound dressing is shown in Figure 21.2.

What must it be like to have a foul-smelling or heavily exudating wound that requires frequent dressing changes and constantly reminds you of a life-threatening disease that you cannot walk away from? This must be recognised and efforts made to sustain or re-establish a sense of dignity and security at a time of vulnerability and dependency:

> Nursing is a metaphor for intimacy . . . Nurses do for others publicly what healthy persons do for themselves behind closed doors . . . [they] are there to hear secrets especially those born of vulnerability . . . and nurses are indelibly identified with those terribly personal times.[12]

Factors interfering with normal processes of wound healing in cancer

The *ageing process* is associated with reduced tissue elasticity, increased likelihood of systemic diseases, impaired immune and inflammatory responses, and generally impaired vascularity. Since cancer is recognised as being primarily a disease of old age, these factors are all likely to complicate wound healing. *Impaired oxygen supply* further compounds the healing process. Phagocytes cannot function effectively when oxygen availability is reduced and as this deficit may arise as a consequence of inadequate lung and cardiovascular function, patients with primary lung cancer or secondary metastatic spread to the lungs may be highly susceptible to delayed wound healing. Chemotherapy commonly results in anaemia, further compromising oxygen availability.

Nutritional status influences wound healing. Efficient wound healing is dependent on the availability of adequate energy, and yet cancer causes

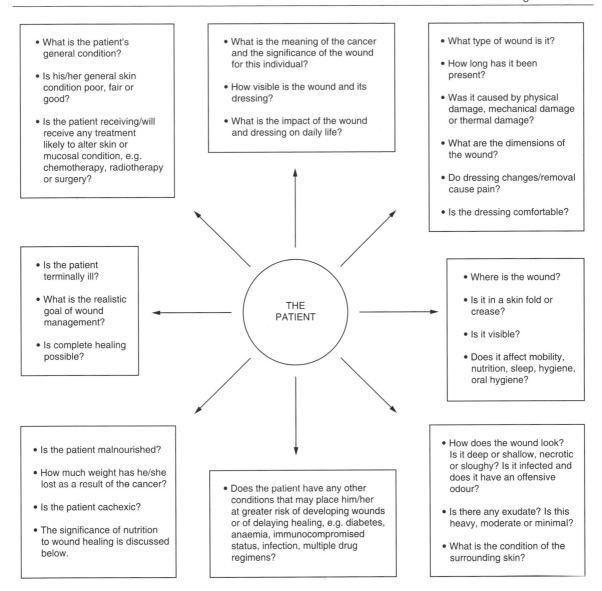

Figure 21.1   A framework for comprehensive assessment.

metabolic demands that greatly exceed energy intake as a result of the demands of the tumour upon the host.[13] Any form of trauma, and particularly a diagnosis of cancer, results in a triggering of a hypothalamic chain of events that culminates in a physiological state known as catabolism, where plasma proteins are utilised to satisfy increased energy demands, at a time when carbohydrate stores are depleted.[14] Of especial relevance for the individual with cancer is the fact that the longer the duration

of injury or stress, the greater the impact on nutritional requirements and extent of catabolism. The nutritional consequences for those who may be ill for months or years are therefore considerable.

Nutritional requirements for the wound healing process include copper, iron, zinc, magnesium, the fat-soluble vitamins A and K, and the water-soluble vitamins B1, B5, and C.[14] In cancer, the risk of malnutrition as a result of anorexia, nausea and vomiting, malabsorption, cachexia, anxiety, and

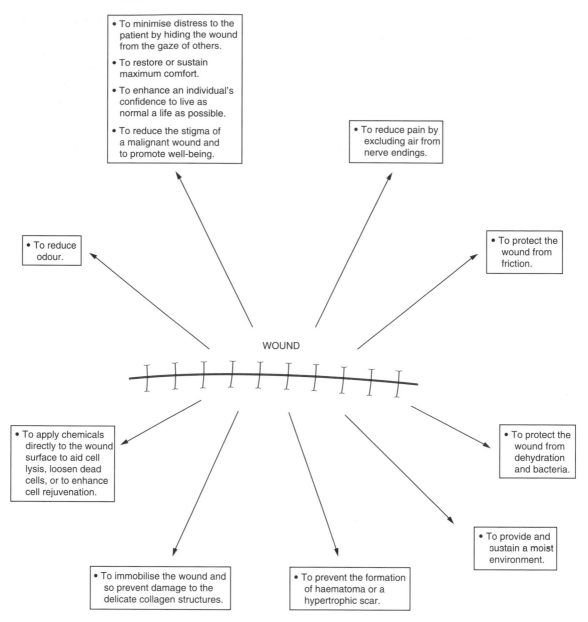

Figure 21.2 Rationale for dressing a wound.[6–8]

depression, leading to increased metabolic rate or reduced intake, as well as tumour-induced metabolic requirements, is great. Undernourishment delays wound healing owing to a reduction in collagen synthesis, while plasma proteins essential for effective wound healing may be utilised elsewhere to satisfy increased energy requirements.[11] The protein demands for tissue repair are consequently unmet. The role of assessing patients' nutritional status and needs for dietary supplements in promoting wound healing is of central importance.

Most chemotherapeutic agents adversely affect dietary intake, often resulting in prolonged periods of reduced food intake. This can lead to weight loss, progressive disability and malnutrition. Nausea and vomiting, diarrhoea, food aversion, and taste changes are but a few of the consequences of chemotherapy, which indirectly impact on wound healing. Similarly, radiotherapy directed at the gastrointestinal tract can result in severe nutritional deficiencies. Malabsorption and malnutrition may arise as a result, as well as severe nausea and vomiting, diarrhoea, and abdominal cramps.[13]

Early detection of potential would infections is important. Signs of inflammation and discharge are commonly relied upon to alert us to potential problems. However, for the individual with cancer, such indicators may be of limited value if treatment has induced neutropenia, if steroids are being taken, or if tumour-related complications result in inadequate inflammatory response. Swelling, redness, and discharge may all be absent.[15] An effective defence system is a critical component of effective wound healing, but for patients receiving a plethora of drugs and treatments that impact significantly upon immunological status and capacity for inflammatory response, the risk of infection and delayed wound healing is considerable. Steroids are especially potent inhibitors of inflammatory response to injury.[15] Anti-coagulants may cause haemorrhage and interfere with clot and scar formation. Chemotherapeutic agents and immunotherapies have the capacity to suppress immune response and to enhance vulnerability to viral and bacterial infection, as well as impairing clotting and healing.[9] Varying degrees of tissue injury arising from radiotherapy can result in the development of an actual wound, which may become the focus for a local infection, or the site of a systemic infection.

Fungating wounds

Of all the lesions experienced by individuals with cancer, perhaps the most distressing for patients, relatives, and health professionals alike are fungating wounds. When malignant tumour cells infiltrate and erode through the skin a wound is said to be 'fungating'.[16] Breast cancer, melanoma, bladder, colon, kidney, ovary, uterus, stomach, head and neck, and lung cancers all have this potential. Fungating breast wounds, however, are reported as being the most commonly occurring.[16,17] Fungating wounds often occur in locally advanced,

metastatic, or recurrent disease, but this is not always the case. They are often characterised by malodorous exudate, whether serous or blood, which may seep out onto clothing, causing extreme distress.[18] Fungating wounds may cause withdrawal from social activities, or daily life, as the persistent odour or heavily exudating wound necessitates frequent dressing changes.[19]

Addressing the psychological impact of a fungating wound, alongside highly skilled physical wound management, is of paramount importance.

The aims of managing fungating wounds are to:

- control tumour growth
- prevent and halt surface bleeding
- where possible, restore skin integrity.[16]

Treatment may include major therapeutic modalities such as chemotherapy, radiotherapy, surgery, hormone manipulation, or a combination of these. Local treatment includes haemostatic agents and topical metronidazole, along with systemic analgesics, antibiotics, or clotting factors as necessary.[20,21] Currently available wound dressings are frequently inadequate for fungating wounds.[22–24] Nursing and multi-disciplinary research, alongside innovative practice developments, are examining strategies for managing these wounds.[17,25,26] Until such time as there are proven data to support the use of a dressing designed specifically for fungating wounds, dressings should be chosen following a consideration of problems identified during a thorough assessment.

Irrespective of the nature of the wound being managed, the rationale for dressing it, the requirements of the wound, and the individual's wishes and expectations form the basis of the decision-making process. Meaningful assessment of outcomes of care and evaluation of interventions employed can only be undertaken successfully following consideration of the processes described above. Once appropriate dressings are identified, planning how the wound can best be managed in partnership with the person and their immediate carers will offer a greater chance of mutual achievement of an agreed outcome. Together can be drawn up a plan of care where wound management is far more than simply a physical affair, reflecting an attempt to respect individuality and circumstance.

Innovations in practice in the management of fungating wounds

Researchers at King's College, London, have undertaken a research project to explore patients' symptoms and experiences of fungating malignant wounds.

They set out to establish how selected dressings, based on maintaining a moist wound environment, control the symptoms and the impact of a fungating wound. The aim was to introduce the concept of an individually moulded wound support system as an accessory, and to observe its effects on symptom control and impact on the patient's daily life.[27]

Key assertions arising from their work to date include the following.

- The assessment of fungating malignant wounds is holistic and multi-disciplinary.
- The patient's perception of priorities for wound management is reflected in the management plan.
- Management outcomes are stated in terms of symptom control at the wound site and reduced impact of the wound in daily life.[28]

References

1. Murphy R.F. (1987). *The Body Silent.* London: W.W. Norton.
2. Goffman E. (1963). *Stigma. Notes on the Management of Spoiled Identity.* New York: Simon & Schuster.
3. Kleinman A. (1988). *The Illness Narratives: Suffering, Healing and the Human Condition.* New York: Basic Books.
4. Gaut D. and Leininger M. (eds.) (1991). *Caring: The Compassionate Healer.* New York: National League for Nursing Press.
5. Flanagan M. (1994). Assessment criteria. *Nursing Times* 31, August–September, 90, 76, 78, 80.
6. Thomas S. (1990). *Wound Management and Dressings.* London: Pharmaceutical Press.
7. Miller M. (1994). The ideal healing environment. *Nursing Standard* 9, 54, 56.
8. Quick A. (1994). Dressing choices. *Nursing Times* 90, 68.
9. Brunner L. and Suddarth D. (eds.) (1992). *The Textbook of Adult Nursing.* London: Chapman and Hall.
10. Winter G.D. (1978). Wound healing. *Nursing Mirror* 146 (Suppl.), 10.
11. Senter H. and Pringle A. (1985). *How Wounds Heal: A Practical Guide for Nurses.* Cheshire: Wellcome Foundation.
12. Fagin C. and Diers D. (1983). Nursing as metaphor. Occasional notes. New *England Journal of Medicine* 309, 116.
13. Holmes S. (1987). Malignant disease: nutritional implications of disease and treatment. *Cancer and Metastasis Reviews* 6, 357–381.
14. Hallett A. (1994). Vital ingredients. *Nursing Times* 90.
15. Cutting K. (1994). Detecting infection. *Nursing Times* 90, 60, 62.
16. Grocott P. (1995). The palliative management of fungating malignant wounds. *Journal of Wound Care* 4, 240–242.
17. Mortimer P. (1993). Skin problems in palliative care: medical aspects. In Doyle D., Hanks G. and Macdonald N. (eds.) *Oxford Textbook of Palliative Medicine.* Oxford: Oxford Medical Publications.
18. Neal K. (1991). Treating fungating lesion. *Nursing Times* 87, 84–85.
19. Clark L. (1992). Caring for fungating tumours. *Nursing Times* 88, 72–75.
20. Reynard C. and Tempest S. (1992). *A Guide to Symptom Relief in Advanced Cancer,* 3rd edition. London: Haigh and Hochland.
21. Hoy A. (1993). Other symptom challenges. In Saunders C. and Sykes N. (eds.) *The Management of Terminal Malignant Disease,* 3rd edition. London: Edward Arnold.
22. Simms R. and Fitzgerald V. (1985). *Community Nursing Management of Patients with Ulcerating Fungating Malignant Breast Disease.* London: Oncology Nursing Society.
23. Bennet M. (1985). As normal a life as possible. *Nursing Times* (Community Outlook Suppl.) 81, 7.
24. Preston K. and Griffen J. (1989). Complex wound management. A case study. *Rehabilitation Nursing* 14, 269–170.
25. Banks V. and Jones V. (1993). Palliative care of a patient with terminal nasal carcinoma. *Journal of Wound Care* 2, 14–15.
26. Boardman M., Mellor K. and Neville B. (1994). Treating a patient with a heavily exudating malodorous fungating ulcer. *Journal of Wound Care* 2, 74–76.
27. Grocott P. (1995). Assessment of fungating malignant wounds. *Journal of Wound Care* 4, 333–336.
28. Moody M. and Grocott P. (1993). Let us extend our knowledge base. Assessment and management of fungating malignant wounds. *Professional Nurse,* June, 586–590.

CHAPTER TWENTY-TWO

Lymphoedema

Angela Williams

The lymphatic system

The lymphatic system is a one-way drainage system that transports a colourless fluid called lymph from the tissues to the blood vascular system (Figure 22.1). The system allows continuous and rapid removal of interstitial fluids, plasma proteins, cells and debris, thus playing an important role in maintaining the physiological environment of the body.

Box 22.1: The lymphatic system

The most peripheral vessels, termed initial lymphatics, undertake the primary function of the lymphatic system, reabsorbing part of the water and electrolytes and most of the proteins that are continuously leaving the blood capillaries and entering the interstitial fluid. The mechanism of the movement of interstitial fluid into the initial lymphatics is uncertain.[1]

These numerous small, thin-walled vessels flow into larger, thicker-walled collecting vessels, which in turn flow into the major lymphatic trunks. The larger vessels transport the collected material through groups of lymph nodes and finally form two large lymphatic trunks called the thoracic duct and the right lymphatic duct, which drain into the large veins at the base of the neck.

The factors responsible for lymph propulsion in lymph vessels include intrinsic contractility, muscular activity, respiratory movements, passive movements, pulsation of blood vessels, and gut motility.[2]

What is lymphoedema?

Lymphoedema is an incurable, progressive condition characterised by chronic swelling, most commonly of a limb and sometimes the adjacent quadrant of the trunk. It is defined as an excess of fluid tissue proteins and lipid causing chronic inflammation and fibrosis due to lymphatic failure. The retention of water is largely through osmotic forces from the accumulated tissue protein. In the majority of cases, chronic oedema will be secondary to circulatory problems, such as venous or lymphatic insufficiencies. It rarely develops from the failure of either the venous or the lymphatic system alone. When the principal fault is the failure of the transport capacity of the lymphatic system, this is termed 'true' or lymphostatic lymphoedema. Other chronic oedemas result from various combinations of lymphatic and venous insufficiency and limb immobility and dependency.[3] All forms of chronic oedema and lymphostatic lymphoedema can occur in cancer, with or without the presence of active disease.

Lymphoedema and cancer

In developed countries, lymphoedema occurs most commonly with cancer or following cancer treatment, due to secondary obstruction or trauma of the lymphatics and venous system. Reliable figures on the size of the problem are largely

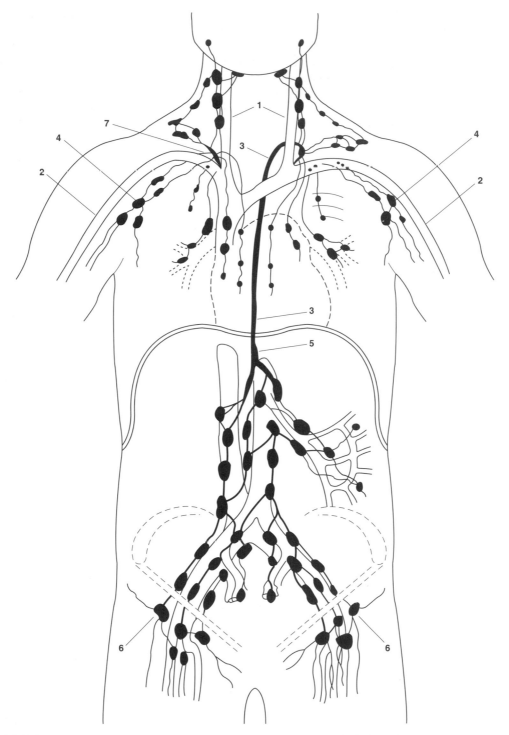

Figure 22.1 Main lymph trunks and lymph node groups in the body (adapted with permission from *Textbook of Dr Vodder's Manual Lymph Drainage*, Vol. 1., *Basic Course*, 4th edition. Brussels: Editions Haug International). (1) Internal jugular vein; (2) subclavian vein; (3) thoracic duct; (4) axillary lymph nodes; (5) cisterna chyli; (6) inguinal lymph nodes; (7) right lymphatic duct.

confined to incidence rates for lymphoedema related to breast cancer and its treatment. Studies of the incidence of lymphoedema following radiotherapy or clearance of the axilla suggest that 25% of women with breast cancer will subsequently develop lymphoedema; this increases to 38% if axillary clearance and radiotherapy are performed.[4] The incidence rates of lower limb lymphoedema in other cancer sites or in advanced disease are unknown.[5]

The pathogenesis of breast cancer-related lymphoedema seems to be a lymphostatic lymphoedema, where the lymphatic system is damaged or obstructed by cancer treatment. Axillary lymph nodes are surgically removed or irradiated and the lymph vessels fail to regenerate. Irradiated, scarred, and fibrotic tissue decreases the transport capacity of the lymphatic system, resulting in pooling of high-protein oedema. However, studies reported in the early 1990s suggest that its development involves factors additional to axillary node and lymphatic vessel trauma.

Box 22.2: Recent studies of the pathogenesis of lymphoedema

Studies by Svensson et al. suggested that obstruction in venous outflow and an increase in arterial inflow are important contributory factors in the pathophysiology of arm swelling, and should considered complicating factors.[6,7]

Bates et al.[8,9] suggested that haemodynamic abnormalities were present, prompting further experimental evaluation of filtration and lymph flow.

Roberts et al.[10] assessed the microvascular architecture and density in the skin of human post-mastecomy oedema, compared to the unaffected limb. The findings tentatively support the view that cutaneous neovascularisation occurs in swollen arms, so influencing fluid load on the lymphatic system.

Diagnosis of lymphoedema

The early diagnosis and treatment of lymphoedema is important if long-term control is to be achieved. Diagnosis is often late, because although lymphoedema can develop immediately following treatment, it may also occur decades later, when the individual has been without active dis-ease for many years and is no longer attending regular follow-up appointments.

Nurses in the hospital and the community have an important role in the early recognition of lymphoedema, as they are likely to come into contact with such women. At the time of treatment, information should be given to women with breast cancer on ways to minimise the risk of developing lymphoedema and on who to contact if they develop swelling.[11] Risk factors for developing lymphoedema are:

- post-operative wound infection/seroma or radiodermatitis[12]
- infections of soft tissue of the arm; tumour on the side of the dominant hand[13]
- obesity.[14]

Diagnosis of lymphoedema is usually made from the patient's history, and from clinical observations. With the exception of the early stages of lymphoedema, when pitting occurs with the application of pressure and the oedema may be reduced by elevation of the swollen limb, lymphoedema does not reduce significantly with elevation or with diuretic administration. Skin problems may also be noted in early stages, as well as in more complicated lymphoedema. These include:

- dry skin
- callosities and corns
- fungal infections
- hyperkeratosis
- acute inflammatory episodes (infective and non-infective)
- contact dermatitis.[15,16]

If lymphoedema is not recognised and treated early, the accumulation of stagnant protein-rich oedema in the skin and upper tissues produces characteristic skin and upper tissue changes. A process of inflammation is stimulated, giving rise to fibrosis and overgrowth of interstitial connective tissue and depression of macrophage activity (phagocytosis). The skin loses elasticity, developing 'papillomatous' dermatitis, with the enhancement of skin folds, loss of hair, and alterations to the nails.[2,17] Stemmer's sign, or the inability to pinch the thickened skin at the base of the digits, is often present and differentiates lymphoedema from other types of oedema. In less typical cases, imaging methods

Table 22.1 Nursing research into lymphoedema[18-23,29-32]

Williams, 1992	Describes the establishment of a community-based lymphoedema service in one district health authority.
Carroll and Rose, 1992	A small study to define the pain present in patients with breast cancer-related lymphoedema and to establish whether conservative management reduces pain during the first 3 months of treatment.
Williams, 1993	Review of the first year of the community-based lymphoedema service.
Woods, 1993	Describes the objectives of a hospital-based service.
Woods, 1993	A study of 40 women with breast cancer-related lymphoedema to explore their perceptions of the condition and factors that may be associated with these perceptions.
Williams *et al.*, 1996	Review of 5 years of an out-patient lymphoedema service and the recommendations for service development.
Sitzia and Sobrido, 1997	A study to consider the measurement of health-related quality of life for patients receiving conservative treatment for limb lymphoedema using the Nottingham Health Profile.
Badger, 1997	A study of the efficacy of multi-layer bandaging and elastic hosiery in the treatment of lymphoedema and their effects of the swollen limb (Ph.D. Degree).
Williams and Williams, 1999	A pilot study examining the compression under a selection of sleeves used in the treatment of breast cancer-related lymphoedema.

such as magnetic resonance imaging (MRI), ultrasound scanning, and *in vivo* visualisation of lymphatic vessels, such as quantitative lymphoscintigraphy, may be used to confirm diagnosis.[3]

Treating lymphoedema

In continental Europe conservative, non-invasive, physical treatments for lymphoedema are well established. The principle of physical therapy is to perform interventions that would normally enhance lymph flow and so maximise remaining lymph transport capacity. It is claimed that swelling can often be reduced dramatically with this therapy, but there is little objective, published evidence to confirm this.[28]

In Britain up until the mid 1980s, treatment approaches were without consensus and largely inappropriate, owing to general ignorance as to the difference between high-protein lymphoedema and low-protein venous oedemas. Treatment using surgery and drugs generally gave unsatisfactory results. The rationale behind the use of the most common treatments (pneumatic compression and elastic hosiery) was often poorly understood by those using them.[29] Provision of treatment was also haphazard and therefore largely ineffective.

In the latter half of the 1980s, it became clear, in particular to nurses working in palliative care and breast cancer, that a sizeable problem existed. Information regarding treatment was sought from continental Europe, thus starting a slow process of learning, developing, and implementing new approaches to treatment. It was not long before the first nursing, out-patient lymphoedema service was established in Oxford, providing diagnosis, treatment, and long-term follow-up to a wide variety of patients. Other specialised nursing and physiotherapy services and clinics were soon set up, together with an increasing awareness of the need for education of all health care professionals about the condition. In recent years, there has been a significant increase in the number of professionals specialising in the management of lymphoedema. The nursing contribution to the development of lymphoedema management in Britain indisputably demonstrates the value of nursing practice and the significance of specialist nursing knowledge in improving patient care. In addition, the more holistic approach to lymphoedema care has suited a nursing philosophy, as opposed to a medical one.[18]

Nursing research in the field has only just begun; the focus to date has been on improving the provision of lymphoedema treatment in community-

and hospital-based services.[18–21] An empirically derived knowledge base with respect to treatment methods and psychosocial experiences is also evolving as a result of nurse-led research.[22,23] As yet, however, there has been little research to evaluate clinical and cost-effectiveness. There are few prospective evaluation studies of lymphoedema management; instead, small studies using various designs have been undertaken, which can at best be considered only as pilot studies and are insufficient to guide changes in clinical practice. Until results from well-conducted studies are available, physical treatment based on Foldi's methods[28] is considered the most appropriate treatment option for lymphostatic lymphoedema.

Physical treatment for lymphoedema

Treatment for lymphoema is determined by the mechanism underlying its formation and the time of its onset. Lymphostatic lymphoedema, as well as various combinations of lymphatic and venous insufficiency (for example, secondary to tumour obstruction and dependency oedemas, can all occur in cancer, with or without the presence of active disease. It is obviously crucial to have an accurate diagnosis of the underlying cause for the oedema and to obtain advice from appropriate health care team members on its management.

The aim of physical treatment is to restore the disturbed equilibrium between the lymphatic protein load and lymph transport capacity, by increasing the latter and so removing excess protein from the tissue spaces,[28] and to address physical problems such as recurrent infection, reduced mobility, and impaired function. Discomfort or pain and secondary musculoskeletal and joint problems may also accompany lymphoedema and need intervention, as does the psychological impact of having a swollen or disfigured limb.[23] Some of these difficulties are illustrated in the quotes that follow.

> Sometimes my leg is so swollen that I cannot bend my knee stopping me from walking and cycling.

> I am unable to get in and out of a bath.

> I cannot wash my hair.

> . . . my arm becomes very uncomfortable if I try to do too much housework or gardening.

> . . . by the end of the day my shoulders and neck ache and it is difficult to get comfortable and go to sleep.

> . . . finding clothes to fit with a swollen arm is difficult and depressing.

> . . . because I am embarrassed and conscious of my leg I won't undress or change in front of anyone, not even family.

The treatment of lymphoedema comprises two phases. The *intensive/drainage phase* comprises skin care, exercise, a form of lymphatic massage, and compression bandaging. It is performed by a therapist over a 2–4-week period. This first phase is aimed at reducing the size of the limb, improving the condition of the skin and subcutaneous tissues, and moulding the shape of the limb to that of a 'normal' one. The second *maintenance phase* is of conservation and optimisation, and comprises skin care, exercise, a form of lymphatic massage and using compression garments. It is taught by the therapist, then continued as daily self-care. Not all lymphoedema patients receive a period of intensive treatment, moving straight into this second phase of treatment. However, the criteria for receiving a period of intensive treatment are not standardised amongst therapists. Badger[15] demonstrated in her research that treatment using hosiery is less effective at reducing moderate to severe lymphoedema (>20% excess limb volume) and restoring shape in the short and the long term than treatment using a period of multi-layer bandaging followed by elastic compression hosiery. This result suggests that a period of intensive treatment is required if the excess limb volume is >20%. Attentive monitoring of the limb must be ongoing, using objective recordings of limb volume measurements and subjective assessments of the limb by the person themselves and by the therapist.

The management of lymphoedema requires motivation and perseverance, since long-term compliance with the daily regimen of care is essential. Adherence to the regimen of daily care and the necessary adjustments to lifestyle that this demands are major problems in many chronic conditions and are a common reason for lymphoedema to deteriorate and reaccumulate in the monitoring phase of treatment.[30] The assessment or measurement of the extent to which compliance or non-compliance with health regimens occurs is difficult. The only study to assess compliance with long-term lymphoedema care is a telephone survey of stable, chronic lymphoedema patients. The study aimed to discover which components of treatment were complied with in the long term, and to ascertain which ongoing problems were experienced by patients. Some of these problems are reflected in the comments below.[31]

> I have to get up nearly an hour earlier in the morning to allow time to put my stockings on after doing the massage and exercises.

> I can't be spontaneous as I have to fit in my self-management routine every day, even on holiday.

> I miss walking in bare feet.

> I no longer go on holiday to hot climates for fear of getting an infection again.

Skin care

Skin care is an important element of the treatment regime. The aims of skin care are:

- to improve the condition of the epidermis and dermis so that they are hydrated, intact, and supple
- to reduce the risk of infection. Protein-rich, static fluid in the tissue spaces is an ideal environment for bacteria to multiply.

Skin care includes:

- good daily hygiene, taking care to wash and dry carefully, especially between the digits
- regular, careful inspection of the skin, observing for changes
- avoiding other sources of skin damage, e.g. sunburn, needles, razors, insect bites
- reducing the risk of cuts and grazes by prompt cleaning and application of antiseptic ointment
- wearing comfortable, well-fitting clothes/shoes
- daily application of bland emollients, avoiding perfumed or lanolin-containing products
- use of appropriate dermatological products for specific skin problems.[32]

External compression

Compression using multi-layer compression bandaging or garments limits blood capillary filtration by raising interstitial pressure, opposing tissue pressure, and improving striated muscle pump efficiency.[3] Multi-layer compression bandaging, as with any other form of therapeutic bandaging, must be applied by therapists with knowledge and training in its application. The technique provides a high pressure during muscular contraction but low pressure at rest. Garments must also be chosen and fitted with advice from a therapist and in some cases from the surgical appliance officer as well. High compression (>40 mmHg) is usually required to maintain control of the lymphoedema. It is vital that health care professionals are aware of who offers treatment in their area and refer appropriately for compression bandaging or garment fitting and supply.

Exercise

Exercise encourages lymph flow through the massaging effect of muscular activity on the lymphatics and surrounding tissues, and promotes lymph flow within the abdominal cavity. Exercise will also benefit joint movement and promote good posture. The optimum exercise an individual should do depends on a number of factors, such as age, sex, occupation, lifestyle, and level of physical fitness. It should be sufficient to favour limb drainage by stimulating lymph flow, but not excessively, so that there is greater arterial inflow. Walking and swimming are excellent activities to accompany specific exercise routines as part of a daily regime. The effect of any exercise is maximised if wearing external compression on the swollen limb while exercising. It is vital to combine relaxation periods with periods of exercise equally. Immobility of the limb is not encouraged.

Massage

In Britain, the most widely used lymphatic massage is a simple form of skin surface massage, used to encourage the movement of lymph along the skin and subcutaneous lymphatics from the swollen, congested areas to normally draining areas, bypassing the lymph system obstruction. This form of lymph massage is based on the principles of manual lymph drainage practised widely in Europe. Massage is used in a daily routine of simple self-massage on the normal lymph-draining areas, commencing centrally at the neck and working towards the swollen limb, but not including the limb itself.[11] Nurses should offer encouragement with continuing daily massage and also some assistance if appropriate.

Summary

The physical treatment of lymphoedema can do much to improve the physical and psychosocial outlook for a patient with this incurable, chronic condition. Increased awareness and understanding by all health care professionals regarding the lymphatic system and the physical treatment methods could augment the development of lymphoedema treatment. Along with this improvement in education and service provision, research addressing the basic clinical issues of treatment must be developed to evaluate treatment clinical and cost-effectiveness.

References

1. Jimenez Cossio J.A. (1994). Physiology of lymphatic oedema. *Phlebology* (Suppl. 1), 19–22.
2. Olszewski W. (1985). *Peripheral Lymph: Formation and Immune Function.* Florida, FL: CRC Press.
3. Mortimer P.S. (1990). Investigation and management of lymphoedema. *Vascular Medicine Review* 1, 1–20.
4. Kissin M.W., Querci della Rovera G., Easton D. and Westbury G. (1986). Risk of lymphoedema following the treatment of breast cancer. *British Journal of Surgery* 73, 580–584.
5. Logan V. (1995). Incidence and prevalence of lymphoedema: a literature review. *Journal of Clinical Nursing* 4, 213–219.
6. Svensson W.E., Mortimer P.S., Tohno E. and Cosgrove D.O. (1994). Colour doppler demonstrates venous flow abnormalities in breast cancer patients with chronic arm swelling. *European Journal of Cancer* 30A, 657–660.
7. Svensson W.E., Mortimer P.S., Tohno E. and Cosgrove D.O. (1994). Increased arterial inflow demonstrated by doppler ultrasound in arm swelling following breast cancer treatment. *European Journal of Cancer* 30A, 661–664.
8. Bates D.O., Levick J.R. and Mortimer P.S. (1992). Subcutaneous interstitial pressure and arm volume in lymphoedema. *International Journal of Microcirculation: Clinical and Experimental* 11, 359–373.
9. Bates D.O., Levick J.R. and Mortimer P.S. (1994). Starling pressures in the human arm and their alteration in postmastectomy oedema. *Journal of Physiology* 477, 355–363.
10. Roberts C.C., Stanton A.W.B., Pullen J., Bull R.H., Levick J.R., and Mortimer P.S. (1994). Skin microvascular architecture and perfusion studied in human postmastectomy oedema by intra video-capillaroscopy. *International Journal of Microcirculation: Clinical and Experimental* 14, 327–334.
11. Reynard C., Badger C. and Mortimer P. (1991). *Lymphoedema: Advice on Treatment,* 2nd edition. Beaconsfield: Beaconsfield Publishers.
12. Britton R.C. and Nelson P.A. (1962). Causes and treatment of postmastectomy lymphoedema of the arm: report of 114 cases. *Journal of the American Medical Association* 180, 95–102.
13. Segerstrom K., Bjerle P., Graffman S. and Nystrom A. (1992). Factors that influence the incidence of brachial oedema after treatment of breast cancer. *Scandinavian Journal of Plastic and Reconstructive Hand Surgery* 26, 223–227.
14. Mozes M., Papa M.Z., Karasik A., Reshef A. and Adar R. (1982). The role of infection in post-mastectomy lymphoedema. *Annals of Surgery* 14, 73–83.
15. Veitch J. (1993). Skin problems in lymphoedema. *Wound Management* 4, 42–45.
16. Jeffs E. (1993). The effect of acute inflammatory episodes (cellulitis) on the treatment of lymphoedema. *Journal of Tissue Viability* 3, 51–55.
17. Casley-Smith J.R. (1992). Modern treatment of lymphoedema. *Modern Medicine of Australia* 35, 70–83.
18. Williams A.E. and Badger C. (1996). The management of lymphoedema: a developing specialism for nursing? *International Journal of Palliative Nursing* 2, 50–53.
19. Williams A.E. (1992). Management of lymphoedema: a community based approach. *British Journal of Nursing* 1, 383–387.
20. Williams A.E. (1993). Management of lymphoedema: a community based approach. *British Journal of Nursing* 2, 678–681.
21. Woods M. (1993). A hospital based service for lymphoedema management. *European Journal of Cancer Care* 2, 165–168.
22. Carroll D. and Rose K. (1992). Treatment leads to significant improvement: effect of conservative treatment on pain in lymphoedema. *Professional Nurse,* October, 32–36.
23. Woods M. (1993). Patient's perceptions of breast cancer-related lymphoedema. *European Journal of Cancer Care* 2, 125–128.

24. Sitzia J. and Sobrido L. (1997). Measurement of health-related quality of life patients receiving conservative treatment for limb lymphoedema using the Nottingham Health Profile. *Quality of Life Research* **6**, 373–384.

25. Badger C. (1997). A study of the efficacy of multi-layer bandaging and elastic hosiery in the treatment of lymphoedema, and their effects on the swollen limb. Unpublished Ph.D. Thesis.

26. Williams A.F. and Williams A.E. (1999). 'Putting the pressure on': a study of compression sleeves used in breast cancer-related lymphoedema. *Journal of Tissue Viability* **9**, 89–94.

27. Williams A.E., Bergl S. and Twycross R.G. (1996). A 5-year review of a lymphoedema service. *European Journal of Cancer Care* **5**, 56–59.

28. Foldi E., Foldi M. and Weissleder H. (1985). Conservative treatment of lymphoedema of the limbs. *Angiology* **36**, 171–180.

29. Badger C. (1994). Pause for thought: nurses use research – don't they? *European Journal of Cancer Care* **3**, 63–66.

30. Cameron K. and Gregor F. (1987). Chronic illness and compliance. *Journal of Advanced Nursing* **12**, 671–676.

31. Rose K.E., Taylor H.M. and Twycross R.G. (1991). Long-term compliance with treatment in obstructive arm lymphoedema in cancer. *Palliative Medicine* **5**, 52–55.

32. Williams A.E. and Venables J. (1996). The management of skin problems in uncomplicated lymphoedema. *Journal of Wound Care* **5**, 223–226.

CHAPTER TWENTY-THREE

Malignant ascites

Nancy Preston

Malignant ascites is a form of lymphoedema that results in 6% of all hospice admissions and can affect up to 40% of patients with metastatic peritoneal deposits.[1] Malignant ascites can be defined as an exudate into the peritoneal space as a result of a malignancy. The primary cancer sites where malignant ascites is most common are ovary, breast, colon, stomach, and pancreas. Any tumour that results in metastatic peritoneal deposits also has a risk of ascites developing. Ascites is common in ovarian cancer; 33% of women diagnosed with ovarian cancer will have ascites at diagnosis and 60% will develop it before they die.

Common symptoms

As fluid accumulates the abdomen becomes distended, giving rise to a range of symptoms including:

- indigestion
- loss of appetite
- altered bowel habit
- abdominal discomfort
- abdominal distension
- changes in body image
- disruption in daily activities and lifestyle
- nausea and vomiting
- ankle oedema, fatigue
- shortness of breath.

Individually, each symptom can be addressed. Indigestion can be treated with regular antacids or even systemic H_2 antagonists. If this is controlled,

appetite might be improved but the ascites squashes the stomach, hence satiety is easily reached. Laxatives can help to maintain soft stool and mild pain killers might be needed for abdominal discomfort. A new wardrobe of clothes may be required as the waistline can increase considerably with ascites. With the change in size, patients' body image may alter. For some, this is not seen as a problem as their lives are predominantly based within the home, but for others this may have far-reaching effects upon femininity and sexuality. As the ascites increases so do the symptoms and this can mean becoming increasingly limited in what is manageable at home. Fatigue, nausea, vomiting, and breathlessness are an increasing consequence of the ascites, and the only way to resolve these problems is to remove the fluid.

Pathophysiology

The causes of malignant ascites are quite distinct from the causes of non-malignant ascites that may result, for example, from cirrhosis of the liver. There are three main causes for the development of malignant ascites:

- lymphatic obstruction
- increased peritoneal permeability
- disruption of the renin–angiotensin system.

Lymphatic obstruction was first noted to be a cause of malignant ascites in 1975.[2] Fluid in the peritoneal cavity leaves via the diaphragmatic lymphatics and ultimately drains back into the main circulation. It has been shown in animals that fluid accumulates after obstruction of the diaphragmatic lymphatics by cancer cells; fluid then builds up and ascites develops.[2] Capillaries are known to be more permeable in someone with ascites and as a consequence more fluid leaks into the peritoneal cavity. Tumours themselves can produce serous fluid and the renin–angiotension aldosterone system may also play a subsidiary role in ascites production. This system is responsible for sodium concentration in the body and a disruption in it may lead to increased fluid retention and exacerbate ascites.

Managing ascites

There is no consensus of opinion as to the optimum way to manage malignant ascites and there appears to be a disparity between palliative care and acute care settings. Palliative care practitioners advocate diuretics and occasional paracentesis, while in acute care attempts to manage ascites may include intraperitoneal therapy, radiotherapy, peritoneovenous shunts, or repeated paracentesis. Reynard and Mannix[1] have produced a helpful flow diagram of decision steps that should be taken when treating a patient with malignant ascites (see Figure 23.1).

Diuretic therapy

Consensus as to the use of diuretic therapy has yet to be achieved. Diuretic therapy has been dismissed by many authors as ineffective in controlling malignant ascites,[3,4] yet others have achieved success in their use with similar patient groups.[5] These discrepancies may be due to differences in prescribed diuretic dosages. Where diuretics have been shown to be effective, higher doses have been prescribed.[6]

There have been no published randomised studies to evaluate the role of diuretics in managing malignant ascites. Diuretics such as spironolactone compete with aldosterone for receptors on the proximal tubule of the kidney, inhibiting the effect of aldosterone.[7] In a series of 15 patients control of ascites was demonstrated in 13 using directics, thereby supporting the role of the renin–

angiotensin–aldosterone system in contributing to ascites formation.[5] The success of diuretics may, however, be due to redistribution of fluid.[6] Using high dose levels of diuretics may result in imbalance of serum electrolytes, but at least one study suggests that this may not be the case. However, a higher incidence of nausea and vomiting related to the use of spironolactone was reported.[5]

In one study, diuretic therapy was used in conjunction with water immersion with ascites resulting from cirrhosis of the liver.[8] Water immersion results in mobilisation of extracellular/ extravascular fluid, improving cardiac output and increasing excretion of salt and water. Restricted mobility in advanced cancer may mean that bathing is impossible, but for those who can this may offer a relaxing method of minimising the distress caused by ascites.

Intraperitoneal therapy

The success of intraperitoneal chemotherapy is likely to be dependent upon the sensitivity of the primary tumour. If a patient is still deemed sensitive to systemic doses of chemotherapy, then they are likely to respond to intraperitoneal doses. Many of those with malignant ascites have chemotherapy-resistant tumours, and those with sensitive tumours may benefit from intravenous administration, as this lessens the risk of infection, bleeding, and chemical peritonitis, which may accompany intraperitoneal use.[9] The side-effects of chemotherapy are, however, lower when administered intraperitoneally.

The use of biological modifiers has been under trial with ascites. In a series of studies using interferon-α2b, control was achieved in five out of 13 patients. All of those who responded positively had ascites only and had no tumour mass.[10] It is much more common with recurrent ascites to have disseminated disease also and the response rate to biological modifiers for this poor prognostic group needs further evaluation. The efficacy of all biological modifiers in relation to ascites is still very much under review.

Batimastat (BB94), derived from a new class of drugs known as the metalloproteinase inhibitors, has been introduced into randomised clinical trials against diuretic therapy in the treatment of malignant ascites. Metalloproteinase inhibitors

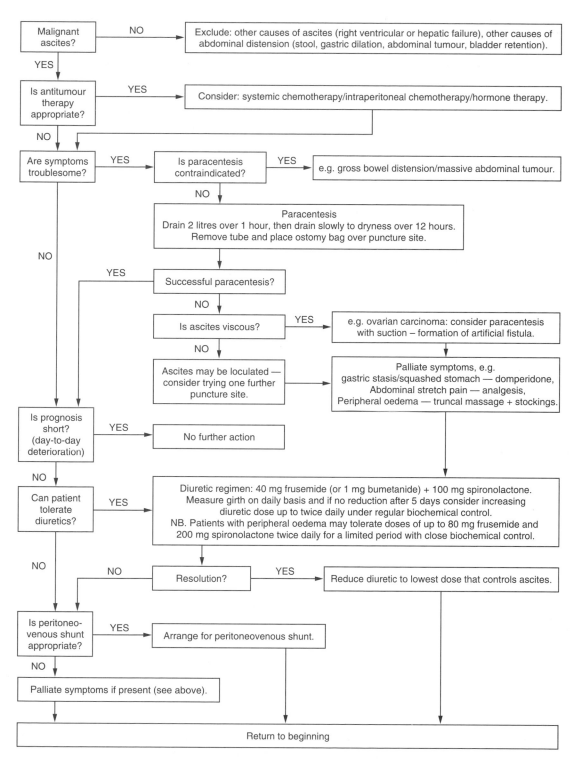

Figure 23.1 Management of ascites in advanced cancer (reproduced with permission from Reynard C. and Mannix K. (1989). *Palliative Medicine* **4,** 45–47).[1]

are primarily aimed at limiting malignant progression. Patients with ascites were chosen to examine this drug because of the success observed in controlling ascites in animal studies.[11] These studies are awaiting completion.

Repeated paracentesis

Anyone with cancer presenting with abdominal distension thought to be due to malignant ascites needs to have this diagnosis confirmed. This is done through cytology, where fluid removed at drainage is examined for malignant cells. Ascites can result from other medical conditions, hence it is imperative to demonstrate that the ascites has occurred due to malignancy. Any drainage of the peritoneal cavity has the risk of bowel perforation. As fluid builds up, so the bowel can float upwards. Insertion of any drainage tube should be carried out with ultrasound guidance, so that the largest area of fluid can be identified and marked for drainage.[12]

Drainage is carried out under local anaesthetic and can be uncomfortable. Further, paracentesis, although offering relief from symptoms, is only temporary and the fluid will reaccumulate. Repeated drainage may result in protein depletion, hypotension, and infection.[13] Many people who have intractable ascites spend their pre-terminal and terminal days in a state that is less than optimal, requiring frequent hospital admissions for drainage.[14]

In an attempt to reduce hospital admissions, a protocol has been evaluated in which a Tenckhoff catheter is left in the abdomen to allow continuous drainage. The catheter site is cared for as a stoma and a stoma nurse monitors care. The researchers felt that this approach was beneficial, although a formal assessment of patients' feelings and symptoms was not recorded.[14] The psychosocial impact of being discharged home with a drainage catheter in place remains unexplored. Future research areas may include the following.

- What are the benefits of being discharged home with a catheter in place, versus delayed discharge and prolonged hospitalisation?
- What educational and supportive care do these individuals require to be able to sustain them at home if that is where they choose to be?

Further investigation is needed into the very real risk of infection and peritonitis. In this study,[14] antibacterial cover was given and only one patient developed peritonitis, while two patients experienced a mild cellulitis. The approach successfully controlled the build-up of ascites in 14 out of 17 patients.

Peritoneovenous shunts

Peritoneovenous shunts were developed for use with intractable ascites as a result of cirrhosis of the liver. This method involves implanting a catheter under the skin running from the peritoneal cavity back into the general circulation, usually via the superior vena cava or right atrium. The two sections are connected by a one-way valve allowing fluid to move in one direction only. Fluid moves upwards owing to changes in intrathoracic and intraperitoneal pressure achieved through normal breathing. A pressure of 3 cm of water is required to open the valve.[15] Patients are asked to wear abdominal binders and to carry out breathing regimes, where they breathe against a pressure for 15 minutes, four times a day, in order to maximise the pressure changes. Peritoneovenous shunts are physiologically based in that they avoid problems of protein depletion. There are two main types of shunt: LeVeen and Denver. Both have been involved in clinical studies with patients with malignant ascites but neither has proved superior.[3] They differ in that the Denver shunt has a valve that can be massaged each day to increase the flow and to push through debris in the catheter that may otherwise occlude it.

Both are usually inserted under local anaesthetic and a review of the literature of studies using shunts on a minimum of 20 patients showed a 65–88% success rate.[9] However, two studies reported little or no benefit and represent a major difference in findings. Further complications following the decision to use shunts are the potentially numerous risks involved. This presents nurses caring for individuals requiring shunts with a significant challenge. Major risks include fluid overload, resulting in pulmonary oedema or heart failure, disseminated intravascular coagulation, infection, and tumour cell infusion.[13] Further, there is the complication of shunt malfunction, where the shunt may become kinked or blocked by debris. Shunts are therefore contraindicated with either bloody or mucinous ascites because of the increased risk of occluding the shunt. One of the largest studies reviewed the success rates of 116 peritoneovenous shunts in 89 patients, and found that 30-day and 60-day mortality rates were 43% and 61%, respectively.[16] They concluded that shunts were not appropriate for this patient group. Although this method may achieve palliation of the symptoms related to ascites, no measurement has been made of recovery from this intervention or of how an indwelling shunt alters an individual's body image and feeling of wellbeing. Clearly, much work needs to be undertaken to examine how nurses can best offer support to someone who is making a decision about whether or not to have a shunt inserted.

Many strategies have been tested for controlling malignant ascites. Unfortunately, there has been no formal assessment undertaken to examine what individuals with ascites themselves feel about these various treatments. The accounts of the two women with ascites below demonstrate the meaning of ascites. The way in which individuals interpret the problem is crucial to how they choose to have their symptom managed. For the majority, malignant ascites occurs at a time when emphasis should be upon minimal intervention and enabling patients to remain as free of hospital admissions and invasive procedures as possible. Evaluation of all methods currently employed, incorporating the perception of outcome from patients, doctors, and nurses, is urgently required. At the Institute of Cancer Research, nursing research is underway to find methods of increasing intraperitoneal pressure in the hope that this might delay the reaccumulation of ascitic fluid following initial drainage, through a non-invasive selfmanaged intervention; the results of this work may be influential in changing current approaches to the management of ascites.[17]

The experience of ascites

A great deal has been written about the various treatments for malignant ascites, although there is no consensus of opinion as to the optimal treatment. No study has as yet formally asked patients about their experience of ascites, or their views on the treatments offered to them. What is apparent from talking to women with ascites is that they have very different experiences. They interpret their ascites according to the meanings they attach to it and its relationship to their prognosis.

Meaning will be dependent upon an individual's own perceptions, which in turn will be influenced by culture, society, and environment. It is possible that ascites was wrongly construed as pregnancy in the past, as implied by Jane Rogers in *Mr Wroe's Virgins*,[18] a story set in the early part of the nineteenth century. The story describes a religious group built up around the teachings and prophecy of Mother Southcote. At the age of 60 she appeared to be pregnant and died during childbirth:

> For she was sixty years of age, unmarried, and had never known a man. Yet she was with child . . . When the time for the child's birth came and passed with no sign of deliverance, her suffering heart broke, letting the captive spirit escape from earthly trials . . . The child born of Mother Southcote was a spirit.

The explanation for her pregnancy may have been malignant ascites as a result of cancer. The pains she suffered could have been those associated with bowel obstruction. When an individual is left without adequate explanation for her ascites, she may believe that the distended abdomen is caused by the presence of tumour. She may fear that the pressure is damaging her organs and it will undoubtedly serve as a daily reminder of the disease. This is illustrated by Jenny's experience (Personal account 23.1).

Personal account 23.1

Jenny is 43. Having been diagnosed for a year with ovarian cancer, Jenny's disease relapsed after first-line therapy. She was prescribed a taxane but continued to be troubled with recurrent ascites. Her appearance was very important to her: Jenny liked to look glamorous. Her husband also dressed well, and they enjoyed an active social life.

Jenny would come into hospital for drainage, when she felt her ascites was gross, when clothes looked awful, and she could no longer cope with the distress caused by her condition. She also associated her ascites with the fear that her chemotherapy was not working. Her ascites was an outward manifestation of the danger her disease posed. Jenny found it very hard to accept that the fluid was not causing her any physical harm, because the feelings she experienced were so great. She would frequently request the fluid to be drained, often when there was insufficient fluid to remove. Her self-image was crucial to maintaining her sense of normality. Her appearance was paramount; it represented the woman she was before becoming a cancer patient. The ascites disrupted this self-image, forcing an unwelcome and painful redefinition of self.

Personal account 23.2

Elizabeth had a different experience of ascites. She was 73, and thought of herself as a survivor, having lived through the war and had seven children. When diagnosed with cancer she thought 'that was it' and was amazed that the hospital could offer any treatment. Everything from then on was a bonus: 'living on borrowed time.' Friends constantly visited her at home; although she rarely left home, she didn't feel embarrassed about her appearance. She thought it funny that people might think 'How can that old girl be pregnant?' She rarely complained of side-effects even though she was often unwell from her treatment.

Her ascites accumulated every 2 weeks, but this did not appear to be a problem for her. She would telephone the ward after 2 weeks telling staff she felt 'a bit uncomfortable'. She would have 10–13 litres of fluid drained. Elizabeth's expectations were markedly different from Jenny's as she saw the ascites as simply an inevitable consequence of her cancer.

Notes on selected cancer sites 23.1: Ovarian cancer

Up to 33% of women with ovarian cancer will present with malignant ascites, and over 60% will develop ascites at some time.[9] Ovarian cancer is the seventh most common cancer in women and an estimated 137 000 cases occurred worldwide in 1980.[19] There appear to be environmental influences upon the development of ovarian cancer. World incidence rates vary according to the population. In Western and Northern Europe and North America the incidence is highest (80–130 per million population), whereas in Japan, China, and India the rates are lowest (30–50 per million population). Japanese migrants to America match the host population, implying that there must be an environmental role to the development of ovarian cancer. Risk factors associated with ovarian cancer are age, race, nulliparity, infertility, history of endometrial or breast cancer, and family history of ovarian cancer.[20] Evidence from one case–control study[21] suggests that pregnancy, breast feeding, and oral contraceptive use induce biological changes that pro-

tect against ovarian malignancy. The slight increased risk in nulliparous women may be due to infertility and subsequent use of fertility drugs. However, there is a great deal of debate concerning the role of infertility drugs as a risk factor for ovarian cancer, and further studies are required.

Screening for ovarian cancer by transvaginal ultrasound and testing for the tumour antigen CA125 is still not specific enough for large-scale screening, particularly in picking up early stage tumours. However, recently a gene thought to be associated with the development of both breast and ovarian cancer has been identified. This gene is known as the BRCA1 gene and trials are underway to discover the incidence of this gene in the ovarian cancer population. The incidence is expected to be quite low because the causes of ovarian cancer are thought to the multifactorial.

Over 70% of ovarian cancers are epithelial in origin. These commonly occur in women aged 65–69 years. Younger women are more likely to be diagnosed with dysgerminomas or teratomas. There are four main histological types of epithelial tumours (adenocarcinomas). Most are serous, mucinous, clear cell, and endometrioid. Tumours are also graded as to their degree of differentiation. Epithelial ovarian cancer usually remains confined to the peritoneal cavity. However, it is divided into four distinct stages.

Stage I disease – confined to ovaries
Ia – confined to one ovary, capsule intact, no tumour on external surface, no ascites.
Ib – confined to one or both ovaries, capsule intact, no tumour on external surface, no ascites.
Ic – confined to one or both ovaries but with ascites or positive peritoneal washings and/or capsule rupture.

Stage II disease – pelvic extension
IIa – extension to uterus or fallopian tubes.
IIb – extension to other pelvic tissue.
IIc – as IIa or IIb plus surface deposits, capsule rupture, ascites or positive peritoneal washings.

Stage III disease – outside pelvis and/or positive retroperitoneal or inguinal nodes
IIIa – confined to true pelvis, negative nodes, histologically proven seedings to abdominal peritoneal surface.
IIIb – greatest peritoneal deposit less than 2 cm diameter.
IIIc – greatest peritoneal deposit more than 2 cm diameter.

Stage IV disease – distant metastases, i.e. lung or positive pleural fluid
Prognosis for ovarian cancer is dependent upon stage at diagnosis, histological type and grade and size of disease remaining following surgery. For patients with operable disease, complete surgery is recommended. This includes a total abdominal hysterectomy, bilateral salpingo-ophrectomy and

omentectomy. However, if a patient is under 25, conservative surgery is usually recommended in case upon histological review she is found to have a dysgerminoma or teratoma. These women have potentially curable cancers and their fertility should be maintained. Unfortunately, the majority of women present with either stage III or IV disease (60–80%) and the following table demonstrates the prognosis for patients at different stages at presentation and recommended treatment:

Stage I	70%	Surgery*
Stage II	45%	Surgery and chemotherapy
Stage III	17%	Surgery if possible and chemotherapy†
Stage IV	5%	Surgery if possible and chemotherapy†

*Certain subgroups have a worse prognosis. While stage I disease usually responds well to surgery alone, patients with poorly differentiated, clear cell stage I disease do not fair so well, with 80% 5-year survival without chemotherapy. In most centres worldwide, stage I disease is usually treated with both surgery and chemotherapy.

†There is some debate as to the role of surgery in bulky disease or inoperable disease. Some authors have shown that surgery offers no survival benefit in this group of patients and only adds to their morbidity.

There are many different regimes and trials of chemotherapy in ovarian cancer. Initial treatment is usually through a combination of chemotherapy agents such as CAP (cyclophosphamide, adriamycin, and platinum) or platinum and taxol. Radiotherapy is usually reserved for treating specific symptoms such as pain or persistent vaginal bleeding.

Unfortunately, most patients succumb to their disease. Bowel obstruction becomes a recurrent problem, which can sometimes be relieved temporarily by an ostomy, but is usually managed conservatively.

References

1. Reynard C. and Mannix K. (1989). Management of ascites in advanced cancer – a flow diagram. *Palliative Medicine* **4**, 45–47.
2. Feldman G.B. (1975). Lymphatic obstruction in carcinomatous ascites. *Cancer Research* **35**, 325–332.
3. Oosterlee J. (1980). Peritoneovenous shunting for ascites in cancer patients. *British Journal of Surgery* **67**, 663–666.
4. Pockros P.J., Esrason K.T., Nguyen C., Duque J. and Woods S. (1992). Mobilization of malignant ascites with diuretics is dependent on ascitic fluid characteristics. *Gastroenterology* **103**, 1302–1306.
5. Greenway B., Johnson P.J. and Williams R. (1982). Control of malignant ascites with spironolactone. *British Journal of Surgery* **69**, 441–442.
6. Reynard C. and Tempest S. (1992). *A Guide to Symptom Relief in Advanced Cancer,* 3rd edition. London: Haigh and Hochland.
7. Herlihy J.T. and Herlihy B.L. (1985). Renin–angiotensin–aldosterone system. *Critical Care Nurse* **5**, 87–88.
8. Fort S., James J.Y., Srivastava E.D., Morris T.J. and Rhodes J. (1991). Water immersion for treatment of ascites in chronic liver disease. *Physiotherapy* **77**, 571–572.
9. Baker A.R. and Weber J.S. (1993). Treatment of malignant ascites. In DeVita, V.T., Hellman, S. and Rosenberg, S.A. (eds.) *Cancer: Principles and Practice of Oncology.* Philadelphia, PA: Lippincott, pp. 2255–2261.
10. Bezwoda W.R., Seymour L. and Dansey R. (1989). Intraperitoneal recombinant interferon-alpha 2b for recurrent malignant ascites due to ovarian cancer. *Cancer* **64**, 1029–1033.
11. Brown P.D. (1993). Proteinase inhibition: a new approach to cancer therapy. *Cancer Topics* **9**, 1029–1033.
12. Ross G.J., Kessler H.B., Clai, M.R., Gatenby R.A., Hartz W.H. and Ross L.V. (1989). Sonographically guided paracentesis for palliation of symptomatic malignant ascites. *American Journal of Roentgenology* **153**, 1309–1311.
13. Kehoe K.C. (1991). Malignant ascites: etiology, diagnosis and treatment. *Oncology Nursing Forum* **18**, 523–530.
14. Belfort M.A., Stevens P.J., DeHaek K., Soeters R. and Krige J.E. (1990). A new approach to the management of malignant ascites; a permanently implanted abdominal drain. *European Journal of Surgical Oncology* **16**, 47–53.
15. LeVeen H.H., Christoudias G., Ip M., Luft R., Falk G. and Grosberg S. (1974). Peritoneovenous shunting for ascites. *Annals of Surgery* **180**, 580–591.
16. Schumacher D.L., Saclarides T.J. and Staren E.D. (1994). Peritoneovenous shunts for palliation of the patient with malignant ascites. *Annals of Surgical Oncology* **1**, 378–381.
17. Preston N. (1995). New strategies for the management of malignant ascites. *European Journal of Cancer Care* **4**, 178–183.
18. Rogers J. (1991). *Mr Wroe's Virgins.* London: Faber and Faber.
19. Cancer Research Campaign (1991). *Ovarian Cancer.* Factsheet 17.1. London: Cancer Research Campaign.
20. Tortlero Luna G., Mitchell M.F. and Rhodes Morris H.E. (1994). Epidemiology and screening of ovarian cancer. *Obstetrics and Gynecology Clinics of North America* **21**, 1–23.
21. Whittemore A.S. (1994). Characteristics relating to ovarian cancer risk: implications for prevention and detection. *Gynecological Oncology* **55** (Suppl.), 15–19.

CHAPTER TWENTY-FOUR

Bone marrow suppression: infection and bleeding

Ruth Dunleavey

The problems of infection and bleeding in cancer may be secondary to the disease process itself or, more commonly, the result of the therapy used to treat it. It has long been the ambition of physicians to produce a chemotherapy agent that is targeted at the malignant cell. By avoiding normal cells, the toxicities currently associated with chemotherapy would be eradicated.

Sadly, the search for such agents has yielded disappointing results. Oncologists have therefore been compelled to employ alternative strategies. To increase their efficacy, conventional agents have been administered at ever escalating doses. The logic behind this is that the greater the dosage, the greater the likelihood that target cells will be reached, albeit at the expense of some healthy cells – less a 'magic bullet', more a 'magic machine gun'.

The most significant casualty of this approach has been the bone marrow. Bone marrow is found inside the long bones of the body and in the sternum, pelvis, and skull. It is here that blood is produced, originating from the 'great, great-grandfather' pluripotent stem cell (Figure 24.1).[1] On dividing, this cell has the unique capacity to produce daughter cells that will mature into either further stem cells or will differentiate into blood. Because of their short half-life, blood cells require constant renewal and divide rapidly. Haemopoiesis is thus exquisitely sensitive to the action of cytotoxic therapy.

Any inhibition of this cell division inevitably results in a reduction in the number of circulating red and white cells and platelets, the consequence of which is anaemia, neutropenia, and thrombo-cytopenia. This section will focus on the last two conditions and the associated problems of infection and bleeding.

The role of the nurse

As cancer therapy evolves, the cancer nurse is encountering the problems of infection and bleeding more and more frequently. Until fairly recently, with the exception of the leukaemias (discussed later in this chapter) the main dose-limiting toxicity in cytotoxic treatment was bone marrow suppression. To a certain extent this remains the case today. However, through the improved management of these toxicities it has been possible to implement high-dose chemotherapy regimes not only for haematological malignancies but also for solid tumours.

Rather than attempting to avoid neutropenia and thrombocytopenia, these are now seen as symptoms to be managed. High-dose therapy and peripheral blood stem cell transplantation (PBSCT) have done much to lift bone marrow suppression out of the BMT unit and into mainstream oncology.

Although cancer therapy has developed, the role of the cancer nurse could perhaps be criticised for not entirely keeping up with the changes. In the face of the potentially life-threatening conditions of infection and haemorrhage, the nurse has traditionally taken a paternalistic, almost custodial role over her patients. There is now a movement away from this approach for three reasons.

First, as mentioned above, the management of these side-effects has improved considerably.

Box 24.1: Peripheral blood stem cell transplantation

Peripheral blood stem cell transplantation (PBSCT) is rapidly replacing conventional autologous bone marrow transplantation in the treatment of haematological and non-haematological malignancies. It is a procedure where 'bone marrow' cells are collected from a patient while they are in remission, then used to support high-dose therapy at a future date.

In the first place, PBSCT requires the administration of intermediate doses of chemotherapy in conjunction with growth factors. It has been found that when the bone marrow begins to recover there is a short period of time during which progenitor cells (stem cells) are mobilised from their normal environment in the bone marrow into the peripheral circulation. These cells can be harvested with the use of a cell sepa-

rator in a process know as leucapheresis. The products can then be preserved and frozen in preparation for transplantation. In this procedure the patient receives a high, myeloablative dose of chemotherapy, but their marrow is rescued by reinfusion of the stem cells.

The advantages of this technique over using bone marrow are threefold:

- the cells engraft more quickly, leading to a rapid recovery of blood count and speedy discharge home from hospital
- it is available to patients unable to undergo a general anaesthetic
- it is cheaper than bone marrow transplantation.

For these reasons, high-dose therapy with stem cell rescue is being offered to a wide range of patients who would previously not have been eligible, such as the elderly and patients with solid tumours (e.g. ovarian cancer, breast cancer).[2-4]

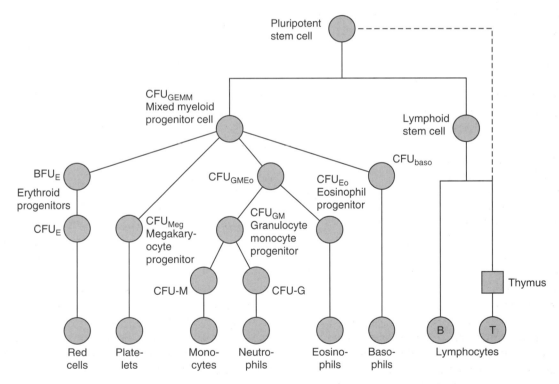

Figure 24.1 Blood cell formation (haemopoiesis) (reproduced with the permission of Blackwell Scientific Publications from Hoffbrand A.V. and Pettit J.E. (1993). *Essential Haematology*, 3rd edition). Diagrammatic representation of the bone marrow pluripotent stem cell and the cell lines that arise from it. Various progenitor cells can now be identified by culture in a semi-solid medium by the type of colony they form. BFU$_E$: burst-forming unit; CFU: colony-forming unit; E: erythroid; Eo: eosinophil; GEMM: mixed granulocyte, erythroid, monocyte, megakaryocyte; GM: granulocyte, monocyte; Meg: megakaryocyte.

Blood products are readily available for transfusion to overcome problems with bleeding. Our increased understanding of sepsis coupled with the availability of more advanced antibiotics enables us to manage infections better before they can become life-threatening.

Secondly, economic changes within the health service make the issue of cost far more evident than in the past. The implication of this is that there is less tolerance for procedures that are unsupported by research. Many centres can be seen to be reviewing their practices in an attempt to promote increased efficiency and eliminate historical rituals that are unsubstantiated in the literature.

Finally, and perhaps most pertinent to nurses, there is a growing recognition that the model of care adopted in the past could be accused of being reductionist. On the whole, there has been a tendency to focus specifically on medical problems such as infection or bleeding, denying the other needs of the patient, which are so fundamental to their general feelings of health and well-being. Increasingly, oncology endeavours to look at the individual holistically, addressing important issues such as quality of life. In Krishnasamy's interesting pilot study of haematology patients, the importance of addressing quality of life issues along with individualised nursing care was repeatedly articulated:[5,6]

> . . . for me the nursing care comes from getting to know me and knowing what I think about my illness . . .

> . . . the nurses . . . I think they just let you hold it all together . . . just hang on . . .

Bleeding disorders

Clinically significant haemostatic abnormalities are thought to affect as many as 15% of cancer patients, with the incidence rising to up to 90% following chemotherapy.[7] These disorders may be the result of either the primary malignancy or the therapy employed to treat it.[8] Normal clotting occurs at the culmination of a complex series of events known as the coagulation cascade. Alteration of any single component in this pathway results in aberrant clotting, which may manifest itself as either thrombosis or haemorrhage.

Clotting defects are multifactorial in their aetiology and may result from secretions from the tumour cell itself or damage to the liver, spleen, or most commonly the bone marrow. The most usual single cause of serious haemorrhage, particularly amongst patients with leukemia, is a low platelet count.[9]

Thrombocytopenia is most frequently the result of chemotherapy, with a nadir count (lowest point) occurring between days 11 and 14 post-treatment. The normal range for platelets is $150–400 \times 10^9$/ml. It is not generally until the count falls below 20×10^9/ml, however, that active measures are instituted. More rarely, thrombocytopenia may be caused through marrow infiltration by the tumour. Bone marrow secondaries are commonly observed in patients with breast cancer, prostate cancer, and the haematological malignancies. Less commonly, they can be seen in a variety of other tumour types including lung cancer and melanoma.[8]

Another cause of thrombocytopenia may be increased peripheral platelet destruction amongst patients with hypersplenism (e.g. lymphoma, chronic lymphoblastic leukaemia), although in such cases the symptoms are usually mild and there is rarely significant bleeding.

Other cancer populations that are particularly susceptible to coagulation difficulties include neutropenic septic patients. This life-threatening condition may be associated with an abnormal clotting profile known as disseminated intravascular coagulation (DIC). This is a hypercoagulable state in which haemorrhage and thrombosis occur simultaneously.[10] It is a syndrome that is particularly associated with acute promyelocytic leukaemia in which bleeding problems are a significant cause of mortality.[11] Other bleeding abnormalities include primary fibrinolysis, microangiopathic anaemia with thrombocytopenia, acquired platelet defects, circulating anticoagulants or inhibitors, or treatment-related bleeding disorders.[8] Local bleeding may occur where a tumour invades a major blood vessel. Sometimes it is the initiation of therapy that promotes bleeding, as the tumour is eroded away but the rich blood supply remains.

The nurse's role in caring for someone at risk of bleeding demands scientific knowledge, coupled with expert interpersonal skills to support these frightening and life-threatening complications.

Management of bleeding

Management involves an attempt to arrest the source of haemorrhage through the application of pressure or of ice. If such steps are insufficient then transfusion of platelets, possibly in conjunction with other clotting factors such as fresh frozen plasma, may be necessary. Tranexamic acid or vasopressin can be administered to assist in the clotting process. Diathermy and packing may sometimes be necessary if other measures fail.

With severe thrombocytopenia in the terminal phase of illness, there is a risk of a major bleed, which would not warrant active resuscitation measures. The experience of living with the Sword of Damocles of a potential bleed hanging above one's head is extremely stressful for patient and family, particularly when being cared for at home. Encouraging patients and their relatives to talk about their fears may help to allay some of the distress experienced:

> . . . having someone you can buzz in the middle of the night and know they . . . will come and sit with you . . .

> I felt so safe that someone was always there.[6]

Bleeding prophylaxis

Education is extremely important in avoiding bleeding. Anyone undergoing chemotherapy treatment needs to be aware of what thrombocytopenia is and when their count is likely to be at its nadir. Provision of information in an accessible form will provide one means of reintroducing an element of self-determination in an otherwise unfamiliar and disempowering environment. It is important to be able to recognise the signs and symptoms of a low platelet count (bruising, bleeding, purpurae, and epistaxis) and to offer counselling about how to modify lifestyle to minimise risk of bleeding. For example, it might be suggested to avoid heavy manual labour and contact sports or to use a soft toothbrush and an electric razor to minimise trauma to the gums and face.[10] Helping patients to voice their frustrations at having to modify established aspects of daily living, and to re-establish priorities for day-to-day living may prove to be especially supportive.[12]

Certain drugs may prolong clotting times and lead to gastric bleeding; for example, steroids and non-steroidal anti-inflammatory drugs. Where possible, these should be avoided, although in real-

ity this may sometimes lead to dilemmas in which the potential risk of bleeding needs to be weighed against important symptom control measures such as pain relief in the terminally ill.

The use of prophylactic platelet transfusions in thrombocytopenia is an issue surrounded by controversy. Fundamentally the size and duration of an improvement in platelet increment is variable and so the benefit of the procedure is not guaranteed. Furthermore, transfusion carries risks. The first risk is that of refractoriness. It is suggested that following as few as one or two platelet transfusions, it is common to become refractory to their beneficial effects;[13] between 15 and 20% of those who are frequently transfused become seriously refractory.[14]

Second, there is the risk of a transfusion reaction. This is relatively common, occurring in 30% of transfusions, and is the result of leucocyte contamination or cytokine release from the transfused product.[13] It is manifested as chills, rigors, rashes and sometimes backache. Not only can this be extremely frightening for the patient, but it also negates any benefit from the transfusion, as the platelets are consumed in the ensuing immune activity. Some units routinely administer steroid and anti-histamine 'cover' pre-transfusion, although the role of the latter is far from proven and warrants further research.[15] The timing of administering cover is also contentious. In recent years there has been increased employment of leucocyte filters. Not only do these minimise reactions but they are also thought to prevent or delay refractoriness and prevent the transmission of some blood-borne infections.[16]

Infection is the third potential complication of transfusion. Recent press coverage describing how large quantities of HIV-positive blood were transfused in France shows the ease with which viral infections may be contracted via this route. Although screening for HIV is now assiduous, other infections, particularly cytomegalovirus (CMV), can pose a serious threat to the immunosuppressed.

Traditionally, prophylactic transfusions have tended to be administered when the platelet count falls below 20×10^9/ml, although this practice has been questioned.[17] A randomised study of women with gynaecological cancer compared prophylactic platelets infusions at counts of 20×10^9/ml and counts of 5×10^9/ml; transfusion at a count of 5 $\times 10^9$ was found to be equally safe.[18]

The decision whether to transfuse prophylactically requires some consideration. It is important to take into account the benefit intended from the intervention. Patients for whom prophylactic platelets are considered are often those with heavily diseased or pre-treated bone marrow whose prognosis is poor. The benefits of transfusion need to be weighed against the fact that they may find themselves spending long periods of time in hospital awaiting treatment, experiencing repeated painful and often difficult cannulations. Furthermore, they are being subjected to the potential of a transfusion reaction or infection.

One final problem with platelet transfusions is that they are costly, in terms of the platelets themselves, the filters necessary to administer them, and the nursing time they take up. There is hope that in future years the need for transfusion will be reduced by the development of a platelet growth factor. Recently, a substance called 'thrombopoietin' has been isolated and has yielded some very promising results in animal experiments. Human trials with this substance are just beginning, the results of which are awaited.

Infection

Recently, a survey of the American Oncology Nursing Society was carried out in order to determine research priorities for forthcoming years.[19] Over 2000 nurses were approached, and one of the top 10 subjects identified was the problem of immunosuppression and neutropenia. Infection amongst the cancer population has now superseded bleeding as the primary cause of death.[9,20] Furthermore, it results in considerable morbidity and may necessitate hospital admission, chemotherapy schedule interruption, and dose reduction.[21]

The human immune system can be divided into two components; the non-specific and the specific. Non-specific immunity refers to the first line of defence against infection and it includes surface membrane barriers and non-specific cellular and chemical defences such as neutrophils, macrophages, and a range of cytokines. The second 'specific' line of defence has the ability to recognise foreign antigens and is able to immobilise, inca-

pacitate, or destroy them. Both systems operate in conjunction with one another.

Lines of defence may be compromised for patients with cancer for a variety of reasons (see below). Chemotherapy and sometimes radiotherapy can disrupt the mucosal surfaces and deplete the neutrophil and lymphocyte count. The depth and duration of neutropenia has been demonstrated to bear a very close correlation with the acquisition of infection, the majority of severe infections occurring with a count below 0.1×10^9/ml.[22] Coupled with this, the hospital environment into which the patient is forced is another source of pathogenic organisms.[23,24]

The potential for infection is further exacerbated by factors such as age, concomitant medical problems (e.g. diabetes, rheumatoid arthritis), and poor nutritional status, as well as the general stress of being diagnosed as a cancer patient.[25] The nurse plays a key role in caring for an immunocompromised individual, primarily being responsible for managing active infection and preventing its further escalation into septic shock, and secondly through promoting a safe environment by instituting appropriate, research-based policies for infection prevention. Finally, and perhaps most significantly the nurse can take on a teaching role, offering education on how to avoid or to manage infection and exploring ways in which individuals can re-prioritise activities during these demanding periods.

Managing acute infection

The key to good management of infection lies with prompt recognition of the early signs followed by immediate action. Because immunity is so impaired amongst this group of people, even a small infection can very quickly escalate into life-threatening septic shock. Septic syndrome is a continuum beginning with a localised infection which progresses to a generalised infection disseminated by the blood (septicaemia).[31] If the body is incapable of mounting an adequate immune response, the result is general vascular collapse (septic shock). Statistics are conflicting and difficult to interpret, but the consensus of opinion suggests that the death rate from septic shock ranges between 25 and 50%, rising to 75% amongst the cancer population and

Box 24.2: Factors predisposing the person with cancer to infection

Disease-related factors
- Defective T-cells found in patients with lymphoma, multiple myeloma and the leukaemias are associated with humoral defence deficits.
- Bone marrow infiltration, tumour obstruction, and erosion.
- Cachexia.
- Stress.
- Extremes of age and poor nutritional status.
- Concomitant disease (renal failure, liver disease, diabetes, cardiac disease).

Treatment-related factors
- Chemotherapy or radiotherapy to the bone marrow cause bone marrow suppression.
- Steroids cause depression of neutrophil chemotaxis, decreased leucocyte adherence, depressed monocyte bactericidal activity, decreased endocytosis, and decreased lymphocyte function.
- Surgery leads to a fall in lymphocytes and is immunosuppressive.
- Invasive procedures such as insertion of an intravascular device provide a route for micro-organisms.
- Some regimens are damaging to mucosal surfaces and can potentiate bacterial translocation.
- Prolonged antibiotic therapy.

Environmental factors
- The hospital environment is potentially hostile because of the large number of micro-organisms it harbours, particularly in inhalational equipment, nebulisers, food sources, contaminated air/water, and through hand-to-hand transmission.[24,26-30]

is greater than 90% if more that one organism is involved.[27,28,31]

Early recognition of infection requires the highest level of nursing skill. Signs may be subtle and listening to the patient and hearing what they are feeling is very important. Symptoms include irritability, confusion, or drowsiness.[27] This may be accompanied by haemodynamic changes, usually involving tachycardia and blood pressure alterations.

The literature tends to classify shock into stages, generally beginning with a hyperdynamic state (warm shock), which progresses to cold shock in which the body's compensatory mechanisms fail and

the patient begins to experience multisystem failure.[29] While of some use in clarifying an extremely complex phenomenon, the pattern of changes associated with the septic syndrome is extremely varied and may not follow any real chronology.

Amongst those 'at-risk', pyrexia should always be treated as indicative of an infection until proven otherwise. Most centres employ a policy of taking blood cultures and other necessary specimens and instituting antibiotics when body temperature rises above 38°C. It is important that these measures commence immediately. More than 70% will respond if antibiotics are given in the first 24 hours, compared with only 22% if they are delayed to the third day following symptoms developing.[32] The management of early bacterial infections has undoubtedly improved considerably over the last decade and this has brought about a change in the pattern of infection in the severely immunosuppressed patient.[33] The result has been that infections from other organisms such as viruses (e.g. CMV), protozoa (e.g. *Pneumocystis carinii*) and fungi (e.g. *Aspergillus*), which tend to arise later in the period of neutropenia, have assumed greater significance.

Prevention of infection: the environment

Much of the literature examining the best environment for immunocompromised patients has tended to concentrate on bone marrow transplant units or haematology wards, where infection is a particularly difficult problem. Most of the studies are medical and many of the results are either inconclusive or conflicting, leading to some confusion.

Three strategies for managing infection in cancer have been proposed; these are described below.[26]

Suppression or elimination of endogenous pathogens
Management of the neutropenia has been significantly improved by a better understanding of the mechanisms through which infections arise.

Schimpff *et al.*[24] analysed the organisms leading to infective episodes among a population of neutropenic patients. They discovered that the vast majority of these were caused by the patients' own commensal organisms. In 47% of cases these were organisms that were acquired during hospitalisation. In the light of this evidence, a number of attempts has been made to render the profoundly immunosuppressed patient free of potential pathogens. These range from sophisticated methods of personal hygiene to endeavours to decolonise the gastrointestinal tract using antibiotics and special diets.

Clean diets vary between institutions but aim to provide the minimum number of pathogens by including only cooked or highly processed foods. Foodstuffs associated with high microbial loads (salad, raw fruit, certain diary products) are eliminated. Once again, the efficacy of such measures is unproven and gut decontamination regimens are unpalatable and unpleasant, with notoriously poor compliance. Many institutions have elected to relax their dietary measures in recent years.[34,35]

Conversely, most centres are in agreement about the importance of good oral hygiene for immunosuppressed patients. Chemotherapy and sometimes radiotherapy can cause serious damage to the oral mucosa. It is hoped that a high standard of oral care will promote symptomatic relief of stomatitis and reduce more widespread sepsis, which occurs as a result of bacterial translocation.[36,37] Another measure that has been extensively researched and shown to have a significant effect on infection rates is effective handwashing.[38] Many studies have highlighted the prevalence of poor hand washing techniques on the ward, although these can be improved through education.[39]

Prevention of acquisition of hospital-associated pathogens

In order to prevent the acquisition of pathogens there has been a logical tendency to isolate individuals in the hope that this will minimise the number of organisms with which they will have contact. Various types of isolation exist, ranging from simple isolation (basically a single room) to highly sophisticated protective isolation units incorporating air filtration devices. The latter are generally restricted to bone marrow transplant units, although many other centres employ a policy of admitting and treating patients in a single room when their neutrophil counts falls below 1×10^9/ml.

Air filtration may incorporate laminar air flow (LAF), usually in conjunction with high standards of sterility. A less strict approach is high efficiency particulate air (HEPA) filtration, in which slightly fewer organisms are eliminated. While air filtration is undoubtedly effective in removing highly pathogenic *Aspergillus* spores, there is controversy about whether it confers any benefit in terms of increased survival.[21,36,40]

The efficacy of isolating patients in the absence of providing filtered air has also been disputed. Nauseef and Maki[41] studied a large group of patients who were neutropenic after chemotherapy and found there was no advantage to nursing them in a single room compared with the general ward (see Research study 24.1). There would also appear to be very little evidence to support other measures aimed at promoting sterility such as using masks, overshoes, sterile gowns, or sterile plates and cutlery when caring for theses patients.[42]

A number of studies has endeavoured to demonstrate the psychological effects of isolation on the patient.[43] This has been a difficult task, in part because of the number of other unpleasant factors confronting these people. Physically they are likely to be feeling unwell, deprived of sleep, in pain and generally vulnerable. Psychologically they have to contend with being away from their loved ones, facing a serious illness and possibly confronting death for the first time. Much of the literature highlights the loneliness and stressfulness of isolation. There is a proportion of people who is unable to tolerate such conditions and break isolation at an early stage in the therapy.[44] How appropriate it is to deprive individuals of invaluable human contact at this time without firm evidence to prove its efficacy is perhaps debatable. While there may be an argument for isolating the profoundly immunosuppressed,[45] this practice is much more ambiguous in the case of individuals who are neutropenic for shorter periods of time, such as those with solid tumours undergoing peripheral blood stem cell transplant:

> . . . it makes you feel like . . . like you're in an institution, where people are just wandering in and out and you really don't matter as an individual.[6]

Furthermore, a proportion is also facing a poor prognosis, therefore the quality of time they spend in hospital is particularly important. Hence there is a movement away from isolation, with centres caring for the immunosuppressed on the general ward and also promoting early discharge and outpatient care.[46] Not only does this remove them from an environment in which there is a risk of colonisation with potentially harmful organisms, but it also acknowledges the significance of psychological well-being in illness.

Russell *et al.*[47] chose to abandon the strict isolation practices in their BMT unit, partly as a result of a nursing strike that depleted staff and rendered such labour-intensive measures inoperable. They failed to demonstrate any increase of infections or mortality as a result. The option to go home during the transplant period even when profoundly neutropenic is now offered routinely.

Research study 24.1: The value of simple protective isolation in patients with granulocytopenia[41]

This interesting piece of research was carried out in Wisconsin between 1977 and 1978. It was conducted by two clinicians hoping to identify whether expensive isolation and disinfection procedures were necessary. Furthermore, they had observed that extreme forms of isolation can have adverse psychological effects on patients and were concerned about the rationale behind such practices.

The study sample consisted of patients either with ALL or aplastic anaemia who had been admitted to hospital for longer than a week. They were undergoing remission induction therapy or treatment for a relapse. Patients were randomised into either protective isolation or given standard hospital care. Protective isolation was defined by the Centres for Disease Control. Their recommendations were for a single room with private toilet and use of clean gown, gloves, and mask for anyone entering. Standard care consisted of an ordinary two-bedded room with a sign on the door reminding people coming in to wash their hands. Neither group was given gut decontamination or sterile food.

In total 37 patients were enrolled on to the study, experiencing 43 episodes of neutropenia in all. Both groups were comparable in terms of age, blood count, therapy and admission time. The study found no statistically significant differences in infection rate between the two groups. Unfortunately, no formal analysis was made of quality of life. However, although the majority of patients was able to tolerate the conditions, even amongst this small sample, two individuals had to break isolation because of psychological distress. Nauseef and Maki[41] concluded:

On the basis of our data, we concluded that simple protective isolation alone, as practiced in most hospitals, offers no appreciable benefits to patients with granulocytopenia in reducing infections or improving the rate of leukaemic remission, and that it does not prolong survival. In view of the added costs and the emotional deprivation that patient and family must endure, its use should be re-evaluated.

For many years it has been recognised that in a very real sense stress can be debilitating both psychologically and physiologically. Through endeavouring to minimise stressful stimuli, the body is placed in a better situation to heal.[28] Furthermore, in recent years there has been a growing recognition that 'cure' is not always the ultimate goal of therapy. Many people undergo treatment in the knowledge that this will not remove the cancer, but it will give them time. It is important that the quality of this time is maximised.

Reversal of host defence defects

The discussion above indicates the ambiguity surrounding the optimal management of the immunocompromised patient. In the light of this debate new management strategies have arisen, illustrating a subtle change of approach. In recent years there have been a number of exciting new developments in cancer therapy. Pharmacologically there have been considerable improvements in infection prophylaxis. Studies have illustrated that very clear benefit can be gained in the prevention of viral and fungal infections by employing agents like acyclovir and fluconazole.[48,49]

Treatment of fungal infections has also been revolutionised by the development of liposomal preparations of anti-fungals such as liposomal amphotericin. These facilitate targeting of the drug to the affected area, allowing the administration of much higher doses without the associated toxicities.[50] Other more innovative approaches have involved harnessing agents of the body's own immunity in order to fight infection.[51] A better understanding of the immune response has allowed us to isolate various cytokines, which can be manufactured artificially. Haemopoietic growth factors such as G-CSF and GM-CSF have proved beneficial in reducing the period of neutropenia leading to a reduction in the number of days with infection and shorter periods in hospital.[52] Other agents also being studied in clinical trials include certain interleukins (e.g. IL2, IL6), interferon, and tumour necrosis factor.[21]

The problems of bleeding and infection remain, but their management is becoming increasingly patient centred. This shift has been made possible through scientific developments and further driven by economic factors. It signifies a change in philosophy whereby the patient is now recognised as an individual. Nursing has a key role to play in continuing the advancement of this ethos of care. No longer is elimination of disease the sole aim of therapy, nor is it necessarily a realistic aim. Instead the issue of quality of life is acknowledged and plays an increasingly central role when planning an individual's care.

Notes on selected cancer sites 24.1: The acute leukaemias

Leukaemia, literally meaning 'white blood' was first identified in 1845 by Virchow.[53] In fact it is more accurately described as a group of disorders characterised by the accumulation of abnormal white cells in the bone marrow.[1] The leukaemias are classified as either acute or chronic and lymphoid or myeloid, depending on which line of haemopoiesis is affected.

Aetiology
Leukaemia can arise at any age but its incidence rises steeply in those over 50. Its aetiology is not fully understood, but a number of factors have been linked with the disease including;

- exposure to radiation
- exposure to certain chemicals, e.g. benzene
- viruses, e.g. T-cell leukaemia lymphoma virus (HTLV1)
- genetic factors – there would seem to be a familial tendency
- chromosomal abnormalities (e.g. Down's syndrome).[1]

Presenting symptoms and diagnosis
Occasionally, diagnosis will be made asymptomatically on a routine blood test, but more frequently patients will present with weakness, fatigue, bruising, and haemorrhage. A large proportion will have an infection. A blood film will sometimes illustrate the presence of leukaemic blasts; however, a bone marrow biopsy is more informative. Remission is achieved only when less than 5% of the marrow is replaced by blasts.

Acute myeloid leukaemia (AML)
This is the most common form of leukaemia found in adults, with a general incidence in the USA of 2–3 in 100 000.[54] The

disease is classified into eight sub-groups according to the French–American–British (FAB) system. This classification relates to the stage in the haemopoietic cascade at which the malignant clone develops.

Acute lymphoblastic leukaemia (ALL)
This is a common form of leukaemia amongst children, with an incidence in the general population of 1–7 in 100 000.[55] A variety of classification systems has been suggested, the most common of which relates to the affected cell type (i.e. T-cell, B-cell, mixed or null-cell). A special concern with ALL is central nervous system involvement, which must be treated prophylactically with intrathecal chemotherapy and radiotherapy.

Treatment
Different regimens are used for each disease, although they tend to use similar drugs. These are:

(a) anti-metabolites (e.g. methotrexate, cytosine)
(b) alkylating agents (e.g. cyclophosphamide, busulphan)
(c) DNA binding drugs (e.g. daunorubicin, mitoxantrone)
(d) mitotic inhibitors (e.g. vincristine)
(e) miscellaneous (e.g. steroids).

Therapy can be divided into stages beginning with remission induction, and an intensive course of chemotherapy, which aims to eradicate as much disease as possible. However, once a remission is achieved, relapse can occur with time and so therapy must be continued. This may be consolidation therapy (basically similar to the remission induction regimen), intensification therapy, or both.[56]

Intensification treatment involves high-dose chemotherapy and radiotherapy. The doses are such that they aim to remove all traces of disease. In the process they also destroy healthy bone marrow, which needs to be replaced through a bone marrow or peripheral blood stem cell transplant. The stage at which to pursue this toxic treatment, if at all, is problematic and surrounded by controversy.[57]

Some regimens also incorporate a consolidation phase in which low-dose oral chemotherapy or cytokines are administered to sustain a remission.

References

1. Hoffbrand A.V. and Pettit J.E. (1993). *Essential Haematology.* Oxford: Blackwell Scientific.
2. Craig J.O., Turner M.L. and Parker A.C. (1992). Peripheral blood stem cell transplantation. *Blood Review* **6**, 59–67.
3. Gale R.P., Henon P. and Juttner C. (1992). Blood stem transplants come of age. *Bone Marrow Transplantation* **9**, 151–155.

4. Henon P.R., Liang H., Beck-Wirth G., Eisenmann J.C., Lepers M., Wunder E. *et al.* (1992). Comparison of haematopoietic and immune recovery after autologous bone marrow or blood stem cell transplants. *Bone Marrow Transplantation* 9, 285–291.

5. Krishnasamy M. (1996). What do cancer patients identify as supportive and unsupportive behaviours of nurses? A pilot study. *European Journal of Cancer Care* 5, 103–110.

6. Krishnasamy M. (1994). *What do cancer patients identify as supportive and unsupportive behaviours of nurses?* Unpublished M.Sc. dissertation, University of Surrey.

7. Goad K.E. and Gralnick H.R. (1996). Coagulation disorders in cancer. *Haematology/Oncology Clinics of North America* 10, 457–484.

8. Rosen P.J. (1992). Bleeding problems in the cancer patient. *Haematology/Oncology Clinics of North America* 6, 1315–1329.

9. Bick R.L. (1992). Coagulation abnormalities in malignancy. *Seminars in Thrombosis and Haemostasis* 18, 353–372.

10. Shuey K.M. (1996). Platelets and associated bleeding disorders. *Seminars in Oncology Nursing* 12, 15–27.

11. Wujcik D. (1996). Updated on the diagnosis of and therapy for acute promyelocytic leukaemia an chronic myelogenous leukaemia. *Oncology Nursing Forum* 23, 478–487.

12. Corner J., Plant H. and Warner L. (1995). Developing a nursing approach to managing dyspnoea in lung cancer. *International Journal of Palliative Nursing* 1, 5–11.

13. Kaushansky K. (1996). The thrombocytopenia of cancer. *Haematology/Oncology Clinics of North America* 10, 431–455.

14. Bayer W.L., Bodensteiner D.C., Tilzer L.L. and Adams M.E. (1992). Use of platelets and other transfusion products in patients with malignancy. *Seminars in Thrombosis and Haemostasis* 18, 308–391.

15. Mollison P.L., Engelfreit C.P. and Contreras M. (1993). *Blood Transfusion in Clinical Medicine.* Oxford: Blackwell Scientific, p. 684.

16. Higgins V.L. (1996). Leucocyte-reduced blood components: patient benefits and practical applications. *Oncology Nursing Forum* 23, 659–667.

17. Napier J.A.F. (1996). *Handbook of Blood Transfusion Therapy.* Chichester: John Wiley, p. 75.

18. Fanning J., Hilgers R.D., Murray K.P., Bolt K. and Aughenbaugh D.M. (1995). Conservative management of chemotherapy-induced thrombocytopenia in women with gynaecologic cancers. *Gynaecologic Oncology* 59, 191–193.

19. Stetz K.M., Haberman M.R., Holcombe J. and Jones L.S. (1995). The 1994 Oncology Nursing Society Research Priorities Survey. *Oncology Nursing Forum* 22, 785–789.

20. Carlson A.C. (1985). Infection prophylaxis in the patient with cancer. *Oncology Nursing Forum* 12, 56–64.

21. Pizzo P.A. (1989). Considerations for the prevention of infectious complications in patients with cancer. *Reviews of Infectious Disease,* Vol. II (Suppl. 7), 1551–1563.

22. Bodey G. (1982). Infections in patients with cancer. In Holland J.F. and Frei E. (eds.) *Cancer Medicine.* Philadelphia, PA: Lea and Febinger, pp. 1339–1372.

23. Schimpff S.C., Scott D.A. and Wade J.C. (1994). Infections in cancer patients some controversial issues. *Support Care Cancer* 2, 94–104.

24. Schimpff S.C., Young V.M., Greene W.H., Vermeulen G.D., Moody M.R. and Wiernik P.H. (1972). Origin of infection in acute nonlymphocytic leukaemia. Significance of hospital acquisition of potential pathogens. *Annals of Internal Medicine* 77, 707–714.

25. Ames B.N. (1995). Understanding the causes of aging and cancer. *Microbiologica* 11, 305–308.

26. Donowitz G.R. (1987). Infection prevention in the compromised host. In Wenzel R.P. (ed.) *Prevention and Control of Nosocomial Infections.* Baltimore, MD: Wilkins & Wilkins.

27. Hartnett S. (1989). Septic shock in the oncology patient. *Cancer Nursing* 12, 191–201.

28. Wilson-Barnett J. (1980). Prevention and alleviation of stress in patients. *Nursing* 10, 432–436.

29. Barry S.A. (1989). Septic shock: special needs for patients with cancer. *Oncology Nursing Forum* 16, 31–35.

30. Carter L.W. (1993). Influences of nutrition and stress on people at risk for neutropenia nursing implications. *Oncology Nursing Forum* 20, 1241–1250.

31. Truett L. (1991). The septic syndrome. *Cancer Nursing* 14, 175–181.

32. Bodey G., Jadeja L. and Elting L. (1985). *Pseudomonas* bacteremia: retrospective analysis of 140 episodes. *Annals of Internal Medicine* 145, 1621–1629.

33. Watson J.G. (1993). Problems of infection after bone marrow transplant. *Journal of Clinical Pathology* 36, 683–692.

34. Somerville E.T. (1986). Special diets for neutropenic patients. Do they make a difference? *Seminars in Oncology Nursing* 2, 55–58.

35. Verhoef J. (1993). Prevention of infections in the neutropenic patient. *Clinical Infectious Diseases* 17 (Suppl. 2), S359–S367.

36. Armstrong T.S. (1994). Protected environments are discomforting and expensive and do not offer meaningful protection. *American Journal of Medicine* 76, 685–689.

37. Carter L.W. (1994). Bacterial translocation: nursing implications in the care of patients with neutropenia. *Oncology Nursing Forum* 21, 857–865.

38. Steere A.C. and Mallison G.F. (1978). Handwashing practices for the prevention of nosocomial infections. *Annals of Internal Medicine* **83**, 683–690.

39. Gould D. (1994). Nurses' hand decontamination practice: results of a local study. *Journal of Hospital Infection* **28**, 15–29.

40. Meyers J.D. (1990). Fungal infections in bone marrow transplant patients. *Seminars in Oncology Nursing* **17**, 10–13.

41. Nauseef W.M. and Maki D.G. (1981). A study of the value of simple protective isolation in patient with panuocytopenia. *New England Journal of Medicine* **304**, 448–453.

42. Mooney B.R., Reeves S.A. and Larson E. (1993). Infection control and bone marrow transplantation. *American Journal of Infection Control* **21**, 131–138.

43. Holland J., Plumb M., Yates J., Harris S., Tuttolomondo A., Holmes J. *et al.* (1977). Psychological response of patient with acute leukaemia to germ-free environments. *Cancer* **40**, 871–879.

44. Collins C., Upright C. and Aleksich J. (1989). Reverse isolation: what patients perceive. *Oncology Nursing Forum* **16**, 675–679.

45. Navari R.M., Buckner C.D., Clift R.A., Strob R., Sanders J.E., Stewart P. *et al.* (1984). Prophylaxis of infection patients with a plastic anaemia are receiving allogeneic marrow transplants. *American Journal of Medicine* **76**, 564–572.

46. Mullen C.A. and Buchanan G.R. (1990). Early hospital discharge of children with cancer treated for fever and neutropenia: identification and management of the low risk patient. *Journal of Clinical Oncology* **8**, 1998–2004.

47. Russell J.A., Poon M., Jones A.R., Woodman R.C. and Reuther B.A. (1992). Allogeneic bone marrow transplantation without protective isolation in adults with malignant disease. *Lancet* **339**, 38–40.

48. Tang I.T. and Shepp D.H. (1992). Herpes simplex virus infection in cancer patients; prevention and treatment. *Oncology* **6**, 101–106.

49. Walsh T.J. and Lee J.W. (1993). Prevention of invasive fungal infections in patients with neoplastic diseases. *Clinical Infectious Diseases* **17** (Suppl. 2), S468–S480.

50. Antrum J. (1996). Meeting the challenge of systemic fungal infections in cancer: nursing implications. *European Journal of Haematology* **56** (Suppl. 57), 7–11.

51. Cunningham R. (1990). Infection prophylaxis in the patient with cancer. *Oncology Nursing Forum* **1** (Suppl. 17), 16–19.

52. Zorsky P.E., Fields K.K., Janssen W.E. and Elfenbein G. (1992). Haemopoietic growth factors in bone marrow transplantation current and future uses. *Haematology Reviews* **5**, 179–197.

53. Maguire-Eisen M. (1990). Diagnosis and treatment of adult acute leukaemia. *Seminars in Oncology Nursing* **6**, 17–24.

54. Stone R.M. and Meyer R.J. (1995). Acute myeloid leukemia in adults. In Abeloff M.B., Armitage J.O., Lichter A.S. and Niederhuker J.E. (eds.) *Clinical Oncology.* New York: Churchill Livingstone, pp. 1959–1976.

55. Frankel H.R., Herzig G.P. and Bloomfield C.D. (1995). Acute lymphoblastic leukemia. In Abeloff M.B., Armitage J.O., Lichter A.S. and Niederhunker J.E. (eds.) *Clinical Oncology.* New York: Churchill Livingstone, pp. 1925–1958.

56. Yeager K.A. and Miaskowski C. (1994). Advances in understanding the mechanism and management of acute myelogenous leukaemia. *Oncology Nursing Forum* **21**, 541–547.

57. Foon K.A. and Gale R.P. (1992). Controversies in the therapy of acute myelogenous leukaemia. *American Journal of Medicine* **72**, 963–979.

CHAPTER TWENTY-FIVE

Compromised nutrition

Mary Pennell

For most people, food, including the buying, preparing, and eating of it, provides a large and generally enjoyable use of time. Food has an important role in any culture. Food is seen as an essential and very normal part of our lives and it might be that the very 'ordinariness' of food has militated against it in cancer care, where research seems to focus on the abnormal: pain, sickness, and interventions such as chemotherapy.

While food may be seen as a normal part of daily living, health carers concentrate on the physical impact of eating difficulties rather than broader social or cultural issues surrounding food and eating. In cancer care, providing replacement meals, usually in the form of either milk- or water-based drinks, is the most common response to someone who has difficulty eating or who has weight loss associated with their disease. This is an expensive approach to intervention, and may not always be the most effective or appropriate response.

Nutrition has also been identified as a difficult problem to deal with by nurses caring for people with cancer in palliative care and community settings.[1] In a retrospective interview study with 207 bereaved carers,[2] there were 144 instances where concerns about anorexia or weight loss were voiced. Of these, 98 said that there had been no real alleviation of the problem, and 46 felt that there had only been moderate relief. This was an area of deep concern to carers, which is not surprising since weight loss is a very visible sign of the insidious disease process and is viewed with real distress, both by people with cancer and by those who care about them. Unlike pain, weight loss was a problem that was not relieved.

Nutrition is a problem affecting almost all cancer patients to varying degrees during their illness. Possible reasons for these are shown below.

Box 25.1: Possible reasons for nutritional deficits

- Poor appetite
- No appetite
- Sore mouth
- Infected mouth
- Dry mouth
- Ill-fitting dentures
- Cannot wear dentures
- Changed taste
- Fickle tastes
- No taste
- Dysphagia
- Pain
- Nausea
- Constipation
- Vomiting
- Fatigue
- Breathlessness
- Metabolic disorders
- Malabsorption
- Having radiotherapy
- Having chemotherapy

- Post-radiotherapy
- Post-chemotherapy
- Enlarged liver
- 'Squashed stomach'
- Smelly wounds
- Own body smells
- Anxiety
- Depression

As with other symptoms or problems associated with cancer, identifying the cause or causes is an important part of devising an effective therapeutic strategy. If eating difficulties are primarily emotional in origin, or result from stomatitis or nausea following chemotherapy, responding by offering food supplements or substitutes will not alleviate the problem. By taking nutrition seriously it may be possible to:

- improve or maintain normality or quality of life
- improve tolerance of treatment
- maintain skin integrity, increase opportunities for wound healing, and reduce the risk of pressure sores
- demonstrate respect for an individual beyond their disease
- acknowledge concerns surrounding nutrition.

Problems of nutrition and cancer

Three major problems associated with nutrition frequently result from cancer. These are anorexia (loss of appetite), weight loss, and cachexia (a condition involving both of the former that is associated with body wasting).

Weight loss

Weight loss commonly accompanies cancer, and in some cancer sites (for example, lung cancer) may be the first sign of the presence of the disease. It is not an early sign of cancer; in fact, significant weight loss is a sign of poor prognosis, independent of performance status (i.e. ability to function or activity level), or stage of disease.[3] In lung cancer, weight loss of more than 10% of total body weight is associated with a poor prognosis.[4]

Weight loss may be due to the effects of cancer itself, poor appetite or intake of food, or cancer treatment. Weight loss is related in part to balance between calorie intake and the body's calorie needs,

and in part to the biochemical demands of the tumour on host tissue.[5] Studies of people with cancer have shown that their energy expenditure is higher than expected for their level of activity, indicating that the effect of cancer is to increase expenditure. This is also related to the extent of the tumour. If a tumour is limited in size, it is likely to be easier to return energy balance to normal. With a large tumour bulk, this may not be possible, as there may be increased calorie consumption by the tumour.[5] Weight loss in cancer is not only a problem of high calorie expenditure by the body. The situation is not the same as a healthy person trying to lose weight, where loss is primarily of fatty tissue. In cancer, loss occurs largely from muscle. This is because tumour cells are unable to use glucose as a source of energy; instead, amino acids drawn from muscle are converted to glucose.[5] Therefore, simple strategies to replace calories may have no impact on the need for muscle wasting to be reversed.

Anorexia

Poor appetite may be the result of one of a number of factors. Sense of taste and smell may be altered, and this is known to be increasingly likely the larger the tumour bulk. Early satiety or a sense of fullness may occur. Delayed gastric emptying is a feature of cancer, due to altered glucose metabolism, loss of muscle in the stomach wall, or treatments such as morphine. Changed glucose metabolism may also result in high blood glucose levels, which cause lack of appetite.[5,6]

Illness, injury, hospitalisation, and surgery are all known to increase the body's nutritional requirements. Because of its toxic nature, cancer treatment further contributes to both nutritional demands and appetite problems. Radiotherapy and chemotherapy reduce appetite through nausea and vomiting, but are also likely to impact on appetite independently of these. These may also be responsible for the development of conditioned food aversions, because of the association of certain foods with the memory of treatment-induced nausea or vomiting. Treatments that may cause local difficulties with eating, such as radiotherapy or surgery to the head and neck, in particular where taste, swallowing, and the production of saliva are affected, contribute to anorexia and weight loss. Specific surgical interventions such as gastrectomy, colectomy, or pancreatectomy also cause problems with food absorption.

Anxiety, depression, fatigue, pain, and emotions contribute to lack of appetite and weight loss. The stress response is also known to have a major impact on both metabolism and appetite.[6]

Cancer cachexia

Cancer cachexia is the wasting syndrome often associated with advanced cancer, and the picture of a wasted ill individual in pain is one often associated with cancer in societal and lay images of the disease. It is also an image left with families and partners of people who have died of cancer. These images can be very powerful, causing lasting and difficult memories, which can complicate loss and make bereavement difficult. While cachexia is not an inevitable consequence of cancer, half of all those with the disease may be affected by it at some point during the disease process.[7] The process of cancer cachexia is unlikely to be reversible, particularly in advanced disease, where tumour burden cannot be reduced or removed, and simple nutritional replacement strategies have little impact. It is, however, possible to help people and their families and carers to understand the reasons behind cachexia, to facilitate expression of feelings associated with it, and help with the expression of grief and feelings surrounding adjusting to a changed self-image. The symptoms of cancer cachexia are shown below.

Box 25.2: Symptoms of cancer cachexia

- Muscle wasting
- Weight loss
- Anorexia
- Oedema due to hyponatraemia
- Rapid onset of fatigue
- Impaired immunity
- Inability to concentrate
- Decreased motor and mental skills[7]

Cancer cachexia results from the process of weight loss and anorexia already described. The process of cachexia is inexorable. The increased energy demands of the tumour and alterations in metabolism increase carbon dioxide production and oxygen consumption. Weight loss and muscle wasting diminish immunity and resistance to infection, and cause weakness and fatigue. These all in turn lead to further anorexia, weight loss, and eventually death.[7]

Nutritional intervention

The goal of nutritional intervention is to maintain or correct nutritional status, particularly when this will facilitate effective definitive therapy or improve quality of life.[7] This is most commonly achieved by giving oral food supplements. Where it is possible to slow or reverse the effects of cachexia, there may be a decrease in fatigue, fewer complications from treatment, improved immunity, and improved feelings of well-being. Nutritional intervention needs to be determined in the context of the overall goal of treatment and care and disease state. De Wys suggests that an important question to ask in determining intervention is 'How much of the nutrient intake goes to the patient and how much to the tumour?'.[5] Where decreased calorie intake is the major cause of weight loss, then nutritional supplements are highly appropriate. Where this is due to increased energy expenditure, increased intake might further increase expenditure by the tumour and still maintain the negative energy balance. Nutritional support in the context of decreased calorie intake and when given with anti-cancer therapy is likely to be effective; however, in the context of palliative care it should be given more cautiously since enhanced nutrition may accelerate tumour metabolism.[5] Care strategy 25.1 outlines nutritional interventions that may be considered.

Enteral feeding may be used when oral intake is not possible. This may be delivered nasogastrically, or through a gastrostomy or jejunostomy tube surgically or percutaneously placed in the stomach or jejunum. The place of parenteral nutrition (feeding via the intravenous route) is controversial. Parenteral feeding can lead to complications such as venous thrombosis, air embolism, infection, and hyper- or hypoglycaemia. While it may be appropriate as an adjunct to surgery, reducing perioperative complications and mortality, or where there is intestinal obstruction or fistula, in someone who is debilitated it can result in fluid overload. When used with radiotherapy or chemotherapy, parenteral nutrition may prevent weight loss and enhance recovery. It is, however, a costly intervention and questions about efficacy are complex. In a study using parenteral nutrition in conjunction with chemotherapy with small-cell lung cancer, while the group of patients receiving parenteral nutrition gained weight, they rapidly lost it again once it was withdrawn, so that no benefit was gained.[8]

Case strategy 25.1: Nutritional intervention in cancer care

For those with little or no weight loss or anorexia at the commencement of treatment (using nutritional intervention aimed at prevention):

- offer counselling regarding maintenance of food intake
  - countering taste changes
  - prevention of nausea and vomiting
  - avoidance of conditioned food aversions
- offer balanced calorie/protein supplements for periods when free of side-effects.

For someone who is unable to eat:

- where the digestive system is intact, or there is disruption in ability to swallow, consider enteral feeding
- if digestive system is not fully functional (for example, in intestinal obstruction prior to surgery), parenteral nutrition may be appropriate.

For those in a palliative care setting or with advanced disease:

- a slightly lower than normal calorie intake may slow tumour growth and prolong survival
- consider an appetite stimulant such as megesterol acetate.

In all situations optimise food intake by:

- encouraging choice of favourite/desired foods
- suggesting eating small meals often
- choosing high protein foods if possible
- providing anti-emetics, analgesia, oral care
- allowing others to cook
- using exercise, wine or apéritifs, relaxation, to stimulate appetite
- using calorie/intake diaries.[3-7]

Wider issues

Food and eating have meaning beyond the immediate need for sustaining physical function, and repair and recovery from illness:

Because of values that go far beyond filling the stomach, eating becomes associated, if only at an unconscious level, with deep rooted sentiments and assumptions about oneself and the world one lives in.[8]

Eating is linked to deep spiritual experiences and social ties, and foods are endowed with metaphorical or symbolic qualities far beyond their nutritional use. The vocabulary of eating is used to describe experience; such language, used in different cultures, reveals unconscious assumptions about food and the world in general. Rituals surrounding eating, from the barbecue to an invitation to dinner, have important social meanings, which extend friendship, or provide settings for business exchange or courtship:

> Eating is symbolically associated with deeply felt human experiences, and expresses things that are difficult to articulate in everyday language.[8]

In the context of illness, in particular cancer, eating, weight loss, and the refusal to eat will therefore have immense significance. Preparing and offering food is a nurturing activity, deeply embedded in family life. Food refused, or the inability to eat, not only has huge significance in relation to health, signalling the imminence of death, but also denies family members an important role in caring. Those unable to eat are alienated from social aspects of eating.

Personal account 25.1

Roger was a 67-year-old man with inoperable cancer of the oesophagus. I met him shortly after his return home having had a Celestin tube inserted. The tube was patent and previous experience suggested that Roger would be able to eat and drink as he wished. The nature of his illness and prognosis had been explained to him on several occasions. His response was 'I really can't swallow this', 'It sticks in my throat when I think about my future, or lack of it.' His drink became largely tea with whisky. He talked a great deal about the food he would eat when he had 'turned the corner', but he never did and never ate.

One day it was clear that there had been a great change in Roger. He sat up in bed and said 'I am going to die' and when I agreed, he said 'I have always known it but I could not take it in, somehow. Now I know, I had such a good breakfast this morning.'

He ate strawberries, cake, soup, and smoked salmon over the next few days, and saw and talked with a constant stream of visitors. He subsequently died at home with his family as they had hoped.

An understanding of both the physiology of nutrition and the unconscious and social significance of food in the context of cancer and its treatment is needed to achieve optimal functioning and symptom management and to facilitate and maintain social and family functioning. Helping someone to manage the everyday activity of eating in a way that reflects their former approach to food may be one of the most effective caring activities that the nurse can offer to someone with cancer.

References

1. Copp G. and Dunn V. (1993). Frequent and difficult problems perceived by nurses craing for the dying in community, hospice and acute care settings. *Palliative Medicine* 7, 19–25.
2. Jones R., Hansford J. and Fiske J. (1993). Death from cancer at home: the carer's perspective. *British Medical Journal* 306, 249–251.
3. De Wys W. (1985). Management of cancer cachexia. *Seminars in Oncology* 12, 452–460.
4. Hespanhol V., Queirozga H., Magalhals A. *et al.* (1995). Survival predictors in lung advanced non-small cell lung cancer. *Lung Cancer* 13, 253–267.
5. De Wys W.D. (1980). Nutritional care of the cancer patient. *Journal of the American Medical Association* 244, 374–376.
6. Bistian B. (1986). Some practical and theoretical concepts in the nutritional assessment of the cancer patient. *Cancer* 58, 1863–1865.
7. Tait N.S. (1996). Anorexia – cachexia syndrome. In Groenwald, Hansen Frogge M. Goodman M. and Henke-Yarbro C. (eds.) *Cancer Symptom Management.* Boston, MA: Jones and Bartlett, pp. 171–196.
8. Weiner R.S., Kramer B.S., Clamon G.M. *et al.* (1985). Effects of hyperalimentation during treatment in patients with small cell lung cancer. *Journal of Clinical Oncology* 3, 949–957.

CHAPTER TWENTY-SIX

Altered self-concept

Mary Bredin

The sense of self is the core of our being, the 'I' that defines a unique, individual, nature. We develop this sense of being largely through our body, and through it we express who we are to the outside world. This self-embodying process unfolds in relation to others, an actual and metaphorical contact that moulds the bodily sense of self. In turn, it influences relationships and shapes our inner experience of self. One's body becomes so familiar as to be unnoticeable unless its comfortable unremarkableness is disturbed by 'tension', by illness, trauma, or disability. Changed experience of the body – when it is permanently damaged, mutilated, incomplete, or spoiled – deeply affects one's sense of self. When that essential familiarity and wholeness is stripped away, feelings of difference, isolation, fragmentation, and a loss of self-worth ensue.

In his article 'The embodied self: personal integration in health and illness',[1] Leonard Zegans explores the confusing way in which self, feelings, and body intertwine:

> To be a self is to experience one's body in a certain way. This implies being able to use one's body to carry out certain intentions in a fluid manner. It also means that the body functions as a medium for receiving and conveying information in a fashion appropriate to one's needs and wishes. Thought, desire, perception, expression, and action can be experienced as one seamless piece. Essential to this harmony and embeddedness of psyche and body is the development of what has been called body schema or body image . . . Often unspoken yet unconscious concerns about the body can interfere directly with the physiological process of healing and the patient's co-operation with treatment.

His perspective is phenomenological (the theory that behaviour is determined by the way a person perceives reality rather than by external reality in objective terms) and he argues strongly for the need of health professionals to recognise the significance of embodiment. The task as he sees it is to help individuals experiencing illness or the impact of physical trauma to adapt to a changed sense of body and self. It is obvious that as nurses we have to be alert to a person's changing feelings and attitudes toward their body – especially during a life-threatening illness such as cancer. How, though, are we to understand their predicament and respond meaningfully? Zegans'[1] emphasis is mainly psychological, but adaptation may call for more than psychological adjustment where the struggle involves a profoundly altered sense of the body.

The separation of body and mind: some clinical consequences

Modern Western medicine has tended to approach illness as the malfunction and breakdown of the human biological system, and treatment as 'fixing' the part of the body that has gone wrong. From this perspective, the 'thinking self' and 'physical body' are viewed as separate[2] – a dualism that is both fundamental in our culture, and particularly pervasive in health care. We learn to understand the body as a fixed object: a material entity determined by the empirical laws of biological science, and characterised by unchangeable inner necessities.[3] This implies that however much we attempt to move beyond the separation of mind and body, and to nurse the 'whole' patient, an implicit division between identified physical symptoms or problems, and psychological distress (whether or not acknowledged) remains. The task-led nature of medicine and nursing tends to reinforce these perspectives.

This paradox cannot be ignored when addressing disrupted body experience, for the bodily distress and emotional experience are obviously *inseparable*. For instance, suppose I once received a wound to my body. The feelings I experienced at the time – the fear, the sense of vulnerability (and the many possible associated feelings, including guilt, anger, blame, despair) – would not have been distinct from associated bodily responses – muscular tensions, altered perceptions, and autonomic arousal. Perhaps, if distress persisted I might eventually talk with a therapist about my feelings. But the usual approaches to psychotherapy and counselling generally would tend not to address the body experience – even though the ongoing distress would quite probably include a bodily component. As Zegans[1] says, the body is in a larger sense 'a vessel of meaning, memory, and intention', yet more than metaphorical distress is involved here, for it is as if the body continues to hold some memory of the wounding experience in the tissues themselves.

In such circumstances it might make sense to meet the body directly through touch, and so respond to the intertwined physical/emotional tensions held within it. Exploring the *meaning* and *memory* held within the body sounds strange, but consider, for example, how when a woman thinks about or touches her lost breast, the meaning and memories there will be deeply bound up with her wounded sense of herself as nurturer, lover, and woman: with her former self and body and what has been lost.

Massage and body image: a rationale for therapeutic intervention

The importance of touch
A growing body of theory and research suggests that touch has an essential influence on physical and psychological development. Touch is the earliest sense to develop in the womb and is a basic behavioural need.[4] Touch continues to be important throughout adult life, and especially so in times of crisis or illness. It has been suggested that the more an ill person's body image is altered, the greater their need for acceptance through touch, since it is the basis for establishing communication, particularly in the realm of emotions.[5]

Touch is one method of intervening in altered body image. By working directly with the body, an individual's perceptions and feelings about it may be changed. The sense of self depends to a degree on the experience of being embodied; behaviour is significantly influenced by the way one adapts to bodily experience. By working with the body, bodily experience can be more directly addressed, and this may help to facilitate behavioural, cognitive, or emotional change in someone who is ill,[6,7] although there is a little empirical evidence to support this.

There has been no systematic research into massage and body image. Nevertheless, there are several reports on the perceived benefits of touch in helping people to cope with altered body image (ABI); for example, McNamara's[8] qualitative study of the experience of 24 massage practitioners working with cancer patients. Notable findings were participants' perceptions that massage helps them to 'be more in touch with their bodies in a positive way,' their beliefs that massage helped them to 'accept and nurture their body', and that it can increase body awareness and improve body image. In another study aimed at evaluating massage with essential oils on cancer patients' perceptions of their quality of life, it was commented that:

> The effect of a caring and knowledgeable individual placing their hands on the body of a patient who for example has undergone physically mutilating surgery could be profound, and represented unconditional acceptance in the minds of some patients.[9]

Body image
Many authors have contributed to our understanding of body image. The earliest and most frequently quoted concept was formulated by the German neurologist Paul Schilder in his book *The Image and Appearance of the Human Body*.[10]

The image of the human body means the picture of our own body which we form in our mind, that is to say the way in which our body appears to ourselves [p. 11].

For Schilder, who was greatly influenced by Freud, body image was not simply cognitive. He emphasised that emotions have a central role in shaping a person's inner representation of their body. A person's body image is also influenced by their social interactions with others. Body image is *subjective,* an inner representation, and may bear no relationship to how a person's body appears to others.[11,12] One might, for example, imagine one's body at different times as fat, thin, ugly, pretty, when in reality one's external physical appearance has not changed. This subjectivity is influenced by cultural norms and social interactions. Its development is, for example, profoundly influenced by the relationships we have with our care providers from infancy onwards, and social influences will affect an individual's body image throughout their life.[13] Individuals therefore not only monitor their appearance in terms of self-satisfaction, but also in relation to others, who act as a social mirror.[14] This means that the impact of a damaged or changed sense of body integrity is influenced by the reactions and behaviour of others.[15] The components that define body image are:[14]

- *perceptions of the body* – perception and experience of the body, through sensations involving the neuromuscular system and through visual appraisal of one's appearance
- *concepts concerning one's body* – thought and language about the body; how we create accounts of the body and describe it in relation to the self
- *attitudes and value systems of the body* – the different feelings and emotional attitudes individuals have towards their bodies, either its separate body parts or as a whole.

Body image and self-concept

A continuing theme in twentieth-century psychology and philosophy has been the debate about the reality of the 'self' or the 'I'. But whether or not it can be said to exist, we nonetheless all experience ourselves as I, and we assume that others do the same. In attempting to define self-concept, Driever[16] explains it as being the answer to the question 'Who am I?'.

In recent years it has become more widely acknowledged that certain aspects of the experience of cancer affect quality of life and make sufferers particularly vulnerable to changes in self-concept.[17] Self-concept can be divided into four compartments:[18]

- the body self (physical function and body image)
- the interpersonal self (psychosocial and sexual function)
- the achievement self (job–role function)
- the identification self (spiritual and ethical beliefs).

A cancer diagnosis is in itself a threat to core beliefs, role interpretations, and role functions; furthermore, its effects and treatment can distort a person's self-concept in a variety of ways. For example, tumour development in different organs or tissues may cause bodily changes, altered body sensations, and unpleasant symptoms; for instance, pain, breathlessness, nausea and constipation. Symptoms may act as a constant reminder of illness and can provoke intense anxiety and emotional suffering, feelings about the body that blur into anguish about existence itself. Tumour growth and the treatments employed to 'fight' the cancer are for many inherently frightening. Not only physically exhausting, and emotionally debilitating, they can potentially alter the body image and self-concept in a variety of ways: the intrusion of a needle to administer treatment; the penetration of the surgeon's knife to cut out cancerous tissue; the restrictive regimes of chemotherapy and radiotherapy with their physical side-effects; the loss of well-being and libido; and the increased dependence on others.[18]

It is not difficult to understand how the experience of cancer can affect body and self, because having a life-threatening illness calls for huge adjustments. The sense that the body is out of control – something to mistrust, to fear and dislike – may grow with a diagnosis of cancer, so that identity, competence, status, and power are all called into question (signifying the damaged self). The loss of control and comfort, of the feeling that tomorrow the body will be much as it was today, can represent a profound threat. Cancer removes the certainty that the body can be relied upon. Every ache, pain, sensation, and body function can become a concern and a reminder of how vulnerable the body and self can be.

Personal account 26.1 explores an approach using a combination of touching and talking to help a woman adapt to her body and self. This work is based on experience and research, working with women experiencing distress and problems with their body as a consequence of mastectomy for breast cancer.[19]

Personal account 26.1

Penny was 45 years old when she discovered a lump in her breast. Her doctor diagnosed a malignant breast tumour; a mastectomy of the right breast and six sessions of adjuvant chemotherapy followed. Penny returned to work 9 months after her original diagnosis.

Penny's partner and teenage daughter were supportive throughout her ordeal. Though relieved when her treatment was over, she was still privately fearful of a recurrence. But she had read in a woman's magazine that women who adopt a 'positive attitude' to cancer were more likely to do better than those who did not. Consequently, when anyone asked her how she was, she would say she felt fine. She tried to believe it herself, although inwardly she felt that her world had changed, and that life could never be the same. Penny had days when she felt extremely low, withdrawn, and tearful.

Penny experienced numbness and coldness of her arm and scar site and phantom sensations of her breast. These unpleasant sensations served as a constant reminder of her physical change. Her body shape had altered; her chest 'went in, instead of out', and she felt 'lop-sided'; her breast scar was red and in her opinion 'ugly'. Initially she could not look at herself and even took her baths in the dark.

I don't like looking at myself, I just put lots of bubbles in the bath, I don't look . . . I suppose to an extent I feel deformed. That's probably the best way to describe it . . . your appearance has changed quite radically. I think it is possibly one of the most mutilating things that a female can have done . . .

Speaking of her reflection in the mirror, she said:

I don't like it, that's not me . . .

To compensate for the change in her body she wanted to improve the rest of her appearance. If she could achieve this she believed she would feel better about herself; other people would not be able to see she was different.

I want to grow my hair long, and lose weight, then I'll feel better in myself because I'll know from the outside it won't be any different.

However by covering up the 'difference' she experienced physically, she masked her distress. As a consequence, although she wanted to talk, she kept her feelings to herself.

If you saw someone walking along and they had just had their leg off you'd think oh they must be feeling . . . I don't want everyone to know I've lost my breast but sometimes I just feel like I've been through so much I want to talk but people don't really want to know, so you keep it all in here to yourself . . .

Before her mastectomy she had felt proud of her body and her breasts; they were also an aspect of her feminine self-concept, bound up with her image of herself as a woman. In her relationship with her partner her breasts had been an important part of her sexual identity and sense of sexual attractiveness. Penny had said after her breast was cut off she felt 'unfeminine' and 'sexually unattractive'. Her sexual relationship with her partner had stopped; significantly, she had showed her breast scar to her partner before she had looked at it herself and then regretted it.

I should not have let him see it because his reaction wasn't what I wanted. I wished really I'd looked at it myself before I'd let him see it because although he said it was all right you could tell by his face it was not, it was shock.

Being unable to look at herself she had showed her partner, hoping for some affirmation that she did not really look 'so bad'. When she showed her breast to him, his expression confirmed her worst fear – that she did look bad. Subsequently, all she could do was to conceal her disfigurement, while her dislike of her body increased. Perhaps in hiding her scars she was also concealing the pain and loss she was feeling, and the inability to express may have heightened her distress. In addition, she felt guilty for feeling upset; after all, she told herself, her treatment had been successful.

The problem extended beyond being simply an altered body image. For the loss of her breast and the experience of having cancer had a wider impact on Penny's self-concept. Inwardly, she realised that she felt different; it was not easy for her to account for this or to explain it in words; she just knew this sense of difference had changed her.

I don't feel the same as I did before the surgery. But nobody can, can they? I mean I don't look any different to the outside world, it's just you are different and there's no getting away from it.

Penny implied that she could cope as long as she kept up an appearance of looking normal by wearing her prosthesis and concealing her sense of physical difference. For example, she said:

When I have my clothes on I can cope because no one needs to know.

Yet despite concealing her breast loss, physically and emotionally she began to feel different – not just to herself but in relation to others. She was more self-conscious, and less confident. It became an effort to socialise as Penny's difficulties in coming to terms with her experience led her to feel increasingly depressed and withdrawn. Living in a culture that promotes images of women with perfect bodies and blemish-free appearances may have contributed to her feelings of alienation and difference.

The intervention of therapeutic massage

Touch is a form of communication that transcends the usual boundaries between human beings. It embodies the experience of being contained, conveying directly feelings of being well-held, cared for and accepted.[19]

Ten months after her mastectomy, Penny came to see me for six sessions of therapeutic massage. Early on in our meeting it became clear that her self-esteem was low. Furthermore, having cancer had disturbed her self-concept; Penny's role a as a mother, provider, lover, and friend had been threatened by her cancer. She had in essence been thrown into 'self-conscious living which is bathed constantly in the shadowy light of death'.[7] The slightest unfamiliar sensation could threaten her with a return of the cancer and she told me she could no longer rely on her body. It had, in her words, 'let her down'. My task was to help her restore her relationship with her body. This in turn might enable her to cope better with the changes she experienced in her body, self, and relationships. My approach involved talking and touch, but it also depended on there being enough mutuality and trust to allow her to talk about unacceptable feelings of physical loss and difference. As we talked, the themes that appeared in Penny's story were of change, uncertainty, loss, and difference at every level of her being. The potential for massage to initiate changes in body perception, and to influence body concept underpinned the approach of my work with Penny.

My intention was to help Penny to re-experience her body in a positive way through the sensation of touch gently applied locally to the area around (but not on) her breasts, i.e. arms, back, and shoulders. (Touch in this sense is only employed with the permission of the recipient.) Penny had described beforehand sensations and body experiences that were traumatic, i.e. mutilating surgery, physical pain, skin numbness, and muscle tension. In a broader sense it enabled Penny to regain a sense of the 'whole of her body'. (We always discussed beforehand where she wanted me to touch: feet, hands, face, whole body, etc.)

An important aspect of body image is the way we conceptualise and create accounts of our body.[14] Yet talking about the unacceptable differences felt as a consequence of breast removal is not encouraged in our culture, nor are these feelings easy to articulate. So I offered Penny the opportunity to talk about her experience of losing her breast, and to express the thoughts, fears, and feelings about her changed body; to re-shape her experience into a more coherent narrative – her body's story. I encouraged her to address her concerns and fears of the cancer returning, her fear of her body being out of her control, of feeling that she was no longer physically attractive to her partner and that she had somehow become different to women whose bodies were still intact. At times when she felt unable to talk, I would hold her literally with my hands allowing her the space just to be with her body and feelings; and it was through touch that I communicated my acceptance of her.

There is a sound theoretical basis for exploring the role of touch after cancer diagnosis and treatment. The availability of a body-centred therapy could meet the need for help with certain aspects of adjustment to changed body image. In particular, it might provide a containment for what had previously been experienced as uncontainable – unacceptable and unspeakable perceptions of a changed body and self. It might offer the opportunity for a person to explore their changed 'untouchable' body, and facilitate the expression of feelings previously hidden because of embarrassment or stigma. However, such an approach should be used with care; some people may benefit from a body-orientated intervention, others not. Further research studies are needed some areas for possible research are shown below.

Potential areas for future research

Research may include identifying:

- patients at risk of body image disturbance
- their experience of the problem
- ways of assessing the contribution of body image problems (quantitatively and qualitatively)
- how to treat these problems effectively and to evaluate their outcome.

The limitations on present resources in health care will undoubtedly constrain innovation. Nonetheless, the experience of cancer is multi-dimensional, and massage could be relevant when the aim is to help individuals to adapt to the bodily and psychological changes it brings. Evolving multi-disciplinary approaches should consider how to include it.

Acknowledgement

I would like to express my thanks and gratitude to David Peters for his help and support in writing this chapter.

References

1. Zegans L.S. (1987). The embodied self: personal integration in health and illness. *Advances* **4**, 29–45.
2. Harré R. (1991). *Physical Being: A Theory for a Corporeal Psychology.* Oxford: Blackwells, pp. 15–35.
3. Lanceley A. (1995). Wider issues in pain management. *European Journal of Cancer Care* **4**, 153–157.
4. Montague A. (1971). *Touching – The Human Significance of the Skin.* New York: Columbia University Press.
5. Barnett K. (1972). A theoretical construct of the concepts of touch as they relate to nursing. *Nursing Research* **21**, 102–110.
6. Pruzinsky T. (1990). Somatopsychic approaches to psychotherapy and personal growth. In Cash T. and Pruzinsky T. (eds.) *Body Images Development Deviance and Change.* London: Guilford Press, pp. 296–315.
7. Fisher S. (1990). The evolution of psychological concepts about the body. In Cash T.F. and Pruzinsky T. (eds.) *Body Images Development Deviance and Change.* London: Guilford Press, pp. 3–19.
8. McNamara P. (1994). *Massage for People with Cancer.* London: Wandsworth Cancer Support Centre.
9. Corner J., Cawley N. and Hildebrand S. (1995). An evaluation of the use of massage and massage with the addition of essential oils on the well-being of cancer patients. *International Journal of Palliative Nursing* **1**, 67–73.
10. Schilder P. (1950). *The Image and Appearance of the Human Body.* New York: International Universities Press.
11. Cash T. and Pruzinsky T. (eds.) (1990). *Body Images Development Deviance and Change.* London: Guilford Press, pp. 337–338.
12. Fisher S. (1990). Development and structure of the body image. In Cash T.F. and Pruzinsky T. (eds.) *Body Images Development Deviance and Change,* Vols 1 and 2. London: Guilford Press, pp. 296–315.
13. Krueger D.W. (1990). Development and psychodynamic perspectives on body-image change. In Cash T.F. and Pruzinsky T. (eds.) *Body Images Development Deviance and Change.* London: Guilford Press, pp. 255–271.
14. Price B. (1994). The asthma experience: altered body image and non-compliance. *Journal of Clinical Nursing* **3**, 139–145.
15. Rafferty D. (1995). Body image: using women who have had breast surgery as a case study. *International Journal of Palliative Nursing* **1**, 195–199.
16. Driever M.J. (1984). Self-concept: theory and development. In Roy C. (ed.) *Introduction to Nursing – An Adaptation Model,* 2nd edition. New Jersey: Prentice-Hall, pp. 255–283.
17. Curbow B., Somerifield M., Legro M. and Sonnega J. (1990). Self-concept and cancer in adults: theoretical and methodological issues. *Social Science and Medicine* **1**, 115–128.
18. Foltz A. (1987). The influence of cancer on self-concept and life quality. *Seminars in Oncology Nursing* **3**, 303–312.
19. Bredin M. (1995). *Mastectomy, body-image and therapeutic massage: a preliminary qualitative study of women's experience.* Unpublished M.Sc. dissertation, Centre for Complementary Health Studies, University of Exeter.

CHAPTER TWENTY-SEVEN

Sexuality and cancer

Siân Dennison

Human beings are sexual in every way all the time. To a large extent human sexuality determines who we are. It is an integral factor in the uniqueness of every person.[1]

Despite a wealth of literature and an increasing quantity of research about cancer and sexuality it is apparent that the subject of sexuality is avoided by health care professionals.[2] Historically, attitudes and beliefs about sexuality have fluctuated according to religious, legal, and political influences; views on sexuality are very much a product of cultural influences.[3,4] Sexuality encompasses who we are within our body, mind, and society. It is closely interrelated with the image we have of ourselves (body image), what we think of ourselves (self-esteem), and how we would like other people to see us. It involves more than sexual desires, activity and orientation; it encompasses touching, intimacy, and the physical closeness of others.[5] It reflects our personality and our role within our families, relationships, work, and society. The importance of sexuality to a person's quality of life is well recognised in cancer care.[6–8] However, many health professionals have not been taught how to cross the boundaries of sexuality, or been prepared to confront and understand their inner self and sexuality, in their own lives and the lives of their patients.

Lawler[9] explored the difficulty nurses face psychologically when dealing with bodily functions that are normally taboo and hidden behind closed doors. Lawler suggests that cultural meanings associated with bodily functions affect the ability of nurses to deal with bodily care, sexuality, and genitalia. She discovered that although nurses were taught how to perform various body care procedures they did not know 'how to manage socially what those procedures entailed, nor how they might respond emotionally to what they had to do' (p. 122).

In the following extract from Lawler's study a female nurse describes her fear and profound embarrassment of having to deal with male nakedness.

I can remember the very first day on the ward . . . begging that they let me do a female one (sponge) first because I couldn't bear thought of pulling down a man's trousers. At that stage I don't think it even occurred to me that my father had genitals. I was that protected from the male anatomy . . . [p. 121].

This difficulty is also evident when nurses have to talk about personal and private parts of the body. In the conversation shown below between a trained oncology nurse and a patient, the nurse is administering an injection of dexamethasone. The nurse is explaining the side-effects of the drug – an itchy or nerve-type sensation in the perineum. Even though the communication of information was difficult, the need to address the issue was recognised, although it took more than one attempt before the patient understood exactly what the nurse meant. While the first nurse was too embarrassed to wash a patient, the second nurse was dealing with sensitive issues about personal and private parts of the body.

Sexuality and sexual functioning can be disrupted as much by the psychological as the physical effects of cancer treatment at any stage of the illness. Even before confirmation of a diagnosis of cancer, psychological and physical effects of the illness can impinge upon a person's sexuality. The devel-

Box 27.1: A conversation between a nurse and patient[10]

Nurse   . . . so I'll give you the dexamethasone first. Now this can give you a really funny feeling all right?

Patient   What sort of funny feeling is that?

Nurse   It gives you like a tingle.

Patient   Oh like I had . . .

Nurse   . . . in your bits . . .

Patient   I don't think I've got any bits left.

Nurse   Oh, you've still got bits there in your bottom, in your rectum, it sometimes gives you a tingle. [The conversation moves on.]

Patient   What bits are affected?

Nurse   Vagina. Sometimes you get a shoot up your vagina and your rectum.

Patient   Oh I see!

opment of symptoms such as abnormal bleeding, lethargy, weight loss, and pain have the potential to cause a negative change in one's self-concept and body image. This ultimately affects a person's self-esteem and self-confidence and in turn impacts on sexual functioning and sexual expression.[11]

During the period of diagnosis and treatment, anxieties and fears may not only lessen the desire for sex but also impact upon a person's sexuality. All sexual functioning may be suspended while the person comes to terms with the threat of the diagnosis.[11,12] There may be uncertainties about the future, the threat to fertility and body image, pain and mutilation. Shame and guilt about the perceived causes, and feelings of helplessness and isolation may increase feelings of anxiety and depression.[13,14]

The interplay between the psychological and physiological elements is described eloquently by one patient:

Sex between us took a long time. I had no self-confidence I couldn't see how my husband wanted me, especially since the maxillectomy with my face red and scarred, plus my hair fell out . . . I just wasn't feeling sexual. I was tired.[15]

The integral nature of self-concept, symptoms, and sexuality is illustrated by the woman's loss of sexual self-confidence and her change in body image from the surgery, alopecia, and fatigue, ultimately affecting the couple's sexual functioning. A study of the experiences of men with testicular can-

cer found that although shock was an initial reaction to the removal of the testis, this was short-lived. Some men were glad to get rid of the testicle because of its discomfort and enlargement. Although some men saw its removal as an insult to their manhood, others very clearly did not. What was most evident in the study was the lack of information given to them about sexual functioning.[12] Table 27.1 lists some possible effects of cancer treatment on sexual functioning.

Cancer can cause a loss of sexual desire throughout the illness experience. Feeling sexually unattractive due to alopecia, nausea, vomiting, and disfiguring surgery is common, as illustrated by the examples above. Women may experience symptoms from premature menopause; for example, hot flushes and vaginal dryness. Effects of radiotherapy such as vaginal stenosis and fibrosis, and changes in breast sensations may also be experienced. Men may experience retrograde ejaculation and erectile difficulties from surgery or radiotherapy.

Studies of the psychosocial and sexual effects of radiotherapy and surgery on women with cervical cancer suggest that symptoms and anxieties experienced by the women negatively affect their feelings of attractiveness and self-confidence; as a result sexual difficulties may persist long after completion of treatment.[16–19]

Psychosexual adjustment following treatment for cancer is dependent on numerous factors: the meaning of the loss (for example, a breast or limb), pre-illness psychosexual functioning, the specific treatment and site of the cancer, and interpersonal relationships.[20,21] The role of the partner and family are important in enabling psychosexual adjustment and reducing feelings of isolation and abandonment.[4,5] Without communication and understanding even the strongest of relationships can be destroyed.[22–24] One woman in Lamb and Sheldon's[11] study of women's experiences of endometrial cancer speaks of the importance of her partner:

I think it [sexual adaptation] depends a lot on the support women get from their husbands. If they can reassure you that whatever happens they'll still love you just as much, or you're just as important, you're just as complete a person as you were before.

Cancer and its treatments can expose and emphasise previous sexual and relationship

Table 27.1 Possible effects of cancer treatments on sexual function

Site of cancer	Surgery	Radiotherapy	Chemotherapy/hormones
Head and neck	Removal of all or parts of the facial and oral structures, laryngectomy	Dysphagia, trismus, changes in salivary texture and amount, taste, skin alterations, loss of voice and normal breathing mechanism	Not commonly given
Breast	Mastectomy, scarring, changes in sensation, prosthesis, reconstruction	Changes in colour, texture, and sensation	Temporary or permanent infertility, nausea, vomiting, alopecia, hot flushes, atrophic vaginitis, weight gain, fatigue
Cervical, endometrial, and ovarian	Hysterectomy, oopherectomy, removal of top third of vagina, infertility, and menopausal changes	Vaginal dryness, stenosis and fibrosis, ovarian failure = menopause, bowel changes, cystitis, skin changes	Temporary or permanent infertility, ovarian failure = menopause, nausea, vomiting, alopecia, weight gain
Vulva	Partial or radical vulvectomy, loss of clitoris		
Testicular	Orchidectomy = infertility, retroperitoneal lymph node dissection = inability to ejaculate or retrograde ejaculation, infertility (temporary or permanent)	Infertility	Temporary or permanent infertility, alopecia, nausea and vomiting
Prostate	Prostatectomy − temporary or permanent erectile dysfunction, urinary incontinence	Erectile dysfunction, transient painful ejaculation, permanent reduction in semen volume	Hormones − castration, hot flushes, loss of muscle tone, changes in hair distribution, erectile dysfunction

difficulties. An insight into the experience of one male patient is described in Personal account 27.1.

Personal account 27.1

John was referred to me by the ward nursing staff, who explained that he was continually talking about his loss of libido and they were finding it increasingly embarrassing. John was married. He explained that he had a very close relationship with his wife and that they loved each other very much. John had a past history of peripheral vascular disease and had

suffered with erectile problems for the past 10 years. His loss of sexual desire had only recently occurred, when he had been diagnosed with cancer and started chemotherapy. He said 'he didn't feel like a man anymore' and felt inadequate because he was unable to satisfy his wife sexually. John told me that he didn't think his wife was as interested in sex as him; however, he was frightened that she might leave him for someone else because of his inability. Conversely, he was certain she would never do this but nevertheless was too afraid to talk through his fears with her.

Identified problems
• Chronic peripheral vascular disease causing erectile problems.
• Loss of sexual desire possibly due to the diagnosis of cancer chemotherapy.

- Anxieties about loss of manhood and concerns about his wife may have perpetuated his difficulties.
- A lack of communication with his wife.

Interventions and recommendations
- Active listening to John's story to identify and pick up cues.
- Provision of information with regard to the causes of loss of desire and the effect of anxieties.
- Discussion of fears and anxieties about talking to wife and the importance of communication.
- Advice regarding specialist referral for erectile problems if desired.

One month later John came back to see me. He told me that they had attempted sex again but with no luck, but he explained that he and his wife had spent the rest of the night crying and talking about how they both felt. John was greatly relieved and contented with the outcome and thanked me profusely.

Most of the 'how to' help with sexual concerns is derived from American literature.[25–27] Within society today there is an expanding awareness of sexuality at all ages; even so, it may not be easy for people to ask for information or help with sexual concerns. One study found that 56% of patients would have liked sexual information but 75% of them would not bring it up themselves.[28] Another study of women undergoing treatment for gynecological cancer found that over half had no sexual counselling before or after treatment, although 89% would have like to have talked to a nurse or doctor about these issues.[2] This suggests that despite increasing societal awareness of sexuality, health care professionals still avoid the subject. Research suggests that many health care professionals are too embarrassed to discuss sexual issues; they may not feel it is relevant to the illness and there is inadequate training. Nurses, are, however, ideally placed to carry out the role as an assessor, educator, confidante, and sometimes counsellor.[25,29]

In order to offer help, a knowledgeable and non-judgemental approach is needed, as well as being comfortable with attitudes and behaviours that are different from one's own. Skilled communication is also required to educate and support the patient and their partner in a positive way. A guide to talking about sexual issues is provided below.

Care strategy 27.1: A guide to talking about sexual issues

As in other areas of communication, there is no definitive formula. Each person is different and the questions you ask will depend on the situation. Therefore the following are only examples of possible courses that can be taken.

Do:
- Create an atmosphere that is comfortable and private.
- Act in a professional and caring manner.
- Acknowledge the sensitivity of the topic and its importance in planning care.
- Spend some time establishing a rapport with the person before moving on to more sensitive issues.
- Be alert to cues, giving them permission to discuss sexual issues.
- Include the partner whenever possible.

Don't:
- Assume anything.
- Pre-judge individuals or relationships.
- Presume they use or understand the same language.

During the nursing assessment ask:
- Do you currently have a partner?
- How is your partner coping with your illness?
- Do you have a close relationship?
- Has the illness affected your relationship in any way?
- Has your sexual relationship been affected by the illness or treatment?
or
- Are you worried about the effects of the treatment or illness on your relationship (intimate or sexual)?[25]

For women:
Ask women about their menopausal status:
- Do you still have periods?
If they are post-menopausal:
- Do you suffer with any symptoms such as hot flushes, weight gain, vaginal dryness or irritation? If so . . .
- Do any of these symptoms affect (intimate) relationship with a partner, or feelings of well-being?

Providing information
Find out pre-existing knowledge about the disease and treatment and what the doctor has told them. Correct any myths and misconceptions and build on previous knowledge. Offer manageable pieces of information and find out what anxieties they have about the illness and treatment:

- What do you understand about your illness or treatment?
- What most worries you about your illness or treatment?

Explain about the effects of treatment generally. Where and how does it affect the body? Many patients do not feel like sex during their treatment because of fatigue, anxieties, or symptoms associated with the illness:

• Do you have any concerns in this area?

For example, with women having pelvic radiotherapy, tell the patient that it will also affect her vagina, that she may experience some discharge. Then proceed to ask:

• Are you sexually active at the moment?
• Do you have any concerns that you would like to discuss?

With patients undergoing chemotherapy, while talking about side-effects such as nausea, vomiting, or alopecia, include the effects on the ovaries, testicles, sexual desire, and sexual functioning. At the end of any conversation ask:

• Is there anything else you would like to ask?

Let them know that they can talk to someone about it and about any specialists that are available. Let patients know that sexuality is a recognised and important part of their care, that it is OK to talk or ask about any concerns they have.

The P.LI.SS.IT model[30] is a guide to the different stages of intervention. It provides a framework for the types of help that can be offered to the person with cancer and their partner. Nurses will differ in their ability to deal with each stage; however, what is most important is that every nurse can address the issue, listen and then refer on if she feels uncomfortable.

P refers to *permission*. This means allowing someone to feel at ease with their own sexuality. In Personal account 27.1, John is given the opportunity to express his concerns about his sexuality, his wife and how she might feel, his loss of libido and erectile difficulties. Simply asking and listening can be reassuring in itself. Not everyone wants to discuss sexual problems, but they need to know they can if the occasion arises in the future. As discussed earlier, the threat of the illness may override issues of sexuality. A crisis such as new diagnosis, recurrence, or treatment setbacks may not be the most appropriate time, so when is?

There is no research to suggest the best time to broach the subject, although there is agreement that discussion should be a routine part of care at diagnosis, treatment, and follow-up.[25] The admission period provides an ideal opportunity to get to know someone, to find out their story and any concerns they may have. The assessment is pivotal to meeting needs; however, lip service is often paid to assessing sexuality. The reason may be because assessment tools tend to divide the body and mind into separate entities, and to begin an intimate conversation relating to a person's sexuality or sexual functioning may be difficult. A more effective approach might be to ask the person to tell their story: 'Tell me about your illness, how it all began'. Through this avenue cues can be picked up, allowing the conversation to be fluid, moving gently from less sensitive topics to issues that are more sensitive.

When giving information it is essential to alleviate anxieties and fears, and talking about the effects of treatment on sexual functioning will provide an opportunity to build upon the discussion. Once treatment is over, getting on with life is a high priority. Resuming sexual relationships, returning to work and socialising once again may be difficult.[16] Support and advice is essential to enable adjustment. Being more forthright but gentle, by asking 'How are things going sexually' is possible, if done sensitively and in private.

LI refers to *limited information*. Providing information should be limited to immediate needs. In John's situation, these include explaining how cancer treatments and anxieties can exacerbate pre-existing problems, helping to reassure him, putting problems in perspective, and reducing anxiety. It also incorporates correcting myths and misconceptions such as 'Is cancer contagious?' or 'Can radiotherapy be sexually transmitted?' Talking about treatment sequelae should include information about possible impairments resulting from treatment, e.g. menopausal symptoms.

SS refers to *specific suggestions*. This includes giving information about strategies to help overcome problems related to the disease or treatment. This might be about the use of dilators and resumption of sexual intercourse following pelvic radiotherapy to prevent adhesions, or prosthetic advice for patients who have had a mastectomy or an amputation. Following reconstruction of the penis, breast, vulva, or vagina, specific advice about what to expect after the operation, and assessment and discussion with regard to expectations and goals, are essential to aid adaptation. Although surgical reconstruction has the potential to improve the body appearance and consequently feelings of masculinity and femininity, function will be altered. Among the changes there will be different sensations and altered appearance. Specific advice may also include using alternative sexual positions for where the vagina or penis may have been shortened, or how to modify present sexual activities when there are symptoms such as pain or fatigue.

IT refers to *intensive therapy*. This is intervention by a specialist in the field or related areas. Nurses need to recognise their limitations and refer on where appropriate. For instance, in John's situation should he have wanted to pursue interventions for erectile difficulties, a specialist in impotence would have been involved. When a difficulty is identified, the nurse needs to know what services are available, and be able to discuss the possible avenues with the patient and to refer on with the patient's consent. Nurses themselves need support to discuss their difficulties and experiences, positive and negative, to build confidence and competence in this area.

Challenging the taboo of sexuality, and overcoming the fears and embarrassment of talking about sexuality can be satisfying and enlightening both professionally and personally. If we as nurse practitioners claim to give holistic care, then sexuality with all its dimensions must be included in our plans of care. Helping and supporting patients to understand and cope with sexual concerns enables one to cross the boundaries of intimacy and view the 'someone with cancer' as a person with individual desires, needs, attitudes, and behaviours. Perhaps that is what we are afraid of; perhaps that is what stops us from talking about sexuality.

Research study 27.1: Early stage cervical cancer – psychosocial and sexual outcomes of treatment[16]

This study describes the psychosexual outcome of 83 women successfully treated with Wertheim's hysterectomy or radiotherapy for stage Ib cervical cancer. Assessments were completed a mean of 97 weeks post-treatment and employed self-report questionnaires and semi-structured interviews.

Sixty-one women were sexually active at the time of assessment and of these approximately 50% reported a deterioration in sexual functioning compared to their pre-illness functioning. Radiotherapy patients were significantly

more likely to report pain during intercourse and loss of sexual pleasure. Eighty-three per cent of patients had been offered a vaginal dilator and all patients reported compliance. More than 40% of patients reported persistent tiredness, lack of energy, and depressed mood. No women were free of worries relating to cervical cancer and fear of recurrence. More than one-third blamed themselves for the disease and the same proportion had lost their self-confidence. More than 25% felt unattractive and older. Psychological factors were highly correlated with subjective physical complaints. More than 40% of patients would have liked more information and counselling. The same number did not want their partners at the clinic consultation. Forty-four per cent felt unable to talk adequately with their partners.

Limitations: as treatment was not randomly assigned, only limited conclusions can be drawn about the relative morbidity of treatment procedures involved.

The research highlights the combined impact of the psychological and physical factors on women's outcome and sexual functioning. It also highlights that women and their partners need more information and support throughout their illness and treatment experience.

Notes on selected cancer sites 27.1: Invasive carcinoma of the cervix

Epidemiology and aetiology

- Invasive carcinoma of the cervix, the sixth most common malignancy in women in the UK, accounts for 4000 new cases of cancer each year and results in around 2000 deaths per annum.
- 75–90% of all cervical cancers are squamous cell, arising from the squamo-columnar epithelium. The remaining types are adenocarcinomas and more rare.
- The definitive cause of cervical cancer is unknown but risk factors include human papilloma virus (types 16 and 18), early age at first intercourse, multiparity, and sexual behaviour, i.e. high number of sexual partners. Smoking, oral contraceptives, and dusty occupations have also been identified as risk factors.

Clinical presentation

- Symptoms present when the integrity of the epithelium is aggravated. Patients with invasive disease may present with post-coital, intermenstrual bleeding, and/or menorrhagia.
- Vaginal discharge is also common and may be scanty, intermittent, or heavy. Patients with more advanced disease may complain of frequency of micturition, pelvic or low back pain. Leg swelling and/or supra-clavicular lymphadenopathy may present in patients with pelvic side-wall disease.
- A speculum examination of the cervix and smear is followed by a referral to a gynaecologist. Further investigations may

involve a colposcopy. A full gynaecological and clinical examination is usually followed by an examination under anaesthetic and biopsy to confirm a diagnosis for staging, planning, and treatment. A cytoscopy and sigmoidoscopy may also be performed.

Spread
Cervical cancer usually spreads by direct invasion to local areas such as the vagina, parametrium, and uterine body. It can also be disseminated through the lymphatic system to pelvic and para-aortic lymph nodes. Blood-borne spread is rare, but is more common in advanced disease and usually spreads to the lungs, liver, and bone.

Staging and prognosis
There are four main stages of cervical cancer with subcategories (International Federation of Gynaecology and Obstetrics, FIGO, Table 27.2).

The incidence and mortality from invasive carcinoma of the cervix are falling and it is suggested that this is probably due to the screening programme.[31] The 5-year survival rate for women with stage I disease ranges from 60 to 80%, stage II 46 to 61%, stage III 15 to 30%, and stage IV 5 to 10%.[32]

Treatment[33]
The choice of treatment depends on age, the patient's condition, stage, tumour volume, and extent of disease.

Stage I–IIa: Early invasive disease should be treated with a cone biopsy where possible, but when this is insufficient to treat the disease a radical hysterectomy and lymphadenectomy should be performed. Both surgery and radiotherapy are equally effective in terms of survival for early stage disease, although surgery should be offered where possible because of the side-effects associated with radiotherapy. Some women may require adjuvant radiotherapy depending on the findings at surgery, therefore careful pre-operative assessment is essential to reduce the number of women who have to undergo both treatments.

Stage IIb–IV: Radical radiotherapy (usually combining intra-cavity and external beam radiotherapy) is the treatment of choice for curative intentions.

- Neo-adjuvant chemotherapy (given prior to radiotherapy and surgery) is not advocated. A review of studies has shown inconclusive results.
- Concurrent chemotherapy (given during radiotherapy): a review of recent studies demonstrates that the use of cis-platin-based chemotherapy can improve survival for women with later stage or bulky disease.

Recurrent disease: Radical radiotherapy may be considered if the treatment has not previously been given. Exenterative surgery may be offered to women with recurrent disease confined to the pelvis. Palliative doses of radiotherapy may also be offered to those with recurrent disease to control bleeding, pain, and discharge.

Side-effects
Radiotherapy. Side-effects can be numerous and the use of concurrent chemotherapy may increase adverse effects. Early side-effects include diarrhoea, nausea, anorexia, skin reactions,

Table 27.2 Modified International Federation of Gynaecology and Obstetrics (FIGO) staging of cancer of the cervix (adapted from Hunter, 1995)

Stage	Description
0	Carcinoma *in situ* (CIS CINII)
	Invasive carcinoma
I	Disease confined to the cervix
Ia	Microinvasive carcinoma
Ib	Tumour >5 mm deep, >7 mm wide
II	Disease beyond cervix but not to pelvic side-wall or to lower third of vagina
IIa	No parametrial involvement
IIb	Parametrial involvement
III	Extension to pelvic side-wall and/or lower third of vagina. Includes cases with hydronephrosis or non-functioning kidney (unless other known cause exists)
IIIa	No extension to pelvic side-wall. Involves lower third of vagina
IIIb	Extension to pelvic side-wall and/or hydronephrosis or non-functioning kidney
IVa	Carcinoma extends beyond true pelvis or involving mucosa of bladder or rectum
IVb	Distant metastases

proctitis, cystitis, and vaginal discharge. Late problems include fatigue, small bowel problems, fistulae, the menopause, and vaginal stenosis and fibrosis leading to a reduction in sexual enjoyment.

Chemotherapy. Side-effects are dependent on the drugs used and may be exacerbated if given concurrently with radiotherapy.

References

1. Stuart G.W. and Suncleen S.J. (eds.) (1979). *Principles and Practice of Psychiatric Nursing.* St Louis, MI: Mosby.
2. Jenkins B. (1988). Patients reports of sexual changes after treatment for gynaecological cancer. *Oncology Nursing Forum* 15, 349–354.
3. Harmatz M.G. and Novak M.A. (1993). *Human Sexuality.* New York: Harper and Row.
4. Weeks J. (1989). *Sex, Politics and Society: The Regulation of Sexuality Since 1800,* 2nd edition. London: Longman.
5. MacElveen-Hoehn P. and McCorkle R. (1985). Understanding sexuality in progressive cancer. *Seminars in Oncology Nursing* 1, 56–62.
6. Webb C. (ed.) (1994). *Living Sexuality: Issues of Nursing and Health.* London: Scutari Press.
7. English National Board (1994). Sexual health education and training: guidelines for good practice in teaching of nurses. *Midwives and Health Visitors Section* 2, 5–27.
8. Fallowfield L. (1992). The quality of life: sexual function and body image following cancer therapy. *Cancer Topics* 9, 20–21.
9. Lawler J. (1991). *Behind the Screens. Nursing Somology and the Problem of the Body.* London: Churchill Livingstone.
10. Dennison S. (1995). An exploration of the communication that takes place between nurses and patients whilst cancer chemotherapy is administered. *Journal of Clinical Nursing* 4, 227–233.
11. Lamb M.A. and Sheldon T.A. (1994). The sexual adaptation of women treated for endometrial cancer. *Cancer Practice* 2, 103–113.
12. Jones L. and Webb C. (1994). Young men's experiences of testicular cancer. In Webb C. (ed.) *Living Sexuality: Issues For Nursing and Health.* London: Scutari Press, pp. 32–49.
13. Smith D.B. (1989). Sexual rehabilitation of the cancer patient. *Cancer Nursing* 12, 10–15.
14. Golden J.S. and Golden M. (1980). Cancer and sex. *Frontiers of Radiation Therapy and Oncology* 14, 59–65.
15. Rhys-Evans F. (1993). *A investigation into functional problems following major oral surgery in head and neck cancer patients and coping mechanisms employed by the patient.* Unpublished M.Sc. thesis, University of Surrey.
16. Cull A., Cowie V.J., Farquharson D.I.M., Livingstone J.R.B., Smart G.E. and Elton R.A. (1993). Early stage cervical cancer: psychosocial and sexual outcomes of treatment. *British Journal of Cancer* 68, 1216–1220.
17. Corney R., Everett H., Howells A. and Crowther M. (1992). The care of patients undergoing surgery for gynaecological cancer: the need for information support and counselling. *Journal of Advanced Nursing* 17, 667–671.
18. Anderson B.L. and Hacker N.F. (1983). Psycho-sexual adjustment of gynaecological oncology patients: a proposed model for future investigation. *Gynaecologic Oncology* 15, 214–223.
19. Morris T., Greer H.S. and White P. (1977). Psychological and social adjustment to mastectomy. *Cancer* 40, 2381–2387.
20. Maguire G.P. (1985). The psychological and social consequences of breast cancer. *Nursing Mirror* 140, 540–547.
21. Fallowfield L. and Clarke A. (1991). *Breast Cancer.* London: Routledge.
22. Lamont J.A., De Petrillo A.D. and Sargeant E.J. (1978). Psycho-sexual rehabilitation and extenterative surgery *Gynaecologic Oncology* 6, 236–242.
23. Shell J.A. and Smith C.K. (1994). Sexuality and the older person with cancer. *Oncology Nursing Forum* 21, 553–558.
24. Gross Fisher S. (1983). The psycho-sexual effects of cancer and cancer treatment. *Oncology Nursing Forum* 10, 63–68.
25. Auchincloss S.S. (1989). Sexual dysfunction in cancer patients: issues in evaluation and treatment. In Holland J.C. and Rowland J.H. (eds.) *Handbook of Psycho-Oncology: Psychological Care of the Patient with Cancer.* Oxford: Oxford University Press, pp. 383–413.
26. Schover L.R. (1988). *Sexuality and Cancer: For the Man Who Has Cancer, and His Partner.* New York: American Cancer Society.
27. Schover L.R. (1988). *Sexuality and Cancer: For the Woman Who Has Cancer, and Her Partner.* New York: American Cancer Society.
28. Vincent C.E., Vincent B. Greiss F.C. and Linton E.B. (1975). Some marital-sexual concomitants of carcinoma of the cervix. *Southern Medical Journal* 68, 52–58.
29. Wilson M.E. and Williams H.A. (1988). Oncology nurses attitudes and behaviours related to sexuality of patients with cancer. *Oncology Nursing Forum* 15, 49–53.
30. Annon J.S. (1974). *The Behavioral Treatment of Sexual Problems.* Honolulu: Mercantile Printing.
31. RCN (1999). *Gynaecological Cancer. Information and Guidance of Nurses.* London: Royal College of Nursing.
32. Hunter R.D. (1995). Carcinoma of the cervix. In Peckham M., Pinedo H.M. and Veronesi U. (eds.) *Oxford Textbook of Oncology,* Vol. 2. Oxford: Oxford Medical Publications, pp. 1324–1349.
33. National Guidance Steering Group (1999). *Improving Outcomes in Gynaecological Cancer: The Manual.* London: NHS Executive, Department of Health.

CHAPTER TWENTY-EIGHT

Anxiety and depression

Meinir Krishnasamy

Sadness and grief are normal responses to many painful life events, but for a significant minority who have cancer, the severe distress experienced may require expert psychological intervention.[1,2] Health care professionals' fear or inexperience of exploring patients' emotional problems has impeded this aspect of cancer and palliative care.

Anxiety

Detecting and managing anxiety in physically ill individuals, and especially those with cancer, can be extremely difficult. Normal fears of death, disfigurement, pain, and disruption in relationships may be especially difficult to distinguish from severe, disabling distress far beyond normal anxiety. Anxiety is the term most commonly used by patients to describe prevalent emotional concerns:[3] feelings of fear, dread, apprehension, a vague sensation or emotion that is difficult to define. In cancer, anxiety is often associated with fear of dysfunction and death. Anxiety is also manifested by physiological changes related to central and autonomic nervous system arousal and neuroendocrine responses.[4]

Despite the universality of its manifestations, there are three main types of anxiety: reactive anxiety, anxiety related to health status, and anxiety related to pre-existing anxiety disorders.

Reactive anxiety is probably the most commonly occurring type experienced by cancer patients. It is a situational anxiety, related to a crisis or a transitional period in the cancer trajectory; for example commencing new treatment, awaiting scan results, or on completion of treatment.[5]

Anxiety related to health status is the second most frequent source of anxiety for patients receiving treatment for cancer.[5] Poorly controlled pain, abnormal metabolic states, hormone-secreting tumours, and anxiety-producing drugs are the most common sources of anxiety of this type. For some individuals a diagnosis of cancer and its many associated complications may reactivate a pre-existing anxiety disorder. The main disorders are classified as phobias, such as agoraphobia and claustrophobia, panic attacks and generalised anxiety disorder and post-traumatic stress disorders.

Between 30 and 40% of people with cancer have been found to report moderate to high levels of anxiety.[6] A diagnosis of cancer may present each individual with a myriad sources of anxiety, some of which are highlighted below. For some, anxiety will be manifested through a variety of physical symptoms:

- restlessness
- insomnia and nightmares
- shortness of breath
- sweating
- tense expression
- poor concentration and memory
- irritability
- worry
- headaches

- nausea and anorexia
- palpitations
- menstrual changes
- hyperventilation
- diarrhoea.

Anxiety in advanced cancer may be a manifestation of many issues. Fears of a painful death, of leaving behind loved ones, fears of dependency, isolation, and stigmatisation are only a few of the stressors confounding the world of the individual with advanced disease. Adjustment disorder, pain, adverse drug reactions, delirium, organic anxiety and other organic mental disorders may also lead to anxiety in an individual with advanced or terminal cancer.[7]

For the individual diagnosed with cancer there are several periods throughout the cancer trajectory that are recognised as being especially anxiety provoking, including:

- confirmation of diagnosis and awaiting test-results[2]
- the period immediately after completion of treatment[8,9]
- long periods at home between follow-up visits[2]
- recurrence of disease.[10,11]

With so many potential sources of anxiety it is difficult to know how best to:

- help to make sense of fears through gentle exploration; for example what fears do symptoms engender – breathlessness and suffocation, depression and insanity, or pain and metastatic spread? Are they realistic fears or are they misperceptions? Are they born out of a sense of isolation?
- gently encourage someone to talk about their illness and its impact on their life, helping them to resolve 'normal' anxieties. At the same time, be watchful for individuals whose anxiety may require a referral for specialist intervention.

Given the likelihood that any number of factors may lead to the onset of anxiety, intervention must be tailored to each individual's unique needs. Pharmacological approaches are outlined below.

Pharmacological management of anxiety and depression[7]

Pharmacological intervention in the treatment of anxiety in cancer and palliative care involves the use of:

- benzodiazepines, e.g. midazolam, lorazepam, diazepam, clonazepam
- non-benzodiazepines, e.g. buspirone
- neuroleptics, e.g. methotrimepramine, chlorpromazine, haloperidol
- anti-histamines, e.g. hydroxyzine
- tricyclic antidepressants, e.g. imipramine
- opioid analgesics.

The main drugs used in the pharmacological management of depression in cancer and palliative care are:

- tricyclic antidepressants, e.g. amitryptyline, dothiepin
- second-generation antidepressants, e.g. trazodone, mianserin
- psychostimulants, e.g. dextroamphetamine
- monoamine oxidase inhibitors, e.g. phenelzine
- lithium carbonate
- benzodiazepines, e.g. alprazolam
- fluoxetine hydrochloride (Prozac). Prozac is an antidepressant, chemically unrelated to tricyclic, tetracyclic or other available antidepressant agents. Its ever-increasing use and anecdotal reports of beneficial effects warrant further investigation in the light of early reports that 5% of patients treated with Prozac complained of symptoms of anxiety, nervousness, and insomnia that led to the discontinuation of the drug. Significant weight loss, especially in underweight, depressed patients may also be an undesirable result of treatment with Prozac, and may be especially significant in relation to malnourished or cachexic patients.

Occasionally, electroconvulsive therapy (ECT) may be warranted for depressed cancer patients with psychotic features or for whom pharmacological intervention carries too many side-effects.

Depression

The incidence of depression has been found to range from 4.5 to 42% in populations of people with cancer and is said to increase as pain, advanced disease, level of dependency, and disability increase.[11,12] Traditionally, health care professionals have presumed that a 'reactive' depression, that is in response to a diagnosis of cancer, is not a 'real' depression, believing that there is an understandable reason to feel depressed.[13] However, this assumption may have dire consequences for the individual struggling to cope alone with feelings of hopelessness and overwhelming sadness.

Personal account 28.1

During a conversation with Tom, a 67-year-old gentleman with small-cell lung cancer, it became clear that he was describing many symptoms of depression. He told me that he was unable to take pleasure in any of the things that used to be so dear to him and had even stopped looking forward to seeing his grandchildren. He had recently begun to stay in bed for most of the morning, even though he was waking very early, saying that on some days he just couldn't see any purpose in getting up at all. These thoughts made him feel guilty and worthless. He explained how caring his family and friends were and how he wished he could make the effort for them. He told me he didn't deserve such loving attention. When I discussed the possibility with Tom that he might be depressed, stressing the normality of his feelings as part of a depressive illness, and their reversible nature, he was able to express an enormous sense of relief. To him, the sense of isolation caused by the depression was, he said, 'almost too much to bear – I thought I was going mad'.

One of the main problems associated with detecting depression in cancer is disentangling symptoms of depression from symptoms of the disease itself or its treatment.[13] Table 28.1 outlines some of the factors that may predispose someone with cancer to depression.

In advanced cancer, the physical manifestations of depression such as fatigue, anorexia, or insomnia are all too likely to be present as a result of the impact of the tumour, making accurate assessment of depression especially difficult.[1,12] The importance of potentiating factors of depression, such as functional limitation or metastatic disease, chronic fatigue or unresolved pain, has clear implications for thorough assessment of depression and the initiation of prompt intervention.

Table 28.1 Predisposing factors for depression[1,14–16, 20]

- A family history of depression or suicide
- A family or personal history of alcoholism
- A previous psychiatric illness, especially depression, also drug abuse or a previous suicide attempt
- Past coping strategies: does the individual employ acceptance–resignation, information-seeking or confrontational coping strategies?
- Patients with advanced disease have a higher incidence of depression than those individuals with newly diagnosed cancer
- Patients with relentless physical symptoms, especially uncontrolled pain
- Medications: corticosteroids, e.g. prednisolone and dexamethasone, cimetidine, diazepam, indomethacin, levodopa, methyldopa, pentazocine, phenmetrazine, phenobarbital, propranolol, and oestrogens. Chemotherapy, especially vincristine, vinblastine, procarbazine, L-asparaginase, interferon, amphoteracin-B are also linked to the onset of depressive symptomatology
- Whole brain irradiation
- Metabolic disturbances, nutritional abnormalities, endocrine imbalance and neurological imbalance

The optimum management of depression has been described as being a combination of supportive psychotherapy, cognitive–behavioural techniques, and antidepressant medications.

Non-pharmacological interventions for anxiety and depression

There is increasing evidence that cognitive–behavioural techniques of managing psychological difficulties are helpful. These techniques have been shown to be easy to learn and to use[17] (see Figure 28.1). A recognition of the growth in use of these techniques has led to a demand for an increase in the research knowledge base of nursing in examining their effectiveness. An in-depth exploration of the various forms of psychological therapies can be found in the *Handbook of Psycho-oncology*, edited by Holland and Rowland.[18]

One of the most commonly used behavioural techniques is progressive muscle relaxation (PMR). PMR involves tensing and then relaxing separate muscles groups throughout the body one after the other. Teaching a patient, family member, or friend

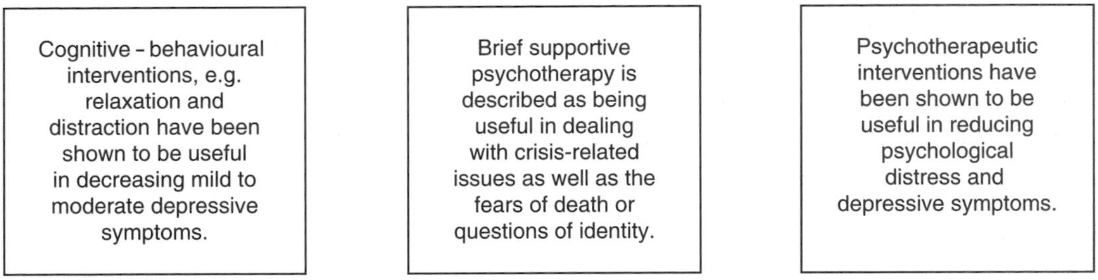

Cognitive – behavioural interventions, e.g. relaxation and distraction have been shown to be useful in decreasing mild to moderate depressive symptoms.	Brief supportive psychotherapy is described as being useful in dealing with crisis-related issues as well as the fears of death or questions of identity.	Psychotherapeutic interventions have been shown to be useful in reducing psychological distress and depressive symptoms.

Figure 28.1 Types of psychological intervention for anxiety and depression.

a relaxation technique is relatively quick and easy and yet the rewards can be significant in both the short and longer term.

Increasingly, massage is being used as a means of enhancing well-being for patients with cancer. However, research findings to date are inconsistent and there appears to be little agreement about the most appropriate research methods to evaluate the benefits of massage therapy in cancer care.[19] There is therefore a significant potential and need for future nurse-led research within this important area of care. For example:

- How effective is massage as a means of helping patients to minimise the distress caused by problematic symptoms, e.g. pain, fatigue, constipation?
- Who needs massage? – A comparison of therapeutic outcomes across different cancer patient groups.
- Researching the benefits of massage – is a triangulation of research methods the most appropriate approach?

In a study of 52 heterogeneous cancer patients, it was concluded that the benefit of reduced anxiety results from a cumulative effect of at least four massage sessions, but the authors also warn that massage can result in emotional release, which requires skilled handling.[19]

The enhancement of patient well-being through maximising beneficial coping strategies is one means of reducing psychological distress. Coping strategies are those processes people use to try to manage real or perceived deficiencies between demands imposed by a crisis such as a diagnosis of cancer and the resources available to respond to it. The two forms of coping mechanisms most commonly referred to in the literature are problem-solving and emotional-orientated strategies.

Problem-solving strategies work in two ways.

- They help to reduce the demands placed on an individual by the stressor, whatever that may be.
- They increase the resources available to deal with a stressor by developing new skills or promoting existing beneficial coping mechanisms.

Emotional-orientated coping is directed at adaptation of emotional response to stress and these mechanisms tend to be used when a situation appears to be unchangeable.

Suicide

Cancer is a chronic illness and for many the dying process can become long and extremely burdensome. The attitude towards suicide for the majority of health care professionals is that it is something to be avoided at all costs, but for many individuals, suicide may reflect an attempt to retain some degree of control or to secure a 'dignified death'.

Despite the fact that people with cancer are at increased risk of suicide relative to the general population, particularly in the terminal stages of illness, there is agreement that very few individuals with cancer actually do commit suicide.[15] Men more than women with cancer have been identified as being at increased risk of suicide relative to the general population. Taking analgesic and sedative drugs is the most common way of committing suicide.[20]

There is growing evidence that people with particular kinds of cancers are at increased risk of suicide. Those diagnosed with lung, pharyngeal, and oral cancers are at particular risk.[15,25] Identifying

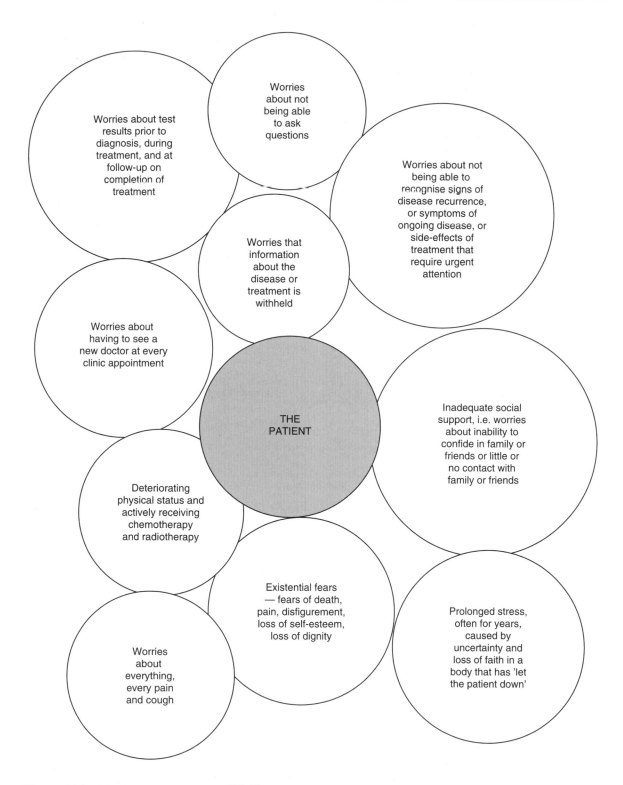

Figure 28.2 Manifestations of anxiety.[2,3,21–24]

reasons why particular individuals or groups may be prone to suicide may allow early, appropriate intervention and help to reduce the risk. The onset of oral, pharyngeal, and lung cancers is often associated with extensive tobacco and alcohol intake. Heavy smoking and drinking may signify a vulnerable group who tend to utilise maladaptive coping skills and as such they may be more prone to suicide as a coping strategy.[25] The disfiguring surgery associated with head and neck tumours, loss of vocal communication for those with pharyngeal tumours, and the marked weight loss and cachexia associated with lung tumours may also contribute to the suicidal potential of these individuals.[15]

As with anxiety and depression there are well-recognised predisposing factors that can help to alert nursing staff to those patients most at risk of suicide. Those with advanced disease and a poor prognosis are most at risk of suicide because of the likelihood of multiple symptoms such as pain, delirium, depression and hopelessness, and fatigue. Feelings of loss of control and helplessness, pre-existing psychopathology, for example, alcoholism, substance abuse, major mental illness, and prior suicide history, also contribute to an individual's heightened risk of suicide.[14,25-28]

Assessment of suicide risk and appropriate interventions based on skilled interaction may often help to prevent suicide.[25] Many of the guidelines for assessment and evaluation of suicide risk in an individual with cancer outlined below are well-suited for use by nurses who are in close day-to-day proximity to those who may be at risk. The principles of assessing risk of suicide are as follows.

- Establish a rapport with the person based upon trust and a non-judgemental approach.
- Invite them to describe their understanding of, and response to, the cancer diagnosis, its treatment and symptoms experienced. It is important that he or she is asked to talk about everything that is important or meaningful. An agenda set by the doctor or nurse may omit the most salient points.
- Be vigilant – is the individual displaying any evidence of depression or delirium?
- Is there any evidence of uncontrolled pain? Does he or she talk of fatigue, exhaustion, feelings of loss of control, hopelessness or helplessness?

- What is the person's past history? Is there any evidence of pre-existing pathology, such as depression or previous suicide attempt? Is there any history of family suicide?

Although nurses are ideally placed to help to find meaning or reasons for suicidal thoughts, as well as an understanding of how serious the patient's intention really is, multi-disciplinary management is essential for the individual who displays serious suicidal intent.

Once again, the contribution of nursing lies with substantiating an appreciation of each individual's needs. Supportive interventions designed to help patients to identify, and respond positively to sources of anxiety and depression where they are able should be offered, or prompt referral for pharmacological, psychiatric, or psychological assessment and care initiated when appropriate.

Some potential future nursing research questions include:

- How effective is progressive muscle relaxation as a means of helping patients to minimise the anxiety of a distressing symptom, e.g. breathlessness, fatigue, nausea and vomiting?
- Can family/friends benefit from psychotherapeutic interventions?
- Nursing interventions known to be effective in helping to manage anxiety in the early stages of illness (for example, relaxation and massage) should be systematically evaluated with patients in the latter stages of their disease.

References

1. Bukberg J., Penman D. and Holland J. (1984). Depression in hospitalised cancer patients. *Psychosomatic Medicine* **46**, 199–212.
2. Lampic C., Wennberg A., Schill J., Brodin O., Glimelius B. and Sjoden P. (1994). Anxiety and cancer related worry of cancer patients at routine follow-up visits. *Acta Oncologica* **33**, 119–125.
3. Stefanek M., Shaw A., Degeorge D. and Tsottles N. (1989). Illness-related worry among cancer patients: prevalence, severity and content. *Cancer Investigation* 7, 365–371.
4. Leigh H. and Reiser M.F. (1985). *The Patient: Biological, Psychological and Social Dimensions of Medical Practice*. New York: Plenum Press.

5. Massie M. (1990). Anxiety, panic and phobias. In Holland J. and Rowland J. (eds.) *Handbook of Psycho-oncology.* Oxford: Oxford University Press, pp. 300–309.

6. Derogatis L.R., Morrow G.R., Fetting J., Penman D. and Piasetsky S. (1983). The prevalence of psychiatric disorder among cancer patients. *Journal of the American Medical Association* **249**, 751–757.

7. Breitbart W. and Passik S. (1993). Psychiatric aspects of palliative care. In Doyle D., Hanks G. and Macdonald N. (eds.) *Oxford Textbook of Palliative Medicine.* Oxford: Oxford Medical Publications.

8. Mullan F. (1985). Seasons of survival: reflections of a physician with cancer. *New England Journal of Medicine* **313**, 270–273.

9. Oberst M.T. and Jones R.H. (1985). Going home. Patient and spouse adjustment following cancer surgery. *Topics in Clinical Nursing* **7**, 46–57.

10. Ormiston M.C., Timoney A. and Qureshi A.C. (1985). Is follow-up of patients after surgery for breast cancer worthwhile? *Journal of the Royal Society of Medicine* **78**, 920–921.

11. Golden R., McCartney C., Haggerty J., Raft D. and Nemeroff C.B. (1991). The detection of depression by patient self-report in women with gynaecologic cancer. *International Journal of Psychiatry in Medicine* **21**, 17–27.

12. Carroll B.T., Kathol R.G., Noyes R., Wald T.G. and Calmon G.H. (1993). Screening for depression and anxiety in cancer patients using the Hospital Anxiety and Depression Scale. *General Hospital Psychiatry* **15**, 69–74.

13. Endicott J. (1983). Measurement of depression patients with cancer. *Cancer* **53**, 2243–2248.

14. Lynch M. (1995). The assessment and prevalence of affective disorders in advanced cancer. *Journal of Palliative Care* **11**, 10–18.

15. Holland J. (1978). Psychological aspects of cancer. In Holland J. and Frei (eds.) *Cancer Medicine,* 2nd edition. Philadelphia, PA: Lea and Febiger.

16. Breitbart W. (1995). Identifying patients at risk for, and treatment of major psychiatric complications of cancer. *Support Cancer Care* **3**, 45–60.

17. Holland J., Morrow G. and Schmale A. (1991). A randomised clinical trial of alprazolam versus patients with progressive muscle relaxation in cancer patients with anxiety and depressive symptoms. *Journal of Clinical Oncology* **9**, 1004–1011.

18. Holland J. and Rowland J. (eds.) (1990). *Handbook of Psycho-oncology. Psychological Care of the Patient with Cancer.* Oxford: Oxford University Press.

19. Corner J., Cawley N. and Hildebrand S. (1995). An evaluation of the use of massage and massage with the addition of essential oils on the well-being of cancer patients. *International Journal of Palliative Nursing* **1**, 67–73.

20. Bolund C. (1985). Suicide and cancer I. Demographic and social characteristics of cancer patients who committed suicide in Sweden, 1973–1976. *Journal of Psychosocial Oncology* **3**, 17–30.

21. Norbeck J. (1981). Social support: a model for clinical research and application. *Advances in Nursing Science* **7**, 443–459.

22. Nerenz D., Leventhal H. and Love R. (1982). Factors contributing to emotional distress during cancer chemotherapy. *Cancer* **50**, 1020–1027.

23. Wortman C. and Conway T. (1985). The role of social support in adaptation and recovery from physical illness. In Wortman C. and Conway T. (eds.) *Social Support and Health.* New York: Academic Press, pp. 281–299.

24. Rodrigue J., Behen J. and Tumlin T. (1994). Multidimensional determinants of psychological adjustment to cancer. *Psycho-Oncology* **3**, 205–214.

25. Breitbart W. (1990). Suicide. In Holland J. and Rowland J. (eds.) *Handbook of Psycho-oncology. Psychological Care of the Patient with Cancer.* Oxford: Oxford University Press.

26. Levin R.B. and Gross A.M. (1985). The role of relaxation in systematic desensitisation. *Behavioural Research Therapy* **23**, 187–196.

27. Faberow N.L., Schneidman E.S. and Leonard C.V. (1963). Suicide among general medical and surgical hospital patients with malignant neoplasms. *Medical Bulletin* **9**, Washington, D.C.: US Veterans Administration.

28. Beck A., Kovacs M. and Weisman A. (1975). Hopelessness and suicidal behaviour: an overview. *Journal of the American Medical Association* **234**, 1146–1149.

CHAPTER TWENTY-NINE

Confusion

Meinir Krishnasamy

Caring for someone who is confused is enormously challenging. It is often painful for all involved as the confusion, like cancer itself, gives rise to feelings of conflict, shame, isolation, and disempowerment in those witnessing its effects:

> . . . cancer appears to have become the metaphor of the deepest fears held about the inevitable disintegration and decay of the body [p. 268].[1]

Confusion, however, all too often places health care professionals in a 'custodial' role, as someone who is confused may no longer 'comply' with therapeutic intent.[2] The moral nature of the nurse–patient interaction is maligned by the onset of a symptom that commonly results in preclusion of self-choice and self-determination. The consequences for nurses' well-being may be profound, as illustrated by Personal account 29.1.

Despite being a common symptom of cancer and occurring with the same frequency as depression, confusion or delirium is poorly recognised by health care professionals.[3] Early symptoms of delirium are often misdiagnosed as anxiety, anger, depression, or psychosis.[4,5] Subsequently, treatment is often delayed until symptoms are severe, causing undue distress to the individual experiencing the confusion and to family and friends witnessing the changes in their behaviour and personality. The necessity for an appreciation of early signs of confusion, and an ability to differentiate those signs from the manifestations of anxiety, depression, and dementia, are important if nurses are to

contribute meaningfully to the management of this difficult symptom.

Personal account 29.1

I'd been caring for Margaret for 5 days. She'd come to the unit so that we could help improve her pain and nausea. Margaret had been diagnosed with metastatic liver cancer 3 months earlier and was now terminally ill. She was very thin, jaundiced, and frightened that her pain wouldn't be relieved. That, she told me had always been her greatest fear, that she would die in pain.

I had first met Margaret when she came to the unit 2 months earlier. At that time, and on subsequent admissions, we had established some degree of trust and I felt that our relationship was based on a mutual affinity, and on her confidence that we would do everything possible to ensure that her death would be as pain free, and as untraumatic as possible. I was unprepared for the confusion that Margaret experienced, despite being aware of her physiological potential to develop delirium. She had liver cancer and all that that entailed biochemically; she had unresolved pain and she was frightened. Nevertheless, I was completely unprepared for how I would feel when she became verbally abusive and paranoid and was therefore ill-equipped to minimise the distress she and her family were to experience throughout this period.

My initial reaction to Margaret's physical abuse was to feel hurt that someone I had worked so hard to establish trust with could now be so hostile. I felt sure that I would be able to communicate and reason with her. Of course I couldn't. I found caring for Margaret very difficult following the sudden onset of her delirium. I was unable to provide her with what she needed most at that time, which was skilful, supportive nursing intervention. I was distressed by her inability to retain self-determination. I found myself forced from a role where we had made decisions together to one in which I now encouraged, coaxed, even manipulated Margaret as she refused medication and food.

Happily, the confusion was promptly resolved by skilled multi-disciplinary care. The contribution of nursing colleagues experienced in the assessment and management of delirious patients and their families taught me a great deal. What, they asked me, did I think family and friends were feeling, if I found Margaret's confusion so painful to endure? Margaret told me later that she was initially aware of the feelings of paranoia and explained that the fear of isolation and destruction was overwhelming. Had I been better prepared to recognise early signs of delirium and developed skills fundamental to the assessment of a confused individual, my ability to support Margaret at this difficult time would undoubtedly have been much improved.

Confusion or delirium (the two words are used synonymously throughout this section) mean a variety of different things, but are most commonly defined as:

'a transient organic brain syndrome characterised by the acute onset of disoriented attention and cognition accompanied by disturbances of psychomotor behaviour and perception'.[6]

Delirium, anxiety, depression, and dementia share many common manifestations, compounding accurate assessment and prompt intervention. Manifestations of anxiety and depression have been described in an earlier chapter and therefore will not be outlined again here. Delirium, however, may be accompanied by any number of concurrent symptoms, including alterations to:

• level of consciousness
• attention
• thinking
• perception
• emotion
• memory
• psychomotor behaviour
• sleep–wake cycle.

Differentiating between dementia and delirium can be extremely difficult because they share common features.[5] A useful *précis* of the key differences between the two conditions is shown in Table 29.1.

Table 29.1 Features of delirium and dementia (reproduced with permission from the American Medical Association from Lipowski (1987). *Journal of the American Medical Association* **258,** 1789–1792)[6]

Features	Delirium	Dementia
Onset	Acute, often at night	Insidious
Course	Fluctuating, with lucid intervals during the day, worse at night	Stable over course of day
Duration	Hours to weeks	Months or years
Awareness	Reduced	Clear
Alertness	Abnormally high or low	Usually normal
Attention	Lacks direction and selectivity, distractibility, fluctuates over course of day	Relatively unaffected
Orientation	Usually impaired for time, tendency to mistake unfamiliar for familiar place and persons	Often impaired
Memory	Immediate and recent impaired	Recent and remote impaired
Thinking	Disorganised	Impoverished
Perception	Illusions and hallucinations, usually visual and common	Often absent
Speech	Incoherent, hesitant, slow or rapid	Difficulty in finding words
Sleep–wake cycle	Always disturbed	Fragmented sleep
Physical illness or drug toxicity	Either or both present	Often absent

Whatever the symptom, delirium, dementia, anxiety, or depression, the single most important factor in effective intervention is skilled assessment.

Identifying those at risk

Anyone with a diagnosis of cancer is at risk of experiencing some degree of confusion due to:

- the emotional turmoil of a diagnosis of cancer and its treatment
- multiple drug regimes. Given the large numbers of medications individuals with cancer commonly require, even the most commonly used drugs may lead to an episode of confusion.

Elderly patients with cancer may have an increased risk of developing delirium as they may be especially sensitive to the potential causes listed below.

- Individuals with a past history of depression may be more likely to experience an episode of delirium as a consequence of a cancer diagnosis.
- Decreased mobility, compromised functional status, poor quality of sleep, and decreased contact with family and friends have all been shown to increase an individual's predisposition to confusion.
- A history of alcohol or substance abuse may also trigger delirium.
- Haematological abnormalities, e.g. microcytic and macrocytic anaemias and coagulopathies.
- General malnutrition, thiamine, folic acid, and B12 deficiencies.
- Paraneoplastic syndromes.
- Metabolic encephalopathy due to organ failure, e.g. liver, kidney, lung, thyroid, or adrenals.
- Electrolyte imbalance, e.g. sodium, potassium, calcium, and glucose.
- Infection.[4,7–11]

Assessment of an individual suspected of developing confusion therefore requires great care and must involve key members of his or her social support network. In Table 29.2 some of factors that might contribute to a confusional state are shown.

One of the most important aspects of caring for an individual who has begun to exhibit signs of confusion is to try to retain a sense of wholeness, of personhood, for as long as possible. As the con-

fusion establishes itself, there may be periods of lucidity when the person will be aware of alterations in their behaviour. Appropriate reassurance at this time that they are experiencing reversible manifestations of the cancer or its treatment will be enormously comforting. Relatives and friends also need to be aware of this information. Explain to them that the confusion is not a sign of mental illness. Someone who is left to contemplate this frightening symptom is likely to become increasingly distressed and subsequently more confused.[12] Family and friends will become increasingly despondent and may even withdraw at a time when most reassurance that they are loved and valued is needed:

> We must work harder at being human all of us: those who are disabled, those who are normal, those who are professional helpers [p. 227].[13]

A brief cognitive assessment, consistently performed, can be used to ensure that confusion is not missed.[8] Non-threatening questions such as 'How have you been feeling?' are a simple and safe way to start the assessment. Once set at ease, questions about address, telephone number, and family member's names can be asked without seeming too intrusive or judgemental. When confused, someone may be easily disadvantaged during an assessment, particularly in an unfamiliar environment. Do they wear glasses or use a hearing aid? Are these available to him or her? Is the environment quiet, well-lit, and free of instruments that might appear threatening or frightening? Have they recently received their first dose of morphine, cyclizine, or any other sedating agents?

Involving family and friends

Family members may often be the only ones aware of subtle differences in behaviour. Family and friends can offer a very important insight into the 'normal' cognitive function and any recent changes in memory or impaired thinking.[8] They may also offer an invaluable insight into the person's awareness and acceptance of their diagnosis and prognosis, highlighting causes for the confusional state that may otherwise remain hidden. For some, the diagnosis of cancer or a prognosis of terminal illness is unbearable, making them become

Table 29.2 Factors for consideration in the assessment of someone who is confused[4,7,8]

- Is there any reason to suspect hyponatraemia, uraemia or hypercalcaemia, or any other metabolic abnormality?

- Does the patient have any respiratory complications?

- Are there likely to be, or is there evidence of current, changes in renal and hepatic function?

- Is the patient in pain?

- Is there any reason to suspect brain metastases?

- When did the patient last pass urine?

- Is the patient constipated?

- Is the patient currently receiving chemotherapy or immunotherapy? – L-Asparaginase, 5-FU, intrathecal methotrexate, nitrogen mustard, procarbazine, and chlorambucil can all cause delirium. Interleukin 2, lymphokine-activated killer cells, and interferon also have a potential to cause confusion.

- Has he/she been started on a new drug within the last 48 hours and what combination of drugs is the patient receiving? – Opiates, non-steroidals, psychotropics, corticosteroids, histamine blockers, hyoscine, oral hypoglycaemic drugs, digoxin, and anti-parkinsonian drugs may all cause confusion.

- Alcohol and diazepam withdrawal can lead to confusional states.

- A chest or urine infection, heart failure, hepatic failure, or renal failure can lead to confusion.

paranoid, withdrawn, and detached. Unable to tolerate the sadness or fear of dying, they may feel that somebody is trying to kill or harm them.[12]

Managing delirium

The most appropriate approach for managing confusion is to identify underlying causes and associated symptoms. Pharmacological management is outlined in Care strategy 29.1. Very few studies have evaluated the effect of non-pharmacological interventions aimed at managing confusion in the cancer population. Most of the psychological and supportive interventions described in the literature are based on anecdote and offer little in the way of research-based practice guidelines. Observation, the use of constraints, a structured daily routine, and minimal room changes have all been reported as being helpful in supporting the confused individual.[8] However, many of these recommendations are believed to arise from current practices, which nurses seem to find unacceptable, ineffective, or impractical.[14]

For the majority of cancer-related symptoms it is possible to offer involvement in decisions about care. Confusion precludes this collaboration. Sometimes the decision involves sedating someone who is quite frail and who it is known may develop a chest infection by virtue of the sleep induced by sedative agents and the resultant inactivity.[12] As a team, along with the family, one of the concepts that may be helpful is to consider whether the time spent awake is of any value. Are they continually muddled and distressed when awake or are there times when they are still able to enjoy being with family and friends? It may be apparent, especially in the last few days of life, that an individual is only settled when sleeping.

If someone who is confused refuses medication, concealing medication in food or drink is inadvisable, as this may serve only to heighten an individual's mistrust when this is discovered.[12]

Terminal restlessness

Cawley and Webber[14] found that nurses repeatedly identify terminal restlessness as a poorly managed symptom that is extremely distressing for family and friends, and often leaves doctors and nurses feeling compromised by the need to sedate patients heavily during the last few days of life. Delirium during the last 24–48 hours of life (commonly referred to as terminal restlessness) may not be reversible and is most probably due to the influence of irreversible processes such as multiple organ failure.[7]

Managing terminal restlessness is an extremely challenging process, compounded by:

- multi-factorial aetiology: one study suggests that a cause is identified in less than 50% of terminally ill patients with cognitive failure[15]
- an often irreversible cause
- inappropriateness of invasive or complex diagnostic assessment.[7]

It appears to be one of the most difficult symptoms to control without also causing sedation in patients with advanced cancer.[11] Traditionally, the treatment of delirium for a terminally ill individual has focused on sedating the patient, which diminishes the possibility of managing any potentially treatable causes; at the same time, unnecessary invasive tests to clarify confusional states in terminally ill patients (i.e. 24–48 hours prior to death) should be avoided, since they may often be of limited value.[16–20] One study reported that researchers were able to identify the cause of delirium in 44% of a group of patients with advanced cancer, noting an improvement in 33% of patients following treatment aimed at identifiable causes.[15] Others suggest that many reversible causes of delirium, even those occurring during the terminal stages of cancer (for example, renal failure, dehydration, hypoxia, or hypercalcaemia), can be identified by a series of simple examinations, including:

- review of medications
- complete blood count
- electrolytes
- urea
- creatinine
- glucose and calcium levels
- pulse oximetry.[18]

Whether these apparently simple medical examinations are acceptable to seriously ill individuals is unknown. The need for sensitive nursing care to help to elicit patients' preferences for their last days and weeks of life is clear.

> ## Care strategy 29.1: Pharmacological management of confusion and terminal restlessness[7,11,21]

- Haloperidol, a neuroleptic, is useful in treating agitation, fear and paranoia. Many patients with delirium can be managed with oral haloperidol but if necessary, the addition of parenteral lorazepam may be more effective in rapidly sedating agitated, delirious patients.
- If benzodiazepines are used in palliative care, oxazepam and lorazepam are the preferred drugs. Adding lorazepam to a regime of haloperidol has been described as a useful means of treating a patient with agitated delirium. However, lorazepam alone has been shown to be ineffective and in some cases was even found to worsen symptoms. Perhaps the only setting in which benzodiazepines in isolation have an established role is in the management of terminal restlessness. In palliative care the cornerstones of therapy are neuroleptic and benzodiazepine drugs.
- Phenothiazines (such as thioridazine, chlorpromazine, and methotrimeprazine) are recommended for severe symptoms when sedation is required. McIver et al.[21] found that small doses of chlorpromazine rapidly relieved the distress of restlessness in terminal cancer and that rectal administration was as effective as intravenous administration, making it a useful drug for patients being cared for at home. At times, however, it may be necessary to sedate patients deeply to control terminal restlessness. Sensitive nursing directed at supporting relatives and friends is paramount at this distressing and difficult time in the patient's illness. Wherever appropriate, patients' wishes for sedation or otherwise will have been gently explored, allowing an opportunity for autonomy of choice right up until the time of death.
- Methotrimeprazine is commonly used to control confusion and agitation in terminal restlessness. However, it causes excessive sedation at a time when patients and relatives have very little time left to spend together. Its potential for causing hypotension and excessive sedation are important limiting factors.
- Midazolam is also used to control agitation. Unlike haloperidol, but similar to methotrimeprazine, midazolam aims only to sedate and will not improve cognition. It should be used when the goal of treatment is quiet sedation only.

Choice of drug must therefore be based on each individual's unique needs. If the intention is to attempt to improve sensory capacity and cognitive functioning, neuroleptic drugs such as haloperidol should be used. When improvement in cognition cannot be achieved, ensuring comfort and minimising distress for the patient and family are paramount.

Notes on selected cancer sites 29.1: Metastatic cancer of the liver[22-26]

The liver is a common site of metastatic disease and may often be the first sign of disease progression when the primary tumour originates elsewhere, or, as in the case of colorectal cancer, may be the only detectable tumour(s). The portal vein drains the abdominal viscera and is the most likely conduit for metastases from tumours of the breast, lung, colon, rectum, stomach, pancreas, biliary tree, and small intestine.

Diagnosis is usually straightforward. An enlarged or tender liver on physical examination, abnormal alkaline phosphatase and transaminases, or abnormal liver scan, sonography or computed tomography (CT) scan of the liver all point to liver metastases.

Metastatic tumours to the liver tend to grow rapidly and their growth and development are dependent upon a number of factors:

- the nature of the primary cancer
- the extent of liver involvement
- the physiological status of the liver parenchyma
- the growth properties of the tumour cells (p. 2201).[22]

Treatment varies depending on the nature and extent of disease in the liver and other sites. For example, patients with lymphomas and testicular carcinoma involving the liver can be cured with combination chemotherapy. Patients with breast carcinoma and small-cell lung cancer may obtain partial remission with chemotherapy, and for patients with colorectal cancer, where spread may be solely or predominantly to the liver, regional treatment may be a viable option.

Standard treatment for resectable colorectal hepatic metastases involves hepatic resection, which may produce a 5-year survival rate in 20–30% of affected patients. Unfortunately, the majority of patients is ineligible for resection. There is some evidence that regional chemotherapy with floxuridine, combined with hepatic resection, may offer superior survival statistics to hepatic resection alone, but no evidence is offered of patients' preferences based upon quality of life issues. Single-agent chemotherapy versus combination chemotherapy, intrahepatic infusion of floxuridine, hepatic artery ligation and portal vein infusion, concomitant hepatic radiation and intravenous 5-FU and radiotherapy alone have all been offered to patients with unresectable hepatic metastases from colorectal cancer. Nevertheless, despite these improvements in early detection of liver metastases, new drug developments, improved surgical techniques and innovative targeted therapies, the prognosis for patients with liver secondaries is very poor. If left untreated, length of survival is estimated between 3 and 24 months.

References

1. Parker J. (1981). Cancer passage: continuity and discourse in terminal care. In Benner P., and Wrubel J. (1989) *The Primacy of Caring. Stress and Coping in Health and Illness.* Wokingham: Addison-Wesley.
2. Lutzen K. (1996). Research in psychiatric settings: some ethical issues. In De Raeve L (ed.) *Nursing Research. An Ethical and Legal Appraisal.* London: Baillière Tindall, pp. 71–84.
3. Fleishman S. and Lesko L. (1985). Delirium in cancer patients: spotting it early, finding the cause. *Primary Cancer Care* 5, 23–27.
4. Zimberg M. and Berenson S. (1990). Delirium in patients with cancer: nursing assessment and intervention. *Oncology Nursing Forum* 17, 529–537.
5. Breitbart W. (1994). Psycho-oncology: depression, anxiety, delirium. *Seminars in Oncology* 21, 754–769.
6. Lipowski Z. (1987). Delirium (acute confusional states). *Journal of the American Medical Association* 258, 1789–1792.
7. Breitbart W. (1995). Identifying patients at risk for, and treatment of major psychiatric complications of cancer. *Support Cancer Care* 3, 45–60.
8. Weinrich S. and Sarna L. (1994). Delirium in the older person with cancer. *Cancer* (Suppl. 1 October) 74, 2079–2091.
9. Holland J. and Massie M. (1987). Psychosocial aspects of cancer in the elderly. *Clinical Geriatric Medicine* 3, 533–539.
10. Fleishman S. and Lesko L. (1990). Delirium and dementia. In Holland J. and Rowland J. (eds.) *Handbook of Psycho-oncology. Psychological Care of the Patient with Cancer.* Oxford: Oxford University Press, pp. 342–355.
11. Steifel F., Fainsinger R. and Bruera E. (1992). Acute confusional states in patients with advanced cancer. *Journal of Pain and Symptom Management* 7, 94–98.
12. Murphy G.E. (1977). Suicide and attempted suicide. *Hospital Practice* 12, 78–81.
13. Kleinman A. (1988). *The Illness Narratives: Suffering, Healing and the Human Condition.* New York: Basic Books.
14. Cawley N. and Webber J. (1995). Research priorities in palliative care. *International Journal of Palliative Nursing* 1, 101–113.
15. Bruera E., Macmillan K., Hanson J. and MacDonald R. (1989). The cognitive effects of administration of narcotic analgesics in patients with cancer pain. *Pain* 39, 13–16.
16. Lichter I. and Hunt E. (1990). The last 48 hours of life. *Journal of Palliative Care* 6, 7–15.
17. Back I. (1992). Terminal restlessness in patients with advanced malignant disease. *Palliative Medicine* 6, 293–298.

18. de Stoutz N., Tapper M. and Faisinger R. (1995). Reversible delirium in terminally ill patients. *Journal of Pain and Symptom Management* **10**, 249–253.

19. Cody M. (1990). Depression and the use of antidepressants in patients with cancer. *Palliative Medicine* **4**, 271–278. Cancer Research Campaign (1988) *Facts On Cancer. Factsheet 2 – Survival in England and Wales.* London: Cancer Research Campaign.

20. Power D., Kelly S., Gilsenan J., Kearney M., O'Mahony D., Walsh J.B. *et al.* (1993). Suitable screening tests for cognitive impairment and depression in the terminally ill – a prospective prevalence study. *Palliative Medicine* **7**, 213–218.

21. McIver B., Walsh D. and Nelson K. (1994). The use of chlorpromazine for symptom control in dying cancer patients. *Journal of Pain and Symptom Management* **5**, 341–345.

22. Niederhuber J. and Ensmiger W. (1993). Treatment of metastatic cancer to the liver. In DeVita V., Hellman S. and Rosenberg S. (eds.) *Cancer. Principles and Practice of Oncology,* 4th edition. Philadelphia, PA: Lippincott, pp. 2201–2211.

23. NCI/PDQ (1996). Physician statement: liver metastases update (August). http://cancer.med.upenn.edu

24. Bozzetti F., Dolci R., Bignami P. *et al.* (1987). Patterns of failure following surgical resection of colorectal cancer liver metastases: rationale for a multimodal approach. *Annals of Surgery* **205**, 264–270: a new approach to cancer therapy. *Cancer Topics* **9**, 1029–1033.

25. Meta-Analysis Group in Cancer (1996). Reappraisal of hepatic arterial infusion in the treatment of nonresectable liver metastases from colorectal cancer. *Journal of the National Cancer Institute* **88**, 252–258.

26. Kemeny M.M., Goldberg D.A., Browning S. *et al.* (1985). Experience with continuous regional chemotherapy and hepatic resection as a treatment of hepatic metastases from colorectal primaries: a prospective randomised study. *Cancer* **55**, 1265–1270.

CHAPTER THIRTY

Rehabilitation and long-term effects of treatment

Jo O'Neill and Kay Leedham

Early detection and improvements in treatment and supportive care have contributed to an increase in cancer survival. The overall 5-year survival rate for all cancers in all groups is 35%. For many cancers in young and middle-aged people, 5-year survival rates are over 50%. A number of long-term survivors has a normal life expectancy. Others, although not cured, live for some considerable time with their disease. Even those who do not have a good prognosis are living longer, with treatment aimed at controlling the symptoms associated with advanced disease.

Increasingly we must consider not only the impact of the cancer diagnosis and the support required by patients dying of cancer, but also the needs of people living with cancer. For some cancers, keeping the disease under control requires extended treatment over long periods. For others, intensive periods of treatment are followed by monitoring and a 'wait and see' policy. In all cases, the psychological trauma of being diagnosed with a serious, life-threatening illness, and the debilitating nature of many cancer treatments, mean that it cannot be assumed that 'life will carry on as normal'. To be meaningful, an increase in survival must be accompanied by an acceptable quality of life for each individual.

Long-term effects of cancer treatment

Until recently, little was known about the long-term impact of cancer on daily living, because unlike the time of diagnosis or the final weeks and days of a patient's life, there is little contact with professionals following completion of acute treatment. Any problems experienced have to be managed alone, and there has been a presumption that this is uncomplicated.

Much information on the long-term effects of cancer treatment has come from the use of two instruments developed by a group working in California: the Cancer Inventory of Problem Situations or CIPS[1] and the Cancer Rehabilitation Evaluation System or CARES.[2] These are self-assessment schedules used in the out-patient follow-up setting, following cancer treatment. Other researchers have developed their own methods of collecting information and some have concentrated on specific groups; for example, women with breast cancer. The problems most commonly identified include:

- fear of recurrence and death, which leads to a pre-occupation with health and somatic symptoms
- concerns about relationships with the health care team, with difficulties in asking questions and obtaining information in medical consultations[3]
- lack of information to explain what is happening and as an expression of support from the professionals involved in patient care[3]
- physical problems, including fatigue, sleep disturbance, nutritional concerns, pain, and long-term side-effects of treatment; for example, radiation fibrosis. The presence of a physical problem increases the likelihood of a psychological problem

- psychological problems such as anxiety and depression, which may be present in up to one-third of people with cancer[4]
- financial worries are a significant concern as many state benefits are designed as short-term provision for the seriously ill but there is little to help the long-term survivor, who may have employment and insurance difficulties for many years
- relationships are often affected by illness. People may be treated differently by friends and colleagues, leaving them feeling isolated and angry. Marital relationships can also suffer, particularly if there were pre-existing communication difficulties. Given all these areas of concern, it is not surprising that many experience a loss of libido and difficulties with sexuality and self-esteem.

Adapting to the stress of living with a cancer diagnosis and uncertainty and fear for the future is difficult.

Definitions of rehabilitation and its application to cancer care

Rehabilitation can be defined as the restoration of the individual to the optimal level of functional ability within the needs and desires of the individual and his or her family, and commensurate with the limits imposed by the disease and its treatment.[5] In cancer care, rehabilitation involves adopting measures to minimise the physical effects of cancer and treatment, helping people to adapt to the changes that the illness brings, and to learn to live with the uncertainty, while also setting personal goals for optimal physical, psychological, social, and spiritual function.

Rehabilitation in cancer care concentrates on adapting and readapting to the changes illness brings. By focusing on adaptation, misconceptions and unrealistic expectations of restoration to a former level of operation are avoided. Dietz[6] outlines four phases of rehabilitation that are relevant to different stages of the cancer trajectory: these are shown below.

In a development of Dietz's ideas, Wells[7] identifies three situations where rehabilitation is important. The first is where there is good life expectancy following treatment and no residual dis-

figurement or disability. Here, the needs may not be physical but counselling may be required to enable movement away from the cancer and sickness role. Health promotion interventions may also be valuable. The second situation is where there may also be good life expectancy but cancer treatment has left physical or psychological disability or disfigurement. Here intensive physical, psychological, and social rehabilitation is needed in order to restore some meaning for being, and to reunite people with those things that made life worth living before they became ill. The third situation is for those for whom treatment has failed or who have relapsed following initial remission. They have a limited life expectancy. The goal of rehabilitation is to enable them to have a good quality of life during the time that they have left.

Box 30.1: Aims of rehabilitation in cancer care[6]

Prevention – the preventive phase of cancer rehabilitation is designed to reduce the impact and severity of the expected disabilities and to assist the individual to learn how to cope with and manage any disability (for example, rehabilitation required after a major surgical procedure such as mastectomy or colostomy formation) to prevent long-term effects such as problems with body image.

Restoration – the restorative phase of cancer rehabilitation is designed to return the patient to a pre-illness level of functioning without residual disabilities from or related to the treatment of disease; for example, after intensive treatment for malignancies with a good prognosis such as leukaemia or lymphoma, where remission/cure is achieved but the patient may find it hard to 'return to normal'.

Support – the supportive phase is characterised by persistence of the disease, a continuing need for treatment and progressive changes in functional ability. The rehabilitation goal is to limit functional changes and to provide support to reduce any disabilities or loss of function; for example, inoperable lung cancer, where the patient may need rehabilitation support to adapt to long-term symptoms such as breathlessness.

Palliation – the palliative phase of rehabilitation is appropriate where there is an increasing loss of function. The goal of palliative rehabilitation is to reduce the complications of the disease process and to provide comfort and emotional support for the patient and family; for example, when a patient is dealing with recurrence or advanced disease.

Opportunities offered by a rehabilitative approach

Assessment and goal setting

Assessment of individual needs and goal setting are key aspects of rehabilitation. A successful rehabilitation programme incorporates many of the skills offered by the multi-disciplinary team; however, it is essential that identification of needs is accurate, that referral is appropriate and that shared realistic goals are agreed. Goals should be centred on the person and selected with them, recognising their unique response to cancer. They should be realistic and aim to promote independence and restore optimal functioning. The intention of a rehabilitative programme is to enhance self-esteem and self-confidence, and to promote a sense of mastery over the situation. Effective communication skills, which help to build rapport, will assist in goal setting by helping the health worker to determine what the person is thinking and feeling about the situation and what their hopes and aspirations in learning to live with cancer are.

Assessment should be focused around functional ability. This means that although the disease process and prognosis are taken into account, the emphasis is to assess the effects of the cancer experience on daily living activities; that is, the extent to which these may be limited by the disease. The goals then set and the interventions planned are aimed towards enhancing the ability to live with cancer in a way that enables people to have quality of living.

Adaptation correlates with effective coping strategies. Most adults have already developed personal resources for coping with stressful life events and it may be helpful to review these and adapt them to their current situation. People vary in the coping mechanisms they employ, but it has been suggested that these tend to be either problem focused or emotion focused.[8] Problem-focused strategies involve the individual in eliciting information and help them to make choices about actions and to seek out new resources and learn self-help skills. Emotion-focused strategies include responses such as denial, blame, and detachment. It is helpful for health workers to recognise the degree to which an individual may be using these strategies to ensure that the care planned reflects the most appropriate help for the individual.

Social support is also a key factor in a person's ability to cope with a stressful event.[3] Effective social support appears to engender a positive effect on physical and mental health. Emotional, informational, and practical support have been identified as important factors in enhancing a person's feeling of well-being. Emotional support is mostly received from family and friends. Health workers can support carers by acknowledging the important role they have, and in recognising the burdens of that role. Assessing informational needs may identify deficits in the understanding of the disease and treatment options; information needs to be given in a format that is understandable and at a pace at which it is possible to digest.

Many volunteer agencies can be called upon to offer a befriending 'listening ear' service or offer practical support, such as help with gardening or shopping. In this way, those people with limited family support or who wish not to depend upon family for all their support can maintain a feeling of independence.

A multi-disciplinary approach

A multi-disciplinary approach to rehabilitation is crucial if a holistic approach is to be achieved using a range of expertise. Team members who may be able to contribute include nursing and medical staff, physiotherapists, occupational therapists, speech therapists, social workers, dieticians, complementary therapists, counsellors, and clergy. In addition, other specialist expertise may be needed; for example, the breast care or stoma nurse.

The nurse's role in rehabilitation

Nurses have a key role in rehabilitation. Collaborative care between patient and nurse should aim to increase feelings of control by giving information, offering choices, or discussing options of care or treatment where appropriate.

Central to effective rehabilitation is the control of symptoms of the disease and consequences of treatment. Nurses should ensure that they have the knowledge and skills to deal with the many complex problems that may be experienced. More research is needed in this area, but some work has already indicated that nursing interventions can minimise the effects of breathlessness, fatigue, and body image problems.

Nursing interventions that facilitate self-help and independence should be planned. For example, education prior to stoma formation or a course of chemotherapy will prepare people for the effects of such interventions and hasten the adaptation process. Encouraging self-medication and participation in identifying discharge needs will also enhance control.

Rehabilitation needs should be viewed within the context of the family. It is important to acknowledge that family members are also experiencing fear and uncertainty and thus experiencing their own difficulties in adapting to the situation.

It is increasingly recognised that adapting to a diagnosis of cancer and learning to live positively with the effects of the disease and treatment may take a considerable length of time, and indeed some people may never reach this position. Individual responses mean that there is no one approach that we as health professionals can advise people to take to enhance adaptation. Some people benefit from attending self-help groups by being able to share experiences with other people who have cancer. Complementary therapies are accessed by an increasing number of people with cancer as a means of relaxation, acknowledgement of their need for nurturing and of doing something for themselves and their bodies. Others seek ways to manage stress by attending stress management courses specifically designed to limit the impact of stressful events, or creative workshops in drama, art, or music to release emotion and to try and make sense of what is happening. Many find satisfaction in discovering hidden talents in craft and painting classes. Often it is through these means that it is possible for them to regain a feeling of self-worth and self-esteem.

The successful outcome of a rehabilitative approach to care is positive adaptation to the changing circumstances imposed by the disease or the treatment. The challenge of rehabilitation is to integrate this approach into mainstream cancer care:

> Rehabilitation is not a functional phenomena; rather, it is a philosophy of care that must be relevant to all health care providers.[7]

Rehabilitation should be an active, ongoing process that begins at diagnosis, continues throughout treatment, and follows for an indeterminate peri-od as long as a need for ongoing support is identified.

Rehabilitation is not about doing things to people but rather about enabling them to do things for themselves. It aims to enable the patient to help themselves and foster hope. Personal account 30.1 demonstrates many of the principles outlined above, presented within patient-centred scenarios.

Personal account 30.1: Assessing the impact of illness on role and lifestyle

George, a 70-year-old retired engineer, was referred to the Community Macmillan Nurse 3 months after a gastrectomy and partial oesophagectomy to remove an adenocarcinoma at the junction of the oesophagus and stomach. All visible tumour had been removed at surgery but the pathology report showed microscopic infiltration at the margins of the dissection. George said that he had expected the diagnosis of cancer and in a way was relieved because he had felt for a long time that there must be a reason for his recurrent oesophagitis and gastric ulcers, although all previous biopsy reports from gastroscopy examinations had been negative.

George had coped well with major surgery, but he was very angry that the tumour had not been diagnosed sooner and he felt the medical staff had been negligent in their management of him. 'They wouldn't get away with mistakes like that in industry', was his comment. He was finding it very difficult to cope with the 'wait and see' policy of follow-up, believing that he should be aggressively tested for recurrence. George monitored his physical state closely and judged any change as a sign that the tumour was regrowing. His anxiety about this was such that much of his conversation with his family and friends was about weight, bowels, diet, and appetite.

Prior to becoming ill, George had been active in a number of local voluntary groups. He was also skilled in DIY and carried out all the maintenance on his house and those of his immediate family. Since surgery George had withdrawn from all these activities. He stayed at home and his visitors were finding it increasingly difficult to sustain conversation focused on George's dissatisfaction with his medical management and the details of his current symptoms.

The nurse allowed George to express his anger at not being diagnosed sooner and the fact that surgery had not been able to remove all traces of the tumour. George knew that it was extremely likely that the tumour would regrow. His anger and anxieties were understandable but they were consuming a lot of his energy and preventing him from 'moving on' to focus on and make use of the time he had. Discussion of his preferred coping style of control and facing difficulties 'head on' allowed George to identify for himself the strengths of this approach when living with a cancer diagnosis and the areas in which he would need additional support from relatives, friends, and professionals. Understanding why he found uncertainty difficult enabled George to cope with it better.

One expression of George's need for control was his concern about his weight. Following surgery he had lost 10 kg, 2 months later he had regained 6 kg, but during the past few weeks he had been unable to achieve any further weight gain.

George's three children lived locally and it was the custom that George, his wife, the children and grandchildren met up together at their parents' house for a meal at weekends.

For the last few weeks George had made the decision not to eat with the family because he 'wanted to concentrate on his eating'. George's children were finding this very difficult to cope with. They had never found their father an easy person to get close to but now it felt as if he was withdrawing altogether. The help of the community dietician was sought to give support and advice about meals and supplements and to help set realistic goals for weight maintenance. George continued to eat his main course alone but he did decide to join the family for dessert and a chat at the end of the meal.

George subsequently realised that since retirement he had found it hard to identify his role within the family, as his wife was much closer to the children and grandchildren, and he could no longer see himself as the 'provider'. George did not want to become a 'burden' to the family as his illness progressed, and he considered it a 'vanity' to presume that they might value his company and presence within the family for its own sake and because they loved him. After talking about his feelings, George decided to resume one of the voluntary activities that he found particularly rewarding. Throughout his illness he found it difficult to seek emotional support from his family.

Adapting to the changes in his role and lifestyle was not easy for George, but by working with the nurse he learned to understand why he found this difficult and was enabled to move on from his initial reaction of anger and withdrawal.

Personal account 30.2: Assessing strategies for coping

Katy, a 32-year-old woman, married with three children, self-referred to a cancer care centre 2 months after diagnosis and treatment for thyroid cancer. She recalled a feeling of complete shock when told the diagnosis and the following 2 weeks, when she underwent surgery, were a very difficult time for her and her husband. The reassurance that there was no evidence of residual thyroid tissue at the time of surgery and that the tumour was a solitary, well-encapsulated nodule, indicating a good prognosis, had done little to allay her anxiety as she could only associate a cancer diagnosis with illness and

death. The need to take thyroxine tablets for the rest of her life was a continual reminder of her illness. These feelings were exacerbated by the need for her to attend a cancer specialist hospital for radio-iodine scans to determine the presence of any residual thyroid tissue not apparent at surgery, or any metastases.

On assessment, Katy identified the areas of particular concern for her. Although able to cope with everyday activities, she expressed fear and confusion about her future and was 'plagued with thoughts of cancer'. She had experienced several episodes of sudden restricted breathing and difficulty in swallowing, with no apparent physical cause. These episodes mainly occurred when collecting the children from school, where she found difficulty in discussing her illness with other mothers. Initially she had been able to discuss her anxieties with her husband and family but now felt it inappropriate to do so, as some weeks had passed since diagnosis.

Helping patients to acknowledge the impact of the cancer on themselves and their families can do much to allay feelings of isolation and maladaptation. Katy expressed an interest in meeting other people learning to live with cancer. She was also keen to read patient self-help booklets, which again reassured her that many other people in her position experience similar difficulties.

Katy identified that her usual way of coping with stressful events was to 'keep busy so you don't have to think about it'. Before the cancer diagnosis she had enjoyed her role as busy housewife and mother and was very involved with school activities. She had returned to this busy lifestyle as soon as she was able but felt she was overactive, 'rushing about and getting nowhere'. She found planning her time increasingly difficult and was feeling very tired.

It was important for Katy to keep up with her activities to ensure that her preferred coping style was being employed and that she was able to fulfil her role in the family. However, she agreed that her ceaseless 'doing' was ineffective and adding to her fatigue. Her goal was to structure her time more effectively and to plan in time for relaxation. She agreed to join a relaxation group to learn some relaxation and breathing techniques, which would help her at home and in particular when experiencing feelings of panic.

After several sessions with the relaxation group Katy reviewed her progress. She had found the relaxation sessions very helpful and had learnt techniques to use at home. These had been particularly useful at her recent hospital appointment. She believed she had begun to find ways to deal with the concerns about the cancer and her future. She had changed her expectations that her life would return to normal for her when she had recovered from the operation, and had realistic concerns and hopes for her future. With help, Katy had gained a new perspective and had developed her own personal coping strategies. She was discharged from the help centre but knew where to access help in the future should there be a need.

Notes on selected cancer sites 30.1: Oesophageal cancer[9]

The incidence of cancer of the oesophagus varies greatly in different geographical areas from 1 in 100 000 to as much as 547 in 100 000. In Europe, the incidence is two or three cases per 100 000 population. In all areas, it is more common in men than in women, but the ratio varies from 2:1 to 25:1. The age groups most at risk are the 60s and 70s and it is rare for an oesophageal cancer to occur in subjects younger than 45.

Aetiology is thought to be multi-factoral and contributing factors identified include alcohol intake, tobacco smoking, and dietary factors, such as very hot food and drinks, preservatives, fungi, mould, and co-carginogens in food. Benign conditions that involve chronic inflammation of the oesophagus such as reflux oesophagitis can progress through dysplasia to carcinoma *in situ* and invasive cancer.

Between 80 and 90% of cancers of the oesophagus are squamous cell carcinomas, of which 50% are located in the mid-thoracic portion of the oesophagus. The remaining 50% are divided equally between the upper and lower oesophagus, with a small number in the cervical oesophagus. Adenocarcinoma is less common but when it does occur it is frequently found at the distal end of the oesophagus, where it joins the stomach. Here, gastric mucosa extends into the oesophagus and chronic inflammations known as Barratt's oesophagus is associated with the development of adenocarcinoma.

The frequent delay in diagnosing oesophageal cancer is due to the fact that there is no specific early symptomatology to differentiate between early stage cancer and benign gastro-oesophageal diseases, such as dyspepsia and gastro-oesophageal reflux. The initial symptom is often a burning sensation in the oesophagus or a feeling of something stuck behind the sternum, both of which feel worse when swallowing food. Dysphagia appears intermittently at first and then continuously so that the patient eats with frequent sips of water. For dysphagia to be felt, at least two-thirds of the oesophageal circumference must be infiltrated by the tumour. It is therefore a later symptom; nevertheless, it is present in over 80% of patients at diagnosis.

Surgery is the treatment of choice as it gives the most relief from symptoms and is the only hope of cure. Approximately 60% of patients are considered suitable for surgery and resection is possible in 34–88% of those depending on the aggressiveness of the surgical technique. The exact procedure depends on the location of the tumour, but it usually requires a double or triple surgical approach. With advances in surgical techniques, operative mortality rates have fallen in recent years, but they remain significant at 5–10%. If it is necessary to include a complete or partial gastrectomy in the operative procedure, then the patient may have to learn to cope with regurgitation, rapid satiety, diarrhoea, and steatorrhoea.

The 5-year survival rate after curative oesophagectomy varies from 15 to 30% on the basis of tumour stage. With no lymph node metastases, the 5-year survival is approximately 50%; in the presence of metastatic lymph nodes it is 13%.

Recent research has investigated the use of multi-modal therapeutic protocols using combinations of radiotherapy, chemotherapy, and surgery. Some studies suggest that pre-operative chemotherapy and radiotherapy may improve prognosis. No benefit has been shown for the routine use of adjuvant pre- or post-operative radiotherapy or post-operative chemotherapy.

A resection is defined as palliative when infiltration of adjuvant structures prevents removal of all the tumour or when microscopic residual tumour is found at the section margins. The 5-year survival rate for palliative resection is 2–5%, with a mean survival of 7–8 months. The initial relief of dysphagia is good, but it recurs as the tumour regrows.

Palliation for the 40% of patients in whom the extent of the tumour at diagnosis precludes surgery, or for those in whom the tumour recurs following, surgery, may be achieved with a wide variety of procedures. These may be used separately or in combination and include radiotherapy (external beam or intralumenal), chemotherapy, laser therapy, intubation, and cauterisation.

Advanced disease is characterised by regional spread and/or distant metastases. The most frequent causes of death are related to regional spread. Dysphagia leads to poor nutrition and cachexia. Inability to swallow saliva, aspiration of food, and infiltration or compression of the bronchial tree lead to bronchopneumonia.

Notes on selected cancer sites 30.2: Thyroid cancer[10,11]

Thyroid cancers are relatively uncommon, but the incidence is slightly higher in females than in males. They can occur at any age but incidence tends to peak between 30 and 50 years. Several aetiological factors have been identified and include exposure to radiation and a high intake of dietary iodine.

Tumours of the thyroid can be divided into three groups:

- tumours arising from the thyroid cells, either papillary or follicular carcinoma
- medullary carcinoma arising from the parafollicular cells
- primary thyroid lymphoma.

Papillary carcinoma accounts for approximately two-thirds of thyroid carcinomas. Most thyroid carcinomas present as an asymptomatic slow-growing nodule. The patient may describe discomfort on swallowing and may have noticed a swelling in the thyroid or in the side of the neck. Some patients may have noticed some hoarseness. Taking the history may reveal an exposure to radiation and progressive rather than sudden growth. Some patients may present with symptoms of metastatic spread, such as back pain.

Investigations may include thyroid scan and needle aspiration for cytology. Following diagnosis, surgical resection is the primary mode of treatment for primary carcinoma and may be either a total or a partial thyroidectomy. Local lymph nodes may also be removed. Occasionally other surgical procedures are necessary, such as tracheal resection and tracheotomy and even more occasionally oesophageal resection, where there is infiltration of these structures.

Post-operative radioactive iodine (^{131}I) following total surgical resection may have the advantage of reducing the possibility of relapse. In patients with metastatic thyroid cancer when surgery may not be indicated, radioactive iodine is usually the initial choice of treatment. This radioactive isotope is taken by the patient in the form of a drink. The thyroid cells take it up from the circulation as if it were normal dietary iodine and are then destroyed by the radioactivity. Patients who may have residual thyroid cells and are receiving an ablative dose of ^{131}I may be given thyroid stimulating hormone (TSH) prior to administration to stimulate the thyroid tissue, thus increasing the uptake of the radioactive iodine.

Since the outcome of treatment is to render the thyroid non-functioning by surgery or by radiotherapy, the patient will become myxoedematous. Thyroxine is given to replace the normal secretion of the gland and thus suppresses TSH secretion. TSH stimulates thyroid function and in the case of malignancy of this gland this should obviously be avoided. Patients are required to have routine blood tests to monitor thyroxine levels.

If the disease progresses, neck node recurrence may be palpable. Lungs and bones are the most frequent sites of distant metastases. Surgery may be considered in patients with bone metastases, which result in orthopaedic or neurological complications. External beam therapy may also be considered for bone metastases. Responses to chemotherapy are limited, but agents such as doxorubicin have been used to palliate patients with progressive metastases, which resist the uptake of radioactive iodine.

Long-term survival is relatively good in comparison with other cancers. Age has been identified as the most important prognostic factor, with older patients having an increased incidence of recurrence and mortality. Patients with well-differentiated papillary and follicular tumours have a similar prognosis, with the worst outlook for those with poorly differentiated cancers.

Lymphoma of the thyroid gland is rare and may develop rapidly. It is most common in people who are elderly and female. Management of the disease is the same as for nodular lymphoma.

References

1. Ganz P.A., Rofessart J., Polinsky M.L., Schag C.C. and Heinrich R.L.A. (1986). Comprehensive approach to the assessment of cancer patients' rehabilitation needs: the cancer inventory of problem situations and a companion interview. *Journal of Psychosocial Oncology* 4, 27–42.
2. Schag C. and Heinrich R.L. (1990). Development of a comprehensive quality of life measurement tool: CARES. *Oncology* 4, 135–138.
3. Dunkel-Schetter C., Blasbank D., Feinstein L. and Herbert T. (1984). Elements of supportive interactions: when are attempts to help effective? In Spacapan and Oskamp S. (eds.) *Helping and Being Helped*, pp. 83–114.
4. Derogatis L.R., Morrow G.R., Fetting J., Penman D. and Piasetsky S. (1983). The prevalence of psychiatric disorder among cancer patients. *Journal of the American Medical Association* 249, 751–757.
5. Romsaas E.P., Julian L.M., Brigg A.L., Wysocki G. and Moorman J.A. (1983). Method for assessing the rehabilitation needs of oncology outpatients. *Oncology Nursing Forum* 10, 17–21.
6. Dietz J.H. (1981). *Rehabilitation Oncology*. New York: John Wiley.
7. Wells R.J. (1990). Rehabilitation: making the most of time. *Oncology Nursing Forum* 17, 503–507.
8. Folkman S. and Lazarus R.S. (1980). An analysis of coping in middle-aged community sample. *Journal of Health and Social Behaviour* 21, 219–239.
9. Peracchia A., Ruol A. and Debesi P. (1995). Malignancies of the oesophagus. In Peckman M., Pinedo H. and Veronsei V. (eds.) *Oxford Textbook of Oncology*, Vol. 2. Oxford: Oxford University Press.
10. Tschudin V. (1988). *Nursing The Patient With Cancer*. London: Prentice Hall.
11. Tubiana M. and Schlumberger M. (1995). Carcinoma of the thyroid. In Peckman M., Pinedo H. and Veronsei V. (eds.) *Oxford Textbook of Oncology*, Vol. 2. Oxford: Oxford University Press.

CHAPTER THIRTY-ONE

Acute events in cancer care

Julia Downing

Improved ability to control many cancers effectively has led to longer survival and altered disease progression. Many individuals are now living with advanced cancer and we are seeing an increase in critically ill cancer patients. Many of the symptoms of advanced cancer can now be controlled, enhancing an individual's quality of life. Spinal cord compression, superior vena cava obstruction, and hypercalcaemia are all consequences of metastatic disease, which can potentially be controlled, but should be recognised as emergencies, to prevent further deterioration in the individual's condition and quality of life where possible.

Spinal cord compression

The spinal column is a common site for bone metastases and a common complication of these metastases is spinal cord compression. Spinal cord compression can be one of the most devastating complications from cancer metastases, for both the patient and his or her family. Its natural course can be relentless, progressing from back pain through to paraplegia and loss of sphincter control in the short-time (e.g. 24 hours), leaving the individual paralysed and incontinent, unless treated promptly. Hence, prompt recognition of the problem and treatment are vital in its management.

Spinal cord compression can present at any time in the cancer trajectory from diagnosis through to the terminal phase of the illness. As many as 5–10% of cancer patients will suffer from spinal cord com-

pression,[1,2] and it is the second most common cause of neurological complications after brain metastases.[1,3] It is caused by the neoplasm impinging on the vertebral column and may be due to a primary malignancy (34%) or a secondary (metastatic) malignancy (66%).[4] The physiology of spinal cord compression is described below.

Box 31.1: The physiology of spinal cord compression[5-8]

Metastatic tumours are usually found in the pedicles of the vertebrae, where they can directly invade the spinal canal, leading to vertebral destruction, blockage of the cerebrospinal fluid, and pressure on the spinal cord. This is the most common cause of cord damage (85% of cases). Intradural metastases are rare and involvement is usually due to primary spinal tumours. Only occasionally will vertebral metastases extend directly into the intradural space. Spinal cord compression can also result from vertebral collapse due to pathological fractures.

Compression of the spinal cord or cauda equina will occur as the tumour in the extradural space increases in size. The resulting impairment of the venous return of the blood from the spinal cord will give rise to oedema in both the white and grey matter, causing the arterial inflow to the cord to be reduced, leading to ischaemia of the nervous tissue. An increase in phagocytic activity is then seen within the spinal cord, leading to demyelination and permanent neurological destruction.

The location of an individual's primary tumour is significant in relation to their chances of developing spinal cord compression, the area of the spinal

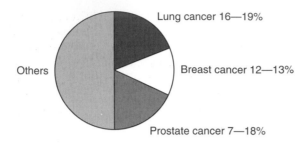

Others: melanoma; renal cell; thyroid; sarcoma; multiple myeloma; gastrointestinal; unknown primary; neuroblastoma in children.

Figure 31.1 Causes and incidence of spinal cord compression by primary tumour type.[6,9]

cord affected, and its subsequent impact on physical functioning. Any cancer that metastasises to the bone has the potential to invade the spine and cause spinal cord compression, although some are more likely to result in cord compression than others. The exact incidence of spinal cord compression from each disease is not clear, although breast, lung, and prostate result in over 50% of incidences of spinal cord compression (Figure 31.1).[8]

Spinal cord compression may occur at any location throughout the spinal column and differing primary cancers are likely to cause cord compression in different areas of the spine:

- 10% affect the cervical region – mainly breast
- 70% affect the thoracic region – mainly lung and breast
- 20% affect the lumbosacral region – gastrointestinal tumours, prostate, and melanoma.[5,10,11]

Variation in the spinal regions affected is due to the proximity of the primary tumour to the spinal region; for instance, 1–12% of individuals with prostate cancer will develop spinal cord compression in the lumbosacral region owing to the close proximity of the gland to that part of the cord.[12] It is important to remember that bone metastases do not necessarily occur in isolation and over 50% of individuals with spinal cord compression have multiple bone lesions.[8]

Signs and symptoms of spinal cord compression
Early detection of spinal cord compression is important as it may cause rapid damage to the spinal nerves. However, individuals will often delay seeking treatment, confusing early symptoms for muscle strain or joint pain. Doctors may also misdiagnose cord compression as arthritis or degenerative joint disease. The signs of spinal cord compression vary and may initially be hard to detect, commencing with back pain, leading on to motor weakness, sensory deficits, autonomic dysfunction and finally bladder and bowel incontinence.[1,3,8,10] Its impact on the patient and their family can therefore be profound. The rate and degree of cord compression are responsible for the different clinical manifestations seen:

> . . . the pain started in April. I enjoy gardening and I thought I had strained a muscle in my back. I did not even think that it could be the cancer coming back and I nearly forgot to mention it to the doctor when I saw him in September . . .

> . . . it [the pain] came right round my chest in a tight band, it felt as if I was being squeezed all the time.

Nursing care is informed by the rapidity of onset of symptoms, the level and degree of cord compression, the presenting symptoms, and type of and response to treatment.[3,6] The individual's specific neurological deficits will determine the nursing care given, though mobility and safety must be important considerations at all times. Information about the goals of treatment, schedule, side-effects, and the prevention and management of side-effects should also be given to the individual. Meticulous and continual assessment of an individual's level of function and mobility is needed,[1] along with interventions to help maintain strength and level of mobility; for example, leg exercises. An interdisciplinary approach is needed, with support from the medical team and physiotherapists.

Back pain is the first and most common presenting symptom of spinal cord compression, with over 90% of patients presenting with it.[2,6,10,13] The onset of pain is gradual and progressive, it is usually dull and aching and is exacerbated by lying flat. The pain caused by thoracic metastases may be bilateral and radiate around the body like a tight band, whereas cervical and lumbosacral pain may be either unilateral or bilateral.[3] The symptoms of spinal cord compression may be gradual, with an individual experiencing pain for several months before the cause is diagnosed, though as the tumour size increases, the physical picture can deteriorate rapidly and suddenly, and severe pain may indicate vertebral collapse followed by rapid paralysis.

For some patients, back pain may be the only symptom of spinal cord compression. Any complaint of back pain should therefore be noted and a diagnosis of spinal cord compression suspected. The provision of cancer care is changing. There has been a shift of care to the out-patient setting, with between 80 and 90% of cancer care now being delivered there.[14] If free from other symptoms, patients may receive the majority of their care in an out-patient department. Back pain is a common non-malignant problem. The necessity for vigilance and an awareness of back pain as a sign of spinal cord compression is therefore of paramount importance.

Motor weakness, although rarely a presenting symptom, is present in about 75% of individuals at the time of diagnosis of spinal cord compression, pain and weakness being the two most predominant symptoms.[6] Individuals will often complain of a heaviness in their limbs, followed by a feeling of numbness in their toes, which gradually ascends to the level of the cord compression. Common sensory loss involves the loss of sensation to pinpricks, vibration, light touch, temperature, and deficits in proprioception.[11] Late signs of cord compression are paraplegia and autonomic dysfunction involving urinary and bowel sphincter control. If treated early enough, individuals need not develop all of these symptoms and may maintain neurological function. If treatment is delayed, however, it is unlikely to be effective and the prognosis is poor. Maranzano *et al.*[15] found that in individuals with untreated spinal cord compression from metastatic disease, 31% were able to walk without support, 16% could walk with support, 43% were unable to walk at all, and 10% were paraplegic. A delay in diagnosing spinal cord compression may therefore result in permanent neurological damage. This has cost implications, both for the patient and their family (for instance, loss of function, loss of independence, loss of role), but also for the health service, as more resources may be needed along with longer hospitalisation.

Nursing care
Nurses have a crucial role in the early detection of spinal cord compression and in the management of an individual's symptoms.[10] However, nursing involvement does not begin with symptomatic detection. An important aspect of nursing practice is to educate individuals at risk of spinal cord compression. Early detection is important in reducing the prevalence of individuals who present with paresis or paraplegia and the burden of suffering,[16] and through education nurses can raise an individual's awareness of spinal cord compression, thus maximising early detection. It is important that health education about spinal cord compression is shared with all individuals who are potentially at risk from it, and not just to those with prostate, breast, lung, and renal cell carcinoma.[4]

Education should focus on explanation of what spinal cord compression is, who is at risk of developing it, what the signs and symptoms are, and what to do if an individual thinks that they might have cord compression.[3] Education should empower the individual, providing him or her with information that will help give back a sense of control. It should not be frightening and hence has to be undertaken in a sensitive manner, allowing time for the individual to absorb information, and to ask any questions they may have. The individual needs to understand the significance of any signs and symptoms, such as unexplained back pain, and the potential outcomes of delay in seeking medical advice:[10]

> I had no idea that this could happen . . . if only someone had warned me I might not be stuck in this wheelchair now . . .

> . . . about a year ago I asked the nurse if there was anything that I should look out for. She told me to watch out for any pains in my back and to let us know if I got any . . . something to do with compression of . . . something . . . I can't remember the term she used . . . but when my back started hurting last month I remembered what she had said and came to see the doctor – it was a good job that I did . . . they say they have caught it early . . .

The treatment of spinal cord compression

Diagnosis
A diagnosis of cord compression is made through both clinical signs and radiological investigations. Investigations such as spinal X-rays, bone scans, computerised tomographic (CT) scans, myelograms, and magnetic resonance imaging (MRI)

may all be used in the diagnosis of cord compression. Bone scans may produce evidence of bone metastases when the radiological appearance is normal,[8] and patients with localised pain, a normal X-ray, and bone scan still have a 50% risk of metastatic disease and so need further investigations, e.g. MRI.[13] An MRI is more sensitive than a bone scan, and is non-invasive, unlike a myelogram. It is also very sensitive diagnostically as it images the whole of the spine and can indicate the presence of cord compression as well as paraspinal masses. However, the individual has to stay still for about an hour in a small confined space, which may not be possible because of pain.[1]

Management

The aim of treatment for spinal cord compression is to recover or preserve normal neurological function, control local disease, provide spinal stability, control pain,[12,17] and prevent regrowth of the tumour at the site of compression.[8] For most individuals, treatment for spinal cord compression is palliative, i.e. it is given with the intention of relieving and preventing symptoms, without looking to eliminate the disease completely.[18] Despite this, treatment should still be given on an emergency basis, as neurological deficits can quickly progress to paraplegia.

Prognostic factors include the extent of neurological damage, rapidity of onset, and the type of malignancy. The rapidity and severity with which neurological dysfunction occurs are more important than the duration of the dysfunction;[3] hence, the goal is to recognise and treat cord compression early, before permanent neurological damage occurs.[4] The type of primary malignancy affects survival time and treatment response. Those individuals with breast, prostate, lymphoma or a primary central nervous system malignancy respond more favourably to treatment than those with other malignancies.[17]

There are three main management options for spinal cord compression: steroids, radiotherapy, and surgery[16] (see below). Chemotherapy is only used occasionally as adjuvant therapy for chemosensitive malignancies such as lymphoma, or in individuals who have relapsed at previously irradiated sites, or are unfit for either surgery or radiotherapy.[17,19] Chemotherapy is also used for chemoresponsive paediatric tumours.[5]

Treatment should not be confined to technological modalities. Spinal cord compression can be devastating to the individual, who is already physically and emotionally compromised by the diagnosis of cancer and its ensuing treatment. Treatment side-effects and disease-related symptoms may be a reminder of the progression of the cancer and feelings of mortality. For some, spinal cord compression may be the presenting symptom, leading to the initial diagnosis of cancer. Spinal cord compression may therefore be synonymous with the knowledge of a shortened life expectancy, having a major psychological impact. Nurses can help the individual to cope with the changes forced on them, by supporting patients in expressing the impact of the devastating effects of spinal cord compression. Patients may feel a loss of control, of mobility, of independence, of being in control of their body or of life itself. Helping to meet the psychological needs of an individual with spinal cord compression is as important to effective care as is helping them to cope with any physical changes.[10]

Box 31.2: Treatment for spinal cord compression[3-8,10,17,20,21]

Owing to a lack of randomised controlled trials into the treatment of spinal cord compression, decisions about appropriate treatment are problematic. Factors that need to be taken into account are the individual's life expectancy, fitness for surgery, any coexistent vertebral collapse, and stability of the spine, along with the radiosensitivity of the underlying neoplasm.

Steroids
- Use is controversial.
- Studies suggest that steroids should be given immediately a diagnosis of spinal cord compression is suspected, before the diagnosis is definite and treatment decisions have been made due to efficacy in decreasing oedema and relieving symptoms.
- Duration of treatment is based on individual response to treatment.
- In the final stage of illness, steroids may be the only treatment given for cord compression.

Radiotherapy
- Radiotherapy alone is a primary treatment for cord compression caused by a radiosensitive tumour.
- It is well tolerated, with minimal side-effects.
- Treatment should be started as soon as possible once the diagnosis has been confirmed.
- The recommended dose is 3000–4000 cGy given over 2–4 weeks.

- Hyperfractionation is often used as larger doses produce more rapid cell kill and are more effective in reoxygenating cells, which is important in solid tumours where the tumour core is hypoxic.
- The treatment field encompasses two vertebral bodies above and below the site of cord compression, though the field may be modified if multiple sites are involved.
- With radiotherapy:
  - up to 70% of those walking at the start of treatment may retain the ability to walk
  - up to 35% of those paraparetic may regain the ability to walk
  - up to 5% of those completely paraplegic may regain the ability to walk.

Surgery
- In the past, surgical treatment consisted of a laminectomy. This allowed decompression and debulking but could cause spinal instability.
- Recent advances are based on the location of the tumour, and tumours anterior to the spine are treated by a vertebral body resection and those posterior by a laminectomy.
- It is only indicated in specific groups due to morbidity associated with surgery for individuals with advanced cancer.
- Surgery should be used:
  - for high-level cervical lesions with risk of respiratory distress
  - where there is pathological fracture or spinal instability
  - with radioresistant tumours
  - for spinal areas that have previously been irradiated
  - where there is progression of disease while receiving radiotherapy
  - when a tissue diagnosis is needed as the primary tumour site is unknown.
- If a patient is relatively fit and has disease anterior to the spine, then he or she has an 80% chance of becoming ambulant after an anterior approach to surgery.
- Radiotherapy may be given after surgery to improve local control.

Strategies for helping patients and their families to cope may include:
- encouraging them to talk about how they feel and listening to them describing the impact of spinal cord compression on their lives
- encouraging them to talk openly together, sharing their fears and sadness
- teaching them and their families how to adapt to new physical limitations by finding innovative ways of helping them achieve realistic goals
- giving them names and contact numbers of health care professionals and support groups, reassuring them that they are not alone and that they do not have to cope independently.

The rehabilitative potential of an individual will depend on their pre-treatment status, i.e. those with a poor neurological status before treatment have less rehabilitative potential than those with a good neurological status. Rehabilitative goals should be set with the individual and their family, and must be both attainable in order to provide motivation, and realistic. Comprehensive nursing care is one of the keys to the management of an individual with spinal cord compression, providing assessment, early detection, symptom management, and rehabilitation.[10]

Superior vena cava obstruction

Superior vena cava obstruction (SVCO) is an uncommon but distressing and potentially life-threatening complication of selected cancers. It occurs in 3–8% of patients with cancer[22] and although it is rarely a true emergency, if left untreated life-threatening complications can occur; for example, airway obstruction.[23,24] Early detection and intervention is therefore important, not only to prevent life-threatening complications, but also to help maintain an individual's quality of life.

The superior vena cava is the major vessel for blood returning from the upper torso, arms, and head to the right atrium of the heart. Obstruction of this vessel can be caused by external compression from a tumour or lymph nodes, by direct invasion of the vessel wall by a tumour, or by thrombosis or fibrosis of the vessel.[5,6,23,25,26] The physiology of superior vena cava obstruction in adults is described below. Superior vena cava obstruction is very rare in children and has a different aetiology.[27]

Over 90% of all cases of SVCO are due to cancer.[31] The most common primary malignant causes of superior vena cava obstruction are lung cancer and lymphoma. Breast cancer is the most common metastatic cause (Figure 31.2). One benign cause of SVCO found in oncology patients is thrombosis formation around a central venous catheter.

SVCO occurs most commonly in patients with a known diagnosis of an intrathoracic lesion. However, some patients may present with superior vena cava obstruction prior to any histological confirmation of the underlying cause.[5] SVCO is largely resolved with appropriate treatment, but

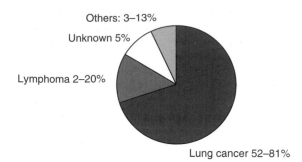

Others: 3–13%

Unknown 5%

Lymphoma 2–20%

Lung cancer 52–81%

Figure 31.2 Causes and incidence of superior vena cava obstruction by primary tumour type.[5,26,29,30]

Box 31.3: The physiology of superior vena cava obstruction[25,27,28]

The superior vena cava is found in the middle of the mediastinum and is surrounded by relatively rigid structures, e.g. the sternum and trachea, and by the lymph nodes that drain the right thoracic cavity and the lower part of the left thorax. It is a thin-walled and compliant vessel, which is easily compressible and therefore vulnerable to obstruction from abnormal growths or by enlarged lymph nodes. Obstruction causes a decrease in venous return to the right atrium, resulting in an increase in venous pressure, venous hypertension, and venous stasis in the head, arms, and upper chest.

When the superior vena cava is fully or partially obstructed above the level of the azygos vein, a collateral circulatory system may develop. This delays the onset of the symptoms of superior vena cava obstruction, as blood is diverted around the obstruction via the collateral system. This compensatory mechanism is confined to the upper body and if the obstruction occurs below the level of the azygos vein, no collateral system will develop, resulting in sudden, severe symptoms.

despite initial improvement it will recur in over 10% of patients.[23] Individuals who have had SVCO previously therefore need to be told about the risk of recurrence, and what they should do if they suspect it.

Signs and symptoms of superior vena cava obstruction

The signs and symptoms of SVCO may develop quickly or gradually. Rapidly developing superior vena cava obstruction may be fatal, whereas gradual onset allows for the development of collateral circulation to shunt enough blood around the

obstruction in order to minimise complications.[6] The severity of symptoms is related to the site, rate, and degree of obstruction.[23,25,32,33]

- Onset is usually insidious and most individuals will experience symptoms 2–4 weeks before diagnosis.[25]
- Early symptoms include vague breathing changes, including a feeling of heaviness or shortness of breath on exertion, headaches, weight gain in a 1–2-week period, upper extremity swelling, and the appearance of veins on the chest or breast.[26]
- In the early stages symptoms may be subtle, yet it is important to recognise symptoms in the early stages. Failure to do this may lead to a life-threatening situation.[32]
- Breathlessness is the most common symptom experienced by a person with SVCO, followed by a feeling of fullness in the head and facial swelling.[23,24,27] Other signs and symptoms include cough, stridor, hoarseness, headache, oedema of the face, neck and arms, cyanosis, distension of the neck veins, and the appearance of dilated collateral superficial veins.[5,27,28] If the obstruction is not treated, neurological signs related to raised intracranial pressure may also be seen, e.g. dizziness, visual disturbances, and occasionally an alteration in mental status.[28] Symptoms may be worse when a patient is prone and may disappear after they have been upright for several hours.[28]
- Patients known to be at risk should be taught about signs and symptoms of SVCO so that they can be aware of them and report them promptly.
- Nurses too need to be aware of the risk factors and signs and symptoms so that early symptoms may be recognised. Identification of, and attention to the population at risk can help to prevent a medical crisis, minimise additional psychological stress for the patient and their family, and possibly prevent hospitalisation.[32]
- As symptoms become more acute they will be frightening to both the patient and their family. Emotional support is vital and anxiety may be reduced by a calm environment, staying with the patient, offering relaxation or visualisation, which may help to distract and comfort the patient, administration of appropriate analgesics

and anxiolytics, and by providing reassurance that the symptoms will improve.[25] The outward manifestations of SVCO can be very distressing to both the patient and their family. Seeing one's loved one struggling to breathe, swollen and cyanotic can be both devastating and frightening, and nurses need to help family and friends to cope with this and to reassure them that things will improve:

> . . . it was horrible seeing him like that . . . his face was all swollen and blue . . . you could hardly recognise him . . . it was such a relief when they told us that the swelling would go . . . I hope it does as I do not want to remember him looking like that!

Clinical identification of SVCO is straightforward as the signs and symptoms are typical and unmistakable[27] and the risk factors known. Diagnosis may, however, be confirmed by chest X-rays, CT scans, MRI, contrast venography and mediastinography – especially where no previous diagnosis of malignancy was known and a histological diagnosis is needed.[25]

The treatment of superior vena cava obstruction
In the past, radiotherapy has been the treatment of choice for SVCO due to its local effects and minimal side-effects, and patients were treated immediately, regardless of the underlying malignancy and irrespective of whether a pathological diagnosis had been made or not. However, more recently, treatment has been based on aetiology and histological diagnosis. If SVCO is the presenting symptom, a diagnosis is reached and treatment is focused on the underlying disease. The goal of treatment is the relief of symptoms and control of the underlying disease.[24,27,32] Some of the underlying malignancies associated with SVCO, such as small-cell lung cancer, non-Hodgkin's lymphoma, and germ cell tumours are potentially curable,[28] hence the need to base treatment on the underlying disease (see below).

Box 31.4: Treatment for superior vena cava obstruction[5,23-28,33]

Radiotherapy
- is the treatment of choice for radiotherapy responsive tumours
- treatment is directed to the thoracic area and mediastinum

- treatment usually starts with 3 days of high-dose radiotherapy (300–400 cGy per fraction), followed by 180–200 cGy daily; the total dose depends on tumour histology and clinical signs
- usually results in symptomatic relief within 3–4 days and an objective response within 1–2 weeks
- provides effective palliation in patients with non-small-cell lung cancer and other less chemosensitive tumours, though prognosis is poor
- is used as initial treatment if histological diagnosis cannot be established and the clinical picture is poor.

Chemotherapy
- is an effective primary treatment for superior vena cava obstruction secondary to lymphoma or small-cell lung cancer. Alone or in combination with radiotherapy, cure rates and long-term survival are superior to radiotherapy alone
- has an adjuvant role with radiotherapy in superior vena cava obstruction caused by tumours such as breast cancer.

Surgery
- is rarely performed in cases of malignant superior vena cava obstruction
- is only considered when other therapies have failed and the patient is expected to survive for a significant period of time.

Stent placement
- may be considered to maintain patency of the superior vena cava until obstruction is alleviated. Expandable wire stents are placed into the obstructed or stenosed part of the superior vena cava under local anaesthetic.

Fibrinolytic therapy
- If obstruction is caused by thrombosis from an intravenous catheter, it can be treated with fibrinolytic therapy, e.g. streptokinase or urokinase and possibly catheter removal.

If SVCO is a sign of progressive disease then other more palliative options may be considered, e.g. use of high-dose steroids in order to relieve inflammation, soft tissue oedema, and respiratory distress.[23,25] Urgent initiation of pharmacological, practical, and psychological management of the consequences of SVCO is needed and nurses have an important role to play in this.[25] In severe cases, when life-threatening complications are seen, radiotherapy may still be given immediately, regardless of diagnosis.[26]

Nursing care
The goals of nursing care include:

- the relief of symptoms and the avoidance of any further complications,[24] e.g. practical steps such as position changes, which may help to alleviate symptoms, avoiding bending forward, which will aggravate the situation, and encouraging patients to remain in bed, sit with their head up, and elevate their arms on pillows, which will help to decrease any swelling and aid breathing. The use of oxygen may help patients who are short of breath.[23,27,33] Frequent assessment of an individual's cardiac, respiratory and neurological systems is needed to ensure recognition of further deterioration due to vascular obstruction

- assisting with medical intervention, e.g. chemotherapy
- providing psychological care and support for patients and their families during what is a highly stressful and frightening experience:[28]

> I was so scared, I couldn't breathe properly and I thought I was going to die . . . it made such a difference when the nurse helped me to get into a better position . . . as well as helping my breathing it also helped me feel safe as I felt that they understood and knew how to help me.

Information about treatment and the resolution of symptoms needs to be given to both the patient and their family. Symptoms such as breathlessness and facial swelling may be easier to cope with if patients are aware that symptomatic relief may be achieved within 24–72 hours of the start of treatment and once resolved, rehabilitation can be rapid.[6] The side-effects of treatment should be explained to help further minimise anxiety. Those patients receiving radiotherapy may experience side-effects such as pharyngitis, oesophagitis, and cough. Side-effects following chemotherapy may be drug dependent. Dietary changes, e.g. having a soft diet, may also need to be made to help to decrease irritation and to aid swallowing.[33]

Individuals with SVCO receiving chemotherapy pose a challenge to nursing staff as variations may be needed in normal methods of administration. Invasive and constrictive procedures should be avoided where possible in the upper extremities, owing to impaired venous return and the potential for bleeding due to the collateral circulation. Administration of vesicants should also be avoided in the upper extremities as SVCO can cause a pooling of the vesicant and inadequate drug distribution, along with possible phlebitis and thrombosis. Maintaining optimum fluid balance is also important during and after chemotherapy, as care needs to be taken to avoid overhydration, which may lead to exacerbation of symptoms.[6]

Hypercalcaemia

Hypercalcaemia is associated with a variety of pathological states, both malignant and non-malignant. Non-malignant causes such as primary hyperparathyroidism, thyrotoxicosis, renal failure, or prolonged immobilisation may also be present in individuals with cancer and nurses need to be aware of these. However, individuals who present with symptomatic hypercalcaemia and weight loss are more likely to have a malignant disorder than not.[34]

Hypercalcaemia is the most common life-threatening metabolic disorder seen in cancer patients,[5,26,35] with between 10 and 20% of all cancer patients developing it during the course of their disease.[35–37] The incidence of hypercalcaemia varies according to the underlying cancer diagnosis, but over half of all individuals who develop hypercalcaemia have squamous cell lung cancer, breast cancer, or multiple myeloma (see Figure 31.3).

Hypercalcaemia is usually progressive and causes unpleasant symptoms such as constipation and dehydration as a result of the role of calcium in maintaining the permeability of cell membranes. Hypercalcaemia can produce symptoms in almost all of the body's organ systems. Effective treatment is available and can result in significant improvement in symptoms for the majority of patients. However, if it is left untreated, it may result in severe dehydration, renal failure, coma, and death. Hypercalcaemia is a poor prognostic indicator. It is often a sign of advanced disease and invariably patients with hypercalcaemia will have bone metastases.[5] Ralston et al.[38] analysed survival data for individuals receiving treatment for hypercalcaemia, and found that 50% died within 1 month of starting treatment and 75% died within 3 months. The cause of death is usually tumour progression, as few patients actually die of the metabolic consequences of hypercalcaemia.[35] The physiology of hypercalcaemia is described below.

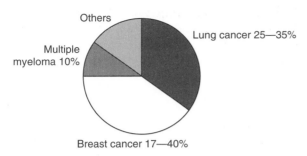

Others: ovarian; cholangiocarcinomas; head and neck;
renal cell carcinoma; lymphoma, gynaecological
malignancies.

Figure 31.3   Causes and incidence of hypercalcaemia
by primary tumour type.[26,35-37]

Box 31.5: The physiology of hypercalcaemia[26,35]

Patients with cancer experience two types of hypercalcaemia:
local, osteolytic hypercalcaemia, and humoral hypercalcaemia
of malignancy. In both instances, there is increased resorption
of bone due to circulatory or local factors.

Local osteolytic hypercalcaemia
This occurs in 20–30% of patients with malignant hypercalcaemia. There is increased absorption of bone as a result of
locally produced factors. These factors, which result in
increased osteoclastic activity releasing calcium from the bone
into the extracellular fluid, have not yet been fully defined.
Patients will have an increase in serum calcium but their serum
phosphate will be normal. They are also likely to have extensive metastatic disease.

Humoral hypercalcaemia of malignancy
This occurs in up to 80% of patients and is usually caused by
the production of a protein called 'parathyroid hormone-relat-
ed peptide'. This causes increased resorption of bone with
reduced bone formation and a corresponding increase in serum
calcium levels and decrease in serum phosphate levels. It does
this by mimicking the effect of parathyroid hormone, which
is a major regulatory hormone that senses changes in serum
calcium levels, increasing its activity when serum levels
decrease.

Signs and symptoms of hypercalcaemia
Ninety-nine percent of the body's calcium is found
in bone and the other 1% circulates in extracellular
fluid.[26,34,39] The normal range of serum calcium is
between 2.13 and 2.63 mmol/l and hypercalcaemia

is diagnosed when the serum level is above 2.75
mmol/l.[36] When measuring an individual's serum
calcium level, a 'corrected' value needs to be calculated, as a low serum albumin precipitates a
deceptively low total serum calcium level. In malnourished cancer patients, a low serum albumin is
common and so an adjusted calcium level is frequently needed:

$$\text{Corrected calcium} = \text{measured calcium} + (40 - \text{albumin}) \times 0.02 \text{ mmol/l.}$$

The clinical presentation of cancer-induced
hypercalcaemia is variable.[34] Symptoms may
occur abruptly or develop over several days to
weeks, determined not only by the level of hypercalcaemia, but by an individual's physical and mental condition and the kidney's ability to maintain
homeostasis.[36]

Mild hypercalcaemia (corrected serum calcium
< 3.00 mmol/l) is usually asymptomatic, although
some individuals may experience nausea and vomiting, anorexia, constipation, thirst, and polyuria. As
the hypercalcaemia becomes more severe, further
symptoms such as dehydration, lethargy, confusion,
disorientation, hallucinations, cardiac arrhythmias, and coma may occur.[5,26] In some instances,
hypercalcaemia has also been shown to lower the
pain threshold in individuals with cancer.[38]
The symptoms of hypercalcaemia can themselves
further compound the existing hypercalcaemia, as
anorexia, nausea and vomiting, and polyuria cause
volume depletion and enhanced resorption of
sodium and calcium by the kidney, causing further
volume depletion and increased serum calcium
levels.[39]

The symptoms of hypercalcaemia can be vague
and non-specific and can easily be confused with
symptoms of other complications, such as brain
metastases, systemic manifestations, or the underlying disease process or side-effects of treatment.[26,36,39]
Nurses therefore need to be alert to the signs and
symptoms of hypercalcaemia so that a prompt diagnosis can be made, allowing prompt treatment, and
promoting an individual's maximum state of wellness and quality of life. Early recognition and
appropriate intervention can successfully reverse
metabolic changes, alleviate symptoms and prevent
irreversible end-organ damage.[37] Psychological

changes and anorexia may be particularly distressing to the patient's family and the patient may be aware of and frightened by mental changes. Nurses are in a key position to educate patient and family about the symptoms of hypercalcaemia and to provide reassurance about the effectiveness of treatment.[39] Education about the purpose and goals of treatment for hypercalcaemia can promote coping by reducing fear and uncertainty, and can help patients and their families to adapt to limitations being imposed by the disease and its symptoms.

> It was heartbreaking seeing him so confused . . . he had always had such a good memory and took a pride in his appearance . . . It was such a relief that they could treat the high calcium levels in his blood, it meant that his confusion went and he was himself again.

Mahon[39] looked at the reasons for hospitalisation in eight individuals over 10 admissions with hypercalcaemia and found that none was admitted with a confirmed diagnosis of hypercalcaemia, but rather because of the symptoms they were experiencing. The most frequently reported symptoms were constipation (30–50%), weakness (60–100%), and anorexia (100%), all of which could have been caused by other disease-related complications, e.g. side-effects of medication, or chemotherapy, or by disease progression. The patients' significant others reported that they had not been informed by either nurses or doctors of the common symptoms of hypercalcaemia and so were not looking for them.

In a study of in-patient and out-patient cancer patients suffering from hypercalcaemia, Coward[40] reported that 88% of individuals were not aware that hypercalcaemia might occur, and 80–95% were not aware of its various symptoms. Nurses have an important role to play in identifying patients at risk from hypercalcaemia and teaching them about early recognition and monitoring of symptoms.[36] Patients and their families should be advised about preventive measures such as adequate fluid and salt intake, how to control nausea and vomiting, and the avoidance, where possible, of immobilisation. Immobilisation tends to increase bone resorption of calcium and aggravates hypercalcaemia, and weight-bearing mobilisation is the most effective way of preventing increased bone resorption due to immobility. However, for those who are unable to mobilise freely, passive exercises can help.[41] The involvement of an occupational therapist or physiotherapist in the care of patients who have restricted mobility is therefore central to effective management.

The treatment of hypercalcaemia

The most effective treatment for hypercalcaemia is therapy directed at the primary malignant disease.[34,35,37] However, hypercalcaemia is most common in patients with advanced disease when control of the disease is no longer possible. When the primary tumour cannot be controlled, treatment for hypercalcaemia is palliative, with median survival being only 1–3 months.[42] The principles behind the treatment of hypercalcaemia are to rehydrate the patient, to enhance calcium excretion by the kidneys, and to decrease bone resorption, thus reducing entry of calcium into extracellular fluid.[34,37]

Treatment involves hydration in order to dilute calcium levels, followed by specific anti-hypercalcaemic therapy. The choice of anti-hypercalcaemic therapy depends on the acuity of the problem, individual variables, e.g. tumour type, renal function, and doctor's preference.[26] In the past, extensive hydration was carried out prior to specific therapy and was the mainstay of treatment.[34] However, most patients now benefit from the early introduction of specific anti-hypercalcaemic therapy, which provides rapid clinical improvement (vital in end-stage disease), with lower overall toxicity and decreased cost.[34] Once rehydration has been established, the use of bisphosphonates, e.g. pamidronate, is the treatment of choice,[34–36,43] although other therapies may be used (see Box 31.6).

There has been debate about when to treat an individual with hypercalcaemia.[35] Some doctors will treat all patients regardless of their clinical features; others will treat only those who are experiencing symptoms. The urgency of treatment depends on the level of serum calcium. Where corrected levels are above 3.5 mmol/l, treatment is considered urgent and when below 3.0 mmol/l, it may be considered less urgent.[35] Patients with asymptomatic mild hypercalcaemia may require only close observation, particularly where therapy for the underlying malignancy has begun, i.e. patients with a previously untreated and responsive tumour such as lymphoma, breast or myeloma. If tumour response is likely to be slow, anti-hypercalcaemic therapy may also be needed initially.[37] The urgency of treatment depends therefore on the serum calcium levels, the symptoms experienced,[36] and the goals of care, as negotiated with the patient.

As hypercalcaemia tends to occur in individuals with recurrent or progressive disease, it may be appropriate in some cases to withhold treatment; for example, in an individual who is in a coma and for whom no further treatment has been planned. However, while treatment may not be beneficial in terms of prolonging life, it can have significant palliative value, controlling symptoms and increasing an individual's quality of life.[35,37] The presence of hypercalcaemia may signify a short life span and nurses have an important role in helping both the patient and his or her relatives, to cope with issues related to death and dying.

With the change in emphasis from long rehydration regimes to shorter ones,[35] patients are spending a shorter time in hospital. This, along with the benefit of bisphosphonates, is promising for individuals who have a poor prognosis and short survival times, as they receive rapid, effective treatment to improve symptoms, allowing early discharge and potentially increased quality of life. Patients requiring care for hypercalcaemia can therefore be divided into those who require urgent in-patient treatment and those who can be managed on an out-patient or day care basis, although patients may require both at different times. The main goals of out-patient treatment for hypercalcaemia are to decrease the need for hospitalisation by preventing worsening of hypercalcaemia or recurrence, thus enabling individuals to remain at home and to feel more in control of their life. This can only happen, however, if clear instructions are given by nurses to patients and their families, informing them of what symptoms to look out for, about how to ensure adequate oral fluid intake, and how to ensure that nausea or vomiting does not lead to further dehydration. Safety issues also need to be explored, particularly with family members, as confusion and disorientation may leave an individual vulnerable and open to injury, both physical (e.g. falling over, not putting out cigarettes) and medical (e.g. taking the wrong medications).[39] Both the individual and their family need to feel secure in their understanding and knowledge of how to cope with

hypercalcaemia, and nurses should ensure that adequate social support is available or is made available to the patient and his or her lay carers.

Box 31.6: Treatment for hypercalcaemia[5,34,35,43,44]

Hydration and diuresis

- Restoration of extracellular fluid is an essential first step in treatment as most patients are significantly dehydrated at presentation. Increased plasma volume improves glomerular filtration and calcium clearance.
- The route of administration depends on clinical status.
- Clinical improvement of mental status and a decrease in nausea and vomiting are usually seen following adequate hydration, often within 24 hours.
- Following the correction of fluid deficits, frusemide may be given to inhibit reabsorption of sodium and calcium by the ascending loop of Henle.

Bisphosphonates

- Pamidronate, clodronate, and etidronate are the most commonly used drugs. They inhibit the release of calcium from the bone by interfering with the metabolic activity of osteoclasts.
- A variety of treatment schedules is used and treatment normalises serum calcium in 70–80% of patients within a week.
- Pamidronate has been shown to be superior to clodronate and etidronate and is given intravenously after 1–2 litres of normal saline.
- If hypercalcaemia reoccurs, these agents can be used again and are safe and efficient for long-term therapy.
- They have poor bioavailability, though clodronate may be given orally as maintenance therapy.

Calcitonin

- It acts on bone to inhibit osteoclastic resorption and on the kidney to promote urinary excretion of calcium.
- It has a rapid onset of action and can be used safely in individuals with renal impairment.
- 80% of patients will show an improvement but it only lasts for between 24 and 72 hours and calcium levels will increase despite further calcitonin.

Mithramycin

- It inhibits osteoclast activity.
- Its duration of response is variable and unpredictable and it is potentially nephrotoxic.

Steroids

- They are most useful in patients whose underlying tumour is responsive to their cytostatic action, e.g. haematological malignancies.
- They decrease the release of cytokines, which can stimulate osteoclast activity.

References

1. Labovich T.M. (1994). Selected complications in the patient with cancer: spinal cord compression, malignant bowel obstruction, malignant ascites, and gastrointestinal bleeding. *Seminars in Oncology Nursing* **10**, 189–197.
2. Byrne T.N. (1992). Spinal cord compression from epidural metastases. *New England Journal of Medicine* **327**, 614–619.
3. Morse L.K. (1992). Spinal cord compression. In Dow K.H. and Hilderley L.J. (eds.) *Nursing Care in Radiation Oncology.* Philadelphia, PA: W.B. Saunders, pp. 237–248.
4. Peterson R. (1993). A nursing intervention for early detection of spinal cord compressions in patients with cancer. *Cancer Nursing* **16**, 113–116.
5. Falk S. and Fallon M. (1997). ABC of palliative care: emergencies. *British Medical Journal* **315**, 1525–1528.
6. Dietz K.A. and Flaherty A.M. (1992). Oncologic emergencies. In Groenwald S.L., Frogge M.H., Goodman M. and Yarbro C.H. (eds.) *Cancer Nursing: Principles and Practice.* London: Jones and Bartlett, pp. 644–668.
7. Holmes S. (1996). *Radiotherapy: A Guide for Practice.* Surrey: Asset Books.
8. Heys S.D., Currie D. and Eremin O. (1997). The management of patients with advanced cancer (III). *European Journal of Surgical Oncology* **23**, 361–365.
9. Sorensen P.S., Borgesen S.E., Rohde K., Rasmusson B., Bach F., Boge-Rasmussen T. *et al.* (1990). Metastatic epidural spinal cord compression: results of treatment and survival. *Cancer* **65**, 1502–1508.
10. Held J. and Peahota A. (1993). Nursing care of the patient with spinal cord compression. *Oncology Nursing Forum* **20**, 1507–1516.
11. Gilbert R., Kim J. and Posner J. (1978). Epidural spinal cord compression from metastatic tumour. *Neurology* **3**, 40–51.
12. Rosenthal M.A., Rosen D., Ragahavan J., Leicester J., Duval P., Besser M. and Pearson B. (1992). Spinal cord compression in prostate cancer. A 10-year experience. *British Journal of Urology* **69**, 530–533.
13. Cascino T.L. (1993). Neurologic complications of systemic cancer. *Medical Clinics of North America* **77**, 265–278.
14. Brown J.K. (1985). Ambulatory services: the mainstay of cancer nursing care. *Oncology Nursing Forum* **12**, 57–59.
15. Maranzano E., Latini P., Checcaglini F., Ricci S., Panizza B.M., Aristei C. *et al.* (1991). Radiation therapy in metastatic spinal cord compression: a prospective analysis of 105 consecutive patients. *Cancer* **67**, 1311–1317.
16. Loblaw D.A. and Laperriere N.J. (1998). Emergency treatment of malignant extradural spinal cord compression: an evidence-based guideline. *Journal of Clinical Oncology* **16**, 1613–1624.
17. Fuller B.G., Herss J. and Oldfield E.H. (1997). Oncologic emergencies: spinal cord compression. In DeVita V.T., Hellman S. and Rosenberg S.A. (eds.). *Cancer: Principles and Practice of Oncology,* Philadelphia, PA: Lippincott-Raven, pp. 2476–2486.
18. Kirkbride P. (1995). The role of radiation therapy in palliative care. *Journal of Palliative Care* **11**, 19–26.
19. Friedman H.M., Sheetz S., Levine H.L., Everett J.R. and Hong W.K. (1986). Combination chemotherapy and radiation therapy: the medical management of epidural spinal cord compression from testicular cancer. *Archives of Internal Medicine* **146**, 509–512.
20. Gilbert R., Kim J. and Posner J. (1997). Epidural spinal cord compression from metastatic tumour: diagnosis and treatment. *Annals of Neurology* **3**, 40–51.
21. Kim R., Spencer S., Meredith R., Weppelmann B., Lee J., Smith J. *et al.* (1990). Extradural spinal cord compression: analysis of factors determining functional prognoses – prospective study. *Radiology* **176**, 279–280.
22. Sculier J.P., Evans W.K., Field R., DeBoer G., Payne D.G., Shepherd F.A. *et al.* (1986). Superior venal cava obstruction in small cell lung cancer. *Cancer* **57**, 847–851.
23. Morris J.C. and Holland J.F. (1997). Oncologic emergencies. In Holland *et al.* (eds.) *Cancer Medicine.* Philadelphia, PA: William and Wilkins, pp. 3337–3367.
24. Morse L.K. (1992). Superior vena cava syndrome. In Dow K.H. and Hilderley L.J. (eds.) *Nursing Care in Radiation Oncology.* Philadelphia, PA: W.B. Saunders, pp. 227–236.
25. Stewart I.E. (1996). Superior vena cava syndrome: an oncologic complication. *Seminars in Oncology Nursing* **12**, 312–317.
26. Shuey K.M. (1994). Heart, lung and endocrine complications of solid tumors. *Seminars in Oncology Nursing* **10**, 177–188.
27. Yahalom J. (1997). Oncologic emergencies: superior vena cava syndrome. In DeVita V.T., Hellman S. and Rosenberg S.A. (eds.) *Cancer: Principles and Practice of Oncology.* Philadelphia, PA: Lippincott-Raven, pp. 2469–2476.
28. Ingle, R.J. (1997). Lung Cancers. In Groenwald S.L., Frogge M.H., Goodman M. and Yarbro C.H. (eds.) *Cancer Nursing: Principles and Practice.* London: Jones and Bartlett, pp. 1260–1290.
29. Belfort M.A., Stevens P.J., DeHaek K., Soeters R. and Krige J.E. (1990). A new approach to the management of malignant ascites; a permanently implanted abdominal drain. *European Journal of Surgical Oncology* **16**, 47–53.
30. LeVeen H.H., Christoudias G., Ip M., Luft R., Falk G. and Grosberg S. (1974). Peritoneovenous shunting for ascites. *Annals of Surgery* **180**, 580–591.
31. Woodyard T.C., Mellinger J.D., Vann K.G. and Nisenbaum J. (1993). Acute superior vena cava syndrome after central venous catheter placement. *Cancer* **71**, 2621–2623.

32. Morse L.K., Heery M.L. and Flynn K.T. (1985). Early detection to avert the crisis of superior vena cava syndrome. *Cancer Nursing* **8**, 228–232.

33. Dunne-Daly C.F. (1994). Programmed instruction: radiation therapy for oncological emergencies. *Cancer Nursing* **17**, 516–525.

34. Warrell, R.P. (1997). Metabolic emergencies: hypercalcemia. In DeVita V.T., Hellman S. and Rosenberg S.A. (eds.) *Cancer: Principles and Practice of Oncology.* Philadelphia, PA: Lippincott-Raven, pp. 2486–2494.

35. Heys S.D., Smith I.C. and Eremin O. (1998). Hypercalcaemia in patients with cancer: aetiology and treatment. *European Journal of Surgical Oncology* **24**, 139–142.

36. Lang-Kummer J. (1997). Hypercalcemia. In Groenwald S.L., Frogge M.H., Goodman M. and Yarbro C.H. (eds.) *Cancer Nursing: Principles and Practice.* London: Jones and Bartlett, pp. 684–701.

37. Ritch P.S. (1990). Treatment of cancer-related hypercalcemia. *Seminars in Oncology* **17** (Suppl. 5), 26–33.

38. Ralston S.H., Gallacher S.J., Patel U., Campbell J. and Boyle I.T. (1990). Cancer-associated hypercalcaemia: morbidity and mortality. *Annals of Internal Medicine* **112**, 499–504.

39. Mahon, S. (1989). Signs and symptoms associated with malignancy-induced hypercalcaemia. *Cancer Nursing* **12**, 153–160.

40. Coward D.D. (1988). Hypercalcemia knowledge assessment in patients at risk of developing cancer-induced hypercalcemia. *Oncology Nursing Forum* **15**, 471–476.

41. Coward D.D. (1986). Cancer-induced hypercalcemia. *Cancer Nursing* **9**, 125–132.

42. Ling, P.J., A'Hern R.P. and Hardy J.R. (1995). Analysis of survival following treatment of tumour-induced hypercalcaemia with intravenous pamidronate (APD). *British Journal of Cancer* **72**, 206–209.

43. Gerrard G.E., Dodwell D.J., Vail A., Watters J. and Overend M.A. (1996). An audit of the management of malignant hypercalcaemia. *Clinical Oncology* **8**, 39–42.

44. Ralston S.H., Gallacher S.J., Patel U., Campbell J. and Boyle I.T. (1989). Comparison of three intravenous bisphosphonates in cancer-associated hypercalcaemia. *Lancet,* 1180–1182.

Part 5

Needs and Priorities in Cancer Care

Introduction

This final section brings together the themes of health and its influences, the need to set priorities in caring, and the relationships between local, international, and global health policy. This is not presented as a coherent, seamless text, but rather as a series of chapters examining needs and priorities in a number of areas. Important to the subjects chosen is to identify needy groups where there are particular challenges to providing care. For this reason children and adolescents, older people, people from minority ethnic groups, and people who are dying have been selected as warranting review as priority groups in need of care. The issues for each are very different; they do, however, represent some of the core factors important as determinants of health: age, social and economic status, race, and gender.

The needs of children and adolescents have been singled out since cancer in childhood, although fortunately rare, is a high-ranking cause of death after accidents. Cancer in childhood represents a rather unique case; it is not a story of disadvantage and neglect, rather one of success. The cancers that occur in childhood are different in character from those in adulthood; many, certainly in younger children, have a congenital origin. As a result of important developments in the treatment of cancer in children these have become curable for a significant proportion of children. These successes are among the most celebrated in the cancer science story, and have been made possible by the organisation of children's cancer services. Owing to the relative rarity of childhood cancers, children's cancer services have been developed as a collective endeavour, with centres collaborating in a national and international research effort; it has therefore been possible to evaluate advances in an efficient and co-ordinated manner. The benefits discovered through studies are now finding a place in practice earlier than would be the norm for adults.

The emotive nature of cancer in children attracts generous donations from the public, further supporting research, treatment, and care. Despite this positive message, cancer in children and adolescents is devastating for parents and demanding for health professionals and requires unique skills. Unusually, this area of care requires a different environment, since it is parents who are the front-line carers, not health professionals; care and often treatment must therefore be mediated through a family-centred model. Adolescents need to be delegated such authority in a controlled and supportive manner; health professionals here must negotiate a delicate and shifting balance between the adult–child, near-adult–parent dynamic that inevitably becomes part of illness. In managing the care for children and adolescents, an eye must also be kept on the future, since it is the very real prospect of cure from cancer that brings with it risks of long-term damage, secondary cancers, infertility, possible learning difficulties, and adult life potentially disrupted by a cancer history.

For older people (those over the age of 65 years) a different picture emerges. Here, genuine concerns over sub-optimal treatment exist, due to older people being characterised as too frail for the demands of cancer treatment and therefore excluded from it or given 'gentle' treatment; or more disturbingly, the question sometimes arises of whether they are considered not to warrant the same intensity of effort as is directed at younger people. A research literature around any aspect of cancer or its treatment in older people is virtually absent, calling into question whether cancer exists as a distinct experience at the extremes of age; we simply do not know.

Likewise, studies surrounding race and cancer are absent, and the issues for people from a whole range of cultural and racial groups within society are little understood. More worrying is the possibility that insensitivity to issues of race, by the majority groups represented by most health carers, could lead to a form of racism in cancer care and treatment, at best because of a crude awareness of the complexity of agendas and influences in a racially diverse society. At worst, there may exist an overt neglect of the needs of people from minority groups.

For people whose disease management may be encompassed by palliative care (that is, they have advanced cancer or are dying), the issues are different. A specific system of care with relatively ample resources exists, founded in the hospice movement, and has now developed into a myriad of services with similar ideals. The issues here are to re-examine the ideals and achievements of this field of care; to explore whether in adopting a different approach to care it has resisted the problems explored in Part 1; and whether palliative care too falls prey to the conflicts and anxieties imposed by the sheer difficulty of caring for people facing death.

The section ends with an exploration of health policy and its contribution to shaping cancer care and the relevance and importance of research into cancer care. Both of these closing chapters address issues of defining priorities in cancer care and in working towards a strategic approach to addressing these. In particular, the potential contribution of nursing to cancer through a nursing research agenda is advocated.

CHAPTER THIRTY-TWO

The needs of children and adolescents

Jenny Thompson

The really unexpected happens so seldom that few of us know how to deal with it. We all move, for most of the time, in a small circle of known possibilities to which we have learned responses. Outside this circle lies chaos, a dark land without guidelines.[1]

Cancer is predominantly a disease of ageing and is very rare in childhood. So when parents, children and adolescents are faced with a cancer diagnosis, their first experience is one of shock and threat. Their world is overturned not just by the unexpected but also by something quite outside their previous experience. The whole family is affected as they are confronted by alien and traumatic situations where medical personnel, their machinery and their medicines appear to take centre stage.[2]

The focus of this chapter is to highlight the differences between the diagnosis, treatment, and care of the child with cancer, as opposed to the adult with cancer; in particular, to examine how children's and adolescents' understanding of a cancer diagnosis and treatment is influenced by their level of cognitive development. It is not the intention here to discuss in detail specific medical treatment programmes or supportive medical care aimed to reduce side-effects of treatment. Such are to be found in a number of relevant texts (for a concise review see 'Recommended reading'). Throughout the chapter reference will be made to the child and the family. In most cases this implies child or adolescent. However, there are issues specific to either the child or adolescent; as these arise they will be discussed under separate headings.

Childhood cancer

Although the incidence of cancer in children and adolescents is extremely low, it remains the second most common cause of mortality following accidents in children over the age of 1 year. Today, two-thirds of children with access to optimal medical treatment and resources are cured, but the different types of cancer have highly variable cure rates. For example, children with Hodgkin's disease, retinoblastoma, and Wilm's tumour all have a 5-year survival rate of 86% or higher, but children with central nervous system tumours, neuroblastoma, and hepatic tumours continue to have a poor prognosis.[3]

In Western populations, around 0.5% of all cancers occur in children aged under 15 years. The incidence rate is typically in the range of 110–130 per million children per year. Childhood cancers exhibit a diversity of histological type and anatomical site and are very different to those observed in adults: the carcinomas of the lung, female breast, stomach, and bowel are all extremely rare among children. Consequently, it is more appropriate for childhood tumours to be classified according to their histology, as opposed to adult cancers that are predominantly grouped by their site of origin. Children's cancers are generally described as belonging to those primarily affecting the haematopoietic system – the leukaemias – while others such as neuroblastoma and bone tumours are referred to as solid tumours.[3]

Paediatric tumours can also be divided into three broad groups. *Embryonal cancers* are due to faulty development of embryonal cells, where there is a proliferation of cells that closely resemble foetal tissue, for example neuroblastoma, rhabdomyosarcoma and nephroblastoma (Wilm's tumour). *Juvenile cancers* arise due to malignant transformation in mature tissue, but are generally unique to the younger age group, such as osteosarcoma, Ewing's sarcoma, and Hodgkin's disease. *Adult-type cancers* rarely seen in children, but histologically identical to adult tumours, include renal cell carcinoma and nasopharyngeal carcinomas.

About one-third of all childhood cancers are leukaemias, and of these three-quarters are of the acute lymphoblastic type (ALL). Between one-quarter and one-fifth are brain and spinal tumours, of which astrocytoma is the most common histological type. The distinctive embryonal tumours (Wilm's tumour, neuroblastoma, retinoblastoma, and hepatoblastoma) account for 15% of registrations. Lymphomas account for a further 11%, with non-Hodgkin's lymphoma (NHL) somewhat more common than Hodgkin's disease.[4]

Different diagnostic groups have distinctive age distributions. The incidence of ALL is highest among children aged 2–4 years. Early age peaks in incidence are also found for the embryonal tumours; indeed for neuroblastoma, retinoblastoma, and hepatoblastoma the highest incidence is found in the first year of life. By contrast, Hodgkin's disease, osteosarcoma, and Ewing's sarcoma show a marked incidence with age that continues into early adulthood. The highest incidence of these cancers is seen in the adolescent population. Overall, childhood cancer is about one-third more common among boys than among girls. The male predominance is greatest in the lymphomas and less marked in leukaemia, brain tumours, and sarcomas of the bone and soft tissue.[4]

The patterns of incidence described are typically those of white populations throughout Europe, North America, and Australasia. There is, however, considerable systematic variation in many types of childhood cancer between different regions of the world and between ethnic groups in the same country.[5] In the USA, blacks have a lower incidence of ALL and the early childhood peak is much attenuated. By contrast, there is little evidence of ethnic variations in the incidence of childhood leukaemia in the UK; in particular, the pattern of occurrence of ALL among blacks and children of South Asian ethnic origin is similar to that among whites, with a marked peak in early childhood.[6]

Little is known about the aetiology of most childhood cancers. Although families of an affected child often link the disease to an environmental factor, such as exposure to smoking, insecticides, or ionising radiation, such a linkage can rarely be confirmed. For some diagnostic groups the high incidence at an early age and the cell type of origin strongly suggest that the causative factors occur before birth or even before conception. As a result, many aetiological studies of childhood cancer have been concerned with exposures occurring during the mother's pregnancy. The relationship between antenatal obstetric irradiation and subsequent cancer in the child was first established over 30 years ago by the work of Stewart *et al.*[7] At that time exposure to diagnostic X-rays in pregnancy was thought to have caused as many as 5% of all childhood cancers. Ultrasound has now superseded X-ray examination in pregnancy and subsequent studies have concluded that there is no increased risk associated with antenatal ultrasound.[8,9]

The role of other environmental exposures in the aetiology of childhood cancer remains far from clear. The only well-established environmental causes in Western populations other than X-ray are intra-uterine exposure to diethylstilboestrol during pregnancy, which was linked with vaginal carcinomas.[10] Viruses are also known to play a role in the aetiology of some types of childhood cancer. It is established that the Epstein–Barr virus (EBV) is associated with Burkitt's lymphoma, and nasopharyngeal carcinoma and the hepatocellular carcinoma usually occur in patients who have had prenatal or early childhood exposure to the hepatitis B virus (HBV).[6]

The analysis of childhood cancer offers a unique opportunity to study not only the cancer phenotype but also the genes that are important in normal embryonic development. Of particular importance was the discovery of a retinoblastoma predisposition gene. Approximately 25–30% of all cases of children diagnosed with retinoblastoma have a family history. In the familial form the retinoblastoma phenotype segregates in an autosomal dominant fashion. That is, it appears as though inheritance of the mutant gene is sufficient for tumorogenesis; thus the offspring of individuals carrying the mutant gene have a 50:50 chance of inheriting it. Another predisposition gene has been isolated for Wilm's tumour and others are beginning to emerge.

The availability of these genes means that mutations in individual patients can be characterised in the tumours. As patterns emerge it is considered possible that particular mutations will be associated with a particular course of the disease, thereby allowing predictions about invasiveness, prognosis, and susceptibility to other tumours.[11]

The increasing complexity of treatments and the necessity for many disciplines to be involved has led to the centralisation of care for children with cancer into specialist units. In caring for children with cancer the primary aim is to cure the child with minimal physical and psychosocial cost to both the child and the family. Thus the approach to care requires the expertise of a multi-disciplinary approach.

In addition to the time trends in survival rates that are attributed to the development of more effective treatment, survival rates were noted to be substantially higher in paediatric oncology centres. The development of specialist units also gave clinicians the opportunity to specialise and to participate in clinical trials. As a result, large numbers of children with cancer are now entered into national and international trials.[12]

Childhood cancer treatments represent one of the great success stories of oncology. Thirty years ago, with the advent of chemotherapy, the first cures of leukaemia in children, previously unheard of, were being recorded.[13] Since that time multi-modality therapy, especially chemotherapy combined with surgery and radiotherapy, has enabled the majority of children with cancer to survive. Children are reported as surviving into adulthood with normal or near-normal life expectancy and productive lives.[13] Thus, it is appropriate that those involved with their care make every effort to maximise survival and minimise the potential physical and psychosocial long-term complications. This goal can only be achieved when there is an exhaustive understanding of the unique differences between the diagnosis, treatment protocols, and approach to care of the child with cancer, as opposed to the adult with cancer.

Box 32.1: Cancer in childhood

- Childhood cancer is rare, affecting 1 in 600 children before the age of 15 years.
- Childhood cancers are classified according to their histology.
- Different diagnostic groups have distinctive age distributions.
- Systematic variation in some childhood cancers occurs in differing regions of the world.
- Childhood cancer is about one-third more common in boys.
- Childhood cancers respond more favourably to treatment than adult cancers.
- Centralisation of care, and advances in combination chemotherapy, surgical and radiotherapy techniques have significantly improved survival rates.
- Established environmental exposures in the aetiology of childhood cancers in Western populations are X-rays, exposure to diethylstilboestrol during pregnancy, and infection with hepatitis B and HIV.
- Predisposition genes in a small number of childhood cancers have been identified.
- There are unique differences between the diagnosis, treatment protocols, and approach to care of the child with cancer as opposed to that of the adult with cancer.

Setting care in context

Knowledge is required by those caring for the child and adolescent of two specialties, paediatrics and paediatric oncology. The complex care required of the child and adolescent with cancer has long dictated a team approach to treatment and psychological care has become an increasingly necessary component. During the earlier years of successful treatment little attention was paid to the impact on the child, the family, and the immediate community. Success was uncommon and in most cases parents were warned of the high risk of death, although the emotional impact of waiting for this to happen was rarely addressed in an open manner.

The special needs of sick adolescents have received greater attention in the last 10–15 years and in the main are attributed to the Western world. The health care needs of this group are slowly being addressed and adolescent medicine as a specialty is emerging. The period of adolescence is now understood to provide a critical example of psychosocial development that is highly subject to severe disruption by the symptoms of and treatment for cancer.

From the moment of diagnosis the child and the family have to face a myriad of practical and psychosocial problems associated with cancer treatments, altered lifestyle, and often a change in ambition. While some of these problems are inevitable, they can be minimised. Knowledgeable professional support is essential to help the child and family retain as much normality as possible.[14]

Essential to facilitating the best possible physical care and psychosocial adjustment of the child with cancer and their family is an in-depth knowledge of child and adolescent development. Factors related to a favourable adaptation to the diagnosis of cancer and treatment include the child's or adolescent's understanding of what is happening to them. The ability of the multi-disciplinary team to address the complex questions of how the consequences of diagnosis and treatment interact with any given child's or adolescent's level of intellectual, emotional and social development is important. A young person's understanding of what is happening and why it is happening will exert a major influence on his or her emotional response to treatment. Similarly, when treatment interferes with normal developmental tasks this needs to be anticipated and remedied.

The importance of those caring for the child with cancer having a theoretical and working knowledge of developmental issues cannot be overemphasised. Without such knowledge decisions about the impact of a cancer diagnosis and subsequent treatment and care for the child and family will be less well informed.

Childhood and child development

To care for the child with cancer there is a need for those involved to understand the ways in which children's needs are understood in relation to children's actual abilities, and the ways that these are perceived and interpreted through concepts of childhood. What does childhood mean? Public opinion, reinforced by philosophical and psychological theories, tends to perceive children as dependent, vulnerable, and lacking maturity to know how they will react to certain situations. A further commonly held view is that children are irrational. Even when it is accept-

ed that children can understand, recall, and recount information, their ability to reason, to evaluate, and to assess information is questioned.[15]

Developmental psychologists, perhaps most influentially Piaget, whose research began in the 1920s, have taught that children understand fragments of knowledge slowly and it is unhelpful to teach children before the prescribed age of readiness. Piaget theorised that cognitive development (which put simply is the ability to reason and think) proceeded through age-related stages, which take place between birth and adulthood. Piaget's interest was not in the uniqueness of individual children but rather in the similarities between children of roughly equivalent age. Through interviewing children and studying his own children he found that at different times during development children appeared to be capable of different kinds of understanding. Piaget subsequently worked out the theory that logical thinking in children developed in age-related stages.

Piaget's theories have been refuted and criticised.[16] One of the main failings of the age stage approach is the failure to recognise the impact of experience upon development. It is claimed that Piaget looked at what children were unable to do rather than what they could achieve if helped by prompts and questions that make sense to them and engaged their interest.[17] Nevertheless, Piaget helped to increase public understanding and respect for children, even though his work is reputed to have overlooked each child's experiences and views. It is therefore suggested that Piaget's stages of cognitive development to symbolic thought should be used as benchmarks, rather than formal expectations.

Other influential work related to child development includes that of Freud, Kohlberg, and Erikson, each of whom suggest that wisdom does not develop until at least adolescence.[18] However, more recent research and everyday evidence shows that young children are capable of cognitive complexity. The example in Personal account 32.1, of a 5-year-old boy who was being cared for at home in the terminal phase of his illness, illustrates this well.

Bluebond-Langner's research[19] with seriously ill young children shows that they can have a mature understanding and can cope with and discuss com-

Box 32.2: Summary of Piaget's stages of children's cognitive development

The sensory–motor stage, age 0–2 years
Children begin to develop an understanding of themselves as separate and distinct from the environment, causality, time, and space. Learning is mainly through the senses and physical activity. Objects in general only appear to exist in terms of what babies can do with them; during the first year objects are simply things to act upon ('Can I suck it?', 'Can I hit it?'). Towards the end of the first year objects appear to become an interesting problem. The baby will spend time looking at, feeling, and exploring an object as if there is an attempt to understand what it is, they appear to ask themselves what is this object, and will search for hidden objects, demonstrating that they know of their existence even if they are out of sight.

The pre-operational (or pre-logical) stage, age 2–7 years
Children at this stage learn much about the physical and social world. Some of this learning is spontaneous, while more is deliberately taught by parents and teachers. This is a time when children are capable of using language and symbolic thinking. This is apparent in their imaginative play. It is a time of egocentric thinking in which children are unable to take the views of others. Pre-operational children start from where they are, and to a greater or lesser extent distort reality in an attempt to make sense of it using ways of understanding they have already developed ('I'm sick and in hospital because I was naughty'). This is also a period when children can only attend to one aspect of a situation at a time.

The concrete operational stage, age 7–12 years
Thinking now becomes logical and children can attend to several aspects of an event at a time. They are now able to look at a situation from the point of view of someone else, and so overcome the earlier egocentrism. Whereas a pre-operational child thinks in absolutes – things are either black or white, good or bad, hurt or will not hurt – children in the concrete operational stage can see things relatively, things can be good or bad, hurt a little, or hurt a lot. Understanding at this stage generally remains in relation to absolute objects, not to events or relationships they have not yet experienced.

The formal operational stage, age 12 years and over
Thinking is now beyond the concrete stage and children can think abstractly and imagine or hypothesise about alternatives. Reasoning about objects, situations or people can be done symbolically without the need for the objects or events to be present or experienced. This is a time when thinking becomes more flexible and concrete, and children are able to combine information from a number of different sources.

plex and painful knowledge. This writer concludes that experience is more salient than age in determining children's understanding. There is a widely accepted view that it is wise not to assume a child is fine just because there is no obvious sign of anxiety or distress. Encouragement to talk and giving a reassuring cuddle may be needed but not requested.

Personal account 32.1

A 5-year-old boy diagnosed with leukaemia had relapsed several times following unsuccessful treatment for his disease and was being cared for at home in the terminal phase of his illness.

He was the only child of elderly parents who believed that he was unaware of his impending death. It was a subject that neither the parents or those professionals involved with his care discussed with him. The child appeared to be 'comfortable' both physically and emotionally and did not ask questions about his situation.

Visiting the home on the day before his death, I noticed that his toys were positioned on the bed in two groups. When I inquired as to how he was feeling he replied, 'Fine thank you'. After a pause he pointed to one group of the toys on his bed and said, 'Those toys you can take back to the hospital, the other toys are going with me when I die.' Giving him a cuddle I thanked him and asked if there was anything else he wanted to talk about.

'Yes', he said, and after a long pause he continued to tell me who was best at giving his medicines through his 'wiggly' (central venous catheter) at the hospital and at home, and which medicines helped most with his 'hurts'. He clearly understood aseptic techniques and was critical of those he felt did not use the correct procedure. He also had a reasonable understanding of the drugs being used to control his pain.

Perhaps developmental theories that refer to age have remained influential because the concept of the ignorant child gradually moving through life towards adult understanding is more comfortable for adults to accept. The child's physical growth is so visible and in most cases obvious that it is easy to use this as a baseline on which to measure children's emotional and mental abilities. In reality, children mature at uneven rates and like adults they can be confident in one respect and not in another. Ability develops unevenly and depends on the experience of the child to a greater extent than the child's age. Another important issue is the widely varying views about childhood between cultures. The level of responsibility accepted by children in developing countries, such as the care of parents and other family members, is generally speaking at odds with the view of children's responsibilities in the Western world.

However, whatever boundaries of childhood are drawn, there remains a broad consensus that children are comparatively more vulnerable than adults, requiring special measures to protect and promote their needs. Certainly young children are vulnerable and their survival depends on the quality of care and commitment provided for them by the adults who have responsibility for them. Nevertheless, as Lansdown[20] argues, the vulnerability that we perceive in children is not an objective definition of their capacity. It is only partially drawn from the biological facts of childhood, and owes much to the social attitudes and perceptions that we impose. Children's vulnerabilities, according to Lansdown[20] and Franklin,[21] derive from historical attitudes and presumptions about the nature of childhood and are a social and political construct, not an inherent or inevitable consequence of childhood.

There may be many theoretical arguments offered as to when, where, how and at what age children should be encouraged to contribute to decisions affecting their lives. Respect for the visibility of childhood and for the value of what children say is not to deny the experience of childhood and the right to be a child. If children are to be encouraged to believe that their views are worth hearing and they can become active participants in society, we should respect their involvement and views from the earliest possible age and assist them to develop the necessary skills to achieve these goals, whether they are sick or well.

Box 32.3: Childhood and child development

- Early developmental psychologists have taught that children understand knowledge at a prescribed chronological age.
- Traditional theories of childhood and children's considered inabilities are now challenged by current research findings and everyday evidence of competent children.
- Children are known to mature at different rates, and ability depends on the experience of the child more than on the child's age.

- Piaget's descriptions of age-related thinking stages in children should be used as benchmarks rather than formal expectations.
- Differences exist between cultures as to the concept of childhood and children's abilities.
- Research with seriously ill young children demonstrates that their understanding is not about abstract concepts but rather intensely experienced illness and treatment.

Adolescence and adolescent development

Ask a number of adults 'What is adolescence and who are adolescents?' and you will get a number of answers. However, it is likely that most will refer to the teenage years and the irritation of teenage behaviour, remarking that they have periods of acting childishly after seemingly achieving acceptable standards of maturity. The terms 'teenagers', 'adolescents', 'youth', and 'young people' are also likely to be used interchangeably.

Adolescence is defined as the process of growing up; that is, the transition of an individual from childhood to adulthood.[22,23] A broadly accepted definition of adolescence is that it represents the period between childhood and maturity, encompassing not only the physical changes of puberty and emerging sexuality but also the emotional, psychological, and social differences between adults and children. Perhaps the most influential approach to adolescence is Erikson's theoretical work on psychosocial development.[24] The period of adolescence has become associated with the process of acquiring identity and is described as a 'task' of adolescence, something that everyone does during this period of their life.

While the onset of adolescence is usually associated with the onset of puberty, the end of adolescence is less clearly defined. It also varies from culture to culture as far as the attainment of independence is concerned. Adolescence is also viewed as a relatively recent concept, one mainly confined to Western societies. In many different cultures there are rites of passage in which the child is initiated into the social roles of adulthood. For males in such cultures psychological and social maturity may only rarely converge. For females, ceremonial transitions such as marriage may be closely linked to physical events such as the first menstruation. Kuykendall[25] refers to this as the social status acquisition approach whereby at various chronological ages individuals gain additional social privileges and status that can be used to define the stage of life they have reached.

This approach is also reflected in modern ideas about the period of adolescence in Western societies that has been influenced by the introduction and extension of compulsory education, by legislation prohibiting the employment of young people under a certain age and the development of services differentiating the adolescent from adults or children.

In 1980, the World Health Organisation considered 10–19 years as the period of adolescence, noting that this age range, which generally encompassed the time from onset of puberty to the legal age of majority, coincided with some population statistics. For the purposes of the International Youth Year, the United Nations defined youth as encompassing the age range 15–24 years. In 1986, the World Health Organisation study group, addressing the issue of young people's health and 'Health for all by the year 2000',[26] adopted a pragmatic approach to the issue of an appropriate age range by merging the two age ranges in the all-encompassing range of 10–24 years. Within this age range, three 5-year subdivisions of 10–14, 15–19, and 20–24 years were considered to be useful, noting that such a grouping facilitates cross-national comparisons of data and experience. For those of us working with adolescents, reference is usually made to periods of early adolescence (12–15 years, when increased awareness of body image, importance of peer relationships, and rebellious behaviour are commonplace); middle adolescence (15–18 years, when physical maturity is almost complete, and there is a realistic self/body image and strong peer relationships are developed); and late adolescence (18–22 years, when concerns for the future and planning for the future become important). However, as with the limitations of using age as a sole indicator of child development, the above age grouping does not acknowledge the discrepancies between age and the biological and psychosocial stages of development or the variations due to personal and environmental factors.

Adolescence is also viewed as a time when young people become alienated from their parents and become influenced by their peers. While it is true that adolescents do have intense emotional interactions with their peers and a need for their approval, this does not mean that they turn away from their parents. However, there is probably no other developmental age that causes as much chaos and muddle within any family unit. This is a time when young people will question the fundamental values of their parents and other individuals, including caregivers. Rapoport,[27] referring to the period of adolescence, supports this view, stating that it is a time for experimenting and testing family and community norms and values. Therefore, it is generally agreed that during adolescence there is a psychological shift in the individual's identity from being bound up with that of the parent to becoming an 'I'. An interesting point about this ego identity shift and the struggle to become independent is that the process is too threatening for the adolescent to go it alone, especially in the early days of adolescent development. Thus, generally they go through the process with their peers, they dress alike, eat the same foods, drink the same things, and have similar hairstyles.[26]

Uncertainties about their own identity and what the future may bring will come to the fore. Their need to compete with their peers and, at the same time to win social approval, is very strong and can place individuals in a situation of painful conflict. Such powerful feelings, which may be experienced for the first time, can lead to bewilderment and stress. It is at a time like this that the adolescent may revert to adopting a more comfortable and tested coping strategy used in earlier childhood years.

It is recognised that the above scenario offers many issues for reflection. However, the purpose of the account is to offer an example of an adolescent's reaction to a potentially bewildering and stressful event by adopting a known coping strategy, which is exhibited in more childlike behaviour. Frustration is one of the most common triggers of normal attention-seeking behaviour in both children and adolescents and the reaction in both is usually similar. They make demands on themselves or others in an attempt to overcome a problem, and if the response is perceived as negative, the child or adolescent is likely to

Personal account 32.2

A 14-year-old boy diagnosed with non-Hodgkin's lymphoma had received his treatment either as an in-patient or an out-patient in a paediatric oncology unit. He had been involved with decisions about the management of his care and appeared to trust and be comfortable with the staff on the unit.

Attending for a routine outpatient appointment, he was found to have low haemoglobin and a blood transfusion was prescribed. As the paediatric unit was unable to accommodate him for this procedure he agreed to have the transfusion carried out in the adult day care area.

During the procedure, a nurse from the paediatric unit visited the adolescent. On reaching the adult area the nurse was confronted by a member of the staff, who stated that she was not happy with the behaviour of the patient from the children's unit and offered the following account:

He has been adjusting the rate of flow of his blood transfusion, I told him not to do it as it was dangerous and I readjusted the flow rate. Later when I returned to see how he was he had changed the rate again. The doctor also explained to the patient that this was unacceptable. Now look at him, we gave him some paints to do some painting as he said that he liked to paint and he has painted his face not the paper. You would think that at his age he would know how to behave, he's not exactly a child.

When invited to give his account of the issues raised, the adolescent offered the following:

Why can't I adjust my transfusion here? I do it on the children's ward, I know it can be dangerous to let it go in too fast. Nobody asked me if I knew what I was doing they just assumed that I didn't. I didn't know what to do, they were treating me like a child.

continue with attention-seeking behavioural responses in an attempt to achieve a quick and acceptable resolution.

This account does, however, raise another issue worth discussing, that is the debate surrounding the provision of separate adolescent units in hospitals. Adolescent medicine in the main tends to fall between the expertise of paediatricians and the expertise of adult medicine, and adolescents are frequently asked to choose between the company of adults or children. Many writers suggest that providing separate adolescent units is the answer to

maintaining the process of adolescence in hospital. Muller et al.[28] offer an alternative view, stating that well-prepared staff with appropriate knowledge and skills about adolescence could provide care whatever the architectural arrangements. These writers do acknowledge that it may be advantageous to offer specialised units and staff, but at the same time they note that it should not be regarded as impossible to maintain optimal support for adolescents where special provision is not an option. They suggest that what is needed is a degree of motivation among staff to develop an understanding of the process of adolescence and to bring this to their patients, whatever the setting.

Box 32.4: Adolescence and adolescent development

- Adolescence is generally defined as the period of transition from childhood to adulthood.
- Early, middle, and late periods of adolescence have their own developmental concerns.
- The onset of adolescence is usually associated with the commencement of puberty and the appearance of secondary sex characteristics.
- The end of adolescence is less clearly defined and varies from culture to culture as far as the attainment of adult independence is concerned.
- The period of adolescence is considered to be a process in which the child is confronted by a number of developmental tasks such as:
  - adjusting to a changing physique and sexual development
  - achieving a sense of independence from parents
  - acquiring the social skills of a young adult
  - achieving a sense of oneself as a worthwhile person
  - achieving a personal set of guiding norms and values.

Cancer and the family

Quality of life issues have assumed increasing importance in discussions about care for the child with cancer and have brought with them the need to consider the whole life constellation around the illness. Leavitt[29] stressed that in order to provide optimal patient care the family needs to be viewed as 'the unit facing illness', rather than simply a refuge or advocate for the patient. One area that has traditionally been considered somewhat more advanced in its understanding and provision of family-centred care is that of the sick child, notably the care of the child in hospital. Much of the impetus to consider the role of the family in illness care evolved from studies carried out in the 1950s and 1960s,[30,31] which began to demonstrate that the isolation of children from their families while in hospital had serious effects on the child's health and well-being. There is now substantial evidence in the literature that the health and well-being of the child's family is also affected when a child is sick, with most of the literature concentrating on families with a life-threatening or chronic illness.[32] Some of the aspects of childhood cancer that make psychological adjustment particularly difficult for family members include the life-threatening nature of the disease, the prospect of uncertain prognosis, and changes in family lifestyles[33] (see, for example, the study by Dermatis and Lesko described in detail below).

Research study 32.1: Dermatis H. and Lesko L.M. (1990). Psychological distress in parents consenting to child's bone marrow transplantation. *Bone Marrow Transplantation* 6, 411–417[34]

Aim of the study
To determine the nature and prevalence of psychological symptomatology in parents of children undergoing bone marrow transplantation and to investigate the manner in which certain psychosocial factors are related to parental distress associated with the informed consent process.

Method
Forty-six mothers and 15 fathers were assessed with respect to psychological distress, coping styles, quality of doctor–patient communication, and recall of bone marrow transplantation information after giving consent for the child to undergo the procedure. Research participants were given the Brief Symptom Inventory (BSI), a self-report measure of psychological distress, and the Ways of Coping (WOC) Checklist. Participants were also asked to complete a researcher-constructed scale concerning the quality of the communication between the doctor and parent during the consent discussion.

Results
Forty per cent of fathers and 60% of mothers exhibited significant psychological distress of a generalised nature. Mothers exhibited a broader range of specific psychological symptomatology, i.e. disturbed thinking and higher levels of depression and phobic anxiety, than did fathers. Consenting

parents who were married exhibited significantly lower levels of global psychological distress than did mothers or fathers who were widowed, separated, or divorced. The quality of the doctor–parent communication was found to be the strongest negative correlate of global psychological distress.

Conclusions
The results indicate that mothers and fathers who gave consent for their children to have bone marrow transplantation exhibited statistically and clinically significant levels of psychological symptomatology. The strongest predictor of parental level of distress was the quality of the communication between the doctor and the parent. This finding suggests that where this was obtained from parents in an unhurried, empathetic and non-threatening manner, lower symptomatology resulted.

Limitations
This was a relatively small sample of parents, especially as the methodology applied to collect and analyse the data was orientated towards a quantitative research approach. There was failure to acknowledge that the finding that mothers' psychological distress was higher than the fathers' fits with clinical observations. Mothers frequently spend more time than fathers with the sick child in hospital, learning to deal with a foreign environment, caring for the child, and permitting the staff to perform frightening and invasive procedures. They also serve as the source of information about medical information to family and friends.

When caring for the child with cancer, part of the care will involve promoting health. Care therefore is concerned not only with the impact of the young person's health on the family but also with the impact of the family on the health of the child. Interestingly, while the implications for the family of a child with cancer are frequently addressed in studies from the 1980s, to date the concept of the family for the most part is not defined. This is perhaps understandable as in Western societies there have been numerous changes over the years in the nature of family life. Many children can now expect to live through periods of marriage, divorce, single parenthood, and remarriage. Substantial numbers of children are likely to live in several configurations of the family; as a result, their experience of family is neither static nor constant.[20] Terkleson,[33] addressing theories of family life, suggests that families are social organisations or units that have specific functions in relation to the developmental and situational needs of their own members, to their own maintenance as a family, and to the maintenance of society. Caregiving, communication, problem solving and decision making are cited as important aspects of family life, no matter what the particular family structure may be. Further, each family needs to be defined by its unique history, culture, and set of values.[35]

Whatever cultural or socio-economic family structure exists, when a child develops an acute or chronic illness various factors change for the family. The balance of daily life shifts as schedules alter to meet the new needs of the child. Parental roles and responsibilities alter in response to the child's changed and changing needs. Extended family members or friends may be called on for emotional support and advice. Other factors, such as sibling needs and financial concerns, may challenge families at the same time. Thomas[35] reminds us that despite a child's medical problems families want to function to the greatest extent possible as normal families. Bishop *et al.,*[36] discussing family/professional collaboration for children with special health needs, state that in contrast to the family, professionals see a child in their care in circumscribed, problem-focused circumstances. Therefore, these writers conclude that it is the family that is the constant in the child's life, while health care services and the personnel within these services fluctuate. They advocate that to keep a focus on the family's central role in the care of the child with special health care needs, it is necessary for health care professionals to recognise and understand the racial, ethnic, cultural, and socio-economic diversities of families.

Box 32.5: Issues for families affected by cancer

- Each family needs to be defined by its own unique history and set of values.
- The life-threatening nature of the child's disease, uncertain prognosis, and changes in family lifestyle contribute to making psychological adjustment difficult for the family.
- Coping and adjustment are influenced by ethnic, racial, cultural, and socio-economic family circumstances.
- The health and well-being of a family are affected when a child or adolescent is diagnosed with cancer.
- The health and well-being of the sick child are affected by the health and well-being of the family.

Approaches to treatment – an overview

Diagnosis

Childhood cancer is usually diagnosed in response to symptoms. This can be problematic as prognosis is primarily related to tumour burden and clinical symptoms may not become evident until the tumour burden is considerable. Pallor, fatigue, and thrombocytopenic haemorrhage are characteristic symptoms of haematopoietic cancers, whereas palpable swelling, pain, and loss of function are usual symptoms of solid tumours. Techniques used in the diagnosis of childhood cancer include laboratory testing of blood, urine, bone marrow aspirates, and other specimens. X-ray examination, ultrasound, computerised tomography (CT) and magnetic resonance imaging (MRI) and other imaging techniques are used to describe the primary tumour and to detect its local and systemic spread.

Treatment

Most childhood cancers, and especially acute leukaemias and lymphomas, respond to various combinations of chemotherapeutic agents. In treating solid tumours, systemic chemotherapy is usually complemented by local therapy with surgery and radiotherapy. In the past, brain tumours have usually been treated with surgery and radiotherapy, irrespective of histology. With attempts to refine radiotherapy techniques and the development of new chemotherapy strategies, it is now considered important that histology is obtained in children if possible. In small children with deep inaccessible tumours, for example in the mid-brain or brainstem, this is often difficult, but stereotactic techniques may be useful. Under general anaesthesia and using a predetermined site based on CT or MRI imaging, the majority of children can now be biopsied with low morbidity.[37]

Because most childhood cancers proliferate and disseminate rapidly, 5-year survival rates before the use of systemic treatment were below 10%. Optimising and standardising systemic combination chemotherapy regimes in the last two decades has led to improvements in the prognosis of most childhood cancers, resulting in a rise in survival rates.[3]

Improved survival rates in some childhood cancers are due to the administration of very high doses of chemotherapy and radiation. This is only possible by infusing harvested bone marrow, either from the child or from a matched donor, following treatment. This procedure is now accepted as standard curative treatment in children with some historically poor prognosis leukaemias and solid tumours. Children undergoing high-dose therapy will face a potentially life-threatening situation, which in terms of management and support provides a challenging and often rewarding aspect of patient care.[37] Bone marrow transplantation (BMT) is the grafting of bone marrow from:

- a matched donor (usually a sibling) or another (allogeneic BMT)
- an identical twin (syngeneic BMT)
- oneself (autologous BMT).

Although the bone marrow is the main source of the haemopoietic stem cells, it is now known that a number of stem cells is present in circulating blood. Children who have received chemotherapy and experience myelosuppression show a marked rise in the peripheral stem cell population as the white cell count recovers. Consequently, if stem cells are collected around this time and stored they can be used to assist in the restoration of haematopoiesis after a child has received megatherapy. The use of stem cells has impressively reduced the duration of neutropenia, which in turn has reduced the number of febrile episodes and promoted earlier healing of the gut mucosa. However, a bone marrow harvest is usually frozen in case the stem cells fail to engraft, thus providing a back-up. This aggressive multi-disciplinary approach to care and the inclusion of children in state-of-the-art clinical trials has led to control of this rare disease, which would be difficult to investigate without the efforts of co-operative groups conducting similar protocols.[3]

Addressing needs – from diagnosis through treatment

When cancer is first suspected, the child or adolescent and family will in most cases be referred to a specialist oncology centre. Throughout all aspects of the child's management and care, nurses and

---

Box 32.6: Medical management of childhood cancer

- Childhood cancers are usually diagnosed in response to symptoms, which may not become apparent until the tumour burden is considerable.
- Various techniques are used to confirm the diagnosis; these include laboratory tests of blood, urine, etc., and imaging techniques such as CT and MRI scanning.
- Systemic combination chemotherapy regimes are used to treat paediatric cancers as most childhood cancers proliferate and disseminate rapidly.
- Solid tumours are treated with systemic chemotherapy and complimented by localised therapy with surgery and/or radiotherapy.
- Brain tumours are routinely treated with surgery and radiotherapy but the addition of chemotherapy is now possible.
- BMT plays a significant role in the treatment of some haematological and solid childhood cancers.
- Aggressive multi-disciplinary treatment and co-ordination of care has resulted in cure for two out of three children.
- Inclusion of children into national and international state-of-the-art clinical trials has led to improved survival.

Care strategy 32.1: Facilitating coping and understanding

To assist the child or adolescent and family to understand and cope with a cancer diagnosis a working knowledge is required of:

- the nature of cancer in children and adolescents
- the differences between adult and childhood cancers
- approaches to medical treatment
- side-effects associated with treatment programmes
- the importance of a team approach to the physical and psychosocial care of the family unit
- concepts of childhood and theories of child development
- concepts of adolescence and theories of adolescent development
- concepts of family and family structures
- cross-cultural variations in childhood and adolescence
- potential impact that the diagnosis and treatment may have on the child or adolescent's developmental process
- potential impact that the diagnosis and treatment may have on the family and individual family members
- long-term sequelae of cancer and its treatments.

---

members of the multi-disciplinary team need to refer continually to knowledge based on the issues discussed in the first half of this chapter.

The needs of parents

Confirming the diagnosis of cancer to a child's family is a necessary but unenviable task.[37] The manner in which the information about the illness is given and the tone set by medical staff and members of the multi-disciplinary team both in the hospital and in the community are of major importance throughout the family's cancer experience. A number of studies investigating the impact of a life-threatening illness, including a cancer diagnosis, conclude that the manner in which procedures were carried out and the way in which news was communicated to the family seemed to be far more important than the specifics of actual treatment.[34,38 39] Initial reactions of parents on hearing the diagnosis for the first time have been universally described in terms such as fear, shock, disbelief, numbness, and feeling guilty. Parents react in this way even when they have strongly suspected the nature of the illness before diagnosis.[37]

In response to the question, 'Can you remember your immediate reaction or feelings after being told of [child's name] diagnosis?', one mother replied:

> It was like having a terrible nightmare that you woke up from and found was true. Our physical reaction was one of shock, feeling weak at the knees and shaky, and of disbelief, we also felt guilty and angry.

Ruccione *et al.*[40] discuss the contents of a letter that a mother of a young boy diagnosed with a spinal tumour wrote to the mother of a girl recently diagnosed with leukaemia:

> The memories of our first days in hospital have been flooding back as I see all you are going through. I look at your faces and see a mirror image of what I looked like. The exhaustion, the fear, the disbelief, the pain and the grief – I was numb . . .

Such statements often heard by paediatric oncology nurses and the paediatric team reflect parents' emotional states after learning that their child has cancer. The illness has come seemingly without warning and for no comprehensible reason. Parents express concern as to the cause of the illness and may question themselves: 'Are we to blame?', 'Is it something we could have prevented?', 'Is it because I smoked during pregnancy?'. Even if they do not verbally express feelings of guilt, parents need to be reassured that they are not to blame.

As feelings of disbelief subside, anger is frequently the next reaction. Anger may be directed at the hospital staff. Nurses must be prepared to accept parental reactions and defences of anger, hostility, and rejection without taking such reactions as a personal assault and without withdrawing themselves from the situation. Reactions to the diagnosis may be further intensified as there may be the necessity to commence treatment immediately, which entails consenting and subjecting the child to intensive and frightening treatment programmes. Another dilemma parents have to face is what or how to tell the child or adolescent about their illness and what to tell brothers and sisters. The effects of the diagnosis will be far-reaching, affecting not only the immediate and extended family but also family friends and friends of the child or adolescent.

What, when, and how to tell the child, adolescent, or siblings about the illness is an issue that generates much debate. Following careful assessment of their level of development and family situation, it is now accepted that children and adolescents have a right to know about aspects of the disease and treatments.

It is clear that the diagnosis and treatment for childhood cancer involve major emotional stresses for parents. To cope with the child's illness parents must simultaneously maintain hope, care actively for the child, and delegate responsibility to medical specialists, develop trust with members of the multi-disciplinary team, and attend to the immediate needs of the sick child and other family members, notably brothers or sisters, and plan for the future.

The watchwords for best patient care are stability and knowledgeable, co-operative teamwork. Family members need to gain a feeling of stability and consistency of care, especially through the early days of treatment. They need to feel that staff are available to provide them with both information and the time to formulate questions. Much time is often needed for parents and families from all socio-economic backgrounds, asking the same questions several times before 'hearing' the answer. Koocher and O'Malley,[39] investigating the psychological consequences of surviving childhood cancer, reported that it was important to families that carers gave a measure of realistic encouragement and hope along with the sense that they were cared about, and that the best possible care would be provided or found for their child. Ruccione *et al.*[40] found that among the most highly rated sources of information were physician, nurse, and social worker. Of these the most consistently highly rated, i.e. with the narrowest range of responses, were the physician and the nurse.

Research study 32.2: Calderwood M. and Koenen L. (1988). Parents' perspectives of paediatric oncology nursing services. *Nursing Management* 19, 54–57[41]

Aim of study
To discover which specific services or behaviours from nurses are important to parents.

Method
A sample of 184 parents was drawn from a list of parents whose children were seen in an oncology clinic. The sample included children with various types of cancer.

A one time only mailed questionnaire was chosen to elicit views. The questionnaire was developed through discussions with clinic nurses, physicians, and administrative staff. Identifying that mail surveys generally have a lower return rate, the questionnaire was designed to make it short, understandable, and easy to complete. The Likert-type questionnaire dealt with two issues: the current clinic situation and the 'ideal' situation.

Results
Sixty-eight questionnaires were returned (37%). As only 64 were complete, data analysis included a 34% response rate. Frequency data were recorded for: mean, median, mode, standard deviation, coefficient of variation (%), standard error and confidence indices of the 0.05 level of probability.

The most striking point was the high rating of items valuing nurses' technical skills and the time spent with nurses. The other highly rated items dealt with the importance of the nurse providing parents with initial survival skills. These included who to call and what to do if they were at all worried about the child. The items rated the lowest dealt with long-term rather than daily survival concerns; this included counselling on behaviour and growth and developmental issues.

Limitations
There was no reference to the length of time since the child's diagnosis. It is known that issues of importance at the time of diagnosis may not be the same as therapy progresses.

The age of the children was not identified. Therefore, it is possible that the sample responses may have been skewed towards care issues relating to a particular age group.

Although the results are significant, the low response rate is puzzling.

The study demonstrates that parents value nurses' technical skills, especially when parents have gained an understanding of the knowledge and skills required to administer complicated and intense chemotherapy regimens.

A phenomenological study[42] using a focused interviewing technique sought to gain knowledge and understanding of parents' experiences and perceptions of caring for their child's central venous catheter at home. Interpretation of parents' accounts revealed three major themes: how parents experienced and dealt with learning to care for the central venous catheter, how parents experienced and dealt with the catheter at home, and how parents dealt with sharing the care of their child's catheter with others. During discussions with parents about the care of their child's central venous catheter, all six parents in the study raised concerns about the differences in knowledge and skills of nurses involved in the care outside the specialist hospital, i.e. in the community or at non-specialist hospitals:[42]

> Well the nurses are much better here [the specialist centre] than at other places, they know what they are doing.

> She [sic] the community nurse never knows much about the Hickman line.[42] I could go to [hospital name] but the care for the Hickman line is nowhere near the standards they have got here [specialist centre]. If I was worried about the line I would ring here because other places you know . . .

The study was carried out in one geographical location, and generalisation of the results could be questioned. However, with the now accepted practice of involving parents in aspects of technical care, over time and through experience parents in any care setting may attain the status of 'expert parent'. As a result, parents become aware of limitations of professionals and enter a stage of 'guarded alliance'.[42]

In the Calderwood and Coenen study (Research study 32.2) the parent's low rating of counselling on child behaviour and growth is interesting, as in clinical practice developmental concerns are seen to be important, although it is noted that these do not generally surface with parents until later in the therapy. This may not seem to be a crucial issue for the parents, but it is well documented and recognised in clinical practice that assisting the child's continuing growth and development physically and psychologically throughout the cancer experience is paramount.

It is essential that parents are helped to find the ability to cope, to provide a supportive environment for the entire family, and to meet the new demands created by the illness. Information about family members, how they interact with each other, their individual family roles, and previous illness experiences and stressful situations enables nurses and other team members to help families to recognise problems and assist them to find means of dealing with them.

Families need to develop a new system that will enable them to find guidelines to help them to cope. These may take many forms and differ as circumstances change but they usually come in some sequence: before anything else there is a need for hard information about the child's condition, parents need to be restored to parenthood, and the team caring for the child should do so by sharing care as human beings.

Care strategy 32.2: Assisting parents to find the ability to cope and restructure their own lives and those of other family members

- Confirming the cancer diagnosis should be a planned event as parents vividly remember how, when, where and the manner in which the diagnosis was given. The approach of the hospital and community team is known to affect the parents' initial and long-term ability to cope.
- Discuss and exchange information about members of the family, their individual roles, and how they interact with each other. Such information enables staff to assess with the parents the possible impact of the disease, and to assist with plans to deal with actual or potential problems.
- Enable parents to gain control of their emotions, giving them time and space.
- Assist parents to regain control over the situation by giving information about the disease, treatment, and side-effects. Information needs to be given and repeated as frequently as parents or other family members require.
- Support parenting roles by acknowledging the skills and knowledge that parents have about the sick child and encourage and negotiate with them to participate in care to whatever level they choose.

The needs of the child

The nature of a child's reaction to his condition is not simply a reflection of how brave or cowardly he happens to be. Proper understanding and management of children with serious illness requires an appreciation of how the illness looks from the patient's point of view.[43]

Information needs of children

What to tell a child who has a life-threatening illness about the diagnosis and approaches to treatment tends to generate much discussion in an attempt to get it right. Certainly if children are to co-operate with frightening, painful, or uncomfortable procedures they must have an understanding of why. The impact of open communication patterns between the family, the child, and carers is clearly important. A known inverse relationship between a child's open discussion of illness and level of depression has been demonstrated: greater openness assists adjustment. There is also clearly a relationship between sharing information on the diagnosis and late psychological adjustment among survivors.[39,44] Children may also have unknown fears and fantasies, which can be more frightening than the realities of the diagnosis and treatment. Such fears and fantasies cannot be adequately expressed in a climate of secrecy.

One study[45] investigating information needs for children with cancer who were between 8 and 17 years of age, found that children want to be fully informed about their disease and its treatment and they do not want information withheld from them. Individually, children and parents considered that they should be given information about prognosis, treatment and all conceivable side-effects, not just those that are likely to occur. Parents, in contrast, wanted to shield their children about prognosis and treatment side-effects. This situation is not uncommon; in meetings with the parents and physician it is preferable that a nurse joins the parents to help them to express their fears and concerns about disclosure. The parents can be informed of the importance of communicating openly and honestly with the child and of the dangers of trying to shield the child from the facts. Bearison[46] states that there are hardly any experiences that can be more frightening for a child than to have cancer. Listening to children talk about their fears is difficult for adults. Thinking that we can protect children is a means of unconsciously trying to protect ourselves, thereby sometimes unwittingly denying children the opportunity to talk about their fears.

There are important differences between the way children understand what they experience and the way adults understand the same experience. These differences are not haphazard but can be predicted by reference to the child's stage of development, remembering that these stages are approximate. It is suggested that information gathering when dealing with children should be put before information giving. Another consideration is that when talking to young children the words used should be chosen carefully, avoiding potentially frightening words like 'cut', which may imply pain.[28]

The use of analogies must also be carefully thought out. Beales, cited in Muller *et al*.[28] gives an example of a young boy with a chest complaint who had not previously given thought to what might be going on inside him. He was far from reassured when the doctor explained that his lungs were like balloons; all the balloons that he had known had extremely short lives, always bursting suddenly and unexpectedly and with a loud bang.

The most constructive approach for any explanation is listening to the child's own explanation. A question such as 'What do you think we can do to make you feel better?' or 'Why do you think you are in hospital?' is an approach that gives an opportunity to confirm to an anxious or uncertain child that certain practices and procedures will help to make things better even if some of the procedures may make them uncomfortable at times.

Interestingly, the issues raised by the children in this study are similar to those expressed by children generally. Concerns about the cause of the disease were mostly expressed in relation to punishment as a result of wrong doing or catching it from someone or something. Siblings also expressed concern about catching the illness and that they may have caused the illness because of a previous disagreement and having thought or verbalised an unkind outcome directed at the brother or sister. For example, children may wish one another dead if they cannot resolve differences. These concerns are also documented in the literature.[25,28,37]

Research study 32.3: Hockenberry-Eaton M. and Minick P. (1994). Living with childhood cancer: children with extraordinary courage. *Oncology Nursing Forum* 21, 1025–1030[47]

Aim of study
To gain an understanding of the personal experience of school-age children with cancer.

Method
A sample of 21 children (11 males and 10 females) with cancer aged between 7 and 13 years was admitted to the study. A purposive sampling technique was used and a phenomenological research method was used to guide the study design and analysis. The interviewer obtained consent from parents and children. Children were asked to participate in a 30-minute audiotaped interview and were interviewed without the parents present.

Results
The children's perceptions of the cancer experience revealed four major themes: knowing, caring, feeling special, and getting used to it. Knowing about the type of cancer and treatment provided a sense of control that was extremely important for the children. However, despite the information given many did not understand why they got cancer and expressed numerous false ideas of disease transmission. One child thought she had got it from her cat or dog. The importance of human caring was emphasised throughout the interviews. Children felt a sense of security and support through human touch. In addition, it was important for the children to have a nurturing environment and to feel special; they also indicated that distraction was an effective intervention.

Limitations
The researchers felt that the small sample and the fact that the sample came from one geographical location may have limited the study's findings. Some may suggest that the cognitive development of school-age children limits their ability to articulate clearly what they perceive and distinguish as being helpful.

Developmental needs

Play and education are considered to be the work of children. Both represent the basis of human development and creativity, not just a way of using up children's time while they grow into adults. The children in Research study 32.3 indicated that distraction was important to assist them in coping with their illness. One such distraction, which is important in the process of development, is the continuation with school and playgroup activities during hospitalisation and at home.

Nurses can play a major role in helping children through difficult situations by implementing distraction methods through play and education.

There are many different types of play, each stimulating the development of a different aspect of a child's life. However, as with the sick child's understanding of what is happening, the particular form of play that engages a child will depend on the level of the child's maturity and individual interest. The potential for play to act as a vehicle for a child to express feelings has long been recognised by psychologists as having value in helping troubled children and has led to the development of play therapy. Play therapy is based on the fact that play is the natural medium of self-expression. It is an opportunity that is given to the child to 'play out' feelings and problems, just as in certain types of adult therapy an individual 'talks out difficulties'.[48] Play therapy is usually defined as directive where the play is guided and interpreted or non-directive where the direction is left to the child.

Play therapists are now considered to be necessary members of the paediatric team. Effective play therapy must give the child complete freedom to play out feelings of frustration, anxiety, insecurity, fear, and bewilderment. The beneficial use of play as a means of helping a child to understand medical procedures and what is happening needs to be considered and incorporated into all aspects of the child's care.

Through play with toys and hospital equipment children can, for example, be introduced to the reasoning for the placement of central venous catheters. Over time, through play and information giving, the child can be helped to gain an understanding of the need for the line. Many also become expert at knowing how the line should be used.

Education is said to be the single most important developmental factor affecting the child's adjustment. The information must, however, be pitched at a level commensurate with the patients' abilities to absorb and comprehend. This may require the use of special educational facilities, frequent repetition of information, or helping parents to learn how to talk openly with their child about the illness.[39]

Considerable progress has been made in assessing and reducing children's distress during repetitive, painful, and unpleasant side-effects of medical procedures, such as bone marrow aspiration, lumbar puncture, or nausea and vomiting and changes in physical appearance. Much of this progress is attributed to the recognition and understanding of the meaning the diagnosis and treatment have for the child. Knowledgeable staff are able to work with the child and family to determine the most appropriate approach to reduce anxiety and to provide a heightened sense of self-control. For example, before subjecting a young child to a course of radiotherapy there is a need to have an understanding of child development, to know the child, to have discussions with the child, parents, play therapist, other members of the paediatric team and the radiotherapy team, before deciding the best approach to getting the child through the procedure with minimal distress. This may be achieved through education and play, by watching another child undergoing the procedure, by giving sedation, a general anaesthetic, or by a combination of any of the above.

Children's involvement in decision making

The growing debate about the status of children and the broader debate around the rights of individuals have influenced the need to ensure that children are given the opportunity to articulate their concerns and to be involved in decision making about their affairs. This situation has been recognised and does not pose too many problems in the day-to-day care of the child with cancer. For example, a child is able to be involved in decision making about activities of daily living, about the most acceptable way of taking medication, about undergoing some diagnostic and medical procedures, and about which play and educational facilities engage their interest. However, there are other decision-making and consent issues that are faltering and uneven. Of particular importance in health care is the right or not of children to consent to medical interventions and participation in research. Arguably the most significant contribution to supporting the child's involvement was the adoption by the United Nations General Assembly in 1998 of the UN Convention of the Rights of the Child.[49]

Care strategy 32.3: Development of appropriate intervention strategies for the child with cancer

- Knowledge of child development
- Knowledge of treatment programmes
- Knowledge of the unique structure of individual families
- Knowledge of individual family dynamics
- Co-operative teamwork, acknowledging skills and knowledge of colleagues
- Knowledge of supportive and relevant literature
- Understanding the importance of play and education
- Using appropriate communication skills that consider the child's developmental level and life experiences
- Flexibility and creativity when communicating with the child, e.g. use of diversional therapy
- Thinking carefully of the words used to communicate with children
- Considering when it is appropriate to use analogies
- Listening to the child and starting where the child is when entering into a conversation
- Involving the child in decision making.

The needs of the adolescent

> Rebelling and pushing out against the injustices that you have suffered in childhood (indeed a sign of hope) shows that the spirit is not broken, that there is an individual in there shouting out 'hey what about me', the beginnings of change, of a sense of one's own needs, of self-worth.[50]

Ettinger and Heiney[51] write that the storm of adolescence may be particularly acute when overlaid with a diagnosis of cancer. As with the child with cancer, the impact of the disease on the adolescent threatens developmental milestones, to add to the psychological concerns raised by the illness itself. Understanding normal adolescent development provides a framework for identifying psychological concerns, predicting problems, and developing appropriate interventional strategies for adolescents with cancer.

Information needs

At the time of diagnosis the adolescent should be informed of the diagnosis and about treatment plans. Such communication helps to establish the trustworthiness of the professional, reduces the possibility of later serious emotional problems, and facilitates future discussions. Concealing the diagnosis is of little value; the adolescent may already be aware of the diagnosis or learn about it elsewhere.[19] Disclosure also prevents isolation, confusion, and stigmatisation. Generally the adolescent, like the adult, should have some control over the information received. Regardless of the potentially beneficial effects of disclosure in most cases, forcing unwanted information on an adolescent is disrespectful and may cause harm.[52] As with children, it is best to be led by adolescents themselves, and they should be asked if they want to know what is wrong with them.

Generally complicated explanations of the illness and how the treatment works are usually meaningless and not well understood.[53] However, adolescents will want to know and can understand what is to be done to them and what effect those interventions will have on their future.

Decision making

The debate about the rights of individuals and adolescents' involvement in consent to treatment and research is much to the fore; this will be discussed later.

Developmental needs

The coping strategy identified in the above study of not thinking about the disease is interesting, as many researchers found denial critically important to the adolescent's adaptation to chronic illness.[55,56] Denial is thought to be part of normal adaptive processes and manifests itself in many different ways. Overcompensation in school activities, and intellectualisation of the disease and treatment is reported as being the adolescent's need to be 'normal'. The need for group identity, the common perception of adolescents that 'nothing will happen to me', and the strong need for autonomy appear to provide the rationale for this coping mechanism. Denial as a coping mechanism may appear irrational or inexplicable on its own, but when viewed in the context of known developmental principles it may be found to be meaningful and provide insight into the psychological functioning of the adolescent. However, denial may prove inadequate and pathological behavioural and responses to stressors are likely to be exhibited. These include hostility, projection of guilt and anger onto others, and withdrawal.[57]

Research study 32.4: Weekes D.P. and Kagan S.H. (1994). Adolescents completing cancer therapy: meaning, perception and coping. *Oncology Nursing Forum* **21, 663–670**[54]

Aim of the study
To explore and describe adolescents' experiences and associated changes in coping strategies during the time period from 3 to 6 months before cancer therapy completion to 6 months after completion.

Method
A convenience sample of 13 adolescents (nine males and four females) with cancer aged between 11 and 18 years was included in the study. The study employed an exploratory, descriptive, longitudinal design. Parental consent and adolescent assent was obtained. A semi-structured interview elicited information regarding the meaning and perceptions of therapy, changes at home, and coping strategies used. The interviews were taped and lasted for about 1 hour.

Results
Three themes emerged from the data: meaning and perception of completing the cancer therapy (task accomplishment, movement towards a normal life); coping strategies before completion of therapy (positive thinking, not thinking about the treatments and 'busyness'); and coping strategies after completion of therapy (negotiation and selective forgetting).

Before completion, therapy was described by 77% of adolescents as invading every aspect of their lives.

Not thinking about the treatments was described by 92% of the adolescents; 'busyness' appeared to be a strategy used to dispel the notion of reduced capability.

After therapy completion, adolescents reported that they could focus on getting back to a normal life. They also made reference to their parents being overvigilant of activities and time spent with friends.

Limitations
The adolescents included in the study came from one geographical area, which may limit the possibility of general application.

As adolescence begins with the onset of puberty, concerns of the adolescent patient with cancer arise from the specific developmental tasks of that age. Concerns may be separated and relate to family relationships, body image and self-concept, loss of control, peer relationships and social isolation, sexuality, and the future. Considering the normal adolescent task of emotional separation from parents, most sick adolescents are often frustrated by the overprotectiveness of parents. Yet they remain ambivalent and want parental comfort when feeling ill, but not when feeling well. They are also concerned about worrying their parents and feel that they need to be strong for their parent.[58]

Cancer treatments result in undesirable changes, and concerns about appearance and altered self-perception are expressed by adolescents, especially as they relate to body image. They also worry intensely about looking different from their peers.[59] Sexuality issues are intertwined with peer relations and body image. There is a dearth of literature on sexuality and the adolescent cancer patient, with most information deriving from anecdotal reports. The author recalls a situation when a 14-year-old male was devastated when he learnt that he was likely to be sterile as a consequence of his proposed treatment. Later when asked what he feared most about being sterile he replied, 'Not being able to have an erection'. It became evident that he was not sufficiently knowledgeable about reproduction and did not separate fertility and impotence. It is therefore important when discussing information of this nature to establish the adolescent patient's current knowledge. However, adolescents may not always be certain of their own values and efforts to discuss intimate issues such as sexuality may meet with hostility. Anger should be accepted as a healthy reaction. Since all individuals have to come to terms with what may or may not be possible for them to achieve, it is better for adults to share problems with the adolescent, rather than trying to solve the unsolvable.

The physical and personal self are perhaps the most important areas of concern for the adolescent and are linked with the major task of identity formation. Adolescents with cancer can be helped with their change in appearance using a practical approach. Stressing the temporary nature of side-effects and linking these problems to the drugs that are responsible will help the adolescent to separate who they are as a person and how they look and feel as a result of their treatment.[60] This information is also valuable for their peers, who may have difficulty acknowledging changes in appearance and 'stay away' from confronting the issue.

Continuation of schoolwork and success in the student role will have a positive impact on self-esteem and implications for future career options. The expectation should be that the adolescent patients will return to school as soon as possible and continue with schooling throughout treatment.

The social needs of the adolescent need to be accommodated and considered both in hospital and at home. Groups of peers visiting in hospital may be viewed by some as being disruptive, and it is possible that this may be so. Adolescent peers require courtesy and a positive approach. Confrontational attitudes by adults are not well received. Brook[22] considers that adolescents' claims that they are misunderstood may be true, since many of the problems of adolescents are actually the problems of the adults who are having to deal with them (see Personal account 32.2).

Care strategy 32.4: Development of appropriate intervention strategies for the adolescent with cancer

- Knowledge of adolescent development
- Knowledge of the adolescent's friends, social activities, goals, and achievements
- Knowledge of family structure and dynamics
- Use of appropriate communication skills
- Listening to the adolescent, respecting and acknowledging their views and opinions
- Being flexible and accommodating towards the need to continue with education, social activities, and peer interaction
- Involving the adolescent in decision making.

The needs of siblings

It is known that having a brother or sister with cancer can have a profound and sustained impact on a sibling. Emotional concerns of being left out, jealousy and resentment of the attention given to the sick brother or sister and fears for their own health are relatively common. Closed communication systems in families may contribute to the development of behavioural and emotional problems.[39]

The effect on siblings will be dependent on the level of development, their age in relation to the sick child, and the family's reactions. It can be frightening for a sibling to witness changes in the

brother's or sister's appearance such as hair loss, weight loss or gain, or limb amputation. As a result of the fears and concerns they are experiencing, siblings may be reluctant to talk to parents as they may become unsure and feel insecure of their position in the family.[61] Siblings should clearly not be neglected by the parents, other family members, or members of the treatment team. They should be offered direct factual information at the time of diagnosis and throughout the course of treatment, be seen as an integral part of the family-centred approach to care, and acknowledged as important participants in the family's life throughout the illness. Enquiring how a brother or sister is and involving them in activities both in hospital and at home will give them a sense of importance and well-being. Involving siblings to whatever degree they want to be involved will also help to provide a real explanation of what is happening and help to address any fantasies that may be more frightening than the real thing.

Consent, decisions, and choices

Debates over the rights of children have had a high profile in recent years, with growing acceptance in national and international law that children are people, entitled to basic human rights. The most significant contribution to this profile was the adoption by the United Nations General Assembly in 1989 of the UN Convention on the Rights of the Child. The Convention has been ratified by 177 countries as of September 1995, a level of support unprecedented in the history of the UN.[20] Article 12 of the convention stresses that all children who are able to express their views must be given the opportunity to participate in decisions that affect them. The right includes decisions made in the private domain of the family and in the public arena of health and education.

A commitment to respect the voice of the child does, however, represent a shift from the traditional understanding of the status of the child in the family and in society. A number of well-worn arguments can be made against involving children in decisions about their care, ranging from developmental theories through to concerns about their lack of ability to comprehend the gravity of important decisions.[62] In the UK, during a consultation exercise undertaken by the Children's Right Development Unit in 1993, 45 children between the ages of 5 and 18 years were approached to discuss their perceptions of how their rights were respected.[63] The children reflected a wide variety of life experiences, but common to the group was a deep sense of frustration that their views and experiences were not taken seriously at home, at school, or by policy makers.

An increased role for minor patients (i.e. those under the legal age of consent, in most cases under the age of 16 years) in medical decision making has been advocated in recent years. Underlying the concept of child assent (refers to acquiescence) are the child's basic right to be informed, and the physicians ethical duty to provide the child with relevant information about their illness and treatment. It is also noted that the child's dissent may be ethically binding in cases of non-therapeutic research or medical procedures that are not considered essential.[45]

Extensive debate about autonomy and the reasons for its importance are not always clear in discussions about children's autonomy. Children may mistakenly be assessed as not having the capacity for autonomy or other personal qualities when they have not be given the opportunity to demonstrate their autonomy. Some practitioners are also sceptical about the rights of children. Claims that 'it has all gone too far' are not uncommon. A popular view seems, to be that the rights of children can only be achieved by denying the rights of others, whether parents or those who work with children.[21] It has to be remembered, however, that not all children want to be involved in decisions about their treatment.[45,64] A general lack of research and experience in this area is likely to compound the views of some health care staff, who believe children are incapable of making decisions and consenting to treatment. There is also a lack of clarity about how to decide whether children are competent and have the capacity to understand the nature of the treatment. Each case needs to be examined in context. Respect for children requires recognition that they may wish to control, share in, or refer decision making. If adults believe that a decision is misguided then they can discuss it with the child in more detail. As with the adult patient, most children if asked do agree to treatment, most commonly because they trust the doctor and their

parents, and believe that the cancer will get worse without the treatment and the treatment will fight the cancer. Involving children in decision making and in the process of consent can be disingenuous if one does not intend to respect a refusal.[52] It can also be argued that a young person, especially one who is ill and under stress, may be more willing to leave decisional authority to their parents. However, if a child or adolescent independently refuses treatment, that refusal should be carefully scrutinised and not hastily overridden.

Every effort should be made to understand the reason for refusal. Leikin[52] advocates that if the refusal has been clarified and addressed and the minor continues to refuse therapy, their level of decision-making competence needs to be examined. There is, however, a considerable lack of clarity about how to decide whether a child is competent. Alderson[64] suggests that competence tests remain subjective and often ask children to show greater levels of competence than the average adult. Such a position and the reluctance of some practitioners to involve young people because of their perceptions of the legal requirements indicate a need for a satisfactory framework for making decisions for children's health. Uncertainty and anxiety lead to some professionals being overcautious about involving children in decision making, even when they agree with the concept.

Another contentious issue is that if a child or adolescent under the age of legal consent refuses treatment for cancer, this may not be considered to be in the 'best interests of the child', as the majority of paediatric cancers responds to therapy. Overriding the child's decision in such cases is usually justified. However complex the issue of consent and decision making, the principle of respect for children's autonomy encourages us to accept that the best people to judge their interests are the children themselves. However, they are compromised if adults withhold information. Children will also often know far more than the adults realise. For example, one child was overheard talking to another in the playroom, saying:

> I heard them using words like 'tumour' and 'malignant' so I looked at these words on the Internet, I then knew that I had cancer. I know what cancer is my auntie got cancer.

Care strategy 32.5: Facilitating understanding and competence

Respecting children's rights requires that they have adequate information appropriate to their level of development, experience, and abilities.

How informed is the child or adolescent about:
- the illness to be treated
- the purpose of the proposed treatment
- the benefits, such as relief of symptoms, i.e. less pain, feeling better
- side-effects, options available, and the implications of not having treatment
- the possible discomforts, such as pain, medications, and scarring
- the time needed for in-patient or out-patient care, disruptions to social activities and school?

Does the child or adolescent show an understanding of the information given:
- by asking questions about its meaning and/or accurately explaining its meaning
- by seeking reassurance about procedures and their benefits
- by answering questions about the information that clearly express an understanding
- by talking about the impact that the treatment might have now and in the future?

Does the child or adolescent need explanations:
- by repeating and rephrasing the information
- by giving more time for discussion
- with drawings, diagrams, books, photographs, play, or medical equipment
- with help from parents, family, peers, other patients, or other professionals?

Death and the dying child

Sadly, today around 30% of children with cancer will die. Most will die from progression of their disease but a small number will die from side-effects of treatment.[65] At this time in the disease process, as at the time of diagnosis, the manner in which information is imparted to families and the emotions that information elicits are likely to remain vivid lifetime memories.[38] Families, notably parents, need to know that although the child is not going to be cured they are not being abandoned. They need to understand that palliative treatment and care will be available and how this can be organised. Survival may no longer be possible for the child but rehabilitative potential is possible, if only for a short while.[39] When planning palliative care it is important to have knowledge of the family, individual family members, cultural and religious views and beliefs, and to be flexible so that families have as much choice and control as possible. The death of a child is one of the most traumatic events that can happen to any family, leaving a permanent mark on their lives.[65]

Children's understanding of death

The issue of how children learn to understand their world and the influence of developmental theories in relation to understanding and illness has previously been examined. A similar approach has been adopted in studying children's concepts of death, with a number of studies indicating that children's understanding is linked to age.[66]

Most of these studies agree that it is difficult for a child under 2 years of age to comprehend fully the meaning of death, the common view being that very young children's response to death is similar to their response to separation. Children over 2 and under 6 years of age are considered to have little knowledge and experience of death, and tend to view it as a reversible state, usually associated with separation and a loss of movement. This age group is also viewed as being unable to separate fact from fantasy: 'Bang, bang you're dead, now get up'. Children over the age of 7 years are said to have a complete or almost complete understanding of death. Adolescents will have a full understanding of death, but this is also a time when young people tend to believe that 'it will never happen to me', take risks in life, and are known to defy death. Therefore, adolescents in the terminal phase of cancer may move from periods of choosing to deny what is happening and getting on with life, to making choices and decisions to forego additional therapy with knowledge and maturity.

A more precise way of categorising children's concept of death is that based upon stages of their cognitive development rather than age alone. Reilly *et al.*[67] studied children's understanding of death in relation to cognitive development. As expected, children at more advanced levels gave more informed answers to questions, and all children between the ages of 5 and 10 years believed in personal mortality. This study and others[19,68] suggest that many children with a serious illness can comprehend death and understand the ideas of their own death. An early study by Spinetta[69] of the dying child's awareness of death found that terminally ill children as young as 5 years were aware that their illness had serious implications, even when they had not been informed by others. This was in striking contrast to their parents' beliefs about what their children knew. Children tend to appreciate more than adults expect, and their level of understanding will influence their concerns and the ways in which to work with them in order to help.[70]

Even when it is considered by professionals that a child is aware of the possibility of dying, there continues to be a need to listen to the child and to be led by the child in conversations. For example, a 7-year-old child with advanced disease stated that 'I'm really frightened of it'. This statement could easily have been interpreted as being frightened of death or dying. When children tell parents and carers how afraid they are it is not uncommon for adults to respond with statements such as, 'there's nothing to worry about, everything will be alright'. These kinds of messages are likely to convey to children that adults do not want to hear about their fears, and may lead to an eventual loss of trust. When the child was asked what was meant by 'it', the child replied, 'having more medicines'. Gently enquiring as to what the child meant indicated to the child that the adult was interested in the child's fears and enabled further discussion. Reluctance to question children's ambiguous expressions and not being alert to their sometimes indirect approaches, such as playing dead with their toys, will only serve to distance the child from the adult. Children recognise the reluctance of adults to talk explicitly with them about their cancer and what is happening, and will use ambiguous expressions to maintain a kind of mutual pretence. Both children and adults need help to overcome their defences.[46] The guiding principle is to avoid lying and to let the child tell you how much to say; children will often end up answering their own questions in their own way. It is important to appreciate the child's perspective and to respond to their questions seriously and sensitively without being too probing or overpowering. Essential to this approach is that it is supported by professionals and parents involved with the child's care. Parents can be helped to communicate with their children in ways other than conversation, as some children will express themselves more readily through play or drawings. Giving parents the opportunity to anticipate awkward situations and to rehearse their response can be helpful. There are times, however, when it appears better to avoid confronting children or adolescents with stark realities and better not to challenge their use of adaptive denial or other psychological means of coping. This is not a statement in support of deception, but simply a statement that the physical and emotional climate of care can be more important than the factual knowledge that the child or adolescent has, or believes. That is to say, the child or adolescent and family members must feel cared about and know that all of their questions will be answered directly and honestly.[39] Whatever strategy is adopted, even the most open, the idea of facing a child's own death with the child is immensely difficult.[66]

Symptom management

Many of the symptoms experienced by children in the terminal phase of their illness give rise to both physical and psychological responses. It is therefore necessary to build up a clear picture of the child's actual and potential problems.

Care strategy 32.6: Issues to be considered when assessing and planning symptom management for children and adolescents with advanced disease

- Nature of the cancer and usual metastatic pattern
- Previous cancer therapies used
- Potential benefits of palliative therapy, e.g. chemotherapy, radiotherapy, blood and platelet transfusion, nerve block, massage, relaxation techniques
- Nature of actual or potential physical symptoms, e.g. pain, nausea, vomiting, constipation, infection, bleeding, or lethargy
- Nature of actual or potential psychological symptoms, e.g. fears about pain, other physical symptoms, change in body image, lack of mobility, loss of control, reduced peer contact, threat to planned goals, and fear of death itself (depends on level of cognitive development)
- Child and adolescent development and concepts of death
- Family structure

- Previously demonstrated child, adolescent, and family coping strategies
- Where care is to take place, i.e. home, specialist centre, local hospital, or hospice
- Appropriate involvement of the multi-disciplinary team in the specialist centre, the child's local hospital, local community, or hospice.

It is important to set realistic goals with parents and the child when symptom management and care is planned. It is possible to provide effective symptom relief for the majority of children, but there are some children who will have severe and resistant problems.[66] One of the worst fears for parents of a child with progressive cancer is that they will suffer pain; such fears are a realistic concern. A study carried out in a paediatric oncology centre in the UK found that of 76 children who died of progressive disease, 87% needed opioid analgesia.[71] This finding is likely to be repeated in other specialist centres where the physiological and psychological benefits of using opioids for severe pain control in children are understood and supported. The use of strong analgesics for pain control in children with progressive disease is known to cause unease with parents and also with professionals who are unfamiliar with their use. As pain control and the use of analgesia play a major role in the management of children with progressive disease, it will be examined here in some detail. A more comprehensive review of pain and other symptom management can be found in 'Recommended reading'.

Pain assessment and measurement

There are many problems associated with assessment and measurement of pain in children and young people, such as their range of cognitive development and their limited means of expression. Varni *et al.*[72] advocate a model of paediatric pain assessment that incorporates biomedical/disease variables, appreciation of cognitive developmental level, measurement of child psychological and social adjustment, and measurement of family environment. Assessment and measurement of children's pain need to consider both the direct and indirect ways in which children may express their discomfort. Direct expression may include the type of cry, how much the child can describe the pain, facial expression, body movement, and how much the child's activities are restricted by the pain. Indirect expression may include hunger, thirst, demanding constant company, becoming withdrawn, unusually quiet or disinterested in favourite activities.

Research into children's pain and its assessment has led to the development of a number of reliable assessment tools.[73,74] For babies, recording systems have been developed that depend on observations of body movement, type of cry and facial expressions. For older children linear analogue scales, pain ladders, and photographs or drawings of ranked facial scales have been used. However, such data on their own will have little clinical relevance without an evaluation of the framework in which children perceive pain, the nature and diversity of their experiences, and their coping abilities.[75]

Generally, experienced nursing and medical staff working with terminally ill children and adolescents tend not to use pain measurement scales, and depend on multi-dimensional clinical observations and the parent's understanding of their own child's reaction to pain. Interestingly, a study that looked at this supposedly unscientific approach to pain measurement found that estimates of a child's physical and psychological pain by several experienced independent observers using a visual analogue scale and behavioural observations correlated well with each other.[76] It is suggested that this approach should not be dismissed, but should serve to promote further research.

In summary, there is a number of principles underlying clinical understanding of paediatric pain.

- Children do suffer pain.
- Children with pain suffer, often silently.
- Assessment of child or adolescent pain requires a multi-dimensional approach.
- The choice of pain relief options needs to be based on advanced learning, research, and teaching.
- The relief of pain should not be physically or psychologically painful.

Pain management

Following pain assessment, a plan of management can be made. This may include a number of approaches, such as palliative radiotherapy, palliative chemotherapy, use of mild to strong analgesia, steroids, antidepressants, anti-convulsants, and psychological approaches. The choice will also depend on what is acceptable to the child and parents; for example, palliative radiotherapy for a very young child may require the use of general anaesthesia. The reason for a period of fasting before the procedure and spending time in hospital during the recovery period will not be understood by a young child. Both situations are likely to cause distress for the child and inevitably the family. Therefore, an alternative, less distressing option for effective palliation would need to be considered.

Analgesia
Most children with progressive disease will develop pain gradually, so can be helped initially with mild analgesia, progressing to moderate or strong analgesia as the pain increases. Important to the prescribing of analgesics is the general principle of regular administration, depending on the length of action of the chosen drug. For mild pain paracetamol is usually the drug of choice. When pain is no longer relieved by regular paracetamol, a mild opioid such as dihydrocodeine can be prescribed. For severe pain, strong opioid analgesics are essential.[66] In the UK, the strong opioids recommended and used most widely are morphine preparations. Many myths and fears continue to prevail concerning pain and the use of strong analgesics, especially in children. Health care professionals who are unfamiliar with the use of strong opioids worry about addiction and side-effects such as respiratory depression. Respiratory depression is uncommon in patients receiving opioids for pain associated with cancer and appears to be no more common in children than in adults receiving comparable plasma opioid levels.[77] Fears surrounding the issue of addiction are usually due to the confusion about physiological and psychological addiction to opioids. Physiological dependence will develop following regular administration, but this rarely presents a clinical problem. If a child's pain, for example, is decreased by the use of palliative chemotherapy then symptoms of withdrawal can be avoided by gradually decreasing the dose of opioids over a number of days. It is reported that there is no evidence that appropriate use of opioids for pain produces psychological addiction.[66] Par-

ents and the child may also have inappropriate fears of side-effects and addiction; it is therefore important to give them time and opportunity to express their concerns, so that explanations can be given.

Where the child is to die
Unlike the adult with progressive cancer, comparatively few children with cancer die in hospital or in a hospice. To be cared for at home in familiar surroundings is almost always the choice of the child and the child's parents and family. The possibility of home care is now a reality owing to the development of community liaison or home care teams in a number of countries; these are usually attached to specialist centres. The expertise of specialist nurses is available to assist and support the child and family, and community-based health care professionals. This support is essential if a child is to die at home as demands upon parents and the community-based team could be overwhelming, as both are unlikely to encounter dying children very often. Specialist nurses working alongside community colleagues are able to assess the child and family for physical and psychological discomfort, and to offer advice on measures to overcome problems. It is important if home care is the preferred choice of the child and family, that they do not feel abandoned by the specialist centre. Families need to know that hospital staff are still available to them, and should they decide to return to the hospital for the child to die, that this can be arranged. In practice this rarely happens; if it does, it is likely to be as a result of a medical emergency such as uncontrollable fitting. In most cases, children die at home with pain and symptoms well controlled. It is worth remembering that what is said, and how carers behave are important factors for parents and family members at this time, as at other significant times in the disease trajectory. There is evidence that parental and sibling long-term adaptation is reduced in families where the child has died at home as opposed to in hospital.[78] If hospital or hospice care is the preferred choice, this should be supported by the team at the specialist centre. As with home care the child and family should know that the plan of management has been carefully considered, is jointly agreed, and is in the best interests of the child and family.

Long-term issues and effects of surviving childhood cancer

The increasing numbers of survivors of childhood cancer provide evidence of the remarkable advances that have been made in paediatric oncology. Commensurate with the rapid advancement of treatment, current estimates suggest that by the year 2000 at least one in 1000 young adults will have been cured of childhood cancer.[79] Survivors may face many difficulties, including growth failure, gonadal damage, radiation and drug-induced cardiac or lung damage, the threat of a second primary cancer, intellectual impairment and problems with re-integration into society (for a concise review see 'Recommended reading').

Koocher and O'Malley[39] report on a 4-year investigation carried out in the 1970s into the psychological, medical, and practical life problems of people who were successfully treated for cancer during childhood. Although this is an early study, it is considered to be one of the most comprehensive investigations undertaken. Overall, this study reported that most survivors lead healthy adult lives, marry and have children, and maintain a quality of life consistent with others in the general population. A healthy adult psychological adjustment, however, is not assured. Virtually all the 117 survivors interviewed used some degree of denial as a coping mechanism, although the population varied widely with respect to adaptive and maladaptive applications of denial. Some of the findings that contributed to psychological concern for survivors were:

- the meaning of residual impairments resulting from cancer therapies
- the prospect for social acceptance and future relationships
- the ease of entry into the workplace
- the ability to obtain health and life insurance
- family communication, and the long-range impact the patterns of openness or secrecy may have on the survivors.

More recently, Apajasalo et al.[80] noted that while sophisticated data on specific problems are available, very little is known about the quality of life of long-term survivors of childhood cancer. Based on previous reports and from their own observations, the researchers hypothesised that the health-related quality of life of adults surviving childhood cancer would be inferior to that of the normal population (see Research study 32.5 for a detailed summary).

Research study 32.5: Apajasalo M., Sintonen H., Simes M.A. et al. (1996). Health-related quality of life issues of adults surviving malignancies in childhood. European Journal of Cancer 32A, 1354–1358[80]

Aim of the study

To establish whether the health-related quality of life of adults who had survived childhood cancer was inferior to that of the normal population, further to attempts to establish whether the health-related valuations of survivors would differ from the valuations of the controls.

Method

A previously validated 15-dimensional questionnaire (15-D), which was considered to cover physical, social, and mental well-being aspects of health-related quality of life, was mailed to 220 survivors. 129 adults who had previously completed the 15-D were chosen randomly as controls. There were no significant differences in the age, level of education, or employment status of the patients and controls. The 15-D measure consisted of multiple choice questions, each representing one health-related dimension, e.g. mobility, vision, hearing, sleeping, eating, depression, distress, vitality, and sexual activity. Analysis of variance, the Mann–Whitney U-test, multiple regression, and correlation coefficients were used to analyse results.

Results

There were no significant differences in the health-related valuations between the survivors and the controls. In statistical terms, the quality of life scores of the survivors were significantly better than those of the controls.

Conclusions

The observed excellent perceived health-related quality of life could be explained in many ways. One explanation may lie in the changes in personality and view of life brought about by the experience of surviving a life-threatening illness. Survivors may find their present life more satisfying and possible defects in their present health status less significant. This is supported by the finding that the most significant differences between survivors and controls were found in the most subjective dimensions, such as vitality and distress.

Limitations

Issues that are recognised by some survivors, such as perceived isolation, abnormal peer or family relationships, self-esteem and body image may not be sufficiently identified through a generic measure. In addition, fear of recurrence, employment and insurance problems, and potential social discrimination may lead to a situation in which survivors may ignore objective symptoms and findings. Denial mechanisms may compensate or overcompensate for the objectively measurable late effects.

In the Koocher and O'Malley study,[39] denial and suppression are noted to be a major coping strategy adopted by survivors. Denial is described as a primitive defence, which might be used in a major way by a child, someone with a mental illness, or someone in a crisis. The mature equivalent, which develops over time from denial, is suppression, the conscious choosing to put aside, not to consider certain disturbing or painful events. Interestingly, although survivors used this coping strategy, most remembered clearly what happened to them.

Perhaps one of the biggest problems survivors have to face is inadequate education of the public, which can lead to ostracisation and discrimination. The ability to obtain employment, life or health insurance, and to serve in the armed forces continues to prove difficult for most. Public information programmes continue to be much needed to dispel the outdated prejudice that the prognosis for childhood cancer is uniformly poor.

Long-term follow-up

Long-term follow-up is now part of the overall management for children surviving cancer. This requires careful handling if patients are to attend, especially during the adolescent years, when the importance of adaptive denial is known to assist psychological coping. Attending for what appears to be an unnecessary appointment may threaten this coping mechanism. One way to overcome the problem is to stress to the individual the seriousness of the illness for which they were successfully treated and to encourage appropriate follow-up and routine health precautions. Health care professionals working with long-term survivors also need to be aware of both subtle and obvious consequences of cancer treatments. The survivor whose puberty is delayed, for example, may experience significant self-esteem problems, which could go unnoticed at a routine medical follow-up.

Recognising that such a symptom can be an issue, a sensitive practitioner can enquire and make referrals as indicated.[39] Therefore, the purpose of follow-up should be to consider the well-being of children with cancer to ensure that they achieve normal or maximal growth, maturation, and psychosocial adaptation. Optimum management requires a multi-disciplinary follow-up service in which a paediatric oncologist, paediatric endocrinologist, and paediatric clinical psychologist contribute. Long-term effects of treatment for childhood cancer are many and varied. Effects due to the toxicity of cancer therapies are currently known and understood; however, new problems may arise due to as yet undescribed toxicity and evolution of tissue damage. Minimisation of these effects can be achieved by vigilant observation and a willingness on the part of clinicians to accept necessary modification of treatment, by early intervention and prevention, and with the co-operation of the multi-disciplinary team. It is suggested that what is needed is that every new protocol should have a section built into it that makes provision for baseline assessment of organ function and psychological status. Well-designed prospective evaluation of treatment effects is also considered to be mandatory.[14] Rather than working to restore lost function, those caring for the child or adolescent with cancer and their family need to work collectively towards preventing or minimising early or late physical or psychological effects. It is not enough to 'mean well' when caring for the child or adolescent with cancer; it is essential to 'know well'.[39]

> A child's life is like a piece of paper on which every passerby leaves a mark.
>
> Ancient Chinese proverb

References

1. Bawden N. (1974). *George Beneath a Paper Moon.* London: Allen Lane.
2. Cooper A. and Harpin V. (1991). *This is Our Child.* Oxford: Oxford University Press.
3. Jurgens H. (1997). Recent advances in childhood cancer. *European Journal of Cancer* **33** (Suppl. 4), S15–S22.
4. Stiller C.A. (1992). Aetiology and epidemiology. In Plowman P.N. and Pinkerton C.R. (eds.) *Paediatric Oncology*

Clinical Practice and Controversies. London: Chapman and Hall.

5. Parkin D.M., Stiller C.A., Draper G.J., Bieber C.A., Terracini B. and Young J.L. (eds.) (1998). *International Incidence of Childhood Cancer.* IARC Scientific Publications No. 87. Lyon: International Agency for Research on Cancer.

6. Voute P.A., Kalifa C. and Barrett A. (1998). *Cancer in Children: Clinical Management.* Oxford: Oxford University Press.

7. Stewart A., Webb D. and Hewitt D. (1958). A survey of childhood malignancies. *British Medical Journal* i, 1495–508.

8. Cartwright R.A., McKinney P.A. and Hopton P.A. (1984). Ultrasound examinations in pregnancy and childhood cancer. *Lancet* ii, 999–1000.

9. Kinnier-Wilson L.M. and Waterhouse J.A. (1984). Obstetric ultrasound and childhood malignancies. *Lancet* ii, 997–999.

10. Voute P.A., Barrett A., Bloom H.J., Lemerle J. and Neidhardt M.K. (1986). *Cancer in Children Clinical Management,* 2nd edition. Berlin: Springer.

11. Stiller C.A. (1992). Aetiology and epidemiology. In Plowman P.N. and Pinkerton C.R. (eds.) *Paediatric Oncology Clinical Practice and Controversies.* London: Chapman and Hall.

12. Nicholson A. (1990). Childhood cancer – an overview. In Thompson J. (ed.) *The Child With Cancer, Nursing Care.* London: Scutari Press.

13. Hammond G.D. (1986). Keynote address; the cure of childhood cancers. *Cancer* 58 (Suppl.), 407–413.

14. Morris Jones P. (1992). Non-endocrine late effects of treatment. In Plowman P. and Pinkerton C.R. (eds) *Paediatric Oncology Practice and Controversies.* London: Chapman and Hall.

15. Alderson P. and Montgomery J. (1996). *Health Care Choices, Making Decisions With Children.* London: IPPR.

16. Siegal M. (1991). *Knowing Children.* Hove: Lawrence Erlbaum Associates.

17. Nicholson R. (1986). *Medical Research with Children, Ethics, Law and Practice.* Oxford: Oxford University Press.

18. Koocher G. and Saks M. (1983). *Children's Competence to Consent.* New York: Plenum Press.

19. Bluebond-Langner M. (1978). *The Private Words of Dying Children.* Princetown: Princetown University Press.

20. Lansdown G. (1995). *Taking Part: Children's Participation in Decision Making.* London: Institute for Public Policy Research.

21. Franklin B. (1995). The case for children's rights: a progress report. In Franklin B. (ed.) *The Handbook of Children's Rights.* London: Routledge.

22. Brook C.G. (1985). *All About Adolescence.* Chichester: John Wiley.

23. Eisen P. (1984). Adolescent coping strategies and vulnerabilities. *International Journal of Adolescent Medicine and Health* 2, 107–111.

24. Erikson E.H. (1968). *Identity, Youth and Crisis.* London: Faber and Faber.

25. Kuykendall J. (1989). Teenage trauma. *Nursing Times,* **83,** 26–28.

26. WHO (1986). *Young People's Health – A Challenge for Society.* Technical Report Series 731. Geneva: World Health Organisation.

27. Rapoport R. and Rapoport R. (1980). *Growing Through Life.* London: Harper and Row.

28. Muller D.J., Harris P.J. and Wattley L. (1986). *Nursing Children Psychology, Research and Practice.* Lippincott Nursing Series. London: Harper and Row.

29. Leavitt M.B. (1989). Transition to illness; the family in hospital. In Gillis C.L., Highly B.L., Roberts B.M. and Martinson I.M. (eds.) *Towards a Science of Family Nursing.* Menlo Park: Addison-Wesley, pp. 262–283.

30. Prugh D.G., Staub E.M., Sands H.H., Kirschbaum R.M. and Lenihan E.A. (1953). A study of the emotional reactions of children and families to hospitalisation and illness. *American Journal of Orthopsychiatry* 23, pp. 70–106.

31. Bowlby J. (1969). *Attachment and Loss,* Vol. 1. New York: Basic Books.

32. Knafl K.A. and Deatrick J.A. (1986). How families manage chronic conditions; an analysis of the concept of normalisation. *Research in Nursing and Health* 9, 215–222.

33. Terkleson K.G. (1980). Toward a theory of the family life cycle. In Carter E.A. and Goldrock M. (eds.) *The Family Life Cycle; A Framework for Family Therapy.* New York: Gardner.

34. Dermatis H. and Lesko L.M. (1990). Psychological distress in parents consenting to child's bone marrow transplantation. *Bone Marrow Transplantation* 6, 411–417.

35. Thomas R.B. (1987). Family adaptation to a child with a chronic condition. In Rose M.H. and Thomas R.B. (eds.) *Children with Chronic Conditions; Nursing in a Family and Community Context.* Orlando: Grune and Stratton.

36. Bishop K.K., Woll J. and Arango P. (1994). Cited in Ahamann E., Family centred care: shifting orientation. *Paediatric Nursing,* March–April, 20.

37. Pinkerton C.R., Cushing P. and Sepion B. (1994). *Childhood Cancer Management.* London: Chapman and Hall.

38. Woolley H., Stein A. and Forrest G.C. (1989). Imparting the diagnosis of a life-threatening illness in children. *British Medical Journal* 298, 1623–1626.

39. Koocher G.P. and O'Malley J.E. (1981). *The Damocles Syndrome.* New York: McGraw-Hill.

40. Ruccione K., Kramer R.F., Moore I. and Perin G. (1991). Informed consent for treatment of childhood cancer: factors affecting parents' decision making. *Journal of Pediatric Oncology Nursing* 8, 112–121.

41. Calderwood M. and Koenen L. (1988). Parents' perspectives of pediatric oncology nursing services. *Nursing Management* **19**, 54–57.

42. Thompson J. (1995). *Parents perceptions of caring for their child's central venous catheter at home.* Open University, NESCOT, MSc dissertation.

43. Beales G. (1983). The child's view of chronic illness. *Nursing Times* **79**, 50–51.

44. Slavin L., O'Malley J.E., Koocher G.P. and Foster D.J. (1981). Communication of the cancer diagnosis to paediatric patients; impact on long-term adjustment. *American Journal of Psychiatry* **139**, 179–183.

45. Ellis R. and Leventhal B. (1993). Information needs and decision – making preferences of children with cancer. *Psycho-oncology* **2**, 227–284.

46. Bearison D.J. (1991). *They Never Want to Tell You, Children Talk About Cancer.* London: Harvard University Press.

47. Hockenberry-Eaton M. and Minick P. (1994). Living with childhood cancer: children with extraordinary courage. *Oncology Nursing Forum* **21**, 1025–1030.

48. Axline V.M. (1989). *Play Therapy.* London: Churchill Livingstone.

49. United Nations (1992). *The Convention on the Rights of the Child.* London: HMSO.

50. Winnicott D.W. (1981). Delinquency as a sign of hope. Cited in Birch D.M. (1996). Adolescent behaviour and health. *Current Paediatrics* **6**, 80–83.

51. Ettinger R.S. and Heiney S. (1993). Cancer in adolescents and young adults. Psychological concerns, coping strategies and interventions. *Cancer* **71** (Suppl. 10), 3276–3280.

52. Leikin S. (1993). The role of adolescents in decisions concerning their cancer therapy. *Cancer* **71** (Suppl. 10).

53. Sussman E., Hersh S., Nannis E., Strope B. and Woodruff P. (1982). Conceptions of cancer; the perspectives of child and adolescent patients and their families. *Journal of Paediatric Psychology* **7**, 253–261.

54. Weekes D.P. and Kagan S.H. (1994). Adolescents completing cancer therapy: meaning, perception and coping. *Oncology Nursing Forum* **21**, 663–670.

55. Kagen L.B. (1976). Use of denial in adolescents with cancer. *Health Society Work* **4**, 70–87.

56. Zelter L., Kellerman J. and Ellenburg L. (1980). Cited in Richie M.A. (1992) Psychological functioning of adolescents with cancer; a developmental perspective. *Oncology Nursing Forum* **19**, 1499.

57. Richie M.A. (1992). Psychological functioning of adolescents with cancer; a developmental perspective. *Oncology Nursing Forum* **19**, 1497–1501.

58. Rudin M., Martinson I. and Gillis C. (1988). Measurement of psychological concerns of adolescents with cancer. *Cancer Nursing* **11**, 144–149.

59. Ohanian N. (1989). Informational needs of children and adolescents with cancer. *Journal of Paediatric Oncology Nursing* **6**, 94–97.

60. Ellis J. (1991). Coping with adolescent cancer: it's a matter of adaptation. *Journal of Paediatric Oncology Nursing* **8**, 10–17.

61. Cairns N.U., Clark G.M., Smith S.D. and Lansky S.B. (1979). Adaptation of siblings to childhood malignancies. *Journal of Paediatrics* **995**, 484–487.

62. Pursell E. (1995). Listening to children; medical treatment and consent. Guest editorial. *Journal of Advanced Nursing* **21**, 623–624.

63. Children's Rights Development Unit (1994). *UK Agenda for Children.* London: Children's Rights Development Unit.

64. Alderson P. (1993). *Children's Consent to Surgery.* Milton Keynes: Open University Press.

65. Gonda T.A. and Ruark J.E. (1984). *Dying Dignified, The Health Professional's Guide to Care.* Menlo Park, CA: Addison-Wesley.

66. Goldman A. (1992). Care of the dying child. In Plowman P.N. and Pinkerton C.R. (eds.) *Paediatric Oncology Clinical Practice and Controversies.* London: Chapman and Hall.

67. Reilly T.P., Hasazi J.E. and Bond L.A. (1983). Children's conceptions of death and personal mortality. *Journal of Paediatric Psychology* **8**, 21–31.

68. Wass H. and Corr C.A. (1984). *Childhood and Death.* Washington, DC: Hemisphere Publishing.

69. Spinetta J.J. (1974). The dying child's awareness of death. A review. *Psychological Bulletin* **81**, 256–260.

70. Lansdown R. and Benjamin G. (1985). The development of the concept of death in children aged 5–9 years. *Child Care Health and Development* **11**, 13–20.

71. Goldman A. and Bowman A. (1990). The role of oral controlled release morphine for pain relief in children with cancer. *Palliative Medicine* **4**, 279–285.

72. Varni J.W., Walco G.A. and Katz E.R. (1989). A cognitive–behavioural approach to pain associated with paediatric chronic pain. *Journal of Pain and Symptom Management* **4**, 238–241.

73. Bayer J. and Wells N. (1989). The assessment of pain in children. *Paediatric Clinics of North America* **36**, 837–854.

74. McGrath P.A. (1990). *Pain in Children; Nature, Assessment and Treatment.* London: Guildford University Press.

75. McGrath P.A. (1989). Evaluating children's pain. *Journal of Pain and Symptom Management* **4**, 198–214.

76. McGrath P.A., DeVeber L.L. and Hearn M.T. (1985). Multidimensional pain assessment in children. In Fields H.L., Dubner R. and Cervero F. (eds.) *Advances in Pain Research and Therapy.* New York: Raven Press, pp. 387–393.

77. Shannon M. and Berde C. (1989). Pharmacologic management of pain in children and adolescents. *Paediatric Clinics of North America* **36**, 855–872.

78. Mulhern R.K., Lauer M.E. and Hoffman R.G. (1983). Death of a child at home or in the hospital: subsequent psychological adjustment of the family. *Paediatrics* **71**, 743–747.

79. Wallace W.H. and Shalet S.M. (1992). Growth and endocrine function following treatment of childhood malignant disease. In Plowman P.N. and Pinkerton C.R. (eds.) *Paediatric Oncology Clinical Practice and Controversies*. London: Chapman and Hall.

80. Apajasalo M., Sintonen H., Simes M.A. *et al.* (1996). Health-related quality of life of adults surviving malignancies in childhood. *European Journal of Cancer* **32A**, 1354–1358.

Recommended reading

Bearison D.J. (1991). *They Never Want to Tell You, Children Talk About Cancer*. London: Harvard University Press.

Bluebond-Langner M. (1978). *The Private Words of Dying Children*. Princetown: Princetown University Press.

Pinkerton C.R., Cushing P. and Sepion B. (1994). *Childhood Cancer Management*. London: Chapman and Hall.

Plowman P.N. and Pinkerton C.R. (1992). *Paediatric Oncology: Clinical Practice and Controversies*. London: Chapman and Hall.

Voute P.A., Kalifa C. and Barrett A. (1998). *Cancer in Children: Clinical Management*. Oxford: Oxford University Press.

Wass H. and Corr C.A. (1984). *Childhood and Death*. Washington, DC: Hemisphere.

CHAPTER THIRTY-THREE

The needs of older people

Christopher Bailey

Introduction: a personal view

For the past 2 years my colleagues and I have been working on a study of people over the age of 60 who have cancer of the colon and rectum. In particular, the study investigates the type of treatment and care older people receive, its effects on their functional status, and whether chronological age makes a difference to the kind of treatment and care older people receive, or should receive. We are still collecting information, so I am not yet able to say what the findings of the study will be. But over the last 2 years I have visited older people with colorectal cancer both at home and in hospital, a rare opportunity to see and hear about the impact of illness and health care in later life.

The first thing to say is that the youngest person I have spoken to was 60 and the oldest 95: at 60 many people are still working, but at 95 few are. While people of 60 and upwards are often described as 'older', it makes no sense to place people in a category like this. I have spoken to people of 90 whose lives are full and varied, and people of 90 whose lives are very restricted. It has become rather a cliché to say it, but there is nothing predictable about the lives of people who have attained a certain age. The same can be said about the needs of older people: it is difficult, if not impossible, to try to understand a person's health care needs properly without going to that person and obtaining information first hand. The question I have often asked myself in the last year-and-a-half is whether we talk and listen enough to older people in the health service. Do we talk and listen enough as a society? Do we talk and listen enough when older people are diagnosed with a disease like cancer of the colon and rectum?

People's material circumstances differ widely, from luxurious to squalid, from homes with magnificent grounds to cluttered apartments with no room to move, where commode, bed, and TV are squashed into one room. People become isolated and despairing in relative luxury as well as in squalor, whether they are at home or in residential care and, more surprisingly, whether they are alone or have a partner. Of course, many older people with cancer lead contented lives, whether or not they are alone. But my impression is that many of the people I have visited are or have been frightened by what has happened to them and would welcome a means of addressing it. This may be as true for those spouses and partners who do not have cancer as for those who do.

Often in later life people's personal circumstances are complicated and demanding in most unexpected ways. One person, while materially and financially well cared for in specially built rooms in the family home, rarely spoke or interacted with other family members, even at meal times, and did not feel able to share the bath so used the sink in his room. Another, while cared for devotedly, was unable to respond or reciprocate because he had become so emotionally isolated. One man, who was in his 70s, was the oldest member of the household as well as the main carer for two or three younger but dependent family members with profound physical and mental problems. Another was the main source of family support for a partner who was in residential care. An elderly woman with cancer cried for the loss of her husband who had died 2 years before, and another recounted the loss of a grandchild 4 years previously before telling me about her surgery.

Cancer can occur in the context of different or difficult lives, which older people often manage with little or no professional support. People who are experiencing fear, loneliness, grief, or the weight of responsibility have the added trauma of cancer and its treatment.

I have found that the most supportive, positive partners and families can experience painful confusion about the nature of a cancer diagnosis, the medical management of the illness, and the likely consequences. Many of the people I have spoken to have expressed powerful fears about the prospect of a colostomy or ileostomy; fewer people have found the practical aspects of stoma care unmanageable. Many, however, have experienced distressing and unexpected stoma 'accidents' or malfunctions, and avoid supermarkets, hotels, restaurants, group holidays or activities, and long journeys because they feel unable to rely on their stoma in these circumstances.

My strong impression, therefore, is that older people with colorectal cancer have a need to reflect upon their illness, treatment, and care before and after their visits to hospital as a means of preparing for it emotionally and practically; reflecting on cancer, though, may mean reflecting on sometimes complicated or difficult lives. I am left with two questions: 'How well does the health service currently respond to this need?' and 'If we see this need as legitimate, what means do we have of responding to it?'

Older people and cancer

Facts and figures

It is no longer surprising to read or hear of statistics demonstrating how the proportion of older and elderly people in the populations of Western countries in changing. Often these figures are quoted in the context of health care, and in particular to illustrate the implications of demographic change for cancer care and treatment.

Victor[1] describes later life in the UK as 'a predominantly female experience', pointing out that 60% of the population aged 65 and over are women, and that in the 85s and over, there are 250 women per 100 men; because women tend to live longer than men, it is more likely for women to be widowed at an earlier age. Burnside[2] points out that in the USA women aged over 75 constitute 74% of the population, and that this group is disproportionately affected by poverty; older women are less likely to have someone to provide their care at home, which, Burnside notes, may be one reason why the majority (70%) of nursing home residents in the USA are women (in the UK, among the 75+ age group women are more likely than men to live in an institutional setting[1]). In the UK 3% of people aged 65 and over live in some kind of institutional setting, though the figure rises to 19% for people aged 85 and over; only 17% of men over the age of 65 live alone, whereas for women the figure is 45%.[1] Writing about the experience of older people with cancer in the USA, McCaffrey Boyle *et al.*[3] highlight the potential consequences of the 'gradual loss of supportive resources' that accompanies the comorbidity and increasing incidence associated with cancer in the elderly:

> Nearly one third of elderly people 65 years of age and over live alone. Most are women who have outlived their spouses and, in some cases have outlived their children and other relatives as well. The difficulties inherent to living alone may be intensified . . . by inadequate external social support networks, possibly resulting in unmet needs for long-term assistance with activities of daily living. These problems may be further exacerbated by loneliness, depression, and limited satisfaction with life.

While many medical and nursing texts use terms such as 'young-old' (65–74 years), 'middle-old' (75–84 years), and 'old-old' (85 years and over), it can be argued that there is little rationale for this categorisation beyond the need to achieve a form of orderliness in health care institutions, statistics, or in society at large. Whatever our age may be, how can we not be part of a process of ageing that encompasses us all equally? The notion of age 'groups' separates us from each other in an artificial way.

In 1993 an advisory report[4] prepared by the European School of Oncology for the European

Community's 'Europe Against Cancer' programme pointed out that while around 15% of the population of Europe is aged over 65, more than 55% of cancers occur in this group. Cancer mortality, as well as incidence, increases with age: American figures indicate that about 67% of all cancer deaths occur in people aged 65 and over.[5]

In the UK, information from the Cancer Research Campaign[6] indicates that in 1991 14% of Europeans were aged over 65, while the estimated figure for 2020 is 20%. This translates to an increase of 17 million people in total, and an estimated increase in cancer registrations of 250 000.

Figures from the Office for National Statistics[7] for 1992 show that out of a total of 258 328 new registrations of malignant neoplasms in England and Wales, 171 415 (66%) occurred in men and women aged 65 and over. About half the cases of the 10 most common malignant tumours in England and Wales occur in men and women aged over 70 years, and about one-sixth occur in people over 80.[8] In the USA it has been calculated that the incidence of cancer increases from 497 per 100 000 in the under-40s, to 2308 per 100 000 in people aged 85 and over.[9]

Treatment issues

It is not surprising given these statistics that age has been described as 'largely a disease of older persons'[10] and 'the greatest risk factor for developing cancer'.[11] There is a clear case to be made for cancer in older people to be treated as a priority both by policy makers and by health care professionals. Yet questions persist about how evenly the attention of policy makers, health care professionals, and researchers is divided between the age groups. The question of whether the nature of malignant tumours changes with age is a vexed one, and the overall picture is mixed:

> Some physicians believe that older people are more likely to have slow-growing cancers than the middle aged or young. Other physicians believe just the opposite . . . It seems that those who believe that slow-growing tumours are associated with old age are correct as are those who believe that rapidly growing tumours are associated with old age. Both are correct, and site and stage are two important determinants . . . groups of old tumours are just as diverse as groups of old people.[12]

Stage at diagnosis may increase with age, especially in cancer of the breast, cervix, ovary, bladder, and melanoma; the finding that there is an inverse relationship between older age and stage at diagnosis in lung cancer and gastrointestinal cancer may be explained by incomplete staging: Hahn et al.[13] point out that the extensive procedures necessary for staging these diseases may not be undertaken consistently in the elderly.

The tendency for older people to have more advanced disease at diagnosis, the increased likelihood that they will be found to have metastatic disease,[9] and the implications that this may have for the effectiveness of any treatment that may be offered, have been cited as evidence for the need to prioritise early detection and screening in the elderly.[14] Faithfull[15] points out that:

> The late presentation and diagnosis of cancers in the older person are frequently cited when considering the possible reasons for the increased mortality of older individuals with cancer. Cancers identified at an early stage are often limited in size and are less likely to have spread to other areas of the body. The advanced stage of disease at initial diagnosis in elderly people decreases the likelihood that optimal treatment will be used and . . . reduces opportunities for cure.

McCaffrey Boyle and Engelking[14] suggest that older people may not seek advice promptly because of their great fear of cancer, and because they may believe that treatment is as bad as or worse than the disease and that death is inevitable. They argue that health care professionals may have a negative attitude towards cancer treatment in the elderly, and that the focus of health services is on sickness, not prevention and early detection. Faithfull[15] concludes that because perceptions of health and illness are such an important influence on people's willingness to come forward for screening or early diagnosis, health services must be prepared to work for a different attitude to cancer in society in order to increase the effectiveness of their early detection practices.

It has been said that cancer in the elderly is poorly treated, undertreated, and poorly understood, and that patients aged over 70 have been excluded from most clinical trials of cancer treatment.[8] The European School of Oncology's report on cancer treatment in the elderly[4] emphatically states that

Table 33.1 Oncology Nursing Society position paper on cancer and ageing (reproduced with permission from McCaffrey Boyle D. *et al.* (1992). Oncology Nursing Society position paper on cancer and ageing: the mandate for oncology nursing. *Oncology Nursing Forum* **19**, 913–933)[3]

1 It is imperative that oncology nurses recognise personal biases towards aging and the elderly that may interfere with the delivery of quality nursing care.

2 It is imperative that oncology nurses advocate cancer prevention and early detection activities for older adults.

3 It is imperative that oncology nurses acknowledge the dynamic and complex interrelationships between cancer and aging that affect cancer nursing care.

4 It is imperative that oncology nurses intervene to prevent or minimise the unique age-specific sequelae of cancer and its management.

5 It is imperative that oncology nurses integrate comprehensive gerontologic assessment into the nursing care of older adults.

6 It is imperative that oncology nurses assess the availability and capability of the support networks of elderly patients and their significant others.

7 It is imperative that oncology nurses increase communication with colleagues about older adults with cancer to enhance problem-solving in a variety of settings and at different points along the cancer continuum.

8 It is imperative that oncology nurses consider age-related factors that affect learning and performance of self-care activities related to the cancer experience.

9 It is imperative that oncology nurses maximise their advocacy role in ethical decision-making relative to quality of life of elderly people with cancer.

10 It is imperative that oncology nurses recognise the effects of health care policy on the nursing care of older adults who have or who are at risk for cancer.

chronological age is not a reliable indicator of frailty and therefore cannot be used for selecting cancer treatment. Instead we should ask, it is suggested, 'Which patients would benefit from which treatments?'[16] In the USA cancer in the elderly has been called the forgotten priority[14] and the elderly with cancer the forgotten minority[17] (though whether older people with cancer are really a minority or not depends on how you define 'elderly').

In 1983 Begg and Carbone[18] analysed 19 studies of chemotherapy for advanced cancer (lung, colon and rectum, stomach, sarcoma, head and neck, melanoma, and ovary) to compare elderly patients (aged 70 and over) with other patients in terms of toxicity, response rate, and survival. They report that the overall picture of toxic reactions 'is one of great similarity between the elderly and non-elderly patients'; differences were observed in haematological reactions with some cancers. They concluded that response rates and survival curves were also similar in both groups. It has been suggested elsewhere that the importance of these findings for clinical practice is limited by the fact that the older patients involved 'may be generally healthier than elderly patients at large'.[19]

Begg and Carbone[18] point out that the older patients in their study were comparable with the younger ones in terms of performance status and other measures. The point is that the value of chronological age alone in the treatment decision-making process for cancer is being put in question. Begg and Carbone did find that with methotrexate and methyl-CCNU the older group of patients experienced significantly more haematological toxicity. They point out that as methotrexate is excreted by the kidneys and renal function in older people is known to be less effective, this finding is unsurprising. Their view overall is that elderly patients should be approached in the same way as younger ones in terms of clinical trials and chemotherapy, unless they have unusual medical problems. Exceptions to this principle include treatment with chemotherapeutic agents that are known to produce greater toxic effects in older patients, and cancers that are known to affect older people differently. Older patients with leukaemia, for example, appear to be more likely to die if they experience sepsis during remission-induction therapy.[20] They also point out that the physiological changes

occurring with age may affect the metabolism or excretion of a drug following administration.

Walsh et al.[20] addressed the subject of chemotherapy in the elderly in 1989. On this occasion, they review the literature in which older patients treated with chemotherapy are compared with younger ones. They point out that some studies have shown that the elderly are less likely than younger patients to receive effective treatment, and that in particular there are indications that the elderly are less likely to receive chemotherapy as part of a course of treatment, even if differences in disease stage and comorbidity are taken into account. They add, however, that their own work suggests that older patients are at a significantly higher risk of haematological side-effects with actinomycin-D, doxorubicin, methotrexate, methyl-CCNU, vinblastine, and etoposide. They conclude that 'a number of drugs have been implicated in causing more frequent episodes of toxicity in older patients' and that there is a 'well-documented difference in response rates between younger and older leukaemia patients':

> However, these appear to be the exceptions. In general, chronological age is only a weak predictor of the likelihood of toxicity or non-response among chemotherapy recipients. Furthermore, what little predictive capacity chronological age does possess is attributable not to the impact of increased age alone, but to the effects of other patient characteristics that often, but not always, accompany longevity.[20]

Newcombe and Carbone[21] interviewed 628 women recently diagnosed with breast or colorectal cancer. Their analysis compared women aged less than 65 with women aged 65 and over. Their findings include:

- no apparent difference in percentage of women with breast cancer receiving surgery as primary therapy
- that women aged 65 and over received radiotherapy and adjuvant chemotherapy for breast cancer less often than the younger age group
- similar proportions of women in both age groups received surgery and radiotherapy for colorectal cancer
- chemotherapy for colorectal cancer was less common in the older age group
- older women were less likely to be referred to an oncologist.

Scalliet *et al.*[22] point out that little is known about tolerance of and indications for radiotherapy in the elderly, though there is no suggestion that age has a major influence on tolerance. They add that, on the basis of the small amount of research evidence available, age does not appear to be related to complications following radiotherapy. The fractionation of radiotherapy in the elderly may be a useful therapeutic avenue to explore as a means of reducing travelling time and increasing rest periods; however, little is currently known about the adverse effects of hypofractionation (larger daily doses to allow more free time) in elderly patients.[22]

In a review of the research literature on surgery and the older cancer patient (65 years and over), Patterson[23] argues that old age alone should not exclude patients from surgery, but that candidates for surgery should be carefully selected and comorbid conditions carefully managed throughout the perioperative period:

> It is not because of age that patients need preoperative attention, but rather because the aged have more deficits and illnesses in relation to their cancer.

They suggest, for example, that with careful planning bowel resections can be carried out in elderly patients with low levels of mortality and morbidity. It is, however, acknowledged that the risks are greater with emergency resections.

In the USA, 25% of new cases of cervical cancer occur in women aged 65 and over. Despite this, about 50% of women in this age group have not received a smear test in the last 3 years.[10] Mor *et al.*,[9] who analysed data from a sample of over 1000 patients with breast lung and colorectal cancer, argue that:

> . . . age-related differences in the receipt of post-diagnostic treatment suggest a deep and pervasive social 'ageism' influencing who receives aggressive treatment.

It has been suggested, however, that age-related differences in the treatment of breast cancer could be due not to age bias, but to differences in what constitutes the most appropriate therapy at a given age: there is little evidence, for example, that chemotherapy benefits older patients with breast cancer,[24] so it should be predictable that fewer older women will receive this treatment. Conversely, if a treatment is known to benefit patients across the age groups, we would expect it to be provided equally if no age bias exists. Guadagnoli *et al.*[24] tested a number of hypotheses of this kind in a study of the treatment of early stage breast cancer in nearly 750 newly diagnosed post-menopausal women. They concluded that 'the use of adjuvant systemic therapy reflects what is known about treatment efficacy'; for example, in women with node-negative disease, no association between age and the use of hormonal therapy (tamoxifen) was found, but there was a negative association between age and likelihood of receiving chemotherapy. They add, however, that:

> . . . although the state of the art suggests that older patients are less likely than younger patients to benefit from chemotherapy, we may not yet have used the best designs to test the efficacy of this therapy in older patients.

Care issues

While there are arguments for and against the presence of an age bias or 'ageism' in the treatment of older people with cancer, there is little doubt that the elderly are the focus of prejudice in our society. The negative view of ageing, it is suggested,[25] springs from the view that growing old involves a series of decrements or losses, so that ageing becomes a process of decay affecting us physically, emotionally, intellectually, and socially. Gross[25] draws our attention to work that suggests that old people experience discrimination socially, in the family, and in employment because they are treated as dull, sickly, or inflexible. In a culture that idealises youth, older adults tend to be viewed uniformly as deteriorating physically and mentally, as being socially isolated, and as being decreasingly productive members of society.[3]

There is perhaps a temptation to associate increasing age with a gradual withdrawing from full citizenship, with all the rights and autonomy that implies; we may on occasion be led into a kind of mental and emotional discounting manoeuvre in our relationships with the elderly that causes us to have fewer expectations and to be less intense in our efforts. We may unconsciously offer less. We can be guilty of behaving as if the rights of older people are somehow easier to ignore: it is hard to imagine, for example, details of diagnosis and prognosis being withheld from younger or middle-aged adults in the way that they sometimes are from older people.

It would be comforting to believe that we have eliminated age bias or ageism in our care of older people, but unfortunately it probably still exists. Sharp[26] argues that elderly patients, particularly those with mental health problems, do not match our idea of the 'ideal' patient: the traditional sick role involves being motivated to get better and co-operating with medical and nursing staff, and patients who do not meet our expectations in this respect are more likely to be disliked, and perhaps represent a threat to our sense of professional authority and therapeutic competence. In 1991 Reed and Bond[27] wrote that:

> . . . the nursing care of long-stay elderly patients in hospital remains a routinised work system within a cure-dominated health care ethos. When cure is not possible it is patients who have 'failed the system'; it is they who are 'hopeless' cases and who 'block beds'.

Nursing, they imply, is partly responsible for perpetuating this system because instead of becoming 'dynamic and self-governing', it still takes its lead from the dominant medical ethos, is dominated by the idea of 'getting through the work', and treats patients as 'work objects'. In their study of nurses' assessments of elderly patients in hospital, Reed and Bond[27] observed nursing activities in a long-term care ward. They comment that assessments:

> . . . did not result in proposals for change in the way the patient was nursed. Changes proposed concerned how the existing routine of care could be implemented more effectively.

They conclude that aiming for cure or rehabilitation in the continuing care setting or with chronically ill patients, essentially the goals of the medical model of care, is of limited benefit to patients and contrary to nurses' own beliefs. They highlight the need for nursing to re-evaluate and make explicit its values for a range of care settings, to acknowledge patients' abilities and the importance of partnership in care, and raise the question of the type of nursing needed to replace the cure-dominated medical model.

Latimer[28] argues that 'older people' as a category is both absurd *and* inescapable: all of us, she says, are part of the process of creating this distinction, in part because of our fear of ageing, which we see as a series of physical losses rather than spiritual gains. She uses an example from her research in

health care to illustrate how we may use the idea that ill-health in old age is biologically inevitable to ease our sense of responsibility for someone: in the light of biological inevitability we see not 'an acutely ill person' but 'an old person' whose illness is outside the domain of the medical ward'.

Latimer tells us that Jessie, who is 91 and has had a massive stroke, is 'refigured' by the ward sister:

> Jessie is . . . put 'outside' one division, a class of patient (the person who is acutely ill), and into another class (that of old person whose difficulties are chronic and the consequence of a natural order of things, a progressive deterioration and decline) . . . there is no possibility of a heroic story of recovery . . . Jessie is a 'blocked bed'.

Koch[29] interviewed 14 patients in her study of nursing care of the elderly in a large (1000-bed) NHS hospital. She identified two common themes in their accounts: 'routine geriatric style' and 'segregation'. Routine geriatric style, a term first coined in the 1970s,[30] is used by Koch to describe the conveyor belt approach to care that she identified in the accounts she collected from patients. Patients, she says, were deprived of care, 'left unwashed, unsafe, and unfed', and felt that they could not draw attention to these issues for fear of making the situation worse. In effect, care was used as a means of controlling patients, of establishing non-negotiable terms for day-to-day life:

> . . . needs became reduced to nursing practices based on hygiene, pressure area care, medications and food, but even these needs were scarcely met.

People, Koch writes, were treated as objects. One patient with metastatic cancer is quoted as saying:

> I am sitting out of bed but I don't want to be here. They just sit everyone out of bed. I have to sit here until they put me back and I don't know when . . . I just sit here until they put me back to bed. I insisted to be put back yesterday, I was so ill. I was told off, they said 'don't dictate to me!'. I said I want to be put to bed, I feel very, very ill. Then sister came.

Koch also feels that patients resented being stereotyped as old (by having the letter 'G' for 'geriatric' on their case notes, for example). 'Old', she says, represented a state of decline and infirmity; patients rejected the idea of incapacity or senility that 'old' evoked. There was unhappiness about being segregated into age-defined groups which,

Koch says, reinforces the standardisation and depersonalisation of care. In fact, she argues, segregation and routine geriatric style go together, one reinforcing the other.

Koch believes that an important reason for the development of a distinctive way of caring for old people is the tendency (that she traces back to the French philosopher Descartes) to view individuals as a combination of mind-in-body, the mind contained within but distinct from the machine-like body:

> . . . the machine or body can be entered, studied, and tampered with in order to be repaired. The body is the object of inquiry. The patient as subject fades into the background and becomes a biomedical object susceptible to medical intervention.

The machine-like body is seen as wearing out over time: Koch's implication seems to be that our age bias or ageism is connected to this, the idea that the older you are the more likely you are to be broken down, no longer productive, and therefore inconsequential. She recommends that geriatric medicine, with its focus on the health of the older person, and gerontology, with its focus on the nature of ageing, should be brought closer together to help to dispel stereotypical and ageist notions; nurses, she says, should examine ageing, dispel its negative images, and 'promote the individual's health status rather than chronological age'.[29]

Harper[31] believes that only acceptance of the mental and physical changes associated with later life as a 'normal and respectable component of the human condition' will enable us to resolve 'the current tension between spirit and body'. As a feminist, she argues that the stigma attached to loss of control over the body is related to the dominance of male notions and expectations of control. In adulthood, she says, women are not accustomed to direct control of bodily functions such as menstruation, lactation, and childbirth. 'It can thus be argued', she says:

> . . . that if absolute control of the body, defined by male experience, was not the overarching notion of adulthood, then the natural lack of control associated with extreme late life would not be so stigmatised.

Feminism, she concludes, may help us to develop a new concept of later life:

> . . . which fully accepts loss of bodily control [and] rejects the stigmatisation of the declining body.

Corner[32] has drawn attention to the importance to nursing care of assessing the physical vulnerability or frailty of the elderly patient with cancer. She identifies a series of indices of frailty to guide assessment, measure outcome, and provide goals for rehabilitation and recovery (see Figure 33.1).

In the same way that chronological age per se is a poor basis for decisions about treatment, the assumption that there is a simple relationship between increasing age and frailty is a poor starting point for planning nursing care. Wenger[33] believes that we expect a high level of dependency in people aged 80 and over and that those who survive into their 80s are seen as a problem. While acknowledging that there are more people in their 80s who are ill and impaired, she argues on the basis of her interviews with people in this age group that only a small proportion are acutely dependent at any one time:

> Some are affected for a short period only; others are never acutely dependent. Most of the over-80s are competent and relatively independent even though impaired.[33]

Conversely, in their study of 1712 patients with cancer aged 65 and over, Havlik et al.[34] found that major comorbidities such as hypertension, cardiac arrhythmias, congestive cardiac failure, and arthritis were quite common, though these results are acknowledged to be preliminary. Rowe and Bradley[35] point out that a decline in cardiac, renal, and respiratory function begins in young adulthood and reaches a plateau at the age of 80 or 90, though levels of haemoglobin and testosterone, for example, are not thought to decline with age.

In 1992 the Oncology Nursing Society in the USA published a position paper comprising ten statements on cancer and ageing (see Table 33.1).[3] It is an important paper, possibly the only one of its kind to date, which provides a focus for debate about a developing body of knowledge and practice guidelines for the care of older people with cancer. In its paper the Oncology Nursing Society highlights some of the obstacles that stand in the way of high-quality nursing care for older people with cancer, in particular our limited understanding of the relationship between

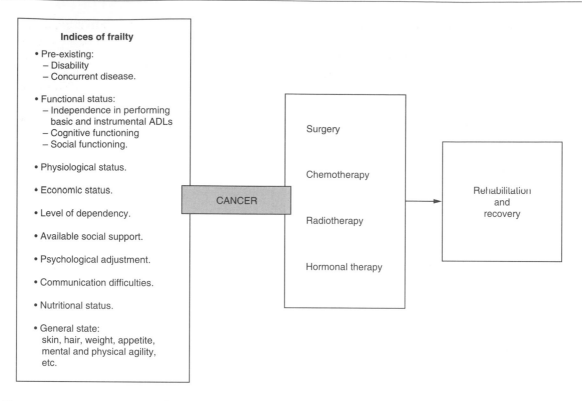

Figure 33.1 Indices of frailty (reproduced with the permission of Blackwell Science Ltd from Corner J. (1993). Some reflections on frailty in elderly patients with cancer. *European Journal of Cancer Care* **2**, 5–9).[32]

cancer and ageing, and our lack of knowledge about the needs of older patients in terms of prevention and early detection, treatment, and rehabilitation.

The issue of prevention and early detection (secondary prevention) for older people has received considerable attention over the years.[36–38] Screening to detect asymptomatic disease or asymptomatic premalignant disease is one of the strategies employed to reduce the prevalence of a disease: the stage of a cancer at diagnosis has an important effect on treatment and survival, so early detection is crucial for all patients including the elderly, who tend to present with more advanced disease. Dellefield[36] identifies three areas of potential difficulty in the early detection of cancer in older people: illness behaviour in the elderly, behaviours of health care providers, and health care system issues. She points out that older people may not be aware that they are a high-risk group, may fear cancer treatment and the consequences of the

disease, and that there may be physical and social factors making it more difficult for older people to access screening facilities. Health care providers may themselves have prejudices about old people and be less likely to act decisively and positively in this area of health care, and health services are typically orientated towards symptomatic disease and cure rather than prevention and early detection. Screening of older people may be complicated by issues relating to the presentation of disease. Weinrich *et al.*[37] suggest that cancer symptoms in the elderly may be general (confusion, weakness, or weight loss, for example) rather than specific, and that elderly people may not realise that a symptom like rectal bleeding is sometimes caused by cancer, and is not always due to haemorrhoids. Dellefield[36] concludes that nurses can make a contribution to reducing cancer morbidity and mortality in older people by actively promoting early detection. Some aspects of screening are, however, a matter of national government policy. In the UK, breast cancer is the most common cause of death from cancer in elderly women, yet women aged 65 and over are not invited for screening (though screening is available on demand). Evidence for the benefits of screening in terms of reduction in mortality for women aged 65–69 years[39] is cited, and though it is argued that for women older than 69 years there is 'no direct scientific evidence that screening mammography will decrease mortality for breast cancer',[39] further trials are needed to provide a definitive answer. In the meantime in the USA, annual clinical breast examination and 2-yearly mammography have been recommended for women aged 65–74 and for women aged 75 and older whose health and life expectancy are good.[38] All women over the age of 65 are advised to continue monthly breast self-examination and to visit their doctor or nurse for further assistance.

McCaffrey Boyle *et al.*[3] summarise the physical and physiological changes that may impair our bodies' various protective mechanisms in later life. Such impairments, they point out, lead to clinical situations that place the older cancer patient at increased risk. They highlight a series of age-related conditions that may have both malignant and non-malignant causes, which are of particular importance for planning and assessment of care, namely: high risk of falls, acute confusion, poor nutrition, alterations in bowel habit and micturition, impairment of the integrity of tissue, skin, and mucous membranes, and alterations in sleep patterns. Initial assessments should therefore:

> . . . establish the natural history of symptoms such as pain, fatigue, diarrhoea, constipation, nausea and vomiting, sleep disorders and so on . . . interventions should be planned to treat or preferably prevent such side-effects.[11]

The effective management of pain in older patients with cancer may be compromised by misconceptions about their pain sensitivity, response to opioid analgesics, and pain tolerance, and there may be a risk of undertreatment, especially if patients are confused or unable to provide detailed information for assessment.[40] In this area of assessment, as in many involving older people, multi-dimensional functional assessment, encom-

passing activities and social, psychological, and physical functioning, is an important source of information about the effects of illness and treatment on a person's life, and can guide diagnosis and choice of intervention, as well as predict outcome and monitor change over time.[3] Constipation is a very common side-effect of treatment with opioid analgesics and should be treated prophylactically and closely monitored.[40] Redmond and Aapro[11] say that clinical experience suggests that fatigue may have a greater impact on the elderly; and they note that mucositis in the elderly with cancer is more severe and has been associated with a mortality rate of 20% in one study of patients aged over 65 treated with 5-fluorouracil and leucovorin. They add that adequate fluid replacement is essential when diarrhoea occurs with mucositis.

As an area of specialisation, the relationship of cancer and ageing and the care and treatment of older people with cancer is still in its infancy. A settled position has yet to be achieved on the criteria for medical decisions which:

> . . . involve a delicate balance between limited life expectancy, risk of treatment complications, and the overall effects of cancer and cancer treatment on the patient's quality of life . . . In elderly cancer patients, life expectancy is a function of age, comorbidity, function, and cancer stage.[41]

At the same time, we must recognise that our perceptions of ageing may lead us to act as if those we categorise as old are less legitimate recipients of a full range of health care resources simply because of their chronological age. As the Oncology Nursing Society position paper[3] puts it:

> Although older adults constitute the majority of people with cancer, clinical trials and the most aggressive approaches to cancer prevention, diagnosis, and treatment have been, for the most part, devoted to younger, healthier subsets of patients with cancer. This discrepancy must be acknowledged and addressed.

References

1. Victor C.R. (1991). *Health and Health Care in Later Life.* Milton Keynes: Open University Press.
2. Burnside I. (1990). The frail elderly: those 85 and over. *Nursing Administration Quarterly* **14**, 37–41.

3. McCaffrey Boyle D., Engelking C., Blesch K.S., Dodge J., Sarna L. and Weinrich S. (1992). Oncology Nursing Society position paper on cancer and ageing: the mandate for oncology nursing. *Oncology Nursing Forum* **19**, 913–933.

4. Monfardini S., Aapro M., Ferrucci V., Scalliet P. and Fentiman I. (1993). Commission of the European Communities 'Europe Against Cancer' Programme European School of Oncology Advisory Report: Cancer Treatment in the Elderly. *European Journal of Cancer* **29A**, 2325–2330.

5. Miller B. (1994). Stat bite: cancer mortality by age. *Journal of the National Cancer Institute* **86**, 257.

6. Cancer Research Campaign (1992). *Factsheet 5.1: Cancer in the European Community.* London: Cancer Research Campaign.

7. Office for National Statistics (1992). *Cancer Statistics: Registrations.* London: Government Statistical Service.

8. Fentiman I., Tirelli U., Monfardini S., Schneider M., Fersten J.F. and Aapro M. (1990). Cancer in the elderly: why so badly treated? *Lancet* **335**, 1020–1022.

9. Mor V., Masterson-Allen S., Goldberg R.J., Cummings F.J., Glicksman A.S. and Fretwell M.D. (1985). Relationship between age at diagnosis and treatments received by cancer patients. *Journal of the American Geriatric Society* **33**, 585–589.

10. Dodd G.D. (1991). Cancer control and the older person. *Cancer* **68**, 2493–2495.

11. European School of Oncology Scientific Updates (1997). In Redmond, K. and Aapro M.S. (eds.) *Cancer in the Elderly.* Amsterdam: Elsevier.

12. Holmes F.F. (1989). Clinical evidence for a change in tumour aggressiveness with age. *Seminars in Oncology* **16**, 34–40.

13. Hahn D.E.E., Bergman L., van Dam F.S.A.M. and Aaronson N.K. (1994). In Fentiman I.S. and Monfardini S. (eds.) *Cancer in the Elderly.* Oxford: Oxford University Press.

14. McCaffrey Boyle D. and Engelking C. (1993). Cancer in the elderly: the forgotten priority. *European Journal of Cancer Care* **2**, 101–107.

15. Faithfull S. (1994). Negative perceptions. *Nursing Times* **90**, 62–64.

16. Yancik R. and Ries M.S. (1994). Cancer in older persons. *Cancer* **74**, 1995–2003.

17. McCaffrey Boyle D. (1996). *Cancer in the Elderly: The Forgotten Minority. Symptom Management Issues in Cancer Nursing.* Philadelphia, PA: Smith Kline Beecham.

18. Begg C.B. and Carbone P.P. (1983). Clinical trials and drug toxicity in the elderly: the experience of the Eastern Cooperative Oncology Group. *Cancer* **52**, 1986–1992.

19. Blesch K.S. (1988). The normal physiological changes of ageing and their impact on the response to cancer treatment. *Seminars in Oncology Nursing* **4**, 178–188.

20. Walsh S.J., Begg C.B. and Carbone P.P. (1989). Cancer chemotherapy in the elderly. *Seminars in Oncology* **16**, 66–75.

21. Newcombe P.A. and Carbone P.P. (1993). Cancer treatment and age: patient perspectives. *Journal of the National Cancer Institute* **85**, 1580–1584.

22. Scalliet P., van der Schuren E. and van den Weyngaert D. (1994). In Fentiman I.S. and Monfardini S. (eds.) *Cancer in the Elderly.* Oxford: Oxford University Press.

23. Patterson W.B. (1989). Surgical issues in geriatric oncology. *Seminars in Oncology* **16**, 57–65.

24. Guadagnoli E., Shapiro C., Gurwitz J.H. *et al.* (1997). Age-related patterns of care: evidence against ageism in the treatment of early-stage breast cancer. *Journal of Clinical Oncology* **15**, 2338–2344.

25. Gross R.D. (1992). *Psychology: The Science of Mind and Behaviour.* London: Hodder & Stoughton.

26. Sharp T. (1990). Old and in the way. *Nursing Standard* **14**, 54–55.

27. Reed J. and Bond S. (1991). Nurses' assessment of elderly patients in hospital. *International Journal of Nursing Studies* **28**, 55–64.

28. Latimer J. (1997). Figuring identities: older people, medicine and time. In Jamieson A., Harper S. and Victor C. (eds) *Critical Approaches to Ageing and Later Life.* Milton Keynes: Open University Press.

29. Koch T. and Webb C. (1996). The biomedical construction of ageing: implications for nursing care of older people. *Journal of Advanced Nursing* **23**, 954–959.

30. Baker D. (1983). 'Care' in the geriatric ward: an account of two styles of nursing. In Wilson-Barrett J. (ed.) *Nursing Research: Ten Studies in Patient Care.* Chichester: Wiley.

31. Harper S. (1997). In Jamieson A., Harper S. and Victor C. (eds.) *Critical Approaches to Ageing and Later Life.* Milton Keynes: Open University Press.

32. Corner J. (1993). Some reflections on frailty in elderly patients with cancer. *European Journal of Cancer Care* **2**, 5–9.

33. Wenger G.C. (1986). What do dependency measures measure? Challenging assumptions. In Phillipson C., Bernard M. and Strang P. (eds.) *Dependency and Interdependency in Old Age: Theoretical Perpetives and Policy Alternatives.* Croom Helm, NH.

34. Havlik R.J., Yancik R., Long S., Ries L. and Edwards B. (1994). The National Institute on Ageing and the National Cancer Institute SEER Collaborative Study on Comorbidity and Early Diagnosis of Cancer in the Elderly. *Cancer* **74**, 2101–2106.

35. Rowe J.W. and Bradley E.C. (1983). The elderly cancer patient: pathophysiological considerations. In Yancik R. (ed.) *Perspectives on Prevention and Treatment of Cancer in the Elderly.* New York: Raven Press.

36. Dellefield M.E. (1988). Informational needs and approaches for early cancer detection in the elderly. *Seminars in Oncology Nursing* **4**, 156–168.
37. Weinrich S.P., Blesch K.S., Dickson G.W., Nussbaum J.S. and Watson E.J. (1989). Timely detection of colorectal cancer in the elderly: implications of the ageing process. *Cancer Nursing* **13**, 170–176.
38. Costanza M.E. (1994). Issues in breast cancer screening in older women. *Cancer* **74**, 2009–2015.
39. Fletcher A. (1995). Breast cancer screening: remember older women. *Geriatric Medicine* **25**, 11–12.
40. Sheehan D.C. and Forman W.B. (1997). Symptomatic management of the older person with cancer. *Clinics in Geriatric Medicine* **13**, 203–219.
41. Bennahum D.A., Forman W.B., Vellas B. and Albarede J.L. (1997). Life expectancy, comorbidity, and quality of life: a framework of reference for medical decisions. *Clinics in Geriatric Medicine* **13**, 33–53.

CHAPTER THIRTY-FOUR

The needs of people from minority ethnic groups

Veronica (Nicky) Thomas

A diagnosis of cancer and the subsequent treatment are the source of much distress and suffering for those afflicted. Culture, beliefs, attitudes, and knowledge significantly affect how people face the problems they encounter. The incidence of cancer is relatively low in ethnic minority groups; nevertheless, cancer is still a major cause of death in these groups. In addition, there are significant numbers in the vulnerable age group for cancer (aged 55 and above),[1] and this means that there will be a significant increase in demand on medical services. Although recognised as a high priority, little research has been done to identify the needs of people from minority ethnic groups.

The experiences of people with cancer from ethnic minority groups have received little attention in nursing textbooks or in oncology literature. The aim here is to highlight specific psychosocial factors that are likely to influence illness behaviour and response to treatment. Knowledge of these culturally based variables should help nurses to organise care more sensitively, and to suggest ways in which needs can be met more efficiently. Nursing people with cancer from black and ethnic minority groups requires flexibility in attitudes, as well as a degree of culturally specific knowledge. Their physical nursing needs do not differ significantly from the majority patient group.

Terminology

The terms 'black' and 'ethnic minority' are used here to refer to all members of minority racial groups in Britain who have different ethnic origin, and cultural and religious beliefs from the majority white population. Although the term 'majority group' is used to refer to the long-established white population, it is recognised that this group represent a multi-ethnic and multi-national population.[2]

Cancer in ethnic minority patients

Epidemiological data point to considerable ethnic differences in mortality from different cancer sites. For example, cancer of the oral cavity and pharynx is higher among those born in the Indian subcontinent, whereas cancer of the cervix, stomach, and lymphatic tissue appears to be high for the population born in the Caribbean.[3] Very few studies have directly examined exposure to cancer risk factors, although research on smoking suggests that this behaviour is negligible among South Asian females.[4] Donaldson and Clayton[5] carried out research that suggests that betel nut chewing among some South Asian populations may be related to the high incidence on mouth cancer, either through the carcinogenic effect of the betel nut itself or through the combined effect of tobacco and betel nut.

Researchers attempting to examine the uptake of cancer prevention services have found ethnic differences in their utilisation. For example, studies on cytology and breast screening have shown that there have been low rates of uptake in inner cities among lower socio-economic groups and ethnic minorities.[4,6] There are also inter-ethnic differences in the extent to which minorities display preventive behaviour. For example, Baxter[7] found that, on the whole, Afro-Caribbean women were more likely to have had cervical smears on their own initiative. They also showed a clearer understanding and were more knowledgeable about breast self-examination and cervical smears. Explanations for low uptake rates for these services have focused on lack of knowledge, and language and cultural barriers.

American studies that have looked at the outcome of cancer have all been conclusive in confirming that the black and ethnic population consistently present with advanced disease and consequently have much lower survival rates.[8–10] For example, a 5-year breast cancer survival study during 1981–1986 revealed a 76% survival rate for white women compared to 63% for African-American women.[10]

The literature tends to concentrate on the diagnostic stage and clinical aspects of treatment, rather than on the experiences of people from ethnic minority groups. However, a study commissioned by CancerLink[7] carried out in central Manchester has provided some insights by exploring the support and information needs of these people with cancer and their carers. The findings revealed a lack of knowledge about the existence of services and reasons for preventive action, communication difficulties, and dissatisfaction with community and hospital-based services. Similarly, another study looking at palliative care service usage by minority groups in Leicester revealed that racial discrimination and poor communication were responsible for considerable amounts of distress.[11]

Attitudes towards cancer

Cancer is a greatly feared diagnosis in society as a whole. Cassileth[12] has argued that cancer is invested with such special meaning that it invokes a unique dread, to the extent that the word 'oncology' was coined in an attempt to avoid frightening the patient. Cancer is perceived as a stigmatised disease and therefore people feel uncomfortable in its presence. One reason for this is cancer's shame-inducing element.[13] Lazare[13] categorised stigmatised diseases in the following ways.

1. They offend others through sight, odour or contagion.

2. They are associated with low social status or poor living conditions.
3. They involve sexual or excretory organs.
4. They are believed to be caused by behaviours that are perceived by others to be weak, stupid, immoral or manifestations of personal failure.

The stigma associated with cancer has diminished over time because more is known about the aetiology; also advances in treatment have given rise to more effective interventions. Nevertheless, stigma exists in black and ethnic minority communities. For example, research has shown that 63% of African-Americans perceive a cancer diagnosis to be equivalent to a death sentence.[14] Bloom[14] also found that a similar proportion believed cancer to be contagious. In the UK, Baxter[7] assessed the knowledge, beliefs and attitudes towards cancer, its causes, prevention, prognosis, and cure among Afro-Caribbean, Asian and Chinese people in central Manchester. The results revealed that cancer is associated with death, incurability, contagion, and feelings of dread. Although cancer is equated with death, the perceived degradation and suffering were even more dreaded than death itself. Afro-Caribbean people were particularly concerned to be in control and to be aware of their surroundings when approaching death. For this reason, they may reject narcotic drugs. Most people believed that cure meant marginally increasing the quality and length of life. Cancer of the internal organs (e.g. lungs) was seen as less treatable than more obvious locations, such as the skin.

In both Italy and Japan there are also strong associations between cancer and death.[15,16] In these countries, giving a patient a diagnosis of cancer is seen as removing hope[17] and therefore represents social death.[15] These beliefs guide medical practices because Japanese doctors do not usually disclose cancer diagnosis to their patients.[16,18,19] Japanese physicians believe that if people knew of their cancer diagnosis they would give up hope and die before too long. A family member is usually told and he or she colludes with the physician by acting 'normally' and by giving a false diagnosis and assurances of recovery. Ohnuki-Tierney[16] provides an example of a man who accidentally discovered his diagnosis and died very soon thereafter.

In a more recent study, Boston[20] looked at the relevance of cultural orientation within a cancer education programme in Canada and found that the word cancer caused a degree of discomfort for Chinese families. During many of the family interviews 'illness' had to be substituted for 'cancer' in order to avoid distress. This need to be protected from the harsh reality of a cancer diagnosis is seen in many other cultures, where physicians and families shield people with cancer from the truth.[21] In the UK and North America, truth telling is considered to be ethically correct and to demonstrate respect for patients' autonomy. However, as Pellegrino[22] has argued, this notion of autonomy is not necessarily always beneficial and consequently it should not be imposed on everyone, irrespective of their cultural beliefs. Autonomy, he believes, also gives the right to delegate one's liberty when this fits one's own conception of beneficence. Such delegation of decision-making authority may be implicit or explicit, depending on the cultural ethos. In Japan, China, some parts of Italy, and other parts of the world, this delegation is culturally implicit.[22] Pellegrino[22] recognises that there are no guidelines available for truth telling or withholding; he does, however, believe that to thrust the truth onto a patient who expects to be buffered is a 'gratuitous and harmful misinterpretation of the moral foundation for the respect of autonomy'. Physicians and nurses must get to know people in their care and their families well enough fully to appreciate their wish for the truth and in this way we will be more likely to preserve autonomy and beneficence.

Since attitudes to health and illness are culturally determined, the model of illness held by people from minority ethnic groups may be quite different to that of the health care professionals caring for them. In many cultures cancer is perceived to be an organic disease, which has spiritual causes such as an evil curse,[23] or it may be seen as punishment for an earlier wrong doing,[20,23] which may include incestuous acts and adultery. Because of this dual construction it is common for some ethnic groups to utilise traditional alternative remedies alongside Western medicine in an attempt to treat cancer. Boston,[20] for example, found that Chinese families considered herbal remedies and certain kinds of foods to be as valuable as the prescribed treatments being offered for cancer in Canada. Similarly, someone who is Nigerian and has cancer may

seek the help of traditional healers, particularly when Western medicine fails to 'cure' their cancer.[23] As Nwonga[23] has argued, the tendency to use alternative health care services when one medical system has failed transcends all cultures. Nurses should be aware of this tendency and adopt a non-judgemental approach when offering advice and support. They should provide information that will offer reassurance that the pain and other symptoms can be controlled. This will give relief and comfort because it provides a new and optimistic concept.[12]

Values and belief systems

In recent years, cross-cultural psychology has identified a number of differences that attempt to provide a framework for explaining culturally specific behaviours. Hofstede,[24] Lin[25] and Rao[26] draw comparisons between the Western and Eastern view of self. According to these theorists, the Western view emphasises independence, self-sufficiency, assertiveness, and competition. Self-fulfilment is dependent on achievement and verbal direct communication is valued. The Eastern view, in contrast, attaches great importance to interdependence, harmony, and co-operation in relationships.

Since values and beliefs influence relationships, it is not surprising that Eastern minority families are organised on an extended family basis. In traditional Chinese families loyalties to parents take precedence over loyalties to spouse and children,[27] and all decision making and problem solving are done by parental authority, which is usually undisputed by younger family members.[20]

Afro-Caribbeans have traditionally held strong religious views and rely very much on these beliefs in times of stress and crisis. In the UK, an anthropological study of beliefs about death[28] revealed that religion and religious beliefs among Afro-Caribbeans had an important role in 'enhancing a sense of belonging, which includes encouraging free expression of emotion'. The ability to express emotions freely is very important to Afro-Caribbeans and contrasts sharply with the more reserved 'stiff upper lip' British attitude. Similarly, an American study of black working classes[29] revealed that the competent families were the ones that retained strong religious Christian values, where biblical concepts determined thought patterns in individual and family lives.

The traditional Afro-Caribbean family is also organised along extended lines. It does, however, differ from Asian and Chinese families in that it encompasses not only those related by marriage or biology, but also many non-related members such as godparents and friends.[28,30]

According to Leininger,[31] effective solutions to health care problems are much more likely when the values and beliefs of patients are considered. In many cultures, illness is often managed within the family, whereas our approach to assessment is usually from an individual standpoint. As discussed earlier, many ethnic minority groups attach great importance to interdependence, harmony, and co-operation in relationships. This, in turn, will influence an individual's 'sick role' behaviour, causing them to be dependent. For example, research has found that nurses experience difficulties in coping with people from minority ethnic groups because of what they perceive to be unwillingness to participate in their own care.[32] Rawlings-Anderson[32] has argued that the rigid adherence to nursing models fostering independence can alienate patients.

Nurses may sometimes feel inadequate when caring for patients from cultures different to their own because, while they feel able to respect cultural differences, they have little knowledge of how these differences can impact on care.[32,33] In these situations, we need to listen sympathetically to what patients are trying to tell us, rather than attempting to impose our conceptual frameworks onto them.[34]

Field *et al.*[35] and Gunaratnum[36] are critical of health service delivery and provision in relation to minority ethnic groups, since too often insensitivity by professional staff results in an unthinking assumption that the white middle-class pattern is 'normal'. Recent approaches to overcome difficulties associated with such care have been criticised for taking a 'culturalist' approach; that is, the assumption that the needs of people from black and ethnic minority groups can be understood in terms of cultural and religious needs. This has resulted in the production of 'factfiles' and 'checklists' of the cultural and religious features of various minority groups[34] and practices around death and dying; for example, Neuberger's *Caring for Dying People of*

Different Faiths. These are inevitably reductionist, treating culture as a constant, unchanging entity, and create sweeping generalisations and stereotypes, rather than recognising variation and idiosyncrasy. They also fail to recognise issues of blending and generational change in multicultural societies such as the UK, North America, and Europe. Gunaratnum[36] argues that, paradoxically, these accounts may serve to create rather than prevent barriers to achievement of genuine, anti-racist multi-cultural caring services.

In her research in the palliative care setting, Gunaratnum[36] found evidence that information resources on cultural and religious practices reinforced professionals' tendency to understand the care of people from black and ethnic minority groups in terms of 'getting it right' or 'getting it wrong', rather than developing genuine sensitivity to and accommodation of individual preference or engaging with personal difference and choice. Gunaratnum[36] argues that these checklists are:

> . . . implicated in mobilising cultural and religious prescriptions as elaborate smokescreens, which de-humanise black and ethnic minority people . . . [while] institutions remain scandalously silent about racism and its effects on professional–user relationships.

Barriers to effective communication in cancer care

There are many barriers that prevent good quality care being delivered to ethnic minority groups; these include lack of knowledge about different needs and lack of education of health care professionals. When we share a common culture with people we can rely on a combination of knowledge, experiences, and empathy to select the appropriate caring response,[37] but it becomes more difficult when we are caring for people from cultures different to our own.[38]

In order to give a reasonable standard of care, nurses should engage in collaborative negotiations with their ethnic minority clients. Collaborative and negotiated care that fully integrates the person's view of care promotes compliance, and is also essential to the planning of treatment.[20] Nurse education has yet to meet the challenge of preparing practitioners to deliver effective and appropriate health care that responds to the needs of ethnic minority groups.

However, there is now compelling evidence to suggest that issues of race and racism and cultural and ethnic information should be an integral part of nursing education programmes, so that nursing care can be therapeutic and effective.[20,32,33,38]

Communication in cancer settings is hampered by the stigma and fear associated with the diagnosis, the treatment,[39] the complexity of the medical information itself and the uncertainty concerning the course of the disease.[40,41] Patients with different levels of comprehension[40] and different preferences for information,[42] and physicians' varying attitudes towards communication[41] are known to restrict the communication process further. Power imbalances between the health care professionals and the patient are said to be another important inhibiting factor.[43] Such disparity is likely to be considerably greater when these differences are increased by language, and socio-economic and cultural divergence. It is well documented that significant numbers of ethnic minority people belong to lower socio-economic classes[44,45] and speak little or no English.[45,46] These deficits naturally serve to exacerbate the problems.

Communication problems and ethnic minorities

There is a paucity of research that evaluates the communication needs of people from ethnic minority groups, but the little existing evidence does highlight some problems. For example, recent evaluation data from a communication skills training course for senior oncologists[47] have revealed that doctors experience great communication difficulties in their work with people who are black or from minority ethnic groups. Similarly, research carried out in the primary and preventive services demonstrates that their underutilisation occurs as a direct result of language barriers.[48–50] Two nurse researchers[32,33] looked at the experience of ward-based nursing care for people from ethnic minority groups in acute medical and surgical wards. Language difficulties were identified as major problems in both studies. Inability to communicate effectively was seen as hindering care and this is evident in the following statements from two of the nurse respondents in the Rawlings-Anderson[32] study:

I think perhaps the difficulty in communication – that's the most poignant thing. Because that influences everything you have to do with the patient and it can cause quite a lot of barriers between you and the patient [Respondent 16].

I don't feel that they get the same care as people who haven't got a language barrier. I think just because of the simple problems that come up – of not being able to express themselves and you not being able to express yourself to them – that's the big thing really, the language barrier [Respondent 4].

It has also been demonstrated that inadequate communication is associated with non-compliance in cancer patients[51] and can increase distress, which impedes recovery. Therefore, if nurses and doctors cannot communicate with people with cancer from black and ethnic minority groups because of cultural and language barriers, a sense of helplessness is created and the patient's psychological distress is likely to be made worse. Currently, no British research has addressed the level of psychological distress of people with cancer from black and ethnic minority groups; however, a recent study involving 117 newly diagnosed, white people with cancer revealed 30% of people experienced anxiety and/or depression serious enough to warrant psychological intervention.[52] In spite of the fact that the oncologist and the white people in this study apparently share a common language and culture, there was a breakdown in communication. This was evident in the finding that the majority of the oncologists underrated the level of distress and consequently felt satisfied with their handling of the interview.

Bilingual health advocates have been used successfully to improve communication and enhance personal control by alleviating anxiety and distress in other areas of health care such as mental health, midwifery, and community.[53–55] A particularly good example of the benefits of bilingual health advocacy is the recent introduction of health advocates within the community.

Bilingual health advocates have been employed at general practitioner (GP) surgeries in order to make primary health care services more responsive and more sensitive to the needs of people from minority ethnic communities.[56] A recent evaluation of the City and East London Family Health Services Authority[55] found a number of beneficial outcomes of health advocacy in the community. They compared GP schemes that employed advocates to those that do not and found significant differences in terms of improvement in the quality of user/professional communications, and improvement in the quality and uptake of health care services and empowerment of people who are ill.

Bilingual health advocates to overcome communication problems in cancer care

Evidence from the community and maternity services suggest that the use of advocates in the acute cancer setting is likely to improve the situation by empowering people, improving the relationships between doctors, nurses, and people with cancer, enhancing the quality of care delivered, and reducing the level of frustration and distress experienced by patients and staff. At present, the range of schemes operating within cancer care settings for people from ethnic community groups is extremely limited, but there is a real need for more widespread use of advocates in acute and palliative cancer care. A number of health authorities has made use of interpreters and family members in order to improve the communication deficits. However, the range and complexity of the problems encountered by nurses and doctors in communicating with ethnic minority patients require more informed intervention than interpreters can provide. Indeed, the Report on the Provision of Specialist Palliative Care for Black and Ethnic Minority Communities, commissioned by the National Council for Hospice and Specialist Palliative Care Services,[1] indicates concern about hospital interpreters because of a reluctance to inform people of their diagnosis and the inaccuracy of their interpretations. A comprehensive training is essential to prepare advocates sufficiently to deal with varied and complex communication issues, and to prepare them to cope appropriately with feelings generated by the stressful nature of the role.

In London a study evaluating the efficacy of bilingual health advocacy among Bengali cancer patients is in its final stages. This multi-disciplinary research (involving this author) aims to determine whether the introduction of appropriately trained advocates in oncology will be beneficial to Bengali cancer patients.

Nurses as patients' advocates

In his article of 1994, Penn[57] put forward an argument for nurses to adopt advocacy roles for people with cancer receiving palliative care. However, I would argue that there is also a need for nursing advocacy in the acute stages of cancer as well. In their review of the literature, Northouse and Northouse[41] identified loss of control as the single most important problem facing people with cancer. Loss of control refers to feelings of powerlessness and helpessness that result from an inability to predict or have an impact on events surrounding one's own illness. Information reduces uncertainty and therefore the provision of accurate information to the cancer patient is an important means of reducing helplessness and enhancing personal control.[58] Nurses can empower people and reduce helplessness by providing accurate jargon-free information. In situations where the person has difficulty understanding English, this process is more likely to be skilfully negotiated with a trained interpreter or health advocate.

Neufeld et al.[59] have shown that a nursing advocacy intervention can help women with gynaecological and breast cancer. In this study, nurses helped women to identify the types of questions to ask in cancer consultations and supported them in obtaining the information they needed. This was shown to enhance significantly the women's level of personal control and degree of involvement in their care. I believe that this type of strategy would be extremely effective for people from ethnic minority groups. Nurses frequently feel helpless and frustrated when they are faced with cultural and language barriers. This type of intervention is a tangible way in which nurses can reduce patients' obvious sense of helplessness, as well as their own feelings of inadequacy.

This discussion has thrown up many more questions than it has answered but, since cancer issues in ethnic minority groups are relatively unexplored areas, this is not surprising. The changes in health care increasingly require hospitals and community units to reassess the services they provide and to ensure that services are free from discrimination, and appropriate and accessible to people from ethnic and minority communities. In order to achieve this objective, a systematic assessment of needs is required. Little is known about the nature of the problems facing people with cancer from black and ethnic minority groups. Research is necessary as it is known that there are cultural differences in pain perception and response among ethnic groups in the UK.[60] More research is also required to address the health education needs of ethnic minority groups. Finally, research interventions such as bilingual health advocacy, which are likely to enhance personal control and reduce distress, should be evaluated in the context of acute cancer care.

The ability to provide support is a key feature of nursing and as such, support of people with cancer is an integral aspect of psychosocial care, irrespective of class, culture, religion, or gender. The importance of sharing relevant culturally based information in the cancer setting is crucial in the provision of adequate support and empowerment for ethnic minority cancer patients. Peters[61] has argued that empowering requires engaged listening. As already discussed, there are language deficits in ethnic minority groups that impede communication. However, in these circumstances, nurses should become more proactive and enlist the help of the hospital advocacy services team, interpreters or link workers to facilitate this process. Davis and Oberle[62] identified six dimensions of the supportive role of the nurse in palliative care, one of these being connecting or 'getting in touch' with the person. Establishing trust is crucial to this activity and, once trust is established, we can achieve a great deal, even in the absence of a common language. This kind of communication is immensely rewarding, as was revealed by some of the nurses in Rawlings-Anderson's[32] study, who experienced great satisfaction when they felt that they had established good relationships despite language difficulties.

Finally, the following is very pertinent to caring for ethnic minority patients:

> Nursing is intimate and particular. Expert communications skills help, and understanding the illness and disease provide unique ways of helping. But there is no way to guarantee the success of caring. Some patients are more accessible and understandable to some nurses than others are. The hallmark of an expert nurse is the recognition of her/his strengths and weaknesses and the ability to shape her or his practice towards strengths.[63]

Box 34.1: Useful information and addresses

The NHS Breast Cancer Screening Programme has developed health promotion resources for women from ethnic minority groups.

CancerLink offers information about all aspects of cancer to black and ethnic minority groups. They also have self-help and support services, which act as a resource to cancer self-help and support groups and individuals throughout the UK. They publish a range of booklets, fact sheets, and audio tapes about cancer in English, Hindi, and Bengali.

Meena Patel is Equal Opportunities Manager at CancerLink, and the address is 17 Britannia Street, London WC1X 9JN, UK.

Share is a national health race project funded by the Department of Health at the King's Fund Centre. The aim is to promote changes in service provision, to disseminate information that will enable good practice to be shared, and to increase awareness of services for black users.

Frances Presley is Information Officer at Share, whose address is King's Fund Centre, 11–13 Cavendish Square, London W1M 0AN, UK.

References

1. Hill D. and Penso D. (1995). *Improving Access to Hospice and Specialist Palliative Care Services by Members of Black and Ethnic Minority Communities.* London: National Council for Hospice and Specialist Palliative Care Services.
2. Smaj C. (1990). *Health Race and Ethnicity: Making Sense of the Evidence.* London: King's Fund Institute.
3. Balarajan R. and Raleigh V.S. (1993). *The Health of the Nation: Ethnicity and Health – A Guide for the NHS.* London: Department of Health.
4. Pilgrim S., Fenton S., Hughes T., Hine C. and Tibbs N. (1993). *The Bristol Black and Ethnic Minorities Health Survey Report.* Bristol: University of Bristol.
5. Donaldson L. and Clayton D. (1984). Occurrence of cancer in Asians and non-Asians. *Journal of Epidemiology and Community Health* 38, 203–207.
6. Hoare T. (1993). *Screening for Breast Cancer in North East and North West Thames.* RHA, pp. 84–89.
7. Baxter C. (1989). *Cancer Support and Ethnic Minority and Migrant Worker Community – A Report.* London: CancerLink.
8. McWorther W.P. and Mayer W.J. (1987). Black and white differences in type of initial breast cancer treatment and implications for survival. *American Journal of Public Health* 77, 1515–1517.
9. Bassett M.T. and Krieger N. (1986). Social class and black and white differences in breast cancer survival. *American Journal of Public Health* 76, 1400–1403.

10. Ries L.A., Hankey B.F. and Edwards B.K. (1990). *Cancer Statistics Review 1973–1987.* Bethesda, MA: US Department of Health and Human Services, Public Health Service, National Cancer Institute Publication 90-2789.

11. Haroon-Iqbal H., Field D., Parker H. and Iqbal Z. (1995). Palliative care services for ethnic groups in Leicester. *International Journal of Palliative Nursing* 1, 114–116.

12. Cassileth B.R. (1983). The evolution of oncology. *Perspectives in Biology and Medicine* 26, 3.

13. Lazare A. (1987). Shame and humiliation in the medical encounter. *Archives of Internal Medicine* 147, 1653–1658.

14. Bloom J.R., Hayes W.A., Saunders F. and Flatt S. (1987). Cancer awareness and secondary prevention in Black Americans: implications for intervention. *Family and Community Health* 10, 19–30.

15. Gordon D.R. (1990). Embodying illness, embodying cancer. *Culture, Medicine and Psychiatry* 14, 273–295.

16. Ohnuki-Tierney E. (1984). *Illness and Culture in Contemporary Japan.* Cambridge: Cambridge University Press.

17. Garro L. (1990). Culture, pain and cancer. *Journal of Palliative Care* 6, 34–44.

18. Feldman E. (1985). Medical ethics the Japanese way. *Hastings Centre Report* 15, 21–24.

19. Long S.O. and Long B.D. (1982). Curable cancers and fatal ulcers: attitudes towards cancer in Japan. *Social Science and Medicine* 16, 237–245.

20. Boston P. (1983). Culture and cancer: the relevance of cultural orientation within cancer education programmes. *European Journal of Cancer Care* 2, 72–76.

21. Surbonne A. (1992). Truth telling to the patient. *Journal of the American Medical Association* 268, 1661–1662.

22. Pellegrino E.D. (1992). Is truth telling a cultural artefact? *Journal of the American Medical Association* 268, 1734–1735.

23. Nwonga I.A. (1994). Traditional healers and perceptions of the causes and treatment of cancer. *Cancer Nursing* 17, 470–478.

24. Hofstede G. (1980). *Culture's Consequences: International Differences in Work Related Values.* Beverley Hills, CA: Sage.

25. Lin T.Y. (1986). Multiculturalism and Canadian psychiatry: opportunities and challenges. *Canadian Journal of Psychiatry* 16, 237–245.

26. Rao A.V. (1990). Indian and western psychiatry: a comparison. In Cox J.L. (ed.) *Transcultural Psychiatry.* London: Croom Helm, pp. 291–305.

27. Boston P. (1993). Culture and cancer: the relevance of cultural orientation within cancer education programmes. *European Journal of Cancer Care* 2, 72–76.

28. Goff S. (1994). Death and unbelonging: beliefs and practices around death of Afro-Caribbean people in London. Unpublished M.Sc. dissertation, Brunel University.

29. Lewis J.M. and Looney J.G. (1983). *The Long Struggle: Well Functioning Working Class Black Families.* New York: Brunner-Mazel.

30. Gopaul-McNicols S. (1993). *Working with West Indian Families.* New York: Guilford Press.

31. Leininger M.M. (1984). Transcultural nursing: an essential knowledge and practice field for today. *Canadian Nurse,* **December**, 41–57.

32. Rawlings-Anderson K. (1992). Nurses experiences of caring for ethnic minority clients. Unpublished M.Sc. dissertation, King's College, London.

33. Murphy K. (1990). Nurses' experiences of caring for ethnic minority clients. Unpublished M.Sc. dissertation, University of London.

34. Parsons C. (1990). Cross cultural issues in health care. In Reid J. and Trompf P. (eds.) *The Health of Immigrants in Australia.* Sidney: Harcourt Brace, pp. 108–153.

35. Field D., Hockley J. and Small N. (1997). Making sense of difference: death, gender and ethnicity in modern Britain. In Field D., Hockley J. and Small N. (eds.) *Death, Gender and Ethnicity.* London: Routledge.

36. Gunaratnum Y. (1997). Culture is not enough: a critique of multiculturalism in palliative care. In Field D., Hockey J. and Small N. (eds.) *Death, Gender and Ethnicity.* London: Routledge.

37. Henley A. (1986). Nursing care in a multiracial society. *Senior Nurse* 4, 18–20.

38. Thomas V.J. and Dines A. (1994). The health care needs of ethnic minority groups: are nurses playing their part? *Journal of Advanced Nursing* 20, 802–808.

39. Sontag S. (1978). *Illness as a Metaphor.* New York: Farrar, Strauss & Giroux.

40. Greenwald H.P. and Nevitt M.C. (1982). Physicians' attitude towards communication with cancer patients. *Social Science and Medicine* 16, 591–594.

41. Northouse P.G. and Northouse L.L. (1987). Communication and cancer: issues confronting patients, health care professionals and family members. *Journal of Psychosocial Oncology* 5, 17–46.

42. Cassileth B.R., Zupkis R.U. and Sutton-Smith M.S. (1980). Informed consent: why are goals imperfectly realised? *New England Journal of Medicine* 302, 866–900.

43. Davis H. and Fallowfield L. (1991). Counselling and communication in health care. The current situation. In Davis H. and Fallowfield L. (eds.) *Counselling and Communication in Health Care.* Chichester: Wiley.

44. Brown C. (1984). *Black and White Britain: The Third PSI Survey.* London: Gower.

45. MORI (1994). *Black and Minority Ethnic Groups in England. Health and Lifestyles.* London: Health Research Unit, Health Education Authority.

46. Stubbs M. (1985). *The Other Languages of England: Linguistic Minorities Project.* London: Routledge and Kegan Paul.

47. Fallowfield L. (1995). Communication training for senior oncologists. *Trends in Experimental and Clinical Medicine* **5**, 99–103.

48. Firdous R. and Bhopal R.S. (1989). Reproductive health of Asian women: a comparative study with hospital and community perspectives. *Public Health* **103**, 307–315.

49. Watt I., Howel D. and Lo L. (1993). The health care experience and health behaviour of the Chinese. A survey based in Hull. *Journal of Public Health Medicine* **15**, 129–136.

50. Naish J., Brown J. and Denton B. (1994). Intercultural consultations: investigation of the factors that deter non-English speaking women from attending general practitioners for cervical screening. *British Medical Journal* **309**, 1126–1128.

51. Maguire P., Tait A., Brooke M., Thomas C. and Selwood R. (1980). Effects of counselling on the psychiatric morbidity associated with mastectomy. *British Medical Journal* **281**, 1454–1456.

52. Ford S., Fallowfield L. and Lewis S. (1994). Can oncologists detect distress in their outpatients and how satisfied are they with their performance during bad news consultations? *British Journal of Cancer* **70**, 767–770.

53. MIND (National Association For Mental Health) (1992). *Guide to Advocacy in Mental Health. Empowerment in Action.* London: Mind Publications.

54. Cornwall J. and Gordon P. (1984). *An Experiment in Advocacy: The Hackney Multi-Ethnic Women's Project.* London: King's Fund Centre.

55. MORI (1994). *Evaluation of Bilingual Health Care Schemes in East London. Evaluation Study.* London: East London Consortium.

56. Baylav A. (1992). Equality of access: are we meeting the challenge. *Primary Health Care Management* **2**, 8–10.

57. Penn K. (1994). Patient advocacy in palliative care. *British Journal of Nursing* **3**, 40–42.

58. Miller S.M., Coombs C. and Stoddard E. (1989). Information, coping and control in patients undergoing surgery and stressful procedures. In Steptoe A. and Appels A. (eds.) *Stress Personal Control and Health.* Chichester: Wiley, pp. 107–129.

59. Neufeld K.R., Degner L.F. and Dick J.A.M. (1993). A nursing intervention strategy to foster patient involvement in treatment decisions. *Oncology Nursing Forum* **20**, 631–635.

60. Thomas V.J. and Rose F.D. (1991). Ethnic differences in the experience of pain. *Social Science and Medicine* **32**, 1063–1066.

61. Peters T. (1987). *Thriving on Chaos.* New York: Knopf.

62. Davis P. and Oberle M. (1992). Support and caring: exploring the concepts. *Oncology Nursing Forum* **19**, 763–767.

63. Benner P. and Wrubel J. (1989). *The Primacy of Caring: Stress and Coping in Health and Illness.* Menlo Park, CA: Addison-Wesley, p. 385.

CHAPTER THIRTY-FIVE

Palliative care and cancer

Mary Pennell and Jessica Corner

Palliative care is a relatively new specialty, recognised formally as a medical specialty in the UK in 1987, and defined as 'the study and management of patients with active, progressive, far-advanced disease for whom the prognosis is limited and the focus of care is the quality of life'.[1] Palliative care as a distinct area of practice evolved from the hospice movement. The concept of a hospice can be traced back to medieval times, although the modern hospice movement is attributed to the work of Dame Cicely Saunders. During her time as medical officer at St Joseph's Hospital in East London, Cicely Saunders developed techniques of giving strong opiate analgesic drugs at regular intervals for the relief of pain, and developed the concept of 'total pain'; this acknowledged the importance of emotional and psychological, as well as physical components of pain. The approach revolutionised the effectiveness of pain relief in advanced cancer. In 1967 Dame Cicely Saunders opened St Christopher's Hospice, a specialised, purpose-built unit devoted to the care and support of dying patients. Since the 1960s, hospice and palliative care have grown into a worldwide movement. The goal of effective pain control for people with cancer anywhere in the world is now a central theme of the World Health Organisation.[2]

The hospice movement grew as a radical and alternative model of care for people who were dying from cancer (and to a lesser extent, other diseases). Over the course of the twentieth century the increasingly technical nature of health care has led to death itself becoming a medical technical event; the boundaries between life and death have become blurred as medical technologies have enabled life to be supported where the body is no longer capable of maintaining itself. Death in the past was largely managed at home, whereas by the 1960s, 70% of deaths occurred in hospitals; this trend continues today. Death has become an event managed by professional carers, rather than the family; seen by some as the great twentieth-century taboo, hidden from daily life in institutions, since death threatens the modern Western belief in youth, health, and personal invincibility. While debate continues over the extent to which death can be constructed in terms of a 'taboo', recognition of death as a subject not acknowledged openly was instrumental in the establishment of the palliative care movement.[3] Palliative care seeks to reverse such trends, foster greater openness about dying, and actively promote high-quality care for people at the end of life.

Hospitals have become the most common setting for institutionalised dying and have been recognised as inadequate in this respect. Unmanaged pain and other symptoms, a lack of openness by health professionals about prognosis and dying, and impersonal care and treatment of the dying and those closest to them, have been shown to be commonplace in hospitals.

In the 1960s in the USA ground-breaking research by Glaser and Strauss[4] and Kubler-Ross,[5] among others, exposed the lack of openness in health care over how an individual comes to understand that they are dying. Glaser and Strauss's work observing types of awareness of dying among men in a veterans' hospital demonstrated that health professionals and relatives conspired to prevent a person knowing that they were dying, and that the organisational culture created and sustained barriers to openness about death and dying. Kubler-Ross[5] undertook what at the time was felt to be impossible; she interviewed over 200 people about their own thoughts and feelings about the fact they were dying. Not only were people frank and open about this, but almost all knew they were dying, regardless of whether or not they had been 'told' this by medical staff. These studies were central in helping to found a movement that supported openness and disclosure in caring for the dying, and coinciding with the development of the hospice movement in the UK, was incorporated into the evolving philosophy of care for the dying.

The palliative care approach

The concept of palliative care for the dying was introduced to broaden care from being confined to those who are imminently dying, to a more home-centred approach. Palliative care focuses on promoting quality of life in people with advanced disease, maximising a person's ability to continue functioning for as long as possible, and supporting family or friends caring for them. Palliative care services are now based in a variety of settings, and offer a range of services (see below). The palliative care approach aims to:

- affirm life and regards dying as a normal, rather than a biomedical process
- neither hasten nor postpone death
- provide relief from pain and other symptoms
- offer assistance to enable individuals to come to terms with their own death as fully and constructively as they can
- offer a support system to help people live as actively and creatively as possible until death
- offer a support system to help family and friends during illness, and following bereavement.[6]

Through this, palliative care has become more 'transportable', and no longer needs to take place in a hospice or palliative care unit, but can be fostered through a philosophy of care, and can therefore exist in hospitals or other institutional settings.

While palliative care started as a form of alternative care, its early financing was derived entirely from charitable donations and it was located within the voluntary sector of health care; increasingly, the goal has been to reintegrate palliative care into mainstream health care settings. This has also created the dilemma of how a movement that had its origins in providing a radical alternative model of care can preserve this agenda when it is increasingly seen as part of mainstream health care, and provided as of right to all who are dying.

Box 35.1: Characteristics of palliative care services

- Offers knowledge and expertise in the control of symptoms associated with advanced cancer, and recognises that symptoms such as pain can have physical, psychological, social, and spiritual components.
- Care is family and home centred.
- Care is delivered by a multi-disciplinary team, including specialist palliative care doctors, nurses, social worker, spiritual advisor, occupational therapist, and physiotherapist.
- Home care, respite care, and day care services are provided, as well as in-patient care.
- Bereavement follow-up services are offered for relatives.
- An educational and research role is recognised.

Evidence for the value of palliative care

Higginson[7] suggests that effectiveness, acceptability, equity and accessibility, and efficiency (value for money) are key indicators of the value of a palliative care service. In two service evaluations undertaken by Higginson and Hearn,[8] one in Ireland, and a second of five palliative care teams in the south of England, pain management was examined as a key indicator of effective care in 695 patients cared for by these services. Seventy per cent of patients were experiencing pain at the time of referral to the palliative care service. After 2 weeks there was found to be a significant improvement in the levels of pain experienced ($P < 0.0001$), indicating that pain had been adequately controlled as a result of the intervention of the palliative care service.

A study in Wales by McQuillan *et al.*,[9] evaluating the effect of establishing a palliative care service at a tertiary referral hospital, used a survey approach. Prior to establishing the service the survey revealed that symptoms of people with cancer and HIV/AIDS were poorly controlled. One year after the new service was introduced, while problems about referral to the service remained the same, fewer patients experienced a worsening of their symptoms as their illness progressed than before. Opioid and non-steroidal analgesic drug prescribing had increased significantly in the hospital, and there was staff satisfaction with the service.

One of the difficulties with palliative care is the problem of acceptability, since the association with terminal care can mean that for some people it is unacceptable, particularly where there is difficulty over accepting a terminal prognosis. In a study by Seale and Kelly,[10] palliative care was evaluated from the perspective of the surviving spouse. The study compared perceptions of care in a London hospice, with care given by hospitals. Those who had received care in the hospice were found to be more likely to know that they were dying, less likely to require emergency admission, and felt that they had received clear communication from professionals. In addition, the environment of care was felt to be more comfortable, visiting was easier, and family members were more likely to have been able to participate in care. Symptom control, however, was found to be equally effective in both hospice and hospital settings[11] and may indicate that over time as knowledge and good practice have been passed on by palliative care teams, care in hospitals may have 'caught up' with hospices in the management of physical symptoms.

Questions over the equity of access to palliative care services have been raised, particularly since it is estimated that only 10% of people with terminal cancer in the UK receive hospice care and yet in this country palliative care services are considered to be well-developed.[12] One reason may be that palliative care services are only available via professional referral, and there may be many barriers to such referrals occurring, such as negative attitudes towards hospice and palliative care, or a reluctance to let go of an individual's care. There may also be evidence to suggest that health pro-fessionals are unaware of an individual's need for palliative care,[13] or are unlikely to refer where the person and their relatives appear to be coping with the situation.[14]

Evidence for the efficiency or value for money of palliative care is limited, partly because this is complex to disentangle from other costs of care, but also because few studies have been undertaken in this area. There is evidence, however, that while palliative care services are more costly than standard in-patient care services, this may be offset by reductions in admissions to hospital and in home visits for uncontrolled symptoms and other problems.[15]

Dilemmas for palliative care

The hospice and palliative care movement has recently been criticised over whether it lives up to the claim of offering a unique and different model of care for the dying. Seale[16] has reviewed studies comparing care in hospice and hospital settings. Data from the North American National Hospice Study,[17] which compared 40 hospice units with 14 conventional settings, indicated differences between hospitals and hospices; in particular, the use of diagnostic investigations and aggressive therapies was greater in hospital settings, and in contrast there was some evidence of greater supportive care being offered in hospices. There is little UK evidence comparing standard care for people who are dying from cancer with palliative or hospice care. The only two comparative studies to be conducted indicate that differences in care are hard to detect; this, however, may be due to difficulties in measuring the outcomes of palliative care. In Kane *et al.*'s[18] trial of hospice versus hospital care, no significant differences were found between the two groups on measures of pain, other symptoms, activities of daily living or psychological morbidity.

In two interview studies by Parkes,[19,20] bereaved relatives were asked about the terminal care received by their family member whose relative had died either at home, in hospital, or at St Christopher's Hospice. Differences existed in feelings about care between the different settings in which care had taken place, in the first study conducted in 1967–69.[19] These differences appeared to have largely disappeared by 1977. This may be due to the fact that palliative care has been absorbed into care of the dying in hospitals and is a mark of the success of the movement. However, some evidence also exists to indicate that a number of hospice and palliative care units may not be as different from hospital care settings as may be claimed. Indeed, those units that are closely related to, or are imbedded within, hospitals, suffer from being unable to establish different organisational systems of care from the host hospital. These units have been found to use more technical interventions for care, to focus on physical care and symptom management rather than emotional aspects of care, and may not actively foster open communication about dying.[21] Seale[16] calls for research to evaluate further differences in care and outcomes for different care settings in order to 'help clarify ideological debates about patient care, and advance our understanding of the practical problems of institutionalising innovations'.

An important concept central to the hospice and palliative care movement is the ideal of facilitating a 'good death'. While what is constituted by 'a good death' carries no single definition or set of features, it has become associated with:

- the ideals of personal knowledge and acceptance of impending death
- care where the dying person and those close to them receive mutual emotional support
- management of the symptoms and problems relating to the dying process so that physical suffering is minimised
- not leaving the person who is dying isolated or alone, and enabling them to complete 'unfinished business'.

The 'good death' as an ideal has helped to transform the care of people who are dying. However, McNamara et al.'s[22] examination of how the 'good death ideal' within a hospice setting has become institutionalised suggests that there is evidence of excessive and unquestioning adherence to this ideal, and this may in turn create problems. Using ethnographic participant observation of nursing in a hospice unit in Western Australia, McNamara et al.[22] observed that certain features of the 'good death ideal' had become so integral to the organisation that this represented a form of 'routine'. The ideal of the 'good death' had been assimilated to the extent that such deaths were required by staff in the

interests of what might be considered socially acceptable, and for the smooth running of the organisation. Nurses were at risk, over time, of developing a rigidity in their views about what constituted a 'good death', so that those who did not conform to this ideal, for example by not accepting their death or hanging on to life, were felt to have 'problems'.

A further area of criticism surrounding the palliative care movement is that of 'medicalisation'. Biswas[23] and Field[24] have argued that the broadened definition of care as 'palliative' signals a move away from care of the dying. The adoption of euphemistic terms such as 'symptom control' and 'palliation' mean that terminal care, or care in the final days or weeks of life has become marginalised, to the extent that there may even be a danger of losing open acknowledgement that someone is going to die. The professionalisation of palliative care as a medical discipline has also meant that care is becoming increasingly technical, dominated by pharmacology, and is assumed to be led by a doctor, marginalising other health professionals.[25]

In the context of cancer care, access to specialist palliative care services and the integration of the palliative care approach into care and treatment settings are core components of good care. Both are required and need to be understood in relation to the critique already offered. The extent to which palliative care has become integral to cancer treatment settings is debatable. One way to explore this might be to ask the following questions of oneself and work setting.

- What is my perception of palliative care?
- At what point in a person's illness would I consider the need for palliative care?
- What is the response of my other professional colleagues to the concept of palliative care?
- What are the usual responses to palliative care from patients and those close to them?

The interface between acute care and palliative care

The relationship between acute cancer care, that is where care is orientated around treating the disease, and palliative care services, is complex. While the need for palliation should be acknowledged as early as possible in the course of illness, the reality is that this is impractical. With the exception of those cancers already at an advanced stage at diagnosis, in many instances it would be inappropriate to introduce palliative care at this stage, and would overwhelm existing palliative care services with the numbers of people who potentially might need help. This then creates a dilemma about the most appropriate time for referral, or for determining when active treatment should be reorientated to more palliative goals. The transition from active to palliative care was the subject of a study by Cawley.[26] Thirty people who had recently been transferred to the care of three different palliative care settings were interviewed. Views of the care they were receiving (i.e. palliative care), how the transition had been communicated to them, their involvement in the decision about transition to palliative care, and their feelings about their disease and situation were explored. The palliative care settings included a palliative care unit based in a specialist cancer treatment hospital, a community/home care team, and a hospice.

For a minority of people, it appeared that the move from an active treatment setting to palliative care had not been openly discussed. This was more common where the referral was made to the palliative care unit based within the specialist cancer hospital, possibly because the change was less dramatic, and did not mean moving out of the hospital where care had always been given. For some, all they knew was that they had been referred to a different consultant. Where this happened, realising they had been referred to the palliative care team was distressing, since they had to work out for themselves that they had reached the end of treatment aimed at curing their disease. Where referral was made to a hospice, this was less likely to happen, since the connotations of the name 'hospice' are with care for the dying. In this instance, for some it meant rapidly coming to terms with the prospect of dying, and for others realising that referral to a hospice did not necessarily mean that death is imminent.

Few of the people interviewed for the study had been involved in decisions over ending active treatment or referral to palliative care. Most came to understand their situation by realising that they were declining by noticing their own physical state and symptoms, and not through discussions with health carers. This study suggests that greater attention needs to be given to the area of communication about progressive cancer and the options open to people where curative treatment may have little to offer.

Adjustment to the knowledge of imminent death

The issues of communication about the transition from active cancer treatment to palliative care represent a further development, or maturing perspective surrounding the difficulties of helping someone adjust to the knowledge of their own imminent death. From the earliest studies, such as those by Kubler-Ross[5] and Glaser and Strauss,[4] researchers have attempted to present a unified theory of this process. Kubler-Ross presented this as a series of emotional responses proceeding in stages from an initial reaction of denial and disbelief through anger, bargaining, and acceptance. Thus the highly influential notion of a developmental psychology of dying emerged. This has subsequently been criticised because it oversimplifies the complexity of emotional responses to knowledge of impending death. It also characterises emotions and feelings one may have about dying as one-dimensional, progressing from denial and finally reaching acceptance, the goal being 'healthy acceptance of dying'. The emphasis has been on a normative model or 'a healthy adjustment', the ultimate goal being to accept one's situation. Subsequently this model has been refined into a three-stage model in which a 'mosaic' of emotional responses may be encountered. These responses include an initial stage (facing the threat), a chronic stage (being ill), and a final stage of 'acceptance'; acceptance, although desirable, is not seen as an essential.

The contribution of Glaser and Strauss was significant in highlighting the importance of the environment in which awareness of dying develops; in particular, how health professionals and family create an environment of open or closed communication surrounding death and dying. These authors also proposed the concept of a 'dying trajectory',[27] in which dying can be characterised by the nature of dying and time over which dying occurs. Four trajectories were defined:

- certain death at a known time
- certain death at an unknown time (this is common for many cancers)
- uncertain death but a known time when certainty will be established
- uncertain death and an uncertain time when the question will be resolved (such as in chronic illnesses).

The awareness context surrounding knowledge of death as imminent (i.e. open or closed awareness, or pretence that death was not imminent) was orchestrated, constructed, and maintained by hospital staff. It is interesting to note that while the goal of palliative care is open acknowledgement of impending death, and to offer support in adjusting to this, Cawley's study[26] indicates that there may still exist contexts in hospital and palliative care settings where full openness cannot be assumed.

Pattison[28] further developed the theory of dying trajectories by defining the 'living–dying interval', commencing at the crisis of knowledge of death and ending at the point of death. Depending on how this trajectory is handled or coped with by the person, dying can be characterised as 'integrated' or 'disintegrated'. Copp[29] argues that in reality, the picture is more complex and both integrated and disintegrated patterns of coping with dying can be seen in individuals (see Figure 35.1).

Theories of coping with dying were largely described early in the development of palliative care, and when open awareness of dying by patients could not be assumed. Copp investigated these in a prospective study of 12 people dying in a hospice, an environment committed to open awareness, by talking to the people themselves in interviews, and in interviews with nurses caring for them. These people were facing death in the trajectory of 'certain death at an unknown time'. Copp[29] found that in these circumstances, there were critical junctures where redefinition of self in the face of impending death was required, as loss of function or status ensued, or in facing physical decline. Physical aspects of dying appeared to play an important part in this process, unrecognised in theories of dying, which have largely focused on psychological adjustment. Both denial and acceptance were used by people who knew they were dying throughout their illness to preserve existing relationships, and avoid the overwhelming threat posed by dying in the context of being openly aware of its inevitability.

In response, nurses' relationships with the dying person were continually defined and redefined, and nurses constantly attempted to gain insight into the feelings and actions of patients in order to interpret how they might most appropriately respond. The nurses' relationships with dying people in this context were characterised by a continual 'encountering' of how facing death was handled by the dying person. Watching and waiting for someone to respond to their predicament, protecting and controlling their physical and emotional state, and holding and letting go were all part of complex strategies and interplay acted out by both the dying person and nurse, as the continual losses arising from the process of dying were faced and dealt with. Nursing was a 'fine balancing act' in this situation. Interestingly, Copp noted that nurses' talk was suffused with an acknowledgement of a mind–self body split as death became imminent; that is, the physical, dying 'body' was increasingly referred to as separate from the body as 'self'. This finding is paradoxical given nursing's contemporary commitment to the embodiment of self where the physical body and 'the self' are seen to be inextricably bound up together and thus not amenable to separate description, as described, for example, in the work of Lawler.[30]

Determining prognosis

The 'fine balancing act' described by Copp[29] is a feature of nursing more generally in advanced cancer, and not just in facilitating emotional and psychological adaptation while facing impending death. Adapting care in this context is difficult because of the unpredictability of dying. The goals of caring (for example, rehabilitation or simply to maintain the status quo), will be determined through an estimate of likely prognosis and the person's own adjustment or acceptance of their predicament. However, estimating prognosis is fraught with difficulties, and there is evidence suggesting that health professionals are frequently wrong in their assessment of how long someone in their care may have to live. Most commonly, errors in predicting prognosis overestimate time until

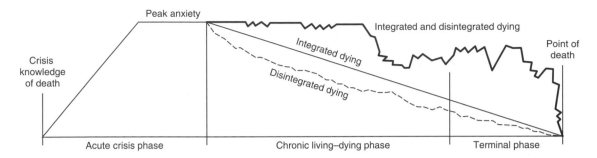

Figure 35.1   Integrated and disintegrated dying with plateaux and declines at different times (reproduced with permission from Copp G. (1996). *Facing impending death: the experiences of patients and their nurses in a hospice setting.* Unpublished Ph.D. thesis, Oxford Brookes University).[29]

death. Co-ordinating appropriate medical treatment, facilitating acceptance, dealing with 'unfinished business', and organising social and community support for someone who may be dying, are critically determined through estimating how long they may have to live, and in balancing this with the person's readiness to face death. This is further complicated at times, when medical and nursing views about prognosis, and therefore the appropriateness of continuing active cancer treatment, are at odds with each other.

A study by Buchan[31] illustrates well the difficulties in predicting prognosis. Buchan set out to explore the accuracy of nurses' estimations of prognosis in the last days of life. Nurses working on two medical wards were asked to identify patients they thought were expected to die within the next few hours or days, as well as to indicate the cues that helped them to make this judgement. This was then compared with the timing of the patients' actual death. The accuracy of these estimates varied considerably. Out of 17 patients who died on the two wards during the study, estimates of prognosis were accurate for only five. The tendency was for estimates to be markedly over-optimistic. Buchan concluded that the study indicated a reluctance to accept that a person was dying. One example was a 64-year-old man suffering from cancer of the lung with widespread metastases. His nursing notes revealed a bed-bound man with spinal cord compression and breathlessness. Despite this, the nursing staff on duty the morning after the man died said that his death had been totally unexpected.

It appeared that the most accurate assessments of prognosis were almost always made by the nurses directly caring for the dying person, and not by the nurse in charge of the ward, even when the nurse in charge was considerably more experienced. The difficulties in facing and predicting imminent death at the very end of life appeared to be great for nurses. If this is the case, then the complexity of ensuring appropriate and timely referral to palliative care services, when this needs to take place weeks or months from death, is likely to be a major barrier to high-quality care for the dying.

Common problems in advanced cancer

An interview study[32] of the bereaved relatives of 2074 people who died of cancer in the UK in 1990 explored the needs and problems of people in their last year of life, and the extent to which these needs had been addressed or relieved by the health care they received. Twenty-nine per cent died in their own home, 50% in hospital and 14% in a hospice. Table 35.1 shows the symptoms experienced in the last year and last week of life. At some stage in the last year of life 88% were reported to have been in pain, 66% were said to have found the pain very distressing, and 61% experienced pain in their last week of life. Pain control was only partial for 47% of those cared for by their family doctor and 35% of those cared for in hospital. Loss of appetite, constipation, dry mouth or thirst, nausea or vomiting, and breathlessness were also common. Although 91% had been in hospital or a hospice in their last year of life, most of the last year was spent at home, where relatives bore the main brunt of care. For one-quarter to one-third of relatives, more help and assistance had been needed with activities of daily living, household chores, and finances. Half reported that they were unable to get all the information they wanted about their relative's condition, and one in five were critical of the manner in which they were told that their relative was dying. This study indicates that despite a relatively well-developed palliative care service in the UK, many people do not appear to receive a high quality of care, and are left with many unmet needs for support and symptom control.

Cancer is associated with unremitting severe pain; however, while 75% of people admitted to a hospice report pain, 25% do not.[6] It is estimated[2] that of one-third of people receiving active cancer treatment experience pain, and more than 60% of those with advanced cancer will experience pain.

Management of pain in advanced cancer is a central goal of palliative care. Pain therapy relieves pain by addressing psychological approaches and modifying pathological processes.

Psychological approaches include offering understanding and companionship and the use of cognitive behavioural therapies to tell the story of the pain, in response to questions such as:

- What did pain mean to you before your illness; what does it mean now?
- What feelings do you have about your pain, yourself as you suffer the pain; are these new or familiar thoughts?
- Is there anything positive you have identified about your pain?

Such questions may give an insight into the emotional impact of pain; once this is known it may be possible to ask 'What part would you like me

Table 35.1 Symptoms reported by respondents as having been experienced by deceased in the last year of life [numbers in parentheses are the totals on which the percentages are based (= 100%)]

Symptom $n = 2074$	Had symptom at some time in last year of life (%)	Had symptom at some time in last week of life (%)	Those with symptom for whom it was 'very distressing' (%)
Pain	88 (2018)	66 (1853)	61 (1704)
Persistent cough	28 (2048)	19 (1991)	34 (554)
Breathlessness	54 (2059)	44 (1988)	50 (1063)
Vomiting or nausea	59 (2023)	36 (1875)	56 (1151)
Dry mouth or thirst	60 (1920)	49 (1758)	30 (1102)
Loss of appetite	78 (2051)	71 (1921)	23 (1515)
Difficulty swallowing	41 (1991)	35 (1913)	52 (776)
Constipation	62 (1886)	41 (1625)	54 (1120)
Sleeplessness	60 (1972)	36 (1771)	34 (1124)
Mental confusion	41 (2057)	33 (1983)	36 (731)
Feeling low or miserable	69 (2007)	47 (1786)	52 (1302)
Anxiety or trouble with nerves	32 (2027)	18 (1924)	47 (615)
Bed sores	28 (2015)	24 (1989)	55 (513)
Loss of bladder control	40 (1999)	35 (1912)	62 (717)
Loss of bowel control	32 (1974)	26 (1893)	74 (555)
Unpleasant smell	25 (2034)	21 (2001)	29 (417)

to play in helping with these thoughts and feelings?' Surprisingly often it is sufficient simply to express such feelings to someone who will hear them, but without making judgements. Where pain in cancer is experienced there may be an associated expectation of bravery, of not making a fuss. Yet for the person who has pain, the desire to weep or tell of the terror that pain brings to mind may be overwhelming, while also perceiving a duty to maintain silence for the benefit of others. By attending to the person behind the pain, there may be a restoration of the person's decision-making capacity.[33]

McCaffery and Ferrell[34] undertook a comparative study considering nurses' attitudes around the issue of pain and management and assessment. Compared with studies of nurses' attitudes undertaken a decade earlier, there were clear signs of nurses possessing greater knowledge in relation to pain management. Nurses still appeared to be fearful of causing addiction, of increasing doses of opioids, and of titrating opioid dose against reported pain, and were reluctant of believe a person's self-reported pain. Questions you might ask yourself in relation to these attitudes are:

- What are my beliefs about the nature of addiction to opioids?
- What are they based on?
- What impact do they have on my response to increased opioid doses?
- Who should take responsibility for planning and undertaking dose titration?
- What factors influence my belief in a person's ability to report pain (age, ability to communicate, physical appearance, behaviour, previous personal pain experience)?
- What is my previous professional experience?

Oreshuk and Bruera[35] made the following recommendations about the introduction and use of adjuvant analgesics in advanced cancer.

- Identify opioids as first-line prescription for the majority of cancer pain.
- Remember opioid responsiveness when titrating drug doses.
- Add adjuvant drugs one at time to avoid combined or enhanced side-effects.

- If a decision is made to use an adjuvant drug, use an effective dose.
- Define outcome measures at the outset of treatment.
- Discontinue adjuvant therapy if not effective.
- Monitor sedation and cognition levels.

Nurses have an important role in managing therapeutic approaches to pain management. Antibiotics as a means of pain control are sometimes denied on the grounds that these may extend the life of a critically ill person. These should not necessarily be omitted if they may relieve pain or other symptoms.

Modification of pathological processes can be achieved through the use of cancer therapies such as radiotherapy, chemotherapy, hormonal therapy, or surgery. The use of radiotherapy in palliative care is well documented[36–38] and can be used to:

- treat bony metastases
- treat bleeding points or wounds
- débride wounds
- reduce tumour bulk prior to surgery
- treat spinal cord compression and superior vena cava obstruction
- increase bone mass proactively.

The place of chemotherapy in active cancer treatment has been examined in detail elsewhere. Recently there has been increased interest in offering chemotherapy as a tool in the palliative management of pain.[39] By reducing tumour bulk, pain can be relieved. Where chemotherapy is used as a palliative measure for pain or other symptoms of advanced cancer, questions concerning its value need to be raised and continually reviewed. If there is an absence of improvement in physical, social, emotional, or spiritual well-being as a result, then it should be stopped. In palliative care, the person is the focus rather than the tumour. There needs to be honesty and openness about the prospects for the treatment, and the right to withdraw from treatment at any time. The timing of chemotherapy needs to be planned around normal activities; for example, if an important family occasion is to take place in a few weeks, then the possibility of hair loss, infection, or general weariness should be raised.

Surgery is used increasingly to alleviate pain and other symptoms, for example in:

- debulking of tumour
- excision of metastases
- insertion of stents
- formation of palliative colostomies
- fixation of fractures.[40]

The rate of healing may, however, be compromised due to the presence of a malignancy or other adjuvant treatment. The use of surgery places a responsibility on nurses to ensure that any consent given follows a true understanding of the procedure and any possible consequences.

Opioid-induced constipation is a common reason for admission in advanced cancer, and is almost entirely caused by inadequate preventive treatment. Opioids reduce peristalsis as well as the sensation of the need to defecate. Other causes of constipation are:

- weakness
- reduced mobility
- problems with communication
- confusion
- reduced food and fluid intake
- altered body electrolytes, e.g. hypercalcaemia
- bowel obstruction
- radiation fibrosis
- existing conditions, e.g. haemorrhoids
- spinal cord compression
- dehydration.

Early prescription of laxatives is essential, and it is assumed that anyone taking opioids should also take a laxative. Oral laxatives are of four main types:

- bulking agents – since these require taking extra fluids they may not be suitable in advanced cancer
- lubricating agents, e.g. liquid paraffin
- softening agents such as lactulose
- muscle stimulants such as senna.

In advanced cancer it is often assumed that a combination of a softening agent and a muscle stimulant should be used. Where the constipation is established or non-responsive to oral medication, rectal measures should be used. Manual extraction is the final option, where there is evidence of faecal impaction or insufficient or absent muscle tone. It is a painful and humiliating process. A fast-acting anxiolytic should therefore be considered and offered 20 minutes prior to the procedure.

Problems with sleep affect at least 50% of people with advanced cancer.[41] The benefits of sleep are wide-reaching and affect the whole person more than might sometimes be recognised. Sleep promotes normal mood and cognitive function, restores healing and immune function and skeletal structures, influences pain thresholds, and provides respite from pain and worry. Family carers may also report sleep disruptions.

The causes of sleep disruption are numerous and include:

- depression
- anxiety
- pain of body, mind, or spirit
- medication, caffeine, steroids, antidepressants
- primary medical condition, e.g. urinary tract infection, respiratory tract infection
- primary sleep disorder
- changes in sleep pattern, e.g. napping in the day
- circadian rhythm changes.

Care strategy 35.1: Possible approaches to helping sleep disruption

- Treat the primary cause wherever possible.
- Use effective pain management.
- Use effective drug management such as prescribing haloperidol for nightmares.
- Provide a comfortable sleeping environment.
- Avoid caffeine in large amounts.
- Warm drinks may tap memories of childhood care.
- Adopt bedtime rituals, such as washing, reading, listening to the radio, or watching television.
- Change the environment so that bed is seen as a place of sleep.
- Listen to/tell anxieties before settling at night.
- Consider a change of mattress to increase comfort.

Other cancer-related problems and nursing interventions for these are comprehensively reviewed in Chapters 17 to 31 and therefore are not addressed here.

Spiritual needs in people who are dying

Spiritual care is often overlooked and is an ill-defined but central part of care for people with advanced cancer.[42] Helping a person to address the spiritual aspect of their lives offers an opportunity to work with the uniqueness of that person. Health carers often declare that they offer holistic care, which by definition must include care of the spirit. In a recent study, people questioned about their care reported that spiritual care was one of the most neglected aspects of care.[43] In an interview study of hospice nurses,[44] 25% said that they did not raise the issue of spirituality unless the person they were caring for did so.

For many people, spirituality is understood to mean religious practice. Cawley,[45] examining the concept of spirituality, suggested that it may be beyond expression in words or a standard definition. Stoll[43] has defined spirituality as:

> . . . a sense of personhood, being concerned with the meaning and purpose of one's existence, and trust in relationships which provide the basis for such meanings.

This may be on two planes: a horizontal plane, where a person finds values that become a focus for life and around which life is organised; and a vertical plane, which suggests movement beyond the horizontal and seeking a relationship with a higher being, whatever form that being has for the person. These may lead to the adoption of religious practices, but this is not automatic. Spirituality is the inner sense of the spirit, which may show itself in religious practice, but does not always do so. Spiritual fulfilment is possible regardless of the plane on which an individual's spiritual nature develops.

Burnard[46] emphasises the importance of nurses' exploring of their own sense of spirituality, so that some understanding can be reached about personal beliefs. It seems self-evident that unless nurses know on what plane their own spiritual nature lies, they will be unable to help others to express this vital element of themselves. A study undertaken in Belgium, exploring the perceptions of 425 health care workers in palliative care settings of aspects of spiritual distress and growth, revealed that nearly half did not perceive discussing spirituality to be part of their role. The study also revealed significant distress amongst nurses.

Stanworth[47] suggests that in our increasingly secular society, few people have a religious vocabulary with which the ultimate concerns of life can be shared. If it is felt that a spiritual language is about a single god or conventional religious practice, this is too narrow and may leave people unable to discuss deeper existential issues. Language is about symbols;[47] one of the challenges of spiritual care is to develop the ability to access subtle areas of language so that areas that may resist expression may be articulated. In these instances it is inadequate to restrict interpretation to surface appearances,[48] including the literal meaning of the spoken word.

Palliative care frequently involves times of transition: for example, finishing treatment aimed at cure and changing to become care orientated. It is likely that people making this transition will reflect on previous times of change, success, or failure in their lives to help to manage their current situation. Stanworth[47] suggests that people have their own individual language of transition, and that it is by attending to such language that true and hidden feelings will be revealed. Patients may repeatedly ask for:

> . . . someone to share the pain of searching, someone who will listen to the frightening dreams and fears, not provide the pat assurances.[47]

This requires personal insight and skilled communication. Cornette[49] reported that the skills needed to manage spiritual distress was the ability to listen and to show empathy and compassion. It may therefore not take specific knowledge, rather being prepared to stay open to what is said, not only in words but also in the silences between words.

Ross[50] suggests that patients' physical problems may make it difficult for nurses to attend to spiritual needs, such as dementia, confusion, or communication problems caused by deafness. The ward environment can also contribute to these difficulties, since privacy and quiet are difficult to find, and low staffing levels make giving time to this area of care hard. However, where a need for care exists these barriers should be overcome and difficulties recognised. In order to offer help with spiritual issues, support in the form of supervision is recommended so that care is not offered in isolation.[46,50] Nurses can maintain a professional detachment in the face of disease because they are not themselves physically ill. However, attending to spiritual issues requires revealing one's own humanity; this is especially challenging. Conversations about spiritual matters may result in the need to rethink personal beliefs and may be painful, mirroring the spiritual distress of the person who is ill or dying.

A study exploring nurses' awareness of spirituality and their confidence in meeting spiritual needs[51] identified how little time nurses spent in addressing spiritual needs, and therefore, training in this area was recommended. To date, this has tended to focus on knowledge of various religious practices related to different religious faiths, and in particular the rituals associated with dying and death. This defines this area of care too narrowly. Ross[50] suggests that there are key factors that contribute to neglect of spiritual care, such as a lack of sense of personal spirit, disillusionment with life's experiences and an unfulfilled personal search for meaning.

Assessment of spiritual needs is an important component of care; these needs are complex and diverse. Spiritual needs include:

- to live in accordance with a personal value system
- to participate in religious rituals
- to express feelings of being loved by others or God
- to express feelings of being forgiven by others or God
- to express love for others through actions
- to seek the love of others
- to seek realistic personal health goals
- to value the inner self more than the physical self.[43]

An important factor in these needs is that they represent normality and also require 'being' rather than 'doing'. Finding meaning in one's situation can be a positive experience for those who have advanced cancer. Ferrell *et al.*[52] noted that some people suffering from severe fatigue as a result of their disease found that their weakened state allowed time to be quiet and contemplative, which was a positive gain, offering an opportunity to find balance in oneself.

Nurses may be reluctant to address spiritual needs explicitly. However, spiritual distress may show itself in a number of ways, for example:

- questioning the value and meaning of suffering
- anger towards an identified supreme being, verbalised inner conflicts about beliefs

- concerns about an individual's relationship with a deity
- questioning the meaning of one's own existence
- nightmares or sleep disturbances
- anger towards representatives of religious practices
- questioning the moral implications or therapies being recommended
- questioning life in its current form
- inability to take part in normal religious practices.

Questions that may be asked while exploring spiritual distress may include:

- What gets you up in the morning?
- How do you usually manage when the world seems bleak and awful?
- Where do you usually find strength?

Helping someone to find reasons to hope may be a concrete way of offering spiritual care. Herth[53] explored hope-fostering strategies amongst people who were dying. These included:

- interpersonal connectedness (the presence of a meaningful shared relationship)
- light-heartedness (feeling of delight, joy, or playfulness shared verbally and non-verbally)
- personal attributes (determination, courage, serenity)
- attainable aims (directing efforts towards some purpose)
- spiritual base (presence of active spiritual beliefs and practices)
- uplifting memories (recalling positive moments or times)
- affirmation of worth (having one's individuality accepted, honoured, and acknowledged).

By contrast, hope-hindering strategies were reported as:

- abandonment and isolation (physical and/or emotional loss of significant others)
- uncontrollable pain and discomfort (continuing overwhelming pain or discomfort despite attempts at controlling these)
- devaluation of personhood (being treated as a person of little worth).

There is some evidence to suggest that people may 'hang on' for a particular event in their lives, and may defy their prognosis.[54] This suggests the powerful effect of hope, particularly where this is affirmed by the positive presence and interest of health professionals.

Bereavement

Palliative care services have traditionally incorporated bereavement care, since assisting those close to someone who has died to come to terms with their loss is in keeping with the aims of palliative care. Many hospice and palliative care services offer bereavement support services, some in the form of counselling, others using volunteers, and others by maintaining contact with relatives of people who have died. However, the presence of these services is also in part due to a commonly held view of grief as a potentially pathological process, which is inherently dangerous to the person experiencing it. Services are orientated towards facilitating the 'healthy' expression of grief by the bereaved, with a view to assisting people to pass through the various stages of grief, and within a defined period of time to return to normal life. Alternatively, they aim to identify individuals at risk of a 'complicated' bereavement and who are therefore at risk of psychological morbidity, or a failure to resolve grief and move on.

Penson[55] describes bereavement as being 'robbed of something valued' and in so doing spreads the net of care wider than the post-bereavement period. When a person is given a diagnosis of cancer, there may be a real sense of bereavement for all sorts of aspects of their lives. In the short term there may be a sense of loss of physical health, known future, income, control over events, role as a healthy person, and other social roles. In the longer term, the losses may include financial security for those left behind, an acceptable body image, and dreams of immortality. When those close to the person hear the news, there may be a similar set of losses experienced, which is termed anticipatory grief. Evans[56] suggests that this is not grief for the final loss of the person, but an ongoing mourning for the many losses being experienced throughout the illness experience. Grief is a cause of real fatigue, which when experienced while trying to offer 24-hour care at home may be especially burdensome and even limit an individual's ability to care.

Because grief is so painful, people often express a hope that experiencing the pain of bereavement in advance will ease suffering afterwards. The evidence is that this may not be so; if anticipatory grief is for current losses, future losses will have to be mourned in due time. However, from a review of studies comparing sudden versus anticipated death, Pedder[57] concluded that people able to anticipate death reported a more bearable period of mourning. This may be due more to the possibility of completing 'unfinished business' than the potential for completing grief working in advance of the actual loss. There is some evidence to suggest that the events surrounding death, and the quality of time spent with a loved person after death, may have a profound effect on the feelings surrounding grief and bereavement. In particular, allowing a relative or friend to spend time with the dead person, giving permission to hold or handle the body, and paying particular attention to the way support is offered around the time of death, are known to assist greatly the feelings and memories surrounding the experience later. Hampe[58] interviewed spouses following bereavement, asking them about their care needs while they were with their dying spouse in hospital. They identified the need to be with the dying person, to feel helpful to them, to be assured that their spouse was comfortable, to be kept informed of the dying person's condition, and to be made aware of their impending death. They also wanted to be allowed to ventilate emotions, to receive comfort and support from family members, and receive acceptance, support, and comfort from health professionals.

Much of our current understanding of grief stems from the writings of Freud[59] and subsequently of Melanie Klein.[60] They described grief as a form of work, whereby investment in the lost person or object must gradually be withdrawn and eventually invested in someone or something else, or the lost person or object becomes internalised, and the loss accepted. This, however, is neither a slow nor an easy process. Subsequent empirical work established, through observation of people who have been bereaved, both physical and emotional reactions during acute grief, and a series of stages through which an individual may pass while coming to terms with loss. For example, Bowlby,[61] observing infants temporarily without their mother, noted that they first appear numb, then display yearning and searching behaviour, and a period of disorientation and crying, before reorganisation of self.

Parkes,[62] following a series of interview studies of the recently bereaved, outlined stages of grief. These stages commence with alarm at the loss, and a period of searching for the lost person. Experiences that temporarily mitigate the pain of grief, such as the intense feeling that the dead person is close, and feelings of anger and guilt towards the lost person, or surrounding the circumstances of their death, are common during the grieving process. Resolution of grief is said to follow when someone is able to gain a new identity and integrate feelings and ideas surrounding the loss within themselves; this is accompanied by feelings of confidence in 'coping' and moving on. Parkes also noted, however, that grief could run an atypical course; it may be prolonged or may not be fully expressed. In these circumstances individuals are at risk of physical health problems, and psychological morbidity such as anxiety or obsessional states and depression. Walshe[63] argued that the stage models of grief have been influential as descriptors of the grief process, but fail to account for the diversity of experience and outcome often seen.

Certain individuals may be at risk of atypical or pathological grief reactions. This may also be determined to some extent by the circumstances surrounding the death. Sudden or unexpected death, traumatic or violent death, or the death of someone where the relationship was difficult or surrounded by ambivalent feelings, are known to be risk factors. Deaths where the person was young, or where the bereaved person is a child or adolescent, are felt to cause more difficult bereavements, and it may be the case that the grief surrounding the death of one's child may never be resolved completely. Stroebe[64] has carried out research into gender differences in mourning. Men and women have been observed to express grief differently. Many men concentrate on dealing with reorganising their life and practical issues, whereas women focus on the loss and pain involved. It has also been noted that physical and psychological sequelae are more common amongst widowers than widows. Stroebe has concluded that focusing on practical issues and feeling the loss are important aspects of mourning; health professionals might usefully therefore help the person to address the side of grieving that they may not be expressing.

Unlike some of the stage theorists, Worden[65] took forward Freud's idea of grief work and proposed four tasks to be completed during bereavement:

- to accept the reality of the loss
- to work through the pain of grief
- to adjust to an environment in which the deceased is missing
- to relocate the deceased emotionally and move on.

The difference between this approach and the stage models is that it may be seen as a more dynamic approach to grief. Whereas the stage models provide descriptors, Worden suggests that the grieving person may have an active role to play.

Personal account 35.1

Working with a woman who had lost both her parents many years earlier, it became apparent that while she continued to feel the pain, there had been no grief work on relocating them and moving on. I suggested that she find ways of relocating her parents in her present context. At our next meeting, she told me with pleasure of the family photos she now had in her house and how she planned to put up a plaque in her parents' memory in the family church. She had not recognised this as a possibility before it helped her to free herself from a log jam of despair, allowing forward movement.

The psychologically orientated theories of grief have been criticised since they focus too much on bereavement as a pathological, rather than a normal event, and exclude social and cultural understandings of grief. Walters,[66] for example, is critical of the idea that grief is about working through emotion, the goal being to move on and live without the deceased. Instead he suggests a sociological model, where the purpose of grief is to construct a biography for the dead person so that their memory can be integrated into the lives of those who go on living. This is achieved through ongoing dialogue with people who knew the person who has died, the difference being that the process is more closely focused on talk than on emotion. Walters recommends that bereavement services should work to facilitate the building of such biographies.

Care for the carers

The ways in which families manage while caring for someone who is dying depend on various factors; for example, the severity of the illness (what level of care is needed), the chronicity of the illness (how long the care will be needed), and the quality of the caring relationship. In addition, an illness such as cancer calls into question the carer's perspective on illness and death, which will also colour their ability to care. Other factors that may influence the way a family, or family member is able to cope with care include the developmental stage of individuals in the family. That is, according to theories of psychological development throughout adult life, different tasks and issues will challenge individuals in different ways, according to their life stage.

There are also stages through which families develop; for example, having young children, or the transition a family must make when children leave home, or other critical times of change such as retirement or redundancy. Existing family problems will cause additional strain at a time of crisis, such as when a family member is ill or dying. The way individual family members or the family as a collective unit cope or manage difficult situations will characterise the way in which caring for a family member is handled. Responses such as fear and denial, attempts at protecting self and other family members from the reality of cancer and dying, create complex dynamics within families that require insight and careful handling on the part of professional carers.[61] There is also evidence that nurses are unwilling to listen to family members' problems.[67] It might be useful to ask the following questions of a family carer:

- What worries you about the illness?
- What is helping most at the moment?
- What else would help you cope?
- What else do you need to know about the illness and treatment?
- What is the worst thing at the moment?

There is evidence to suggest that where some sense of hope is maintained for family carers this is helpful. Herth[68] studied 25 adult family caregivers in order to identify strategies that maintained hope for them while they were caring. These included:

- being part of a sustaining relationship
- cognitive reframing; for example, trying to see the situation in realistic terms, accepting the here and now
- time refocusing, a decision to focus on the present and to see the future in terms of good events such as a family meal out
- focusing on attainable expectations, setting achievable goals and being flexible enough to change these if the situation warrants it
- maintaining spiritual beliefs; for example, a belief in a power greater than oneself
- finding ways of balancing energy expended with energy available.

Hope was hindered by being isolated, the experience of concurrent losses, or poorly controlled symptoms, when either the family member or professional carers could not successfully ease symptoms, especially pain, continuous vomiting, diarrhoea, or agitation.

Palliative care, the role of the nurse

Davis and Oberle[69] interviewed a community-based palliative care nurses on a number of occasions, asking her to draw on the experiences of working with 10 patients and families. The interviews in total amounted to 25 hours of conversation. The taped conversations were analysed and six discrete but interwoven themes were identified. These were then presented as six dimensions of the role of the nurse in palliative care. These are shown below.

The dimensions described by Davies and Oberle need to be seen as interwoven. In current health care contexts the pressure to give care can be so great that at times only 'doing for' rather than the totality of the nurse's role in caring for the dying is emphasised.

Surviving care

Working with dying people is immensely demanding.[70] Over-commitment to people who are dying is a risk for nurses and may lead to 'battle fatigue'. Fisher[71] has explored the possibility of staff growth through sensitive handling of the losses that constantly occur in any ward or care setting. Many nurses become very close to the people they care for, and yet have to act as though the death has no

Box 35.2: Six dimensions of the role of the nurse in palliative care

- *Preserving integrity*
  Looking inward
  Valuing self
  Acknowledging one's own reaction
- *Valuing*
  Global valuing – having respect for the inherent worth of others and a predisposition to look for this worth in others
  Particular valuing – understanding the uniqueness and abilities of each individual
- *Connecting*
  Making the connection – establishing credentials, explaining roles, getting baseline information, and explaining how to contact the nurses when necessary, spending time, finding a common bond and establishing rapport
  Sustaining the connection – being available, spending time, sharing secrets, giving of self, being available
  Breaking the connection – usually at death
- *Finding meaning*
  Focusing on living
  Acknowledging death
- *Doing for*
  Being a team player
  Taking charge – symptom management, lending a hand and making arrangements
- *Empowering*
  Facilitating
  Encouraging
  Mending
  Defusing
  Giving information

personal meaning for them. Care fatigue through repressing feelings of closeness or the need to grieve following the death of a person blurs the perception of daily concerns and effective working.[71,73] Strategies to help to prevent this include active stress reduction combined with increased awareness of the feelings and events surrounding caring for dying people. These need to be addressed at both an individual and an organisational level. A commitment to acknowledging this and to reflecting on care while also offering support and 'time out' for recovery or grieving are essential to maintaining the ability to work within emotionally demanding care settings, and in particular in caring for people who are dying of cancer.

References

1. Doyle D. (1993). Palliative medicine: a time for definition? *Palliative Medicine* 7, 253–255.
2. WHO (1990). *Cancer pain relief and palliative care.* Technical Report, Series B04. Geneva: WHO.
3. Walters T. (1993). Modern death: taboo or not taboo? In Dickson D. and Johnson H. (eds.) *Death, Dying and Bereavement.* London: Sage.
4. Glaser B.G. and Strauss A.L. (1965). *Awareness of Dying.* Chicago, IL: Aldine.
5. Kubler-Ross G. (1969). *On Death and Dying.* New York: Macmillan.
6. Twycross R. (1997). *Introducing Palliative Care,* 2nd edition. Oxford: Radcliffe.
7. Higginson I. (1993). Quality, costs and contracts. In Clark D. (ed.) *The future of Palliative Care.* Buckingham: Open University Press, pp. 30–51.
8. Higginson I. and Hearn J. (1997). A multicentre evaluation of cancer pain control by palliative care teams. *Journal of Pain and Symptom Management* 1491, 29–35.
9. McQuillan R., Finlay I., Roberts D., Branch C., Forbes K. and Spencer M. (1996). The provision of a palliative care service in a teaching hospital and subsequent evaluation of that service. *Palliative Medicine* 10, 231–239.
10. Seale C. and Kelly M. (1997). A comparison of hospice and hospital care for people who die: views of the surviving spouse. *Palliative Medicine* 11, 93–100.
11. Seale C. and Kelly M. (1997). A comparison of hospice and hospital care for the spouses of people who die. *Palliative Medicine* 11, 101–106.
12. Douglas C. (1992). For all the saints. *British Medical Journal* 304, 479.
13. Nash A. (1993). Reasons for referral to a palliative nursing team. *Journal of Advanced Nursing* 18, 707–713.
14. Pugh E.M. (1996). An investigation of general practitioner referrals to palliative care services. *Palliative Medicine* 10, 251–257.
15. Rafferty J., Addington-Hall J., Macdonald L. *et al.* (1996). A randomised controlled trial of the cost-effectiveness of a district co-ordinating service for terminally ill cancer patients. *Palliative Medicine* 10, 151–161.
16. Seale C.F. (1989). What happens in hospices: a review of research evidence. *Social Science and Medicine* 28, 551–559.
17. National Hospice Study (1986). *Journal of Chronic Diseases* 39, 1.
18. Kane R.L., Wales J., Bernstein L., Leibowitz A. and Kaplon S. (1984). A randomised controlled trial of hospice care. *Lancet* i, 890–894.
19. Parkes C.M. (1979). Terminal care: evaluation of an in-patient service at St Christopher's Hospice, Part 1: views

of surviving spouses on effect of the service on the patient. *Postgraduate Medical Journal* 55, 517–522.

20. Parkes C.M. and Parkes J. (1984). 'Hospice' versus 'Hospital' care – re-evaluation after ten years as seen by surviving spouses. *Postgraduate Medical Journal* 60, 120–124.

21. James N. (1989). Emotional labour: skills and work in the social regulation of feelings. *Sociological Review* 37, 15–42.

22. McNamara B., Weddell C. and Colvin M. (1994). The institutionalization of the good death. *Social Science and Medicine* 39, 1501–1508.

23. Biswas B. (1993). The medicalisation of dying. In Clark D. (ed.) *The Future of Palliative Care.* Buckingham: Open University Press, pp. 132–147.

24. Field D. (1994). Palliative medicine and the medicalization of death. *European Journal of Palliative Care* 3, 58–62.

25. Corner J. and Dunlop R. (1997). New approaches to care. In Clark D., Hockley J. and Ahmedzai S. (eds.) *New Themes in Palliative Care.* Buckingham: Open University Press.

26. Cawley N. (1997). *The experiences of patients with advanced cancer undergoing a referral to palliative care: a phenomenological study.* Macmillan Practice Development Unit, Institute of Cancer Research, London.

27. Glaser B. and Strauss A.L. (1968). *Time for Dying.* Chicago, IL: Aldine.

28. Pattison E.M. (1977). *The Experience of Dying.* Englewood Cliffs, NJ: Prentice-Hall.

29. Copp G. (1996). *Facing impending death: the experience of patients and their nurses in a hospice setting.* Unpublished Ph.D. thesis, Oxford Brookes University.

30. Lawler J. (1991). *Behind the Screens: Nursing, Somology and the Problem of Body.* Melbourne: Churchill Livingstone.

31. Buchan J.E.F. (1995). Nurses' estimations of patients' prognoses in the last days of life. *International Journal of Palliative Nursing* 1, 12–16.

32. Addington-Hall J. and McCarthy M. (1995). Dying from cancer: results of a national population-based investigation. *Palliative Medicine* 9, 295–305.

33. Cain J. and Hammes B. (1994). Ethics and pain management: respecting patient wishes. *Journal of Pain and Symptom Management* 9, 160–165.

34. McCaffery M. and Ferrell B. (1997). Nurses' knowledge of pain assessment and management: how much progress have we made? *Journal of Pain and Symptom Management* 15, 151–158.

35. Oreschuk D. and Bruera E. (1997). The 'dark side' of adjuvant analgesic drugs. *Progress in Palliative Care* 5, 5–13.

36. Holmes S. (1996). *Radiotherapy: A Guide For Practice,* 2nd edition. Dorking: Asset Books.

37. Kirkbride P. (1995). The role of radiation in palliative care. *Journal of Palliative Care* 11, 19–26.

38. Kaye P. (1994). *An A–Z Pocketbook of Symptom Control.* Northampton: EPL Publications.

39. Oliver G., McIllmurray, M., Aston V., Harding S. and Donovan G. (1997). Active palliative anti-cancer therapy. *International Journal of Palliative Nursing* 3, 232–233.

40. McNamara P. and Sharma K. (1996). Fracture in palliative settings: a study of management and outcome. Report of Palliative Care Research Forum, Durham, 1995. *Palliative Medicine* 10, 57–63.

41. Satera M. and Silbefarb P. (1996). Sleep disorders in patients with advanced cancer. *Progress in Palliative Care* 4, 120–125.

42. Stoter D. (1996). Spiritual care. In Penson J. and Fisher R. (eds.) *Palliative Care for People with Cancer,* 2nd edition. London: Arnold, pp. 158–168.

43. Stoll R. (1989). The essence of spirituality. In Carson V.B. (ed.) *Spiritual Dimensions of Nursing Practice.* Philadelphia, PA: W.B. Saunders, pp. 4–23.

44. Bowman M. (1995). *The Professional Nurse.* London: Chapman and Hall.

45. Cawley N. (1997). An exploration of the concept of spirituality. *International Journal of Palliative Care* 3, 31–36.

46. Burnard P. (1993). Giving spiritual care. *Journal of Community Nursing* 1, 16–18.

47. Stanworth R. (1997). Spirituality, language and the depth of reality. *International Journal of Palliative Care* 3, 19–22.

48. Kearney M. (1992). Palliative medicine – just another speciality? *Palliative Medicine* 6, 39–46.

49. Cornette K. (1997). For whenever I am weak, I am strong. *International Journal of Palliative Care* 3, 6–8, 10–13.

50. Ross L. (1997). The nurse's role in assessing and responding to patients' spiritual needs. *International Journal of Palliative Care* 3, 37–41.

51. Narayanasamy A. (1993). Nurses' awareness and educational preparation in meeting their patients' spiritual needs. *Nurse Education Today* 13, 196–201.

52. Ferrell B.R., Grant M., Dean G.E., Funk B. and Ly J. (1996). 'Bone tired': the experience of fatigue and its impact on quality of life. *Oncology Nursing Forum* 23, 1539–1547.

53. Herth K. (1990). Fostering hope in terminally ill people. *Journal of Advanced Nursing* 18, 538–548.

54. Flemming K. (1997). The meaning of hope in palliative care patients. *International Journal of Palliative Care* 3, 14–18.

55. Penson J. (1995). Caring for bereaved relatives. In Penson J. and Fisher R. (eds.) *Palliative Care for People with Cancer,* 2nd edition. London: Arnold, pp. 269–281.

56. Evans A. (1994). Anticipatory grief: a theoretical perspective. *Palliative Medicine* **8**, 159–166.

57. Pedder M. (1995). The role of the nurse in bereavement care. *Progress in Palliative Care* **3**, 219–223.

58. Hampe S.O. (1975). Needs of the grieving spouse in a hospital setting. *Nursing Research* **24**, 113–120.

59. Freud S. (1984). On mourning and melancholia. Reprinted in *On Metapsychiatry, the Theory of Psychoanalysis.* London: Penguin Books.

60. Klein M. (1940). Mourning and its relationship to manic depressive states. *International Journal of Psychoanalysis* **21**, 125.

61. Bowlby J. (1981). *Attachment and Loss.* London: Penguin Books.

62. Parkes C.M. (1986). *Bereavement: Studies of Grief in Adult Life.* London: Penguin Books.

63. Walshe C. (1997). Whom to help? An exploration of the assessment of grief. *International Journal of Palliative Care* **3**, 132–137.

64. Stroebe M.S. (1998). New directions in bereavement research: exploration of gender differences. *Palliative Medicine* **12**, 5–12.

65. Worden J. (1983). *Grief Counselling and Grief Therapy.* London: Routledge.

66. Walters T. (1996). A new model of grief: bereavement and biography. *Mortality* **1**, 7–26.

67. Munroe B. (1996). Terminal illness and the family. In Ford G. and Lewin I. (eds.) *Managing Terminal Illness.* London: Royal College of Physicians, pp. 55–62.

68. Herth K. (1993). Hope in the family caregivers of terminally people. *Journal of Advanced Nursing* **15**, 1250–1259.

69. Davis B. and Oberle K. (1990). The dimensions of the supportive role of the nurse in palliative care. *Oncology Nursing Forum* **17**, 87–95.

70. Earnshaw-Smith E. (1987). We don't need to be God after all. *Palliative Medicine* **1**, 154–162.

71. Fisher M. (1991). Can grief be turned to growth? Staff grief in palliative care. *Professional Nurse* **12**, 178–182.

72. Mathers P. (1995). Learning to cope with the stress of palliative care. In Penson J. and Fisher R. (eds.) *Palliative Care for People with Cancer,* 2nd edition. London: Arnold, pp. 296–308.

73. Vachon M.L. (1987). *Occupational Stress in the Care of the Critically Ill, the Dying and the Bereaved.* New York: Hemisphere.

CHAPTER THIRTY-SIX

Health services and cancer care

Sue Hawkett

Health service provision for cancer care is developed and delivered in a number of different environments. As cancer continues to be a major health problem across the world, it is important to examine the different ways in which countries develop strategic plans to reduce the risk of cancer and organise the delivery of care. There are, however, many factors that will determine how this is achieved. The cultural, epidemiological, social, and economic factors are just some of the considerations that will drive the priorities and planning of health care provision in each country.

At the ninth International Conference on Cancer Nursing held in England in 1996, the theme was 'Creating the Future'. In pushing any frontier there must be vision, commitment, enthusiasm, and a clear understanding of international, national, and local demands on health care. This message was delivered at the conference by strategists, educationalists, and clinicians, who repeatedly emphasised the importance of influencing policy makers in shaping and driving health care services forward. It is recognised that the interaction between expert professional advisers and those responsible for developing policy is vital. Policy informed by clinical experts, and its implementation driven by committed professionals is more likely to be translated into improved, effective, and lasting health care.

Cancer nurses, in particular, are well versed in this principle. The fact that such international conferences are established and respected, with thousands of delegates attending, is evidence of the influence that cancer nursing has exerted worldwide. Such international conferences are frequently attended by the host government health minister, who openly acknowledges the influence of nurses in policy development and health delivery. However, influencing strategic change relies on a number of dynamic factors, all of which nurses understand both instinctively and professionally.

Dynamic influences on health care provision

Critical mass of expertise – this, translated into expert practice based on research evidence and clinical care, underpins the development of health policy. Traditionally 'critical mass expertise' has been represented by uniprofessional groups. However, those who have the responsibility for developing health policy are concerned with providing the best possible care within the available resources. They are concerned with the totality of care provided by a health care team. Increasingly in Western countries, policy makers and purchasers of health care are reluctant to support a purely uniprofessional view.

Throughout the history of health care, however, one of the greatest influences, which cannot be ignored, is the dynamic of the doctor–nurse relationship. It has often been pivotal to change. Although this will always be the case, personal relationships between all members of the health care team are central to the delivery of health care both between professionals and between professional and patient. Therefore, successful health care delivery is dependent on inter-professional respect, willingness and ability to work together.

The nature of the work undertaken by different health professionals means that inter-professional boundaries are constantly shifting. As knowledge increases, coupled with technical and organisational complexity, traditional boundaries are eroded. Also pushing at these boundaries are users of health care, who have increased expectations of the service.[1] It is also becoming evident that within many health care teams there is a greater understanding of the roles of colleagues and therefore greater sharing of expertise.[2]

Good quality care needs to be delivered at a reasonable cost, which might involve care by a less trained person or someone with limited but focused training, supported and supervised by professionals with expert knowledge and expertise. Cancer care has many examples of innovative development, which has brought together the combined skills of a multi-professional team in delivering high-quality cancer care across the world.

Challenges

We have not, however, arrived! There is a long way to go in developing truly collaborative practice, which becomes an international model. The international conference on cancer nursing is an example. When will we see multi-professional conferences replacing these? Nurses, like other professionals, are reluctant to 'let go'. One reason for this may be that they often feel that they suffer from being classed as 'soft' and relegated to the end of conference programmes after all the 'hard' scientific papers have been given and most of the doctors have left.

There is tremendous scope for shared educational learning. As professional boundaries shift, so should our education. There are, of course, core elements belonging to the body of knowledge of any profession that remain sacrosanct. There are also, however, considerable areas of mutual interest, overlap, and duplication. This was to some extent recently identified by the Department of Health for England in a letter issued to the Health Service.[3] In this letter, the National Health Service Executive recognised the need for better integration of medical and non-medical workforce planning. It explained about moves to achieve greater multi-professional team working, together with blurring of traditional roles and responsibilities, which would require a more integrated approach to planning medical and non-medical education and training.

Agents for change

Policy makers are those who have an overall macro view and contribute towards decisions about health care resources. The allocation of these resources will be influenced through convincing professional advice based on sound evidence that the resources spent will provide the greatest outcomes for the investment.

At the ninth International Conference on Cancer Nursing, Richard Lamm, Director of the Centre for Public Policy and Contemporary Issues, University of Denver, posed some challenging questions on worldwide health needs and provision. Infinite needs have run into finite resources. How do countries set limits in health care? How do we ensure that resources are allocated where they will buy the most health?

How do we ensure value for money, in providing care that is at the same time appropriate, accessible, and of good quality? Can helpful lessons be learnt from developed countries over the last 30 years? Any lessons learnt, however, must be put within the context of the particular epidemiological, social, and political factors of that country.

It would be unwise to place the whole responsibility and power at the feet of governments and policy makers. Any central dictate is only as good as the commitment and enthusiasm of those who are able to deliver the care. Policy makers will always appear to those 'on the ground' as distant, out of touch, and unrealistic. Those charged with the responsibility of identifying priorities and planning the health care of the local population will grapple with the challenge of gaining the best possible care within their allocation from government. Those who provide the clinical expertise in caring for people with cancer will often feel that they could do so much more if given greater resources.

The relationship, however, between the macro and micro delivery of care, is a dynamic one. Because the 'chain' is so long from the point of policy development and implementation to the actual care received, it is not surprising that each part feels remote from the other. The opportunity to influence is often lost because of a lack of understanding about the role and function of each level.

Understanding some of the complexities facing some countries in providing health care and gaining a wider view will in itself empower nurses to seize opportunities to influence care at both a strategic and a local delivery level. In order to gain some appreciation of these issues, I look first at the European Community's 'Europe Against Cancer' programme, followed by a description and analysis of the current cancer policy for England and Wales.

Europe

The report from the Commission on the state of the health of the European Community (EC)[4] identifies cancer amongst the major diseases of adult life and as one of the main causes of death (along with accidents) for children between 1 and 14 years.

In response to its own epidemiological and social trends, each country needs to have a co-ordinated and assertive approach to the prevention and treatment of cancer. Although there will be regional differences in trends and the actual organisation of health care, there are nevertheless significant benefits from shared databases and collaborative research across Europe.

In order to address these issues in a common manner, action by the European Community has been undertaken. Article 129 of the EC treaty requires that 'the Community shall contribute towards ensuring a high level of human health provision' and commits the EC to contributing to disease prevention in all its aspects through Community action.

In Europe, cancer is the main cause of death for adults and accounts for four out of 10 deaths. Lung cancer continues to be the most frequent cause of death in men, although numbers are rising in women. Breast cancer is the most common cancer in women and is rising in most EC countries. The causes of breast cancer continue to be poorly understood. Cervical cancer causes about 7500 deaths in women in the EC each year. Cancer of the ovary causes twice as many deaths as cancer of the cervix. Stomach cancer causes about 5% of cancer deaths in the EC each year.

European action plans

In responding to these problems and as part of the co-ordinated approach the *Europe Against Cancer: the Second Action Programme (1990–94)*[5] included:

- an anti-smoking campaign
- action to improve eating habits
- development of systematic screening and early diagnosis for breast and cervical cancer
- contribution to directives for protection against carcinogenic agents
- the European Code Against Cancer
- development of a European network on cancer data.

The European Code Against Cancer, developed by the European Community Committee of Cancer Experts, set out 10 principles that reduce the risks of some cancers and cure others if detected early. It is claimed that, if universally adopted, the code should lead to a reduction of about 15% in the number of deaths from cancer in the Community by the year 2000.

On 29 March 1996 the European Parliament and Council of Ministers approved a third action plan to combat cancer within the framework for action in the field of public health (1996–2000).[6] The Community, in their commitment to implement the plan, instigated a number of actions. In brief, these were:

- data collection and research
- information and health education
- early detection and screening
- training, quality control, and guarantees
- establishing common objectives
- standardisation and collection of comparable and compatible data on health, including the development and strengthening of the European network of cancer registers
- programmes for exchange of experience and of health professionals and for the dissemination of the most effective practices
- creation of information networks – European-scale studies and dissemination of the results

- compilation of reports to monitor the measures taken
- exchanges of experience on quality control of the early detection of the disease and the prevention of its development, including palliative methods and contributions for selecting priorities in cancer research and transfer of basic research into clinical trials.

To support the implementation, a new management committee consisting of two members designated by each member state was set up by the European Commission. Arrangements were put in place for non-member countries and international organisations to be involved in the implementation.[6]

An example of how aspects of the action plan have been put into practice is illustrated by the *European Guidelines for Quality Assurance in Mammography Screening.*[7] In this document, the function of the European Network of Reference Centres (EUREF) is described. The EUREF is the European network of reference centres for breast cancer established by the Europe Against Cancer programme. Its office acts as a training, co-ordinating, and documentation centre. The office is charged with the responsibility of responding to and co-ordinating quality assurance training and monitoring the progress of the programme. In this way, screening programmes can be set up, supported, and evaluated to ensure consistency of approach at an agreed level of quality across Europe.

European cancer nursing

As cited above, the Second Action Plan for Cancer spanned 1990–94. In this action plan a great deal of work was done in co-ordinating and sharing good practice in cancer education. In 1991 the European Oncology Nursing Society (EONS), in conjunction with the European Commission's Europe Against Cancer programme (EAC), published *A Core Curriculum for a Post-Basic Course in Palliative Nursing*[8] and a year later *Core Curriculum for a Post-Basic Course in Cancer Nursing.*

These curricula were adopted by many European countries (except for Luxembourg, France, and the UK) in ensuring that knowledge and skills were taught at a consistent standard throughout Europe. This work was referred to in the report of the sub-committee on palliative cancer care (see below).

Although the core curriculum was not adopted in the UK, mainly because of pre-existing courses approved and accredited by nursing statutory bodies and some universities, a network was established with a steering group to monitor the provision and quality of cancer courses.

The European Oncology Nursing Society has taken three strands of cancer nursing education forward. These are concerned with cancer care curricular content in pre- and post-registration courses and advanced cancer nursing courses.

Their work has been strategic and comprehensive. Having produced the post-registration core curriculum for cancer and palliative care, a 5-year follow-up survey has been undertaken.

In addressing pre-registration courses, a European conference was held. As a result of this conference, it was agreed that guidelines should be developed for pre-registration courses across Europe. This has now been achieved.

Palliative cancer care

In 1990 a survey was conducted by the European Commission as part of an exchange of experiences in palliative care under the 1990–94 action plan. The aim was to identify palliative care provision in the member states and to recognise that palliative care was an integral component of cancer care.[9] The survey showed that only some 5% of people with cancer received care in a palliative care unit in 1989. This percentage fell to under 1% if the UK was excluded. It was estimated that 20% of people with cancer in the UK received treatment in a palliative care unit.

Unlike the UK, where the concept and initial practice began as early as 1967, palliative care is a relatively recent area in the other member countries. At the time of the survey, however, there was a rapid development of palliative care in six countries; two had recently set up centres, one had developed a system based on voluntary services, and two had not yet established a unit.

Following this survey, a working group of experts was constituted to prepare a report.[10] The report described palliative care in order to establish some agreed understanding of the term and made recommendations for education and training and the widespread implementation of palliative care.

The sub-committee recommended that national governments should promote integration of palliative care into their health care systems 'in order to ensure an optimal quality of life for patients', as also recommended by the World Health Organisation.[10] The main areas in which the committee made recommendations were:

- education and training
- implementation and monitoring
- finance.

The report supported the concept of education and training being available for all health care professionals, irrespective of where they were practising, with the recommendation that it should form a compulsory part of all undergraduate courses. The working group also recommended that continuing education and training be provided for all health care professionals practising palliative care. National cancer and other relevant organisations were identified as having a key part to play in raising the awareness of the general public of the member states through publicity campaigns. In the UK, Macmillan Cancer Relief is an exceptional example of how such organisations can influence policy makers and providers of care.

The sub-committee considered how palliative care should be implemented and monitored in the EC. The essence of the deliberations is summarised below.

- Palliative care should be an integral part of services offered by National Cancer Institutes (the UK Expert Group recognised this).
- Impediments that unnecessarily restrict the availability of morphine and other important drugs used in palliative care should be removed.[10,11]
- Patients should receive good palliative care at home, in hospital or in other institutions.[12]
- Volunteers should be trained to work alongside but under the supervision of professional health care workers.
- All major cancer centres should evaluate the adequacy of their palliative care facilities and services (recognised by the UK Expert Group).

With regard to resourcing issues for the implementation of the recommendations, the sub-committee said that health care finance, both public and private, should cover the costs of palliative care, irrespective of that care setting. They also recom-

mended that funding be made available for education, training, and research. As a result of this recommendation, a special fund was set up to support educational programmes and 'site visits' to other countries for 4 years from 1992. Many educational initiatives have taken place across Europe as a result of this particular recommendation.

In 1990 the British government announced an additional allocation of £8 million to enable health authorities to contribute more to the voluntary hospice movement and similar organisations. This allocation had risen to £35.7 million by 1994–95.[13,14]

The Europe Against Cancer programme has made a significant impact on health care provision, education and training, research, treatment, and care of cancer patients across Europe. It is, however, only possible to evaluate the true effect by reviewing cancer statistics in each country. In the UK the *Health of the Nation*[15] initiative, which began in 1992, set out a strategic plan to promote health and prevent disease in four major cancers for which the toll in terms of ill-health and death is high and where prevention measures and health education could reduce the mortality and morbidity significantly. This was done with the government's long-term objective to reduce the mortality and morbidity caused by all cancers. Prevention is recognised across the world as a key element in the fight against cancer. The UK actively supports the Europe Against Cancer programme in its aims to reduce the number of deaths from cancer by 15% by the year 2000, through prevention, public information and education, training, and the co-ordination of research. The Health of the Nation strategy and its successor, Our Healthier Nation, continue to be part of that overall initiative.

UK approach

There are over 200 different types of cancer. More than 200 000 new cases are diagnosed in England and Wales each year. One in three people will develop cancer at some time in their life, and after coronary heart disease, cancers are the most common cause of death in England.

Cancer is particularly predominant in older people: 65% of new cancers registered and nearly 75% of deaths are in the over 65s.

Table 36.1 Deaths (England and Wales, 1996): all malignant cancers – 13 092[16]

Men		Women	
All cancers	**71 855**	**All cancers**	**66 237**
Lung	19 874	Breast	11 098
Prostate	8 782	Lung	11 077
Colon	5 021	Colon	5 524
Stomach	4 252	Stomach	2 526

Health of the Nation[15]

In summary, the key targets set for four cancers as part of the UK strategy for the reduction of cancers were as follows.

Lung
- Reduce death rate for lung cancer by at least 30% in men under 75 and 15% in women under 75 by 2010.
- Reduce prevalence of cigarette smoking in men and women aged 16 and over to no more than 20% by the year 2000.
- In addition, at least 33% of women smokers to stop smoking at the start of their pregnancy by the year 2000.
- Reduce consumption of cigarettes by at least 40% by 2000.
- Reduce smoking prevalence in 11–15-year-olds by at least 33% by 1994.

Breast
- Reduce rate of breast cancer deaths in the population invited for screening by at least 25% by 2000 (from 1990).

Cervix
- Reduce incidence of invasive cervical cancer by at least 25% by 2000 (from 1990).

Skin
- Halt year-on-year increase in incidence of skin cancer by 2005.

In considering the above in the light of the European initiative, it is interesting to see how one country (England) approached the health promotion and education aspects of cancer, the progress of which is now described.

Health of the Nation – progress

Lung cancer continues to be the most common cancer among males, accounting for 25% of all registrations of malignant neoplasms (excluding non-melanoma skin cancer), and the third most common cancer in females, accounting for 11% of all malignancies.

Smoking continues to be a major risk factor for lung cancer and therefore its reduction has been a major Health of the Nation target. Figures show that adult smoking rates in England continue to fall, although smoking among 11–15-year-olds has increased. In February 1994 the government published Smoke-free for Health: An Action Plan to Achieve the Health of the Nation Targets on Smoking. As part of this action plan, a 3-year national smoking education campaign costing £13.5 million was launched, aimed particularly at parents. Children whose parents smoke are twice as likely to smoke than the children of non-smokers.[17]

Reducing deaths from breast cancer is a major Health of the Nation target. The breast screening programme in England has been described as a success story. Set up by the government in 1987, it was the first country in the European Community and one of the first in the world to launch a nationwide breast cancer screening programme based on computerised call and recall. Since then the targets set by the programme (except for the detection of small cancers) have been exceeded. All screening centres have completed their first round of screening and are now inviting women for their second screen after an interval of 3 years. Over a million women attend the NHS breast screening programme annually, which is an uptake of 72%. In 1994–95 this rose to 77%. Some 15 000 cancers were detected by the programme during the first full round of screening in England.

The Health of the Nation target for invasive cervical cancer has already been met. Cervical cancer deaths fell by over 30% between 1988 and 1995. The cervical screening programme began in 1988 and was the first in the European Community. Screening is a health priority for women aged 20–64, who are encouraged to have a cervical smear at least every 5 years.

The achievement of the skin cancer target is entirely dependent on the general public being aware of the risks of ultraviolet (UV) exposure and changing their behaviour. The Health Education Authority in 1994 launched a 'Sun Know-How' campaign promoting the messages to stay out of mid-day sun, taking care not to burn, to cover up and wear a hat. Evaluation showed that during 1994 87% of adults were aware of some publicity about sun and skin cancer and 51% saw the UV forecasts.

The UK, however, although addressing health promotion and education, considered that more could be done. The general public raised concerns about the provision of cancer services. In addressing this, the chief medical officers for England and Wales convened an expert multi-professional group to advise them.

Putting the problem into context

In order to put in context the cancer policy that emerged as the result of the recommendations of the expert group, it is important to trace the changes that have taken place in the National Health Service (NHS) in England. The past 8 years have seen major organisational re-structuring to support the implementation of the White Papers – *Working for Patients* (1989),[18] *Health of the Nation* (1992),[15] *Caring for People* (1989),[19] *The New NHS – Modern and Dependable* (1997),[20] *Our Healthier Nation* (1998),[21] and *A First Class Service* (1998).[22]

As a result of the health service changes in 1991, the then district health authorities (DHAs) were charged with the responsibility of assessing the health needs of their population. They were then to contract with service providers to meet those demands in an effective and balanced manner, taking into account the views of the population they served. In developing primary health care services, general practitioners (GPs) were given the opportunity to become 'budget holders'. This has enabled GPs to assess the needs of their patients and contract directly with service providers for care.

Both DHAs and GP fundholders, however, had to take account of available resources when contracting services and GPs were only able to contract for certain services. There was, however, a number of pilot projects enabling GPs to purchase all care, which included cancer and palliative care. This project is undergoing an evaluation, which was due to be completed in 1998.

The purchasers or commissioners of health care have been encouraged to integrate primary and secondary care purchasing, to support the drive towards decentralisation in the NHS, and to develop stronger health authorities better able to champion the interests of local people.[23] This integration was further supported by three subsequent White Papers – *A Service with Ambitions* (November 1996),[24] *Choice and Opportunity* (October 1996),[25] and *Primary Care: Delivering the Future* (December 1996).[26]

With the merger in 1996 of DHAs and family health services authorities (FHSAs) to become health authorities (HAs) and the closer working relationships with GP fundholders and local authorities, the potential for effective purchasing power was enhanced. Such agencies have the ability to take a strategic view of the resource requirements for cancer and palliative care (as for other services), thus identifying gaps and preventing over-provision and duplication. A possible danger of such large purchasing authorities is that of size, making it difficult to maintain effective communication between service providers and purchasers. The cancer policy emerging from the expert group's recommendations sought to reduce that danger.

Clinical nurse cancer specialists have a significant role to play in facilitating links between purchasers and providers of cancer care and in providing expert advice. In order to achieve this, nurses need to transfer knowledge from an operational level to a strategic framework and to provide advice to commissioning agencies.[25] There has been a number of most successful initiatives, where cancer nurses have been supported in providing professional advice in the strategic planning of cancer services.

Further major government initiatives

As mentioned above, further government initiatives focused on integrating primary and secondary health care. This was encapsulated in the three White Papers – *A Service with Ambitions* (November 1996),[24] *Choice and Opportunity* (October 1996),[25] and *Primary Care: Delivering the Future* (December 1996).[26] Each has an impact on the organisation of cancer and palliative care services.

A Service with Ambitions (November 1996)[24] reaffirmed the government's commitment to the NHS on the basis of its founding principles of universal, high-quality care available on the basis of clinical need. The paper sits alongside *The Health of the Nation* (1992)[15] and *Caring for People* (1989)[19] as the third part of an overall health and health care strategy.

Primary Care: The Future – Choice and Opportunity (October 1996)[25] and *Primary Care: Delivering the Future* (December 1996)[26] brought together the proposed strategy to provide and resource a high-quality, integrated health service, organised and run around the health needs of individual patients. These papers outlined opportunities that would support the integration and co-ordination of cancer patients between acute care and community. So often it is in the community that a patient begins and completes his or her 'journey'. Also of particular note in these papers were the opportunities outlined for nurses working in primary care for personal, professional and career development. These opportunities have been strengthened further through *The New NHS, Modern and Dependable* (1997).[20]

Each year, the government issues medium-term priorities for the NHS. These are specific objectives, which provide key indicators of progress towards achievement. They are defined in such a way that at each level of health care provision agreement can be reached on how these will be achieved and by what measures. These objectives include promoting clinical effectiveness and HAs are asked to consider potential for action in areas of national priority, which in 1997–98 included *The Health of the Nation* and the reconfiguration of cancer services. Greater emphasis was given to this in *The New NHS* (1997)[20] and in *Our Healthier Nation* (1998).[21] *The New NHS* guarantees that everyone with suspected cancer will be able to see a specialist within 2 weeks of their GP (family doctor) deciding that they need to be seen. The target for these arrangements will begin with those with suspected breast cancer by April 1999. *Our Healthier Nation* (1998)[21] suggests that the death rate from cancer amongst people aged 65 should reduce by at least one-fifth by 2010.

A policy framework for commissioning cancer services

Care and treatment for cancer patients form a substantial part of NHS work in primary and secondary care sectors (around 7% of NHS resources). At the moment, treatment is provided in general hospitals and specialist cancer centres. Palliative care for people dying from cancer is also provided by the voluntary sector through individual hospices and national charities like Marie Curie Cancer Care and Macmillan Cancer Relief.

In response to concerns about variations in treatment across the country or a 'cancer lottery', an expert group on cancer was convened to advise the Chief Medical Officers for England and Wales. As a result of this work, a strategic framework for the future development of cancer services, based on the advice of the expert group, was described in the report *A Policy Framework for Commissioning Cancer Services*.[27] This was launched in April 1995, following wide consultation, and had general support from health care professionals and users of the service.

The report was produced partly in recognition that in the UK there were apparent variations in recorded outcomes of treatment. Patient care was at the centre of these new proposals. The key principles emphasised the need for greater public and professional awareness to help the early recognition of symptoms of cancer and to make sure that all patients had access to high-quality care to ensure maximum possible cure rates and best quality of life. Wherever possible, it was recommended that care should be provided as close to the patient's home as possible, with patients, their families and carers being given clear information about their condition so that they could understand about treatment options and outcomes.

The report recommended that cancer services should be organised at three levels.

1. Primary care should be the focus of care. GPs should be better informed about available diagnostic and treatment services to make appropriate referrals and be informed promptly about the outcomes of tests and of any treatment. Subsequently, this was reported in the white papers on primary health care.
2. Cancer units would be created in many local hospitals. These would be of a sufficient size to

support a multi-disciplinary, multi-professional team with the expertise and facilities to treat the more common cancers. A lead clinician would co-ordinate cancer services and develop treatment protocols between primary care, cancer units, and cancer centres to ensure a network of care of a high standard.

3. Cancer centres situated in larger hospitals would treat the less common cancers and support cancer units by providing services not available in smaller hospitals, including radiotherapy.

The report stressed that palliative care should be an integral part of cancer care and not be associated exclusively with terminal care. The report recommended that each district should have a specialist palliative care resource for both primary care and hospital-based services. This concept was further developed in a specific Executive Letter (EL) on Palliative Care – this being the first EL to address direct care and provision and definitions of palliative care (EL(96)85).[12] This was followed in June 1998 by a Health Service Circular on Palliative Care (HSC 1998/115),[28] which stressed the importance of palliative care becoming mainstream in hospitals and that palliative care skills and knowledge were appropriate for those suffering from other life-threatening illnesses.

Implementation of the recommendations contained within the policy framework

A great deal of work was soon underway in the NHS towards the implementation of the strategic framework.

Key elements in this were:

- regional mapping of current patterns of provision of cancer services
- regional/local development of process for implementation
- identification of cancer units and cancer centres
- agreement of explicit contracts between purchaser and provider for the provision of cancer services
- development of a plan for improving the availability and quality of data
- central implementation.

Central implementation

Although the strategic framework was devolved to regions in England and Wales, a number of central co-ordinating measures was also put in place. Following the launch in April 1995, regional co-ordinators in each of the regions in the two countries were appointed who subsequently formed a national network meeting with Department of Health officials. In addition, a national network of nurses working as regional advisers taking the lead for overall non-medical interests in each of the regions was set up. In each region, implementation groups were organised to co-ordinate the new provision of cancer and palliative care services. The national networking groups provided an overview that enabled mutual concerns and issues to be addressed and prevented unnecessary duplication of effort.

As the implementation progressed, so further guidance was issued by the NHS Executive: (EL(96)15),[27] (EL(96)66,[29] and (EL(96)85.[12]

EL(96)15[27] was issued on 15 March 1996, giving more detailed guidance for HAs on the implementation of the cancer strategic framework, building on the substantial work already in hand within the NHS. The guidance included recent evidence, where it was available, on the benefits of specialisation within cancer sites and projected timescales for enacting change.

Cancer site-specific guidance

Simultaneously, to support work being taken forward regionally, the NHS Executive commissioned work to prepare evidence-based guidance in a rolling programme of work, starting with the more common cancers.

The work was taken forward by a sub-group of the NHS Executive's Clinical Outcomes Group. The group was multi-professional and chaired by Professor Bob Haward (Professor of Cancer Studies, Leeds University). The group's remit was to help purchasers and providers to identify cancer units and cancer centres by making recommendations on the characteristics of a centre or a unit. These would include:

- minimum throughput compatible with a high-quality service, including where appropriate

guidance on the clinical management of cancers
- ways of measuring the quality of care delivered, including measures of outcome.

Breast, lung, and colorectal cancers were considered in the first tranche, with breast cancer being used as a pilot for the development of guidelines for a wider range of cancers.

Improving Outcomes in Breast Cancer was published in July 1996 (EL(96)66).[29] This represented the first in the series of guidance documents on services for the more common cancers. Guidance on colorectal cancer[30] and lung cancer[31] has been published and guidance on gynaecological cancers will follow.

The recommendations in the guidance formed a set of priorities that helped purchasers and providers of care to focus on areas most likely to make a difference to the outcomes. The guidance was explicit about the nature and strength of the evidence on which the recommendations were based and was published in two volumes:

The Manual set out recommendations on a series of 11 topics, including patient-centred care, rapid and accurate diagnostic services, patient follow-up, palliative care, and effective inter-professional communication.

The Research Evidence presented summaries of the evidence relevant to each of the topics covered in The Manual.

Palliative care

It is interesting to track the way in which palliative care has developed in the UK in recent years and in particular in England. As mentioned above, a significant proportion of palliative care has been provided by the voluntary sector. With the 1991 NHS reforms enabling HAs to identify and purchase health care for their local populations, so contracts were developed with the voluntary sector. This was supported initially by specific allocations from central government to HAs for palliative care services (as mentioned above). This has since been integrated into the HAs' general purchasing intentions for palliative care across their district. As part of the

government support, HAs were encouraged to match funds raised by the voluntary sector. This was a national target and did not apply to individual providers and, as contractual arrangements became firmer between the sectors, ceased to be appropriate (EL(96)85).[12] Clark carried out a study of how the NHS reforms had affected the hospice movement.[32] The study included a postal survey of all UK in-patient hospices and palliative care units for adults and 12 case studies of a representative cross-section of these. Among the voluntary sector hospices who replied to the questionnaire, the mean income for NHS contracts was 38% of the total. This was compared with NHS 'hospices', who received 91% mean income from contracts. The overall view from the study was mixed and contradictory but Clark suggested that:

> . . . the message from our research is optimistic and favourably inclined to the beneficial impact of purchasing. Indeed the majority mood is positive.[32]

The influence and contribution to development and establishment of palliative care made by the voluntary sector hospices cannot be ignored.

Hospices provide specialised palliative care and support for terminally ill people and their families. Services provided (mainly to patients with cancer, motor neurone disease, and AIDS) include in-patient care, day care, home care, and counselling.

Most hospices are in the voluntary sector. At January 1996 there were 207 hospices operating in the UK with a total of 3097 beds, with 557 provided by 50 NHS units. There were over 225 day units, 383 home care teams, 168 hospital support nurses, and 101 hospital support teams. In England alone, there were 171 hospices, with a total of 2599 beds, 308 home care teams, 89 hospital support teams, and 191 day hospices). Some of these are part of larger national voluntary bodies (Marie Curie Cancer Care, the Sue Ryder Foundation), but most are locally based individual charities. There are two umbrella organisations: Help the Hospices and the National Council for Hospice and Specialist Palliative Care Services. The latter, which represents services in England, Wales and Northern Ireland, has made a significant impact both in a co-ordinating role between the many arms of the movement within the voluntary sector and NHS, and also in influencing government health policy.

Increasingly, as mentioned before, palliative care is an essential and integral part of effective cancer care. It can be provided in a variety of settings – in the community, hospital, hospice, and nursing home. It is, however, from hospices that much of the knowledge, skill, and motivation for change has emanated in supporting cancer patients and their families.

Palliative care more than any other is a multi-professional activity, which crosses professional boundaries between health and social care. The needs of patients facing a life-threatening illness are multi-faceted and may be shaped by a variety of personal, social, and cultural factors. Palliative care principles can support people at different points of their illness and need not be confined to the terminal stages.[33]

The National Council for Hospice and Specialist Palliative Care Services defined palliative care in its document 'Specialist Palliative Care: A Statement of Definitions' in a most helpful way, which has been endorsed by the government in guidance to purchasers of health care.[12] The National Council has made the following distinctions.

- Palliative care is the active total care of patients and their families by a multi-professional team when the patient's disease is no longer responsive to curative treatment.[31]
- Palliative care is a broad term, which covers provision in both community and in-patient settings. Services may be NHS or voluntary, multi-professional or uni-professional; and may be provided by individuals or teams. Some services will meet the definition of specialist palliative care services, others may not; they are all staffed by professionals who have extensive experience and/or additional training in aspects of palliative care, some up to specialist level.
- The palliative care approach aims to promote both physical and psychological well-being. It is a vital and integral part of all clinical practice, whatever the illness or its stage, informed by

a knowledge and practice of palliative care principles.
- Specialist palliative care services are those services with palliative care as their core speciality. Specialist palliative care services are needed by a significant minority of people whose deaths are anticipated.
- Palliative care, as the World Health Organisation has recognised, is the active, total care of patients whose disease no longer responds to curative treatment, and for whom the goal must be the best quality of life for them and their families.
- Palliative care is now a distinct medical and nursing speciality in the UK. It focuses on controlling pain and other symptoms, easing suffering, and enhancing the life that remains. It integrates the psychological and spiritual aspects of care, to enable patients to live out their lives with dignity, as well as offering support to families during both the patients' illness and their own bereavement. Bereavement follow-up for families and carers should be provided initially by local palliative care/hospice teams or community nurses. Identification of further needs for support or complex grieving may require the involvement of specialist services or trained counsellors.[32]

All of these principles were firmly embedded into the framework for cancer services and have been included in the implementation of the policy.

Cancer nursing services

The Royal College of Nursing Cancer Nursing Society recognised the important opportunity that the framework for cancer services presented for the patient, health care professionals and not least the nursing profession. In response, it set up a working group to examine the type of cancer nursing services that should be shaped in the light of the proposed framework. This was encapsulated in the document *A Structure for Cancer Nursing Services* (1996),[34] which was commended by the Secretary of State for Health for England at the ninth International Conference on Cancer Nursing. In summary, the report recommended the following.

- People with cancer should have access to nurses with appropriate experience and skills.
- Specialist cancer nurses, with their mix of inter-personal skills, knowledge, and expertise, should also be involved in the purchasing side of health care.
- Consideration should be given to whether aspects of education and training in cancer care should be multi-disciplinary and multi-profes-sional.
- Specialist nurses working in cancer centres and units should have attained first degree level or master's level education in cancer care.
- When the size of the patient population does not merit the cancer unit providing all special-ist nursing expertise, liaison with a cancer centre should be ensured and joint posts considered.
- Cancer nursing research should focus not only on disease and treatment but also on the impact of the disease on the patient and family.

The recommendations, however, need to be placed in context and facilitated by nurses at dif-ferent levels of health care provision in order for the implementation to become a reality.

The influence of expert clinical advice on purchasers of health care has already been discussed. More than any group, nurses have close daily contact with users of health care services. Nursing services account for approximately 25% of the total NHS budget and 80% of direct care is delivered by nurses. Research has shown that Chief Executives of HAs and NHS Trust hospitals recognise that the experience and skills that nurses possess are crucial to effective purchasing.[35] Grasping this potential and building on the research evidence, a region in England identified eight cancer nurse specialists and actively involved them in the selection of cancer units. The nurses were given initial training to ensure consistency of assessment across the units and subsequent sessions to identify common themes regarding nursing issues for the implementation of the units. The programme also looked at ways in which nurses can be best supported to make policy-level contributions.

Specialism – professional issues for nurses

A Policy Framework for Commissioning Cancer Services[27] reviewed the evidence supporting spe-cialisation of care as a means of improving cancer treatment outcomes. The debate that ensued identified that improving outcomes in cancer care had many facets. It was not just a matter of a sin-gle professional with expert skills. Although this was important, so too was the combination of this expertise working with a multi-professional team of trained, skilled, and experienced staff. It was stat-ed[27] that other facets of specialism included the facilities available and the number of patients treat-ed. Although the evidence is not clear as to which of these facets is responsible for improved out-comes, treatment from a multi-disciplinary, multi-professional team composed of those with a special interest in the treatment of a specific can-cer is desirable.[36] A specialist cancer nurse has a sig-nificant role to play in these teams.

In their report,[34] the Royal College of Nursing differentiated between a nurse working in a spe-cialty and a specialist nurse. The distinction was made by describing nurses providing everyday care to cancer patients in wards and departments in can-cer units and centres. These nurses would be in practice-based positions requiring limited in-depth knowledge and experience. They would draw on the expertise and support of specialist nurses.

Specialist nurses are those who have acquired higher and advanced level cancer qualifications and possess in-depth specific knowledge and skills. They would provide an expert resource for their col-leagues working in any care setting, as well as practical intervention for specific cancer-related problems within their specialty.[37]

Education for cancer nurses

As has been described earlier, cancer education and training for medical and non-medical staff became an important issue in the implementation of the framework for cancer services. Here, as with other areas, the influence and voice of cancer nurses are important. The RCN Cancer Nursing Society has recently published *Guidelines for Good Practice in Cancer Nursing Education* (1996),[38] which aims to provide expert and research-based standards for cancer nursing education. This, with its parallel work *A Structure For Cancer Nursing Services*,[34] supports the need for patients to have access to, and to have their care supervised by, specialist registered nurses with appropriate training. It was generally acknowledged that the proposed changes in service delivery would require a flexible responsive approach in education.

Responsive education

The advances in technology require increased skills and knowledge and greater support for the non-specialist. The shift within health care generally from acute to primary care results in greater demands on the primary health care team. These demands are increased with the development of faster referral routes into and out of specialist cancer services. In order for these services to be effective, there must be robust communication and co-ordination. Education therefore needs to respond by looking at opportunities for multi-professional education, courses which are modular, flexible, and delivered at the required academic level by teachers who are credible in clinical practice.

Fewer than 1% of registered nurses are estimated to have any specialist cancer training.[39] The impact that specialist nurses have on the emotional and physical well-being of cancer patients is considerable.[40–43] Their place in specialist cancer teams cannot be disputed,[27] and their contribution to strategic planning is recognised but underutilised. The framework for cancer services in England and Wales[27] provides an excellent example of how nurses can come to grips with the intricacy of health policy, strategic planning, and management of cancer services. Such nurses require appropriate training. Therefore, the challenge to educationalist and practitioner alike is considerable.

In 1996 the English National Board for Nurses, Midwives and Health Visitors undertook a national curriculum review of their cancer courses to ensure that they were matching the changing pattern of cancer nursing and care. The review was supported by a multi-professional steering group. This was just one example of the way in which statutory, voluntary, professional, and government organisations caught the vision of the cancer policy and sought to contribute to its successful implementation.

Resources

To implement such a strategy has resource implications. The Department of Health stressed that the implementation would take some years to allow for any changes in the provision of services and medical and nursing training. In the interim, however, the need for increased education and training programmes for medical and nursing staff was examined.[3]

It was estimated in 1996 that NHS current spending would grow by £1.3 billion in 1996–97 and, together with efficiency gains, would enable the NHS to make further improvements in cancer services.

Summary

The changes in the NHS in England have been considerable in recent years. Cancer and palliative care are an integral part of these changes, further supported by specific government policy.

The success of this policy will finally be dependent on the vision, commitment, and enthusiasm of those who prize their clinical expertise in cancer and palliative care. Cancer nurses are part of that group and have a role to play in ensuring that the right structures are put in place, with nurses having adequate training not only to provide but also to lead the service in the future.[34]

References

1. The National Cancer Alliance (1996). *'Patient-Centred Cancer Services?' What Patients Say.* Oxford: National Cancer Alliance.
2. Hopkins A., Solomon J. and Abelson J. (1996). Shifting boundaries in professional care. *Journal of the Royal Society of Medicine* **89**, July 96.
3. Department of Health for England (1996). *Education and Training Planning Guidance,* EL(96)46. Copies obtained from Mrs Jane Hare, Tel. 0113 254 6121.
4. Commission of the European Communities (1995). *Report from the Commission on the State of Health in the European Community, COM(95)357 Final.* Brussels: Commission of the European Communities.
5. International Agency for Research on Cancer (1990/94). *Europe Against Cancer – European Code Against Cancer.* Luxembourg: Office for Official Publications of the European Communities.

6. European Parliament and European Council (1996). Decision no. 646/96/EC of the European Parliament and of the Council of 29 March 1996, adopting an action plan to combat cancer within the framework for action in the field of public health (1996–2000). *Official Journal of the European Communities No. L 95/9.*
7. European Commission (1996). *European Guidelines for Quality Assurance in Mammography Screening.* Luxembourg: Office for Official Publications of the European Communities.
8. International Society of Nurses in Cancer Care (1991). *A Core Curriculum for a Post-Basic Course in Palliative Nursing.* Manchester: Haigh and Hochland.
9. Doc. No. DGV E 1/6601/93. *Survey on Palliative Care in Europe.* Europe Against Cancer. European Commission.
10. Doc. No. DGV E 1/6002/93. Report of a sub-committee on Palliative Cancer Care. Europe Against Cancer. European Commission.
11. National Council for Hospices and Specialist Palliative Care Services (1994). *Guidelines for Managing Cancer Pain in Adults.* London: National Council for Specialist and Palliative Care Services.
12. Department of Health for England NHS Executive (1996). *A Policy Framework for Commissioning Cancer Services: Palliative Care Services,* EL(96)85 Leeds: National Health Service Executive.
13. Department of Health (1990). *Funding for Hospices and Similar Organisations,* EL (90)P/10. London: Department of Health.
14. Department of Health NHS Management Executive (1994). *Contracting for Specialist Palliative Care Services,* EL/(94)14. Leeds: National Health Service Executive.
15. Department of Health for England (1992). *Health of the Nation: A Strategy for Health for England.* London: HMSO.
16. Office of National Statistics (1997). *Deaths Registered in 1996 By Cause, and By Area of Residence,* monitor DH2 97/1. London: HMSO.
17. National Council for Hospices and Specialist Palliative Care Services (1995). *Specialist Palliative Care: A Statement of Definitions,* Occasional Paper 8 October 1995. London: National Council for Hospices and Specialist Palliative Care Services.
18. Department of Health for England (1989). *Working for Patients.* London: HMSO.
19. Department of Health for England (1989). *Caring for People.* Heywood, Lancs: Health Publications Unit.
20. Department of Health for England (1997). *The New NHS, Modern and Dependable.* London: HMSO.
21. Department of Health for England (1998). *Our Healthier Nation, A Contract for Health, A Consultation Paper.* London: HMSO.
22. Department of Health for England (1997). *A First Class Service. Quality in the New NHS.* London: HMSO.
23. Department of Health for England NHS Management Executive (1993). *Purchasing for Health: A Framework for Action. Speech by Dr Brian Mawhinney.* Heywood, Lancs: Health Publications Unit.
24. Department of Health for England NHS Executive (1996). *A Service With Ambitions.* London: The Stationery Office.
25. Department of Health for England (1996). *Choice and Opportunity. Primary Care: The Future.* London: The Stationery Office.
26. Department of Health for England (1996). *Primary Care: Delivering the Future.* London: The Stationery Office.
27. Department of Health for England NHS Executive (1996). *A Policy Framework for Commissioning Cancer Services,* EL(96)15. Leeds: NHSE.
28. National Health Service Executive (1998). *Palliative Care,* HSC(1998)115. Wetherby: Department of Health.
29. Department of Health for England NHS Executive (1996). *Improving Outcomes in Breast Cancer: Guidance for Purchasers,* EL(96)66. London: Department of Health for England NHS Executive. (Further copies from Health Literature Line.)
30. Department of Health for England NHS Executive (1997). *Improving Outcomes in Colorectal Cancer: Guidance for Commissioning Cancer Services,* EL(97)66. Wetherby: Department of Health.
31. Department of Health for England NHS Executive (1998). *Improving Outcomes in Lung Cancer: Guidance for Commissioning Cancer Services,* HSC 1998/114. Wetherby: Department of Health.
32. Clark D. (1995). Hospices to fortune. *Health Service Journal* **23**, 30–31.
33. Hawkett S. (1995). In Richardson A. and Wilson-Barnett J. (eds.) *Policy Issues and Provision of Cancer Service in Nursing Research and Cancer Care.* London: Scutari Press.
34. RCN Cancer Nursing Society (1996). *A Structure For Cancer Nursing Services.* London: RCN Cancer Nursing Society.
35. Department of Health for England (1994). *Building a Stronger Team: The Nursing Contribution to Purchasing.* Heywood, Lancs: Health Publications Unit.
36. World Health Organisation (1990). *Cancer Pain Relief and Palliative Care,* World Health Organisation Technical Report Series 804. Geneva: World Health Organisation.
37. Selby P., Gillis C. and Howard R. (1996). A new model for cancer care: evidence for benefits from specialised care. *Lancet* **348**, 313–318.
38. RCN Cancer Nursing Society (1996). *Guidelines For Good Practice in Cancer Nursing Education.* London: RCN Cancer Nursing Society.

39. Corner J. (1996). Nursing vital to cancer care – comment. *Nursing Standard,* **10** (35), 17.

40. Smith J.E. and Waltman N.L. (1994). Oncology clinical nurse specialists' perceptions of their influence on patients outcomes. *Oncology Nursing Forum* **21**, 887–893.

41. Wilkinson S. (1991). Factors which influence how nurses communicate with cancer patients. *Journal of Advanced Nursing* **16**, 677–688.

42. Corner J., Plant H. and Warner L. (1995). Developing a nursing approach to managing dyspnoea in lung cancer. *International Journal of Palliative Nursing* **1**, 5–11.

43. Heslop A.P. and Bagnell P. (1988). A study to evaluate the intervention of a nurse visiting patients with disabling chest disease in the community. *Journal of Advanced Nursing* **13**, 71–77.

CHAPTER THIRTY-SEVEN

Research and cancer care

Jessica Corner

Research is a dynamic process, through which knowledge is generated about and for any given field of activity. It can also be seen as an important force for change, given that the goal of research is constant improvement and discovery. The need for research into cancer, its treatment and care is unquestionable. It is a moral and ethical duty to ensure that patients are receiving optimal treatment, and that their needs are established, understood, and catered for; also that the various forces and conditions that create the construction of cancer treatment and care are more clearly understood, so that these can be redefined and taken forward as appropriate. This may be by conducting studies into the biological and genetic causes of the disease, developing and evaluating new treatments, or researching new and better ways of caring for patients. In nursing, there is increasing interest in how research can be used as a means of developing practice in a way that is more immediate than relying on practitioners to read the results of published studies. For this to become a reality, research and practice must be integrated in clinical settings and with practising nurses.

Research has always played a prominent part in the management of cancer. Since a very large number of patients remains incurable and the aggressive nature of cancer treatment continues to have a major impact on quality of life, those working in the specialty of oncology have constantly sought to identify more effective cancer treatments. Researchers from other disciplines such as psychology and sociology have studied the emotional and social consequences of cancer to both the sufferer and family or friends. Nurses too are increasingly using and undertaking research; in particular, they are studying the needs of patients and nursing effectiveness in relieving problems related to cancer or its treatment.

More generally, health care reforms internationally are driving changes in the management of research and its funding. This in turn affects research into cancer treatment and care. There is a recognition that in health care, research needs more planning and a strategic direction. In the past, the topics and research questions identified have been in the main developed by 'enlightened individuals', frequently driven by the interests and skills of an individual or a research team, rather than by what is needed for the health services, or what might be identified as the greatest problem area by patients. This has resulted in a tendency to research only the 'rare' or 'interesting', rather than more direct questions about the way everyday health care is practised. Internationally, countries are working to identify priority areas of research for funding, so that studies can actively contribute to improving services for patients. The Europe Against Cancer programme, for example, is an initiative of the member states of the European Community, which aims to reduce the number of cancer deaths by 15% by the year 2000. Research studies have been commissioned by the programme as well as from central European research funds, which will help to achieve this aim.

In the UK, major reform of the way research is viewed within the National Health Service has taken place. A research and development (R&D) directorate was established at the Department of Health, with the specific remit to commission priority-driven research aimed at the needs of the health service and not solely at the 'cure' of disease. This has brought about a fundamental change in the way that health services research is viewed. It represents the first attempt in the UK to establish a coherent research and development infrastructure to support the promotion of health and the provision of health care. The programme is intended to develop knowledge that can provide a basis for improvements in the approach taken to health care by managers, health care professionals, and users of health services.[1] Key features of the programme are shown below.

Box 37.1: Key features of the NHS R&D strategy[1]

- A systematic approach to identifying and setting R&D priorities in which staff and users of the service are being asked to identify important issues confronting them and, in partnership with the research community, to characterise and prioritise these problems as a basis for seeking solutions.
- Staff are not only invited to set the agenda for research but will, in future, be better placed to use the output of research more effectively. Information systems are being established to ensure the systematic transfer of up-to-date research results to users in the service in an accessible form.
- The research community has a new opportunity to work closely with managers and clinicians in the service to identify obstacles caused by lack of information and to identify existing knowledge or new research that can directly help the service.
- The programme of applied research involves researchers from a wide range of disciplines in medicine, nursing and the basic social sciences, bringing a multi-disciplinary team together to consider issues from a variety of perspectives using a wide variety of methodological approaches.
- The R&D strategy aims to place the NHS in the position of a discriminating user of technology. Through the advice of the CRDC Standing Group on Health Technology, the NHS will be able to ensure that practice reflects research-based knowledge and that new health technologies in need of assessment do not find their way prematurely into routine use.

The research and development strategy involves not only commissioning studies, but also establishing a national database of ongoing research, and supporting systematic reviews of studies already undertaken so that best evidence for practice can be ascertained, and from which guidelines for clinical practice can be written, the fundamental principle being establishing relevant research findings within everyday practice. The interdisciplinary nature of the strategy is of great importance to nurses, since they are an integral part of all decision-making processes and in identifying priority areas for research. Uni-disciplinary research is no longer encouraged; instead, it is felt that research should be conducted in interdisciplinary research teams. This does not preclude nurses from leading research teams, and a number of nurse-led projects has been funded by the programme.

Cancer was identified early on as a priority area for the commissioning of research studies. The priority areas identified for cancer are shown below. These priorities, derived by consensus from a multidisciplinary community of health care professionals and researchers, have radically altered the research agenda away from a basic science and treatment orientation for much of research, to more wide-ranging studies encompassing quality of life and service issues. It is hoped that this will have an important effect on the nature of research undertaken on cancer.

Research and cancer treatment

Clinical trials and cancer

Clinical trials of new treatments have been the mainstay of research in cancer care and are a dominant part of the environment of cancer centres. Cancer treatment is largely experimental, and research is a driving force behind much of service development. Unfortunately, little attention has been paid to the impact this has on care, or the treatment packages on offer to patients. Because of the experimental nature of much cancer treatment, many people will have their treatment while involved in a clinical trial, particularly if they are being treated in a specialist cancer treatment centre. Cancer nurses are therefore frequently involved in administering experimental cancer treatments to patients, or talking through issues surrounding clinical trials and experimental treatments with patients and their families. Cancer nurses can find themselves having ambivalent

Box 37.2: Priority areas for research into cancer[2]

- Ways of effecting, maintaining, and evaluating behavioural changes, leading to a reduction in smoking at all ages.
- Factors influencing delayed presentation by patients (e.g. psychosocial) and variations in onward referrals by physicians to oncology specialists.
- Factors influencing the accrual of patients into cancer trials (including why clinicians are reluctant to enter patients into multi-centre trials).
- Studies designed to explain variations in disease outcomes, particularly in relation to variations in patterns or practice.
- Comparison of care for common cancers (e.g. lung, breast, colorectal) in specialist and non-specialist treatment settings with respect to psychosocial and clinical outcomes and the relative costs of managing each step of disease progression.
- The clinical utility of second-line chemotherapy in advanced cancers, particularly its comparison to best supportive care.
- Optimal management strategies for unrelieved symptoms, including pain and non-pain, in cancer patients.
- The most appropriate and cost-effective model of service delivery and level of provision of palliative care services, including the role of nurse practitioners.
- The early natural history of cancers that may particularly lend themselves to screening to reduce mortality (e.g. prostate, oral, and skin cancers).
- The most cost-effective way to provide information to meet the needs of cancer patients, their families, health care professionals, and the public.
- The roles of adjuvant, neo-adjuvant, and combined modality treatments for primary common cancers.
- Cancer treatment of the elderly, including clinical outcomes and cost-effectiveness.
- The value of integrating quality of life data and data on costs in the measurement of outcome in prevention, treatment, and care of cancer patients and their carers.
- What prevents terminally ill people from dying at home, if they so wish, and how general practitioners and their teams may access information to help them to care more effectively for their patients at home.

attitudes to such experimental treatments, and the ethics of patient involvement in clinical trials. Nurses working in cancer therefore need to have an understanding of the issues surrounding clinical trials and cancer and of an individual's rights regarding participation in these.

Clinical trials are the means by which the efficacy of a new treatment is established. Since new treatments for cancer are continually being developed, it is necessary to determine whether existing established treatments should be replaced by these new developments. The ultimate goal is to improve the rates of disease remission, survival, and quality of life. Increasingly, cost and economic evaluation are also becoming an important feature of clinical trials, since cancer treatment is costly and governments are requiring tangible, measurable benefits of treatment to be assessed against the costs.

Clinical trials for new treatments are conducted in three phases (see below). The principles on which each is based are somewhat different, as are the dilemmas. The principles that justify such studies are a careful assessment of the likelihood of achieving a medical advance versus any risks to the person undergoing treatment. This is most difficult in phase I and II trials where the likelihood of benefit to those participating, who already have advanced disease and where standard treatments have already failed, is minimal, whereas the likelihood of adverse effects could be significant. There is a need for participating subjects to have given informed consent to all aspects of the study, including potential adverse effects and without pressure, or the fear that their care might be adversely affected if they refuse to participate.[3] In addition, studies must be governed by the 'uncertainty principle', that is there must be genuine uncertainty as to the therapeutic effectiveness of the treatment, and a likelihood that this can be determined through the trial.[4]

Phase III trials are larger studies usually involving a comparison of a new drug or treatment with an existing treatment. People who are identified as eligible to take part are considered to be representative of the wider population of those with the same condition and are known as a sample. Those agreeing to take part are then usually allocated at random to receive one or other of the treatments. Participants are then studied over time to examine how they fare according to certain identified outcome criteria. Common outcome indicators are: tumour response (reduction in size of the tumour, classified either as non-response, partial response, or complete response, i.e. no evidence of tumour following treatment); length of survival; toxicity or side-effects experienced.

Box 37.3: Clinical trials

A clinical trial is a planned experiment designed to elucidate the most appropriate treatment for future patients with a given medical condition. Results based on a limited sample of patients are used to make inferences about how treatment should be conducted in the general population of patients who will require treatment in the future.[5] Clinical trials involving new drug, chemotherapy, or radiotherapy treatment for cancer are classified into three phases.

Phase I trials
Conducted to determine drug safety, bio-availability, and drug metabolism, usually through dose escalation studies in which patient volunteers are subjected to increasing doses of the drug. There is little or no likelihood of benefit to the patient and therefore patients consenting to take part are really doing so for the benefit of future patients.

Phase II trials
Small-scale studies of the effectiveness and safety of a drug. Different doses of the drug are given to different groups of patients to help to identify the therapeutic dose and activity of the drug. Again, patients are usually invited to take part in a phase II trial when other more conventional treatments have failed, therefore there may be only a small likelihood of the patient benefiting.

Phase III trials
New drugs with known effectiveness are compared with standard treatment regimes in a trial of a large number of patients. Patients are usually randomly allocated to the different treatments under comparison. Efficacy of different treatments is evaluated using outcomes such as disease response, survival, and changes in performance status, which is a crude measure of an individual's functional state on a scale from 0 (representing fully mobile and functional) to 4 (completely dependent, or moribund), as well as quality of life and economic effects or costs.

Quality of life

Quality of life is a relatively recent addition to outcome assessment in clinical trials of cancer treatments. In the past, studies were criticised because they did not sufficiently take into account the individual's experience of treatment.[6] Researchers conducting early clinical trials of new treatments were preoccupied with increasing the survival rates of invariably fatal cancers. Progress in the treatment

of such cancers (for example, leukaemia in childhood, and testicular cancers) led to other factors such as the physical and long-term cost of treatment to the individual becoming a greater priority. In addition, the requirement to seek the patient's viewpoint has increasingly been recognised and there is criticism of a failure to respond to this in cancer trials.

A wide variety of quality of life measures has been developed for use in clinical trials. Quality of life tools address one or all of a number of domains of the potential impact cancer and its treatment may have on an individual. These are as follows.

- *Physical well-being* – perceived and observed bodily function or disruption (for example, pain, nausea and fatigue). It encompasses the degree to which the individual is experiencing disease symptoms, treatment side-effects and general physical problems.
- *Functional well-being* – the ability to perform activities of daily living such as walking, feeding, bathing and dressing oneself; taking part in social activities and ability to work.
- *Emotional well-being* – usually assessments are made of the extent of psychological morbidity from anxiety and depression.
- *Social well-being* – the extent of social support needed and available, disruptions to family functioning, intimacy and sexual functioning.[7]

Quality of life studies have shown a wide variety of disruptions caused by cancer treatment; some of these have been helpful in determining the relative value of different treatments. An example of this is the collective evidence of studies on the differences for women having mastectomy as opposed to conservative surgery for breast cancer, such as lumpectomy. Fallowfield[8] has collated a number of studies, which seem to show that conservative treatment may not yield the lower rates of psychological morbidity anticipated from the less physically mutilating treatment. Rather, Fallowfield suggests that this is a more complicated issue; in studies where they were given a choice over their treatment, women fared better regardless of the type of surgery they received. It is the cumulated evidence from studies using quality of life measures that allows insights into such aspects of treatment to be explored.

The difficulties in making the assessment of quality of life part of all clinical trials and a meaningful and practical tool for clinical practice are well recognised. These may raise ethical dilemmas; for example, measuring quality of life in clinical trials may identify problems that are not then acted upon; there are difficulties in obtaining complete data on all patients; and interpretation of the results of studies, and the validity and reliability of quality of life instruments are problematic.[9]

Some criticism of the measurement approach to quality of life has been expressed in the nursing literature.[10] Established measures of quality of life have pre-determined the aspects to be measured for the patient; these are usually in the form of a series of items to be rated by the patient. The problem with this is that it does not allow for the unique and individual experience of cancer and its related problems to be expressed. This means that it is impossible to know whether the items selected for inclusion in the tool, or the scores yielded for that individual, truly represent their quality of life. This is an issue of validity in measurement. Benner[10] argues for studies using a phenomenological approach to the study of quality of life. Such studies attempt to access the individual experience, through the person's own eyes, using in-depth, open-ended interviews, from which detailed accounts of experiences can be derived. According to Benner, it is only by undertaking such studies that real insight into patient needs and agendas can be gained. In phenomenologically orientated studies, the domains of inquiry would be somewhat different to those identified by Cella[7] and would encompass:

- the changing experience of the body
- changing social relationships as a result of illness
- changing tasks and demands of different stages of the disease process and disease trajectory
- predictable responses and effective coping strategies for treatment side-effects and sequelae
- the particular – what the illness interrupts, threatens, and means to the individual.[11]

Faithful[11] has combined both a phenomenological perspective and a well-established quality of life tool (the EORTC QLQ-30[12]) in order to gain deeper understanding of the symptoms patients experience when undergoing pelvic radiotherapy for cancers of the bladder and prostate. This allowed data on both symptom severity using the EORTC QLQ-30 scale and detailed information about the meaning of symptoms and their impact on patients' lives to be gathered. The use of a standard measure such as the EORTC QLQ-30 was useful in that it made comparisons with other patient groups possible, and was useful as a measure of change within this group of patients over time. However, open-ended interviews allowed the researcher to develop much deeper understanding of the needs and difficulties that they were facing. Combined method approaches such as this have a lot of potential for nursing research.

Economic evaluation

With the growing pressure on health services internationally to contain escalating health care costs, economic evaluations of all new cancer treatments are increasingly being demanded by health planners. These evaluations are designed to give information on the cost-effectiveness of such treatments, and to enable comparisons with existing best methods of management. The introduction of new treatments therefore increasingly will have to be justified in relation to their costs, in terms of both quality of life for individuals receiving them, and the economic costs. Techniques for the economic evaluation of treatments vary. These may take the form of:

- *cost-effectiveness studies* – undertaken to compare different health care interventions with different consequences, and comparing the different levels of effectiveness of these with their costs
- *cost-utility studies* – for example, calculating quality of life-adjusted years or QALYs. Here the analysis takes into account a trade-off between length and quality of life as a result of different treatments
- *cost–benefit studies* – where all the consequences of interventions, the changes in length and quality of life, and their expense are expressed in financial terms.

From these it is possible to assess whether the total value of the extra benefits from one intervention exceeds the extra costs involved if it is also more expensive. In reality, economic evaluation is complex, and many factors influence the validity of cost and benefits in relation to new and existing cancer treatments; they are, however, going to become an increasingly common factor in health care research, and nurses need to become familiar with considering economic issues when scrutinising research into cancer treatments and in undertaking their own research.

Ethical issues in cancer research

All research raises ethical issues about the manner in which a study is conducted, and the checks and safeguards for individuals involved, or who may be affected by the research itself or its findings. This is particularly the case when the research involves vulnerable individuals such as patients with cancer or their families and carers, and where the research may involve the experimental use of new treatments. The principles on which research involving human subjects should be based were laid down in the Declaration of Helsinki in 1964.[13] These reinforce the necessity for the justification of all research in terms of the balance of the potential benefits to the person involved as a research subject against inherent risks, and identify the importance of informed consent. This means that the potential subject must be adequately informed of the aims, anticipated benefits and hazards of the study, and that consent is freely given to their involvement in it. Such consent must be given voluntarily, without pressure or incentive to take part; subjects should also understand that they can withdraw from the study at any time, and that non-participation will not prejudice their treatment or care in any way. In most instances, this consent would be required to be given in writing and witnessed by an independent observer.

Participants in research also have rights that need to be protected by the researcher, such as the right to anonymity, confidentiality of any data about them used in the study, the right to receive optimum treatment and not to be disadvantaged in any way by their participation or non-participation, and the right to withdraw from the study or experimental treatment. These rights equally need to be protected in studies involving experimental cancer treatments known to be toxic, as well as in apparently less hazardous studies, such as interviews with

individuals about their disease and needs for care. Studies using qualitative research methods, such as tape recording of in-depth interviews with participants, are increasingly being recognised as having ethical implications, and are potentially exploitative of vulnerable individuals.[14]

Studies involving patients or patient data are required to be scrutinised by a hospital ethics committee. This is a body set up by the hospital, health authority, or university that has medical, non-medical, scientific, nursing, lay, and legal representation. Researchers are required to submit detailed proposals or protocols of the research study to the committee. These should include sufficient detail for the following to be made clear to the committee:

- the scientific merit of a study (since inadequate research is also unethical)
- the potential hazards and risks to the patient
- the means by which informed consent will be obtained
- copies of written information for patients regarding the study
- assurances over the protection of anonymity, confidentiality, and other rights of any individual taking part in a study.

In addition, the committee requires that researchers declare any potential conflict of interest they may have in conducting a study, such as receiving payment by a pharmaceutical company for undertaking the work, if this could encourage bias in interpreting the results of a study.[15,16] Clinicians undertaking studies involving the evaluation of a new drug or other treatments are also subject to stringent monitoring and registration requirements, depending on the country in which the research is taking place. There are also international systems in place for the notification of adverse effects of experimental drugs and treatments.

While there is increasing scrutiny of research into new cancer treatments through local ethics committees, the nature of cancer treatment is such that much treatment offered, particularly in specialist centres, is experimental. This means that nurses working in cancer care will frequently find themselves caring for patients who are participating in clinical trials, and they may be asked to administer experimental treatments. Nurses can find themselves questioning the ethical basis of such treatment trials, and at times may feel ambivalent over their involvement. The ethical issues surrounding clinical trials have been the subject of much discussion and debate. Hazel Thornton, a woman diagnosed with breast cancer, was asked to take part in a trial of different treatments for ductal carcinoma of her breast. As a result of her experience she has actively campaigned for greater involvement of patients in the design of such trials. Personal account 37.1 contains an excerpt of Hazel Thornton's[17] writing on this, which gives insight into the dilemmas people with cancer may face in giving consent. The work of Luker et al.[18] suggests that more than half of women diagnosed with breast cancer would adopt a very passive role in decision making about their treatment if given a choice. This makes it difficult for nurses to understand their own role in working with patients undergoing experimental treatment. Professional bodies for nursing give some guidance here; for example, the Royal College of Nursing[19] advises that in acting as a witness to a patient giving informed consent, nurses should 'satisfy themselves' that this has been freely given and that the patient understands what they are giving consent to and any risks involved. In the event of the research being seen to have an adverse effect on the subject, the nurse has an obligation to intervene by informing the researcher and appropriate person in authority.

Increasingly, some of these issues are being addressed through the involvement of cancer patients in the design and monitoring of clinical trials. This trend towards the 'user as commissioner' allows co-operation and shared responsibility in planning and designing clinical trials and in particular in the preparation of information for participants so that it is clear and assists decision making. As Hazel Thornton[20] says,

> . . . this approach demonstrates a new attitude to research that is not imposed on the patients, but which has been devised and executed as an expression of the appreciation of the ideal that, as this research is for the patient, the patients have been allowed to exercise their responsibility by participating in designing and planning trials which might more clearly express their desired outcomes, thereby providing trials in which they might be pleased to participate.

Personal account 37.1: Extract from Thornton H. (1992). Breast cancer trials: a patient's viewpoint. *Lancet* **339, 44–45 (reproduced with permission)[17]**

The practice of 'informed consent' before inclusion in randomised controlled trials is well known. My invitation to participate in such a trial is well known. My invitation came 2 weeks after an operation to remove an abnormal piece of breast tissue. I was handed a leaflet that explained the need for the DCIS trial and which listed the treatment options. The booklet *Living with Breast Cancer*, published by the UK Health Education Authority, was given to me and I was advised to telephone the British Association of Cancer United Patients (BACUP) to obtain information on radiotherapy and tamoxifen. I was asked to come back in 2 weeks with my decision and was assured that, if I declined, my aftercare would not be affected.

A lay person's dilemma is clear. A woman is given a diagnosis that she has never heard of before and a leaflet indicating four widely differing treatment options: no further treatment, a 4–5-week course of X-ray therapy to the breast, one tamoxifen tablet daily for 5 years, or both radiotherapy and tamoxifen. This scenario begs the question: What is informed consent?

I sought every means to inform myself during the next 2 weeks about DCIS and its treatments, and about randomised controlled trials. I quickly became aware that without the facts of my case, e.g. size of DCIS, volume of tissue removed, state of marked excision margins, histological sub-type, and oestrogen receptor status, it would be impossible to speculate on the likely effects of the four treatments on offer. I was fortunate to have excellent sources of information.

My instinctive reaction against radiotherapy for this non-invasive condition was reinforced by several experienced and well-informed doctors and radiotherapists . . . radiotherapy is included in two out of the four treatment options in the trial; my feeling was that, because I was unwilling to undergo radiotherapy, I could not take part in this study . . . Without the supplementary information that I was able to obtain myself, I cannot understand how a woman can properly judge the proposal that has been put to her. Even with such information it is a haphazard assessment for the lay person. I was astonished that . . . women were asked to co-operate in a study where the range of treatments was so wide. To suggest that randomised controlled trials are necessary and to ask your average woman-in-the-street to have to decide whether or not to take part at the moment she has just been told she has a carcinoma would seem to be asking just too much.

Nursing research and cancer care

The enormous potential for nurses to undertake research in cancer care is obvious. The number of nurses working in cancer settings, and the move of basic and post-basic nurse education into the higher education setting has meant that nurses are increasingly becoming equipped to conduct studies into areas of their practice. The growth of advanced practice and nurse specialist roles, where systematic evaluation of practice and service innovation are inherent, will increasingly require nurses to undertake research as part of their roles. The number of nurses undertaking PhD study continues to grow, and therefore internationally there is a network of nurses in key positions who can play a pivotal role in instigating programmes of research and facilitating others to initiate studies. The need for research into aspects of cancer care is ever more apparent. Nursing needs an evidence base for its practice, not just to provide information on how best to provide effective care, but also to offer evidence for the need for specialist nursing intervention at a time when the value of all health care settings and interventions is being called into question.

Over the last 20 years, a number of attempts has been made to identify priorities for the focus of nursing research in cancer care. Oberst's[21] priority setting study using the Delphi technique was the first to attempt to do this systematically. A panel of 575 nurses was surveyed and asked to identify priorities for cancer nursing research. A list of problem statements was generated from the responses, which was then returned to the panel members to rate in terms of the value to nursing research and patient welfare these may have. In two further rounds of the survey, consensus was reached over the items and their ranked order. For areas with the greatest potential for improving patient welfare, items relating to problems surrounding physiological responses to cancer treatment, especially chemotherapy, and relief of patients' physical discomfort, including pain, were given highest priority. Items judged to have the highest value to practising nurses surrounded the need for organisational support systems for the practitioner, and educational and communication needs. A replication study of Oberst's work was conducted by the

Western Consortium for Nursing Research.[22] Broadly similar areas of priority were identified. The top five combined areas are shown below.

Box 37.4: Priority areas for cancer nursing research[22]

1. Find ways to prevent and/or treat stomatitis from chemotherapy.
2. Determine needs of health professionals for education related to pain management.
3. Evaluate the effectiveness of patient teaching in relation to patient compliance, maintenance of self-care, and coping.
4. Evaluate the use of relaxation, imagery, and biofeedback techniques in decreasing anticipatory nausea, side-effects of treatment, or in enhancing quality of life.
5. Determine effective methods for prevention and control of chemotherapy-induced side-effects.

The authors of the Western Consortium study were critical of the amount of progress that had been made in cancer nursing research since Oberst's study 10 years earlier. They examined the accumulated nursing research evidence for the priority areas: with the exception of pain management, limitations were identified in the research in each of the other four areas. Small sample sizes and inadequate research designs in studies undertaken severely limited their usefulness, as did the complexity of interventions evaluated. Little evidence of programmes of research or of multi-centre studies was present.

The most recent research priority setting survey has been that of the USA Oncology Nursing Society's membership conducted in 1994.[23] For the survey 93 items were listed under seven major categories: symptom management, care delivery issues, psychosocial aspects of care, special populations, continuum of care, health promotion behaviours, and treatment decision making. In addition, respondents were asked to identify the type of research needed. A total of 773 questionnaires was returned, making a response rate of only 36%. The items remained relatively consistent. This survey, however, also highlighted the demand for intervention and research orientated towards the outcomes of care, as the most frequently needed types of research. This survey reflects the fact that increasingly nurses are relying on the results of research to guide their practice and to develop and improve their nursing interventions. Advanced practice was identified as the eleventh ranked priority area for research, which also reflects the development of nursing into specialist and nurse practitioner roles.

The realisation of the criticisms of nursing research, as overly descriptive and lacking clear ongoing programmes of study, led a group of UK nurses to take a somewhat different focus. Supported by the Cancer Research Campaign, a British charity, two meetings were held, to identify through a process of consensus development the issues and difficulties in promoting nursing research activity in cancer care. The first step in this process was to agree a working definition of nursing research in cancer care, and priority areas for research, then to make recommendations about possible means of promoting high-quality research. The outcome of these meetings was reported.[24] Nursing research in cancer care was felt to focus on:

> . . . the impact of the disease and its treatment on the individual and his or her family, and the efficacy of nursing care in alleviating/ameliorating disease or treatment induced problems and needs.[24]

As such, it has a distinct and complementary orientation to medical research, which largely concerns itself with the assessment of disease outcome in response to treatment using endpoints such as duration of survival, tumour response, treatment toxicity, and cost versus quality of life estimates. In contrast, nursing research has focused on the consequences to the individual with cancer and its treatment at any stage of the disease process, and on investigating the most effective methods of providing supportive care.

Two broad areas of research were felt to encapsulate nursing practice in cancer care and therefore should be the focus of research activity. These were:

1. Patients, problems, systematic methods of assessment, and studies related to the management of these.
2. The experiences and needs of patients, survivors, close relatives, and significant others, and methods of facilitating coping and adjusting to cancer.

The group strongly recommended that research into cancer care should be promoted by the development of ongoing coherent programmes of research by groups of nurses according to agreed priorities. Centres conducting such research programmes would also be in a position to offer research training. Programmes of research could be built using a framework similar to that of clinical trials for anti-cancer agents, using multi-phase studies, which incorporate theory-generating and exploratory/descriptive phases, before moving onto more traditional intervention studies, for example:

Phase 1 Exploration of a problem (e.g. descriptive studies of the level and nature of fatigue following chemotherapy or the symptom of breathlessness in lung cancer)

Phase 2 Development and piloting of an intervention/problem management strategy

Phase 3 Formal evaluation of the intervention, using clinical trials, evaluation research, and multi-centre studies.[24]

It has, however, been recognised that there is a number of barriers to nurses developing a strong research base in cancer care. Payne[25] identifies constraints such as a lack of research training in basic and post-basic nursing education. Neither Bachelor's nor Master's programmes in nursing could really be described as offering anything more than an introduction to research. Real research training in other disciplines is not considered to start until higher degree level, such as in Ph.D. programmes. Until there is a 'critical mass' of nurse researchers qualified at doctoral level internationally, nursing research in cancer care is unlikely to develop fully. Payne[25] identifies the lack of funding available for nursing research, the difficulty of access to skilled research supervision, and the lack of time in busy clinical posts for research as significant constraints. She also argues that there is no money or status to be gained for the majority of nurses who might contemplate undertaking research, and a powerful anti-intellectual ethos apparent in some parts of nursing may militate against its development. Despite these difficulties for nursing in establishing its research base, a range of work has been conducted that continues to be highly influential for practice, and suggests an important future for nursing research in cancer care.

Core tasks of research for cancer nursing practice can be listed under five headings.

1. Systematic reviews of the current state of knowledge/evidence in any given area.
2. Studies that develop and test research instruments and measures, or research approaches.
3. Development of detailed understanding of cancer-related problems or client needs.
4. Evaluation of existing or new practices aimed at enhancing care or alleviating problems.
5. Detailed evaluation of existing and new services in cancer care.

A range of research methods and techniques has been used in studies; these vary according to the particular question the study aims to answer and the orientation of the researcher.

Systematic research reviews

Reviewing the literature to ascertain the current state of knowledge and level and type of research that has previously been undertaken in any given field is a traditional precursor to undertaking any study. Over recent years, there has been growing interest in the use of more systematic techniques of research synthesis. Traditional reviews, conducted by a single researcher describing and giving a critical overview of previously conducted research, have a number of problems. They are inherently open to bias since the reviewer can be highly selective in both the studies chosen for the review and the level of detail and critical evaluation presented. In addition, one of the most problematic areas of reviewing the literature lies in the area of determining what actions should be taken as a result of a collective body of evidence from the totality of studies conducted. This is particularly the case when decisions are being made about the effectiveness of treatments or new interventions. For this reason methods of systematic review have been developed. Systematic reviews are also heralded as a means of getting research findings into practice, since the findings of larger volumes of studies can be examined and recommendations made for practitioners.

Integrative review and meta-analysis techniques use statistical procedures to combine the findings of a collective body of studies. These techniques allow judgements over the quality and strength of the findings of individual studies to be weighted and then these weightings can be taken into account for the statistical analysis.[26] Theoretically the results of a carefully conducted meta-analysis are much less open to bias on the part of the reviewer than more traditional methods. However, these techniques are not without their critics.[27] The quality of any systematic review lies in the coverage of the review. What is important is the confidence one has in the retrieval of all studies in a given area. This may mean accessing unpublished studies, since it is known that a large response bias exists towards the publication of studies that show a positive effect of treatment or intervention, rather than a negative one. The latter are much more likely to be rejected or never submitted for publication.

Searching the literature is a difficult and complex process. On-line computer searching using databases such as Medline and CINAHL is known to yield very low retrieval rates (some estimates suggest between 30 and 50% of published studies).[28] Retrieval is much improved by supplementing searching with hand searching journals and retrieving studies referenced by other authors. The second area of difficulty lies in the judgements made about studies during analysis. Determining effect, size, and quality of studies is difficult, and often inadequately reported by the original authors.

These techniques yield the most useful data when a large volume of studies focused on intervention and/or outcomes exists. Since a dearth of research exists in cancer nursing, systematic reviewing can be problematic. However, it was used by Smith et al.[29] to examine American oncology nursing research. Of 428 research studies retrieved over a 10-year publication period, 90% were purely descriptive and therefore not amenable to meta-analysis techniques. Forty-two intervention studies were, however, of sufficient quality to examine this way. Using the meta-analytic technique, cancer nursing interventions were found overall to be significantly effective, with membership of the intervention group improving success by 22%.

Richardson[30] has used a rather different review technique to explore the current understanding of the nature of fatigue in cancer. This literature is descriptive, rather than focused on interventions.

However, Richardson has retrieved the body of work existing in the field and has presented all studies available in tabular form, allowing comparison of methods, research instruments, and findings to be compared across existing studies. This provides a very useful synthesis for clinical nurses and researchers.

Studies that develop and test research instruments and measures, or research approaches

In order for cancer nursing research to develop, further methodological work is essential to develop measures for use in studies focused on patients and/or carer outcomes, and detailed work needs to be undertaken on research approaches and designs most suited to answering the kinds of questions nurses are asking. Traditionally, nursing has looked to the methods employed by related disciplines such as biomedicine, psychology, and sociology. In some instances nurses have developed research instruments specifically for use in nursing studies; in others, research designs and instruments have been taken from other established health disciplines and applied to nursing situations.

Quality of life is one area in which cancer nurses have been active, and a number of quality of life measures has been developed by nurses; for example, Holmes and Dickerson's Symptom Distress Scale.[31] Mast[32] has reviewed quality of life research in cancer nursing and has found work using unidimensional scales where quality of life is measured as a single dimension, studies that treat it as a multidimensional entity in which these are measured within a single instrument, and studies that have used multiple separate scales. More recent studies show a trend towards the development and use of scales specific to different cancers, and towards evaluating the outcomes of nursing interventions.

Quality of life research in cancer is a large and growing field; in the main, nursing research has had little impact to date on this field more generally, and measures developed by nurses have in most instances not been used more widely by researchers from other disciplines. This raises the question of whether there is a need for measures developed specifically for nursing research, since it will not be possible directly to compare results obtained from these with studies conducted by other health professionals who use standard measures. One frustration for nursing is, however, the lack of research instruments available to assess outcomes in areas of nursing interest, since these frequently combine physical, functional, and psychological aspects of any given problem. This has led nurses to seek alternative approaches to acquire information and insight into the lives of people who are ill, through the use of qualitative research methods.[10]

Development of detailed understanding of cancer-related problems or client needs

Since one of the most important areas of focus for nursing research is the problems and needs of people with cancer, imposed either by the disease itself or as a result of treatment, nursing research in cancer care has concentrated on a whole variety of different problems. Pain management and fatigue are two prominent examples. There is now a growing body of research into the problem of fatigue in cancer, which is led by nurses. Studies have been undertaken to develop measures and assessment tools for the problem,[33] as has work to define and understand the term in the context of cancer. Other studies, such as those by Richardson and Ream[34] and Glaus,[35] have used different approaches to gather data to give insight into the symptom and its pattern during chemotherapy, and have compared fatigue in patients with cancer with reports of fatigue amongst healthy individuals. Furthermore, ongoing work is underway to explore and evaluate possible interventions to alleviate the problem, and there also exist international collaborations for dissemination of information discovered from fatigue studies and from multi-centre studies. Initiatives such as the American Oncology Nursing Society's FIRE™ project and the European 'Action on Fatigue' project are examples of such work.

A second area of work is a more general approach to attempting systematically to identify needs amongst the cancer population, and comparing these with service provision. These studies are known as needs assessment studies. Cancer nurses are beginning to undertake such studies; for example, Meinir Krishnasamy is currently undertaking a needs assessment of lung cancer patients in the UK. This study is surveying a large sample of patients, their relatives or carers, and their family doctors, to identify from their perspective the problems they have and their current access to health care for these. It is hoped that data from this study will be useful to health planners and policy makers. As such, this kind of study is likely to act as an agent for change, particularly for groups of patients such as those with lung cancer, who have been rather neglected by service provision.

Evaluation of new or existing practices aimed at enhancing care or alleviating problems

Cancer nursing research is increasingly being used to evaluate nursing interventions, so that there is an emerging evidence base for the specialty, although in reality this is new and emergent. Much of the research into cancer nursing to date has been descriptive and focused on delineating patient problems and/or describing nursing approaches and inadequacies in relation to these. There is, however, a growing number of examples where knowledge is being generated about practice.

An example of this is our work on breathlessness in lung cancer.[36,37] We set out to develop and evaluate a nursing approach to the management of breathlessness in lung cancer using the research process as a vehicle for this. We reviewed the literature to examine the problem of breathlessness, and to identify strategies used in other fields, such as chronic pulmonary disease rehabilitation, to identify possible intervention approaches. We then conducted a pilot study, which recorded the experiences of patients with breathlessness and randomly allocated a small group of consenting patients either to attend a nursing clinic where a therapeutic approach to breathlessness was offered, or to be followed up as a control group. This pilot study allowed the intervention strategy to be developed and articulated, as well as producing some useful evaluation data indicating that this approach was promising. The approach has now been evaluated more formally in a multi-centre randomised controlled trial in six centres around the UK. Data from this second study have confirmed the findings from the initial study, and further replication work is ongoing in Australia and Canada. The research process offers a useful framework for the development and evaluation of cancer nursing as a therapeutic endeavour.

Detailed evaluation of new and existing services

This area of research encompasses a wide range of studies; for example, work evaluating nursing roles and practices. Wilkinson's[38] work on factors that influence how nurses communicate with cancer patients reflects a body of earlier work on the quality of care delivered to patients revealed through a number of studies of nurses' communication skills. Davis and Oberle[39] have studied the role of the specialist palliative care nurse and reported this case study in their influential paper. Watson et al.[40] have given good evidence for the effectiveness of breast care nurse specialists. Other studies have evaluated new types of nursing service.

An area that is currently very important is studies evaluating new, extended roles for nursing in the cancer arena. McCorkle et al.[41] used a randomised clinical trial of home nursing for lung cancer patients, in which 166 patients were assigned to either a specialist cancer home care nurse, care from regular home care nurses, or an office-based care group. Patients receiving home care were shown to have less symptom distress and greater independence than the office care group. A range of studies is also ongoing into the effectiveness of nurse-managed care in a variety of situations, such as monitoring patients undergoing radiotherapy, and follow-up for patients with lung and breast cancer. In these studies, nurse-managed care is being compared with conventional medical care for outcomes such as quality of life, symptom management, and cost. These studies are likely to be influential in the further development of the nursing role in cancer care.

Methodological issues for nursing research in cancer care

In the process of developing research into cancer care, as with many other areas of health care, nurses have found themselves questioning the methodological traditions on which prevailing research has been based. Traditional research methods, exemplified by the randomised controlled trial employed in much of health care research, have been felt to be too narrow and limiting to answer the kinds of questions nurses have wanted to pose about the nature of the experience of having cancer, the needs of patients, or for evaluating nursing interventions. As in the wider field of social sciences this has led to a schism and the emergence of opposing methodological camps, according to the research methods felt to be most valid. This is seen at its most extreme in the 'quantitative versus qualitative methods debate'.[42] Unfortunately, the model of measurement, prediction, and causal inference upon which quantitative and experimental research relies does not easily fit a world where health, illness, recovery, and participation in care are frequently the variables one is attempting to measure. This has led a number of nurse researchers to reject the paradigm of the natural sciences as the only truly 'scientific' method. Such quantitative methods are most commonly represented by experimental research, where causal relationships between variables are examined and controlled, and observations are quantified and analysed to determine statistical probabilities and the certainty of a particular outcome. Instead, qualitative methods are advocated, which seek to examine phenomena in context, generating theory from the actor's perspective, and encouraging study designs where the researcher and subject are part of a two-way process in which understanding develops in the development of theory.

Over the past 20 years important contributions to cancer care have been made by nurses using methods derived from both schools. Bryman[43] is critical of the 'quantitative versus qualitative methods debate' since the literature has until recently concentrated on the distinct and incompatible nature of these two methodologies, rather than on the value of particular research techniques in answering specific questions. According to Bryman, the discussions also confuse the epistemological (issues relating to the philosophical principles on which research methods are based) and technical aspects of data collection and analysis. The epistemological arguments have tended to exaggerate the differences between the method types, rather than suggest where each may be relevant.

These issues have been played out in cancer research, with quantitative methods being predominant in medical research with clinical trials research, and in psychological research using standardised measures of anxiety, depression, and quality of life. The distinction between the 'hard' science pursued by medical clinicians and the 'soft'

science pursued by nurses has exaggerated further the idea of methodological encampments occupied by distinct professional groups, and frequently issues of power, status, and funding are played out in the debate.

Many researchers are now trying to move beyond such polarised views of research by encouraging greater eclecticism in methods, and greater fluidity and flexibility in methods adopted for a given study, which should be determined by the specific question being pursued and the methods most suited to answering it.[44] It is also increasingly recognised that qualitative methods encompass a wide range of particular research methods, each with its own tradition and philosophical origins. So studies derived from ethnographic, phenomenological, or ethnomethodological schools will be quite different in approach, even though they may all use qualitative methods. This means that researchers need to be quite clear about the particular approach they are using in any given study.

Qualitative methods have been championed to a large extent by nurses, who have been attracted to the use of material gained through the use of in-depth, semi-structured interview techniques to gain deeper insight into the experiences and needs of cancer sufferers.[10] These methods, although providing insightful and moving accounts of what it is like to receive a diagnosis of cancer and to undergo cancer treatment, are in themselves problematic, and have been criticised by Bailey.[45] The notion that such methods offer a superior means by which to access the 'true' meaning of experience of cancer, and that researchers can access this in some way through post hoc analysis of interview data, is an unlikely one. Bailey argues that all research needs to become much more consensual and collaborative in nature, with researcher and participant together focusing on the actions required in order to allow their situation, and health care more widely, to move forward.

Critical for nursing research in cancer care is that rigorous methods are utilised to pursue questions relevant to the experience of patients with cancer and their carers, and to the practice of nursing. Nurses need to be confident in conducting such studies, and in being members of, and taking on leadership roles in, multi-disciplinary research teams. The research agendas in health care have in the past been heavily dominated by basic scientists and medical clinicians. Increasingly, these agendas are changing so that they are directed to questions surrounding effective health care and the needs of individuals and client groups. Nursing has an important and central role to play in determining the direction such research agendas take, and in conducting the research generated as a result. Cancer patients and their families and carers also have a vital role in this process; nurses could also play a significant role in making this possible for them because of their close and intimate role in their care.

Nursing research and practice development

Recently, practice development has been adopted as a goal for researchers, to encourage researchers in nursing to act responsively towards the needs of practising nurses, so that they use research to develop their practice and effectiveness. Macmillan Cancer Relief, a UK-based cancer charity, has funded a major practice development initiative and established Macmillan Practice Development Units at the Centre for Cancer and Palliative Care Studies in London and at the University of Manchester. The goal of research undertaken in these units is to identify key areas for investigation with practising nurse specialists in cancer and palliative care, and then to develop research studies that both target areas where practice itself can be taken forward, and actively engage nurses in the research process itself. This means that nurses may become part of research in a much more immediate way than simply waiting for research results to be published. Studies emerging from the Practice Development Units both inform practice (for example, by conducting research reviews), and create and develop knowledge for practice in a collaborative way. Nurses themselves and patients are therefore seen as participants in the research process.[46,47]

Studies in the programme develop in a series of stages, from in-depth exploration of specific problems faced by patients with cancer, such as breathlessness or fatigue in advanced cancer, through deeper understanding of these problems, to develop approaches to practice that might more adequately address the needs of those experiencing them. Interventions are evaluated both locally, and

with regard to their transferability to a range of care settings in multi-centre studies. Wherever possible, specialist nurses are asked to take part in these evaluation studies so that they are actively involved in the process of practice development through research, and not just recipients of its end-product. The features of practice development research using this approach are:

- consensus with consumers of research over questions to be asked and the design of studies aiming to answer these
- collaborative inquiry (with both nurses as clinicians, and patients and carers as consumers as partners in all stages of the research process)
- radical deconstruction and reconstruction of health care situations and problems for consumers of services. During this process all the features of the problems and the context in which these arise and are treated and cared for, are taken apart. All elements are examined for their ability to help or hinder healing, adjustment or alleviation, alternative approaches to the problem developed, and the environments in which such problems are managed adapted
- creative use of methods of dissemination, such as practice reviews, and practitioner as partner researcher in multi-centre studies.

Cancer care research and the future

Throughout this book, there has developed an extended critique of current approaches to the management and care of people with cancer, and an examination of the contribution cancer nurses can make to the environment of care and the nature of care delivered. There are numerous opportunities for nurses to change the culture of care for cancer and to play a central role in any reformulated system that may emerge. Central to such change and development is research, which can act as a powerful force to initiate change, and to offer evaluations of existing and new systems of care. For this to happen, however, nurses need to become much more effective users of research, and to become recognised as expert researchers themselves. For it is research that generates the knowledge on which all systems of care rest.

The prevailing knowledge base is derived from information generated from clinical trials and the biomedical tradition. Currently, there is a dearth of high-quality nursing research focused on intervention, or new and different models of care, and of research with a true consumer focus. While this situation is improving, cancer nurses need to be much more proactive. Important agenda-setting work has been undertaken in cancer nursing research. This has been to some extent overtaken by the multi-disciplinary health services research agenda. Nurses cannot afford to remain outside this, but need to seek positions of power and leadership within it. Only then will there be a flow of funding to support programmes of nurse-led research. What is needed now is for the nursing research agenda in cancer to be placed centre stage, and for it to be seen as aimed at radical change, so that the potential for nursing research to change the agenda for cancer care in general can be realised.

References

1. Department of Health (1993). *Research for Health.* London: Department of Health

2. Department of Health (1994). *R&D Priorities – Cancer: Report to the NHS Central Research and Development Committee.* London: Department of Health.

3. Tattersall M.L. and Jones R.J. (1992). Issues in informed consent. *In* Williams C.J. (ed.) *Introducing New Treatments for Cancer.* Chichester: John Wiley.

4. Stenning S. (1992). 'The Uncertainty Principle': selection of patients for clinical trials. *In* Williams C.J. (ed.) *Introducing New Treatments for Cancer.* Chichester: John Wiley.

5. Pocock S.J. (1983). *Clinical Trials: A Practical Approach.* Chichester: John Wiley.

6. Clark A. and Fallowfield L. (1986). Quality of life measurement in patients with malignant disease: a review. *Journal of the Royal Society of Medicine* 79, 165–169.

7. Cella D.F. (1994). Quality of life: concepts and definitions. *Journal of Pain and Symptom Management* 9, 186–192.

8. Fallowfield L. (1990). *Quality of Life: The Rising Measurement in Health Care.* London: Souvenir Press.

9. Hopwood P. (1992). Progress, problems and priorities in quality of life research. *European Journal of Cancer* 28A, 1748–1752.

10. Benner P. (1985). Quality of life: a phenomenological perspective on explanation, prediction and understanding in nursing science. *Advances in Nursing Science* 8, 1–14.

11. Faithfull S. (1995). 'Just grin and bear it and hope that it will go away': coping with urinary symptoms from pelvic radiotherapy. *European Journal of Cancer Care* 4, 158–165.

12. Aaronson N.K., Ahmedzai S., Bergman B., Bullinger M., Cull A. *et al.* (1993). The EORTC QLQ–C30: a quality of life instrument for use in international clinical trials in oncology. *Journal of the National Cancer Institute* 85, 365–376.

13. World Medical Association (1964). *Declaration of Helsinki: Recommendations Guiding Medical Doctors in Biomedical Research Involving Human Subjects.* Helsinki: World Medical Association.

14. Smith L. (1992). Ethical issues in interviewing. *Journal of Advanced Nursing* 17, 98–103.

15. Royal College of Physicians (1990). *Guidelines on the Practice of Ethics Committees in Medical Research Involving Human Subjects.* London: Royal College of Physicians.

16. World Health Organisation (1982). *Proposed International Guidelines For Biomedical Research Involving Human Subjects.* Geneva: World Health Organisation.

17. Thornton H. (1992). Breast cancer trials: a patient's viewpoint. *Lancet* 339, 44–45.

18. Beaver K., Luker K.A., Owens R.G., Leinster S.J. and Bejner L. (1996). Treatment decision making in women newly diagnosed with breast cancer. *Cancer Nursing* 19, 8–19.

19. Royal College of Nursing (1998). *Research Ethics: Guidance for Nurses Involved in Research or any Investigative Project Involving Human Subjects.* Standards of Care Series. London: Royal College of Nursing.

20. Thornton H. (1995). Passive patient or involved participant? *British Psychosocial Oncology Newsletter,* March.

21. Oberst M.T. (1978). Priorities in cancer nursing research. *Cancer Nursing* 3, 281–290.

22. Elgner L. (1987). Priorities for cancer nursing research: a Canadian replication. *Cancer Nursing* 10, 319–326.

23. Stetz K.M., Haberman M.R., Holcomb J. and Jones L.S. (1994). Oncology Nursing Society Research Priorities Survey. *Oncology Nursing Forum* 22, 785–789.

24. Corner J. (1993). Building a framework for nursing research in cancer care. *European Journal of Cancer Care* 2, 112–116.

25. Payne S. (1993). Constraints for nursing developing a framework for cancer care research. *European Journal of Cancer Care* 2, 117–120.

26. Cooper H.M. (1984). *The Integrative Research Review.* Beverly Hills, CA: Sage.

27. Eysenck H.J. (1984). Meta-analysis: an abuse of research integration. *Journal of Special Education* 8, 41–59.

28. Dickerson K., Scherer R. and Le Febvre C. (1995). Identifying relevant studies for systematic reviews. In Chalmers I. and Altman D.G (eds.) *Systematic Reviews.* London: BMJ Publishing.

29. Smith M.C., Holcombe J.K. and Stullenberger E. (1994). A meta-analysis of intervention effectiveness for symptom management in oncology nursing. *Oncology Nursing Forum* **2**, 1201–1210.

30. Richardson A. (1995). Fatigue in cancer patients: a review of the literature. *European Journal of Cancer Care* **4**, 30–32.

31. Holmes S. and Dickerson J. (1987). The quality of life: design and evaluation of a self assessment instrument for use with cancer patients. *International Journal of Nursing Studies* **24**, 15–24.

32. Mast M.E. (1995). Definition and measurement of quality of life in oncology nursing research: review and theoretical implications. *Oncology Nursing Forum* **22**, 957–964.

33. Piper B., Lindsay A. and Dodd M. *et al.* (1989). The development of an instrument to measure the subjective dimensions of fatigue. In Frant S., Tornquist E. and Champagne M. *et al.* (eds.) *Key Aspects of Comfort: Management of Pain, Fatigue and Nausea.* New York: Springer.

34. Richardson A. and Ream E. (1996). The experience of fatigue and other symptoms in patients receiving chemotherapy. *European Journal of Cancer Care* **5** (Suppl.), 24–30.

35. Glaus A. (1996). A qualitative study to explore the concept of fatigue/tiredness in cancer patients and healthy individuals. *European Journal of Cancer Care* **5** (Suppl.), 8–23.

36. Corner J., Plant H. and Warner L. (1995). Developing a nursing approach to managing dyspnoea in lung cancer. *International Journal of Palliative Nursing* **1**, 1–11.

37. Corner J., Plant H., Warner L., A'Hern R. and Bailey C. (1996). Non-pharmacological intervention for the management of breathlessness in lung cancer. *Palliative Medicine* **10**, 299–305.

38. Wilkinson S. (1991). Factors which influence how nurses communicate with cancer patients. *Journal of Advanced Nursing* **16**, 677–688.

39. Davis B. and Oberle K. (1990). Dimensions of the supportive role of the nurse in palliative care. *Oncology Nursing Forum* **17**, 87–94.

40. Watson M., Denton S., Baum M. and Greer S. (1988). Counselling breast cancer patients: a specialist nursing service. *Counselling Psychology Quarterly* **1**, 25–34.

41. McCorkle R., Benoliel J.Q., Donaldson G., Georgiadou E., Moinpour C. and Goodell B. (1989). A randomised clinical trial of home nursing care for lung cancer patients. *Cancer* **64**, 1375–1382.

42. Corner J. (1991). In search of more complete answers to research questions in quantitative versus qualitative research methods: is there a way forward? *Journal of Advanced Nursing* **16**, 718–727.

43. Bryman A. (1988). *Quantity and Quality in Social Research.* London: Routledge.

44. Pope C. and Mays N. (1996). Qualitative methods in health and health services research. In Pope C. and Mays N. (eds) *Qualitative Research in Health Care.* London: BMJ Publishing.

45. Bailey C. (1996). *Derrida, de Man, Habermas: implications for qualitative analysis of interviews in cancer nursing research, a methodological study.* Unpublished M.Sc. dissertation, Institute of Cancer Research, London.

46. Bailey C. (1996). Ethical issues in multi-centre collaborative research on breathlessness in lung cancer. *International Journal of Palliative Nursing* **2**, 95–101.

47. Krishnasamy M. and Plant H. (1998). Developing nursing research with people. *International Journal of Nursing Studies* **35**, 79–84.

Index